# THE NETTER COLLECTION OF MEDICAL ILLUSTRATIONS

3rd Edition

## Digestive System

### Part II—Lower Digestive Tract

VOLUME 9

*A compilation of paintings prepared by* **FRANK H. NETTER, MD**


*Editor*

**James C. Reynolds, MD**
Professor of Clinical Medicine
Co-director, Neurogastroenterology and Motility Program
Division of Gastroenterology and Hepatology
Department of Medicine
Perelman School of Medicine at the University of Pennsylvania
Philadelphia, Pennsylvania

*Senior Associate Editor*

**Peter J. Ward, PhD**
Professor of Anatomy
Department of Biomedical Sciences
West Virginia School of Osteopathic Medicine
Lewisburg, West Virginia

*Associate Editors*

**Suzanne Rose, MD, MSEd**
Professor of Medicine
Senior Vice Dean for Medical Education
Perelman School of Medicine at the University of Pennsylvania
Philadelphia, Pennsylvania

**Missale Solomon, MD**
Gastroenterologist
GastroHealth Maryland
Catonsville, Maryland

**Christopher Steele, MD, MPH**
Assistant Professor of Medicine
University of Connecticut School of Medicine
Farmington, Connecticut

*Additional Illustrations by*

***Carlos A.G. Machado, MD***

**CONTRIBUTING ILLUSTRATORS**

John A. Craig, MD
Tiffany S. DaVanzo, MA, CMI
DragonFly Media
Paul Kim, MS
Kristen W. Marzejon, CMI
James A. Perkins, MS, MFA


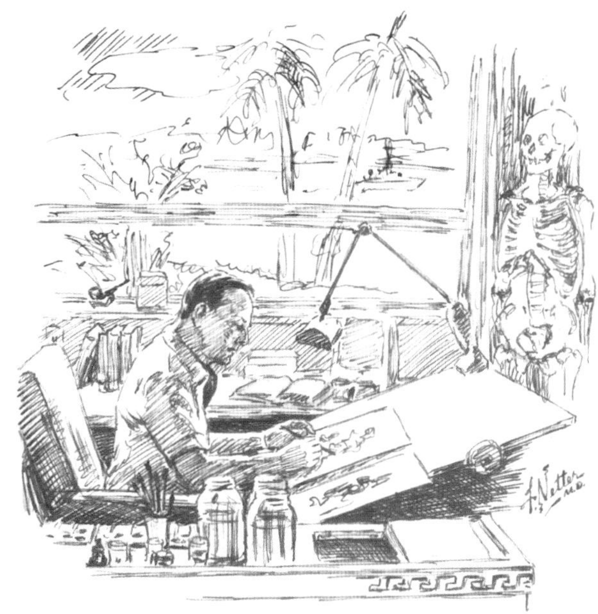

*Self portrait by Dr. Netter*

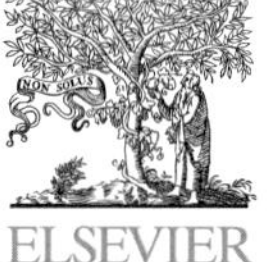

ELSEVIER

ELSEVIER
1600 John F. Kennedy Blvd.
Suite 1600
Philadelphia, Pennsylvania

THE NETTER COLLECTION OF MEDICAL ILLUSTRATIONS:
DIGESTIVE SYSTEM, PART II: LOWER DIGESTIVE TRACT,
VOLUME 9, THIRD EDITION ISBN: 978-0-323-88131-9


**Notices**

Knowledge and best practice in this field are constantly changing. As new research and experience broaden our understanding, changes in research methods, professional practices, or medical treatment may become necessary.

Practitioners and researchers must always rely on their own experience and knowledge in evaluating and using any information, methods, compounds, or experiments described herein. In using such information or methods they should be mindful of their own safety and the safety of others, including parties for whom they have a professional responsibility.

With respect to any drug or pharmaceutical products identified, readers are advised to check the most current information provided (i) on procedures featured or (ii) by the manufacturer of each product to be administered, to verify the recommended dose or formula, the method and duration of administration, and contraindications. It is the responsibility of practitioners, relying on their own experience and knowledge of their patients, to make diagnoses, to determine dosages and the best treatment for each individual patient, and to take all appropriate safety precautions.

To the fullest extent of the law, neither the Publisher nor the authors, contributors, or editors, assume any liability for any injury and/or damage to persons or property as a matter of products liability, negligence or otherwise, or from any use or operation of any methods, products, instructions, or ideas contained in the material herein.

*Publisher:* Elyse O'Grady
*Senior Content Strategist:* Marybeth Thiel
*Publishing Services Manager:* Catherine Jackson
*Senior Project Manager/Specialist:* Carrie Stetz
*Book Design:* Patrick Ferguson

Printed in India

Last digit is the print number: 9 8 7 6 5 4 3 2 1

***"Clarification is the goal. No matter how beautifully it is painted, a medical illustration has little value if it does not make clear a medical point."***

*—Frank H. Netter, MD*

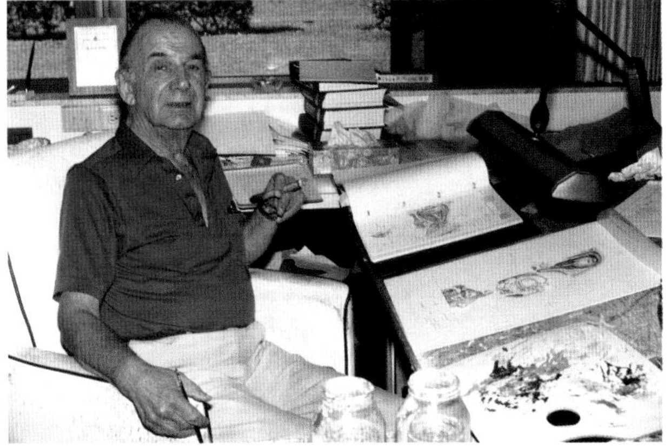

Dr. Frank Netter at work.

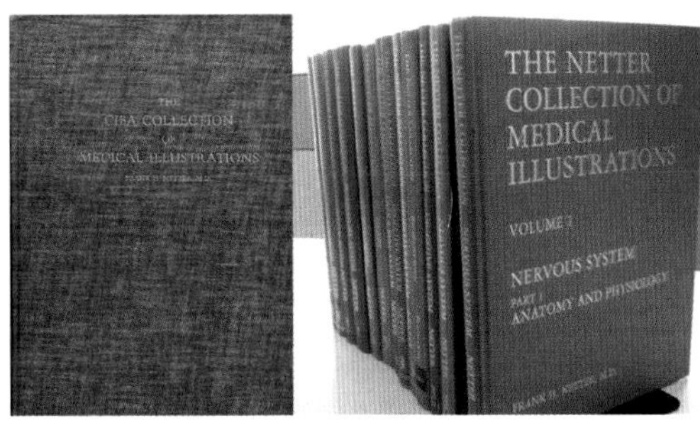


The single-volume "Blue Book" that preceded the multivolume *Netter Collection of Medical Illustrations* series, affectionately known as the "Green Books."

**Dr. Frank Netter** created an illustrated legacy unifying his perspectives as physician, artist, and teacher. Both his greatest challenge and greatest success was charting a middle course between artistic clarity and instructional complexity. That success is captured in *The Netter Collection,* beginning in 1948 when the first comprehensive book of Netter's work was published by CIBA Pharmaceuticals. It met with such success that over the following 40 years the collection was expanded into an 8-volume series—with each title devoted to a single body system. Between 2011 and 2016, these books were updated and rereleased. Now, after another decade of innovation in medical imaging, renewed focus on patient-centered care, conscious efforts to improve inequities in healthcare and medical education, and a growing understanding of many clinical conditions, including multisystem effects of COVID-19, we are happy to make available a third edition of Netter's timeless work enhanced and informed by modern medical knowledge and context.

Inside the classic green covers, students and practitioners will find hundreds of original works of art. This is a collection of the human body in pictures—Dr. Netter called them *pictures,* never paintings. The latest expert medical knowledge is anchored by the sublime style of Frank Netter that has guided physicians' hands and nurtured their imaginations for more than half a century.

Noted artist-physician Carlos Machado, MD, the primary successor responsible for continuing the Netter tradition, has particular appreciation for the Green Book series. "*The Reproductive System* is of special significance for those who, like me, deeply admire Dr. Netter's work. In this volume, he masters the representation of textures of different surfaces, which I like to call 'the rhythm of the brush,' since it is the dimension, the direction of the strokes, and the interval separating them that create the illusion of given textures: organs have their external surfaces, the surfaces of their cavities, and texture of their parenchymas realistically represented. It set the style for the subsequent volumes of *The Netter Collection*—each an amazing combination of painting masterpieces and precise scientific information."

This third edition could not exist without the dedication of all those who edited, authored, or in other ways contributed to the second edition or the original books, nor, of course, without the excellence of Dr. Netter. For this third edition, we also owe our gratitude to the authors, editors, and artists whose relentless efforts were instrumental in adapting these classic works into reliable references for today's clinicians in training and in practice. From all of us with the Netter Publishing Team at Elsevier, thank you.

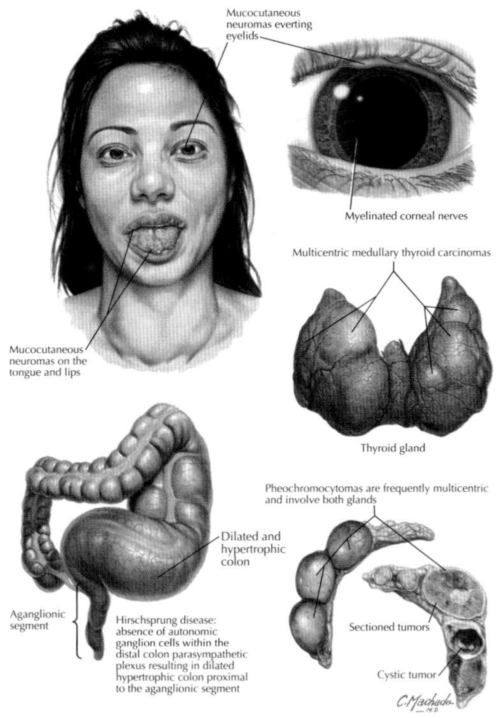


An illustrated plate painted by Carlos Machado, MD.

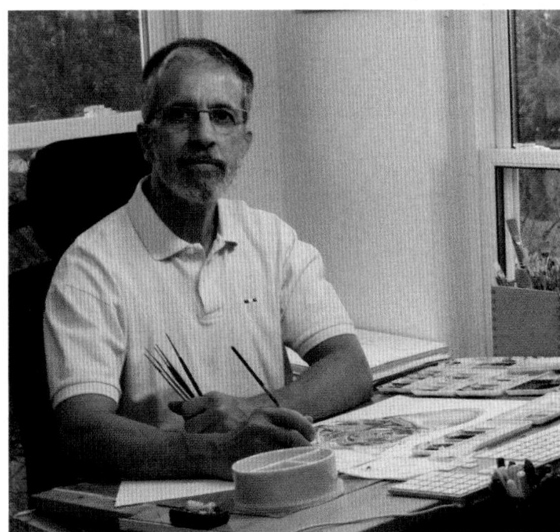

Dr. Carlos Machado at work.

**The Netter Collection**
OF MEDICAL ILLUSTRATIONS
3rd Edition

- Volume 1: **Reproductive System**
- Volume 2: **Endocrine System**
- Volume 3: **Respiratory System**
- Volume 4: **Integumentary System**
- Volume 5: **Urinary System**
- Volume 6: **Musculoskeletal System**
- Volume 7: **Nervous System**
- Volume 8: **Cardiovascular System**
- Volume 9: **Digestive System**

# ABOUT THE EDITORS

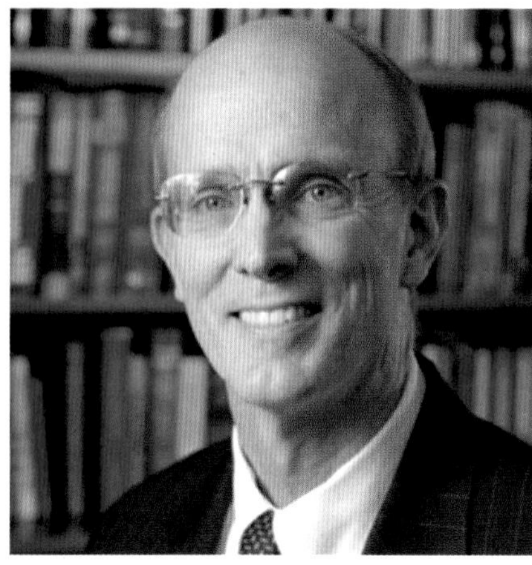

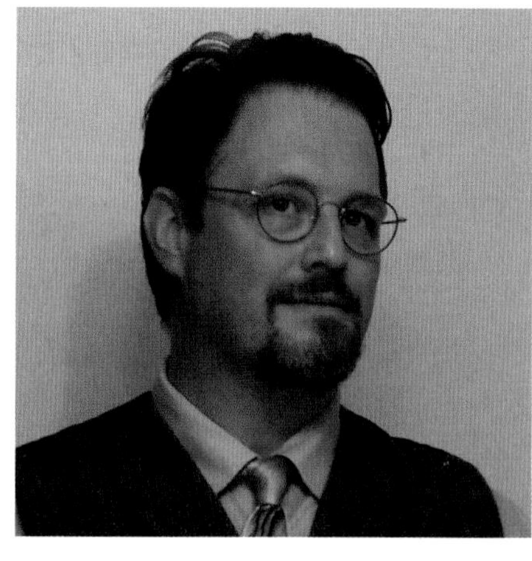

**James C. Reynolds, MD, Editor,** is professor of clinical medicine and the Co-director of the Neurogastroenterology and Motility Program, Division of Gastroenterology and Hepatology, Perelman School of Medicine at the University of Pennsylvania in Philadelphia.

A native of Florida, Dr. Reynolds graduated from Florida State University and received his medical degree from the University of Florida, where he was president of his class and received several honors, including admission to Alpha Omega Alpha (AOA) as a junior, the John B. Gorrie Award as the student with best promise for outstanding future performance, and research awards. He completed his residency at Cornell University at New York Hospital and Memorial Sloan Kettering Cancer Center. He then completed a 3-year fellowship at the Hospital of the University of Pennsylvania. He joined the faculty at the University of Pennsylvania, where he became program director and associate chief of the division. He remained funded by the National Institutes of Health (NIH) and other national organizations for his research into the effect of neuropeptides on gastrointestinal motility. In 1990 he became chief of the Division of Gastroenterology, Hepatology, and Nutrition at the University of Pittsburgh, where he was a tenured associate professor of medicine and cell biology. He was co-director of the Centers for Digestive Health and an associate professor of medicine and cell biology. In 1996 he became professor of medicine with tenure and chief of the Division of Gastroenterology and Hepatology at MCP Hahnemann University, now the Drexel University College of Medicine. He held this position and that of program director from 1996 to 2008. In those 12 years he held numerous leadership roles in the hospital and college of medicine. He was elected vice president of the university physicians practice plan (Drexel University Physicians) and served in this role from 1999 to 2007. From 2006 to 2008 he served as president of the medical staff at Hahnemann University Hospital and was a member of the board of directors of the hospital. He became interim chair of medicine in 2002. In 2005 he was named the June F. Klinghoffer Distinguished Chair of the Department of Medicine. As chair, he has led the department to a fivefold increase in clinical billing while doubling faculty size and extramural research income. In 2016 he returned to Penn to become director of the Neurogastroenterology and Motility Program, where he continues today.

Dr. Reynolds is a member of the editorial board of *Digestive Diseases and Sciences* and is a reviewer for many other journals. He has published more than 100 manuscripts in peer-reviewed journals and has coedited five books. He has received numerous honors, including Phi Beta Kappa, AOA, and Physician of the Year in 1995 by the Greater Pittsburgh Chapter of the Crohn's and Colitis Foundation of America, and has been recognized as the most outstanding gastroenterologist in Pittsburgh on two separate occasions by *Pittsburgh Magazine*. He has also been named among Philadelphia's "Top Docs" 10 times by *Philadelphia Magazine*. He has received teaching awards in both basic and clinical sciences from the University of Pennsylvania and Drexel.

Dr. Reynolds is board certified in internal medicine and gastroenterology and hepatology by the American Boards of Internal Medicine. His primary clinical interests are in the early detection and prevention of cancer, complications of gastroesophageal reflux, and gastrointestinal motility disorders.

**Peter J. Ward, PhD, Senior Associate Editor,** is professor of neuroscience at the West Virginia School of Osteopathic Medicine in Lewisburg, West Virginia. He grew up in Casper, Wyoming, graduating from Kelly Walsh High School and then attending Carnegie Mellon University in Pittsburgh, graduating with a BS in biology in 1996. He began graduate school at Purdue University, where he first encountered gross anatomy, histology, embryology, and neuroanatomy. Having found a course of study that engrossed him, he attended and helped to teach those courses in the veterinary and medical programs at Purdue. Dr. Ward completed an MS in molecular biology and then began a PhD program in anatomy education. In 2005, he completed his thesis and joined the faculty at the West Virginia School of Osteopathic Medicine (WVSOM) in Lewisburg, West Virginia. There he has taught gross anatomy, embryology, neuroscience, histology, and the history of medicine. Dr. Ward has received numerous teaching awards, including the WVSOM Golden Key Award and the Basmajian Award from the American Association of Anatomists, and has been a finalist in the West Virginia Merit Foundation's Professor of the Year selection. Dr. Ward has also been director of the WVSOM plastination facility, coordinator of the anatomy graduate teaching assistants, creator and director of a clinical anatomy elective course, and host of many anatomy-centered events between WVSOM and two Japanese colleges of osteopathy. Dr. Ward has also served as council member and association secretary for the American Association of Clinical Anatomists. His research explores how professional students learn effectively, how medical history is taught, as well as identifying connective tissue structures and how these can impact patient health. In conjunction with Bone Clones, Inc., Dr. Ward has produced tactile models that mimic the feel of anatomical structures when intact and when ruptured during the physical examination. He created the YouTube channel *Clinical Anatomy Explained!* where he presents the anatomical sciences to a broad audience and promotes the importance and excitement of understanding how the human body works. Dr. Ward is the author of *Clinical Anatomy Explained: Netter's Integrate Musculoskeletal System*, which was published in 2022. He has served as the Senior Associate Editor for the previous three volumes of *The Netter Collection: The Digestive System*, second edition. He is a contributor to *Gray's Anatomy* and is one of the editors of *Netter's Atlas of Human Anatomy*. In his spare time he enjoys reading and teaches martial arts at the Yatagarasu Dojo in Lewisburg, West Virginia. He is exceedingly lucky to be the husband of Sarah Koressel and father to Dashiell and Archer Ward, who make him proud every day.

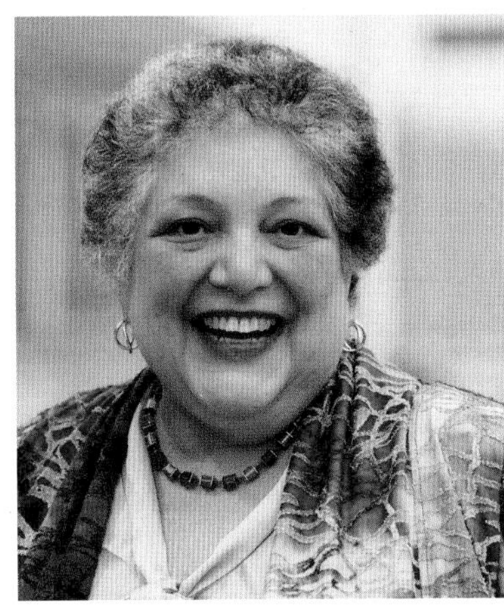

**Suzanne Rose, MD, MSEd, Associate Editor,** serves as Senior Vice Dean for Medical Education at the Perelman School of Medicine (PSOM) at the University of Pennsylvania. In this role, Dr. Rose oversees undergraduate medical education (UME) and continuing medical education (CME) with additional contributions to graduate medical education (GME). Serving on the dean's leadership team, Dr. Rose oversees an education council to coordinate education across all programs at PSOM as well as to collaborate with other schools in the university. The focus of the PSOM UME is on learners and their future service to science, patients, and our communities. The approach is one of compassionate education with rigor and high expectations of PSOM learners while providing support and a focus on wellness.

Prior to her arrival in 2018, Dr. Rose was Senior Associate Dean for Education at the University of Connecticut and led the creation of the innovative lecture-less MDelta Curriculum. She also served for 13 years at Icahn School of Medicine at Mount Sinai in various leadership capacities. She previously held positions at Weill Cornell Medical College (1996–1997) as the Director of Motility and the second-year pathophysiology course and at the University of Pittsburgh (1990–1996), where she ran the second-year GI course. She also assumed leadership roles in the gastroenterology fellowship programs at both Pittsburgh and Cornell.

Dr. Rose's clinical interests are in pelvic floor dysfunction and GI disorders in women. She has served in many leadership roles in the American Gastroenterological Association (AGA), including education councillor on the governing board. She convened all six GI societies to create end-of-training entrustable professional activities, cocreated the first subspecialty academy for educators in this country, served as codirector of the AGA Future Leaders Program, and was appointed course director for the postgraduate course (2017). In addition, under the AGA's auspices, she convened a task force to review maintenance of certification requirements, with whom an impactful, scholarly paper suggesting alternatives that were relevant and aligned with adult learning theory was published. Dr. Rose was awarded the AGA Distinguished Educator Award (2016). She has prepared many educational products, including slide sets and problem-based learning cases, and has edited the textbook *Gastrointestinal and Hepatobiliary Pathophysiology.* She edited her second book, *Constipation: A Practical Approach to Diagnosis and Treatment,* published in 2014. Dr. Rose is sought out for workshops and talks on women's issues in medicine, lifestyle concerns, mentoring, coaching, and networking.

In her role in medical education, Dr. Rose completed a 2-year term as cochair of the Northeast Group on Educational Affairs (NEGEA) of the Association of American Medical Colleges (AAMC) and served as the chair of the group on educational affairs of the Association of American Medical Colleges. She received the inaugural NEGEA Distinguished Service and Leadership Award in 2015.

Dr. Rose received her bachelor's degree from the University of Pennsylvania in Russian language and literature, followed by a master's degree in education from Penn. She spent the summer of 1976 at Leningrad State University. She taught high school for 2 years and was a park ranger at the Grand Canyon before completing postbaccalaureate studies at Columbia University. She graduated from Case Western University School of Medicine as a member of the Alpha Omega Alpha Honor Society and completed her internship and residency there. She went to the Cleveland Clinic Foundation (CCF) for her GI fellowship, including the chief fellow year (as the first woman chief fellow at CCF). Dr. Rose has been married to Rabbi Kenneth Stern for over 40 years, and their living apart/together status has ended with her husband's recent retirement. She is a mother and mother-in-law and is "Nana" to three adorable grandchildren. Her son is a lawyer (working for the Department of Energy), her daughter-in-law has an executive leadership role in the travel hospitality business, and her daughter is a higher education professional who is also pursuing an online doctoral degree in education at Vanderbilt University. She has collected turtles since she was 6 years old, with a collection of over 2000 turtles (everything from a coffee table to jewelry), and she enjoys snorkeling in the Cayman Islands, throwing parties, being with family, and reading.

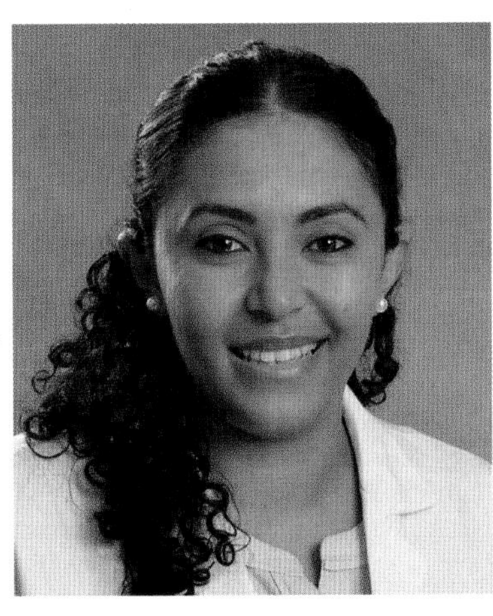

**Missale Solomon, MD, Associate Editor,** is currently a Managing Partner at GastroHealth in Maryland and was previously an assistant professor at Drexel University College of Medicine where she served as the Director of Nutrition and Small Bowel Disorders in the Division of Gastroenterology and attending gastroenterologist in the Drexel Adult Cystic Fibrosis Center. She received her medical education at Jimma University in Ethiopia and later attended Drexel University College of Medicine for her internal medicine residency and gastroenterology fellowship. She is the recipient of the 2014 Nestle Nutrition Clinical Fellowship and the Developing Innovative Gastroenterology Specialty Training (DIGEST) grant offered by the Cystic Fibrosis Foundation. Dr. Solomon's clinical practice focuses on nutritional disorders related to gastrointestinal dysfunction and women's digestive health. Dr. Solomon and her husband live in Columbia, Maryland, with their two children.

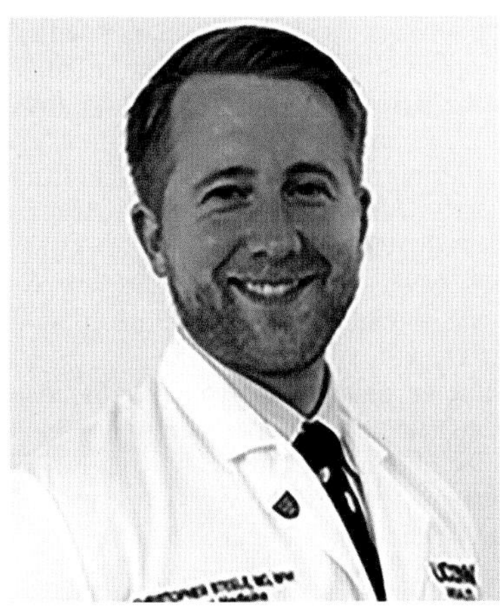

**Christopher Steele, MD, MPHS, Associate Editor,** is an assistant professor of medicine at the University of Connecticut School of Medicine and a practicing academic hospitalist. He received his medical education from the University of Connecticut School of Medicine and attended Johns Hopkins for his internal medicine residency training. Dr. Steele currently holds the title of the educational liaison, in which he works with both undergraduate and graduate leadership to improve the learning experience for residents and medical students. Dr. Steele's academic interests are in health equity and improving the way we deliver healthcare for the medically vulnerable. He is the cofounder of the University of Connecticut Health Leaders (UCHL) program, where he trains volunteers to screen and address social determinants of health for patients seen in both outpatient and inpatient settings. Dr. Steele and his wife live in Simsbury, Connecticut, with their three children.

# PREFACE

The opportunity to continue to promote the extraordinary educational value of the exquisite art of Dr. Frank Netter in a state-of-the-art update of this classic series has been an honor for me and my esteemed associate editors. Dr. Netter's images have brought insightful value to students for over 6 decades and have been updated again to enhance the continued benefit of this publication for future generations. This edition of *Digestive System* has been rewritten and renewed to include cutting-edge science and state-of-the-art endoscopic, pathologic, and radiographic images, along with Netter's ageless drawings and images that provide insights that foster students' and practitioners' understanding of the anatomy, physiology, and pathophysiology of all eight regions that make up the fascinating and complex digestive system.

Frank Netter, MD, described by the *Saturday Evening Post* as the "Michelangelo of Medicine," continues to be an icon in medical education. The insightful imagery of his medical illustrations provides value for students at all levels of experience who seek insights into the structure and function of digestion in ways that few other texts have in the history of medical education. His vision for these texts—integrating factual information with visual aids—provides unparalleled insights. Though born at the onset of the 20th century, his background mimics many modern medical students—beginning his education in the arts before becoming a scientist. By following his mother's wishes to move beyond art and into medicine, Frank Netter used his passion and brush to communicate the science and the art of medicine in unparalleled ways. In distinction to anatomy texts that offer images of structure only, Netter's paintings also brought incredible insights into the pathophysiology of disease. Just as important, in ways unsurpassed by any other text, he and his dedicated disciples have illustrated how patients are affected by the suffering caused by disease. In all three of these revised parts of *Digestive System,* new artists committed to the style and value of Dr. Netter's illustrations and led by Carlos Machado, MD, have modernized both the science and the art of his illustrations in all aspects of the digestive system.

This update of the digestive system's anatomy and disease has taken a new approach to communicate the complexity and integrated beauty of this fascinating organ system. The classic images Dr. Netter drew were preserved whenever possible and altered only as necessary. Dozens of modern radiographic and endoscopic images have been added to all sections in all volumes. The first section in both Parts I and II summarizes shared aspects of the digestive system. Each subsequent section is dedicated to a specific organ and reviews normal anatomy and physiology, pathology, pathophysiology, and disease presentation and treatment.

Each section has been written by authors who were chosen for their dedication to teaching the fascinating aspects of the digestive system. I had the honor of choosing incredibly distinguished associate editors with whom I have had the pleasure of working throughout my career. In each case they have published expertise in their respective organ system and have demonstrated their commitment to and skill in medical education. Their knowledge and insights bring updated scientific understanding of disease mechanisms and current treatments that will convey understanding of the largest and most complex organ system that is unparalleled by other texts. In each section, Dr. Peter Ward updated each of the subsections on normal anatomy and physiology. He has worked hard to preserve the original pictures of Dr. Netter while ensuring the accuracy of the text based on current terminology and science.

In Part I of this three-part set, I sought to provide insights and an overview of the upper digestive tract. Michele A. Young, MD, previously the chief of gastroenterology at the University of Arizona's Veterans Administration Hospital in Phoenix and now serving as Chief of Staff at the New Jersey VA Health Care System, has written the first organ-focused chapter on the complex anatomy, physiology, and pathophysiology of pharyngeal and upper esophageal functions. New insights into imaging and physiologic understanding of the complexities of swallowing are provided. David A. Katzka, MD, distinguished professor of medicine at New York Presbyterian, Columbia University Irving Medical Center, where he is director of esophagology and the Swallowing Center, revised the section on the esophagus as one of the world's authorities on the topic. New insights into diseases that are common today but were not known at the time of the first edition, including Barrett esophagus and eosinophilic esophagitis, are beautifully illustrated and discussed. Part I closes with a section by Henry Parkman, MD, a renowned gastric physiologist and physician from Temple University, where he serves as vice dean for research. Dr. Parkman brings a special new focus on the neurophysiology and electrical physiology of normal gastric function and disease.

I review common anatomic, physiologic, and clinical aspects of intestinal disorders in Section 1 of Part II. In Section 2, Dr. Missale Solomon offers a beautifully written treatment of normal and abnormal disorders of the primary digestive organ, the small intestine. In Section 3, one of modern gastroenterology's eminent educators and senior vice dean for medical education at the Perelman School of Medicine, University of Pennsylvania, Suzanne Rose, MD, MSEd, in collaboration with Christopher Steele, MD, MPHS, discuss the complex and fascinating aspects of physiology and pathophysiology of the colon.

Part III reviews the normal physiology and pathophysiology of the liver, biliary tract, and pancreas. Grace Li-Chun Su, MD, a distinguished clinician and scientist, chief of the Gastroenterology Section of the VA Hospital of the University of Michigan, has exquisitely updated the section on the liver in a way that will bring great insights into this, the largest solid organ in the body. John Martin, MD, a premier physician from the Mayo Clinic, provides wonderful modern images of the biliary tract in Section 2 as well as descriptions of its many associated disorders. Section 3, on pancreatic function and disease, is written by one of the world's premiere scientists and clinicians on pancreatology, David Whitcomb, MD, PhD, director of the Center for Genomic Studies at the University of Pittsburgh.

I would like to express my gratitude for the talented and dedicated contributors to this wonderful update. First and foremost, thanks must be given to Dr. Netter posthumously for providing the initial version of this text and its wonderful illustrations. I especially want to thank the associate editors and other contributing authors. I also want to thank the amazing artists who work with the publishers, Jim Perkins, Tiffany DaVanzo, Kristen Wienandt Marzejon, and especially Dr. Machado, for their talents and commitment to preserving the magnificent style and imagery of Dr. Netter's drawing. I want to thank my editors at Elsevier, Marybeth Thiel and Elyse O'Grady, for their expertise, patience, and support. Finally, I want to thank my loving wife for more than 4 decades of unwavering support of my efforts to make contributions to the field of gastroenterology, which never ceases to fascinate and challenge me.

**James C. Reynolds, MD**

# INTRODUCTION TO THE FIRST EDITION

The general outline for The CIBA Collection of Medical Illustrations calls for eight to ten volumes, each of which is designed to cover the anatomy, pathology, and essential physiologic aspects of one of the various systems of the human organism. When planning the volume on the digestive system, it was decided that, because of its scope, the volume should be divided into three separate parts. Part I was to deal with the upper alimentary tract from the mouth through the duodenum; Part II with the lower alimentary tract from the jejunum through the anal canal, the abdominal cavity, and the fetal development of the gastrointestinal pathway; and Part III with the liver, biliary tract and pancreas. For various reasons I did not undertake these sequentially but first prepared Part III and then Part I. When these two books were completed, I thought that the most difficult problems were behind me. Consequently, as I began this second part of Volume 3, I felt the relief of a long-distance swimmer who, having battled perseveringly against a strong current, senses the tide turning in his favor and believes that, despite his fatigue, the remainder of the course will be relatively easy. Imagine my chagrin to find, as I "paddled" furiously among the conflicting eddies of knowledge dealing with the lower digestive tract, that the "swimming" here was even more difficult than it had been in the upper alimentary canal.

Fortunately, however, in this portion of the course I had the support of a valiant "team," who had struggled with me through Part I of this volume. In the Introduction to that part, I wrote about the personal pleasure and scientific help received from my contacts with Professor G.A. G. Mitchell of Manchester, England; Dr. John Franklin Huber of Temple University, Philadelphia; Dr. Nicholas A. Michels of Jefferson Medical College, Philadelphia; Professor Gerhard Wolf-Heidegger of the University of Basle, Switzerland; and Dr. William H. Bachrach of the Veterans Administration Center, Los Angeles. In working on this book, my appreciation of these men and of the tremendous help they have given has been multiplied many times.

In addition, I have had the good fortune to make new associations which have proved equally enjoyable and advantageous. Notable in this respect was my collaboration with the São Paulo (Brazil) University Group—Dr. José Fernandes Pontes, his brother Dr. José Thiago Pontes, Dr. Mitja Polak, Dr. Daher E. Cutait, and Dr. Virgilio Carvalho Pinto.

To Dr. Polak, in particular, I must express my sincerest appreciation, not only for his work in connection with those plates for which he was specifically the consultant but also for his coordinating activities on behalf of the entire group. The spirit of cooperation among this group was exemplified by the way other members of the Faculty of Medicine of the University of São Paulo generously contributed of their time and knowledge. Specifically, I must mention Dr. Mario R. Montenegro of the Department of Pathology, Dr. Luis Rey of the Department of Parasitology, Dr. Fernando Teixeira Mendes of the Section of Hematology and Cytology, and Dr. Godofredo Elejalde, Bacteriologist.

From the Brazilian group I learned much about the diseases of the gastrointestinal tract. I learned also to admire their knowledge and their sound and progressive medical thinking. In particular, I was gratified by their devotion to the project we had in hand and by the assiduity with which they pursued it.

Finally, I am grateful to Dr. Pontes and his associates for their efforts to acquaint me with the many wonderful cultural and social features of Brazil. In particular, its architecture and its music will remain among my most treasured memories.

In preparing those plates concerned with congenital anomalies and those demonstrating the anatomic complexity of the peritoneum, it became strikingly evident that, for a better understanding of these topics, a short review of the essential steps and phases in development would be indispensable. The next problem, naturally, was centered around the question as to how deeply we would have to go into detail to present a coherent narrative of the normal developmental processes and to clarify the deviations which lead to the most frequent congenital anomalies. Dr. E. S. Crelin, thanks to his many years of teaching experience and his acquaintance with the mentality of student and physician alike, knew exactly what and how much embryology we would need in order to provide the basic background for all the topics touching upon intestinal development and its anomalies. It was a rare pleasure to have Dr. Crelin as consultant, not only because of his interest in the task before us and the stimulation he conveys but also because his critical attitude did not permit the omission of any important detail, in spite of the inevitable condensation.

As the specialty of proctology developed during the past few decades, it became important to obtain a more exact knowledge of the anatomy of the anorectal region. The older anatomic concepts did not suffice either for an understanding of the pathology of the region or for the development of improved operative techniques based on physiologic principles. This led to new investigations of the subject, undertaken by a number of men, largely spearheaded by the group at St. Mark's Hospital in London. In this country, Dr. Rudolph V. Gorsch of New York City was one of the pioneers in this work and is one of the leading students of the subject. His painstaking and meticulous studies were always carried out with an eye to practical application of the knowledge gained. It was through perusal of his publications, particularly of his classic book, *Proctologic Anatomy,* that I came to the conclusion that he was the man who could best help with this subject. This decision proved to be correct, and I enjoyed unraveling with him the most modern concepts of the anorectal regions, the perineopelvic spaces, the sphincters, and the various related structures.

In the section dealing with the diseases of the small and large intestine, I encountered topics which, because of their almost totally surgical character, required special handling. For certain of these—volvulus, intussusception, and the surgical aspects of ulcerative colitis—Dr. Cuthbert E. Dukes, the distinguished pathologist at St. Mark's Hospital in London, recommended to us the brilliant young surgeon Dr. H. E. Lockhart-Mummery. His knowledge of the conditions on which we worked is all-encompassing, and his ability to restrict the discussion to its essentials was illuminating.

The enormous progress made in the handling of infants with serious congenital anomalies of the digestive tract similarly required the cooperation of a surgical expert. Dr. C. Everett Koop of The Children's Hospital in Philadelphia has made emergency surgery of the newborn his special field of endeavor. The benefit derived from discussing with him, and preparing under his guidance, the plates which appear at the beginning of Section XII was indeed remarkable, and I can only hope that his clarity in describing the pathophysiologic situations and the essential points of the surgical procedures is adequately reflected in the paintings.

When we came to "hernia," though it is, strictly speaking, a disease of the abdominal wall, the editor and I decided to devote a special section to it, because it is so important and so much of an entity. The consultant for this topic was Dr. Alfred H. Iason, a man who has studied the subject in all its phases, who has written voluminously concerning it, and who has had vast operative experience in the field. His monumental volume, *Hernia,* is widely known.

Intestinal obstruction and the "acute abdomen" proved to be unique subjects because of the vastness of the fields they encompass. These two topics touch on almost every condition covered in this book, but what was needed was a cross-sectional view, a reclassification of the material in such a manner as to be helpful to the student and practitioner. For aid in these problems, I called on a close friend, Dr. Samuel H. Klein of New York City. Because of his vast surgical experience and knowledge, his keen analytical mind, and his understanding of the teaching approach, he was ideally suited for the task at hand. In order to get another point of view for the task of abridgment, Dr. Klein called in an associate, Dr. Arthur H. Aufses, Jr. Together, we worked out the plates which appear on pages 188 to 192.

Paroxysmal peritonitis is an entity of relatively recent recognition, and for the plate on this subject I fortunately was able to obtain the collaboration of Dr. Sheppard Siegal of New York City, who had much to do with the identification of this condition.

Gastrointestinal physiologists and clinicians have for some time suspected that the ileocecal junction acts not purely as a flap valve but as a physiologic sphincter or pylorus. It remained for Dr. Liberato J. A. Di Dio of the University of Minas Gerais, Belo Horizonte, Brazil, to demonstrate a more appropriate concept of the structure of this valve and its function. Dr. Di Dio, who was in New York at the time I was working on this subject with Professor Wolf-Heidegger, most graciously explained to us his findings and showed us drawings and photographs of his dissections and also his remarkable motion picture of the function of the valve in vivo. The illustrations on page 52 are based on his material.

Our concept of the structure of the epithelial cells of the intestine has been greatly modified in recent years, and the help of an expert in this field was needed when it came to the making of the illustration on page 50. This subject is most important today because of the interest in absorption and malabsorption. I am therefore most grateful to Dr. S.L. Palay of the Laboratory of Neuro-anatomical Sciences, National Institutes of Health, Bethesda, Maryland, who has personally made most extensive electron microscopic studies of these cells and who graciously gave me of his time and his knowledge.

A number of illustrations in this volume were originally made in consultation with Dr. Jacob Buckstein of New York. They were first issued in individual brochures and later in The CIBA Collection of Medical Illustrations, published in 1948. These plates appear in Section X, Plates 1, 2, 3, 6, 7, 8, 25, 28, and 29; in Section XII,

Plates 16, 18, 23, 30, 34, 44, 45, 46, and 49; in Section XIII, Plate 4; and in Section XIV, Plate II. Some of them are reproduced here in their original form, others with modifications. I wish to thank Dr. Buckstein for his help with these plates.

Also from an older series of pictures stem Plates 9 to 14 in Section XIII, dealing with abdominal injuries. I am most grateful to Dr. Michael E. De Bakey, under whose guidance these pictures were developed in 1945, for his kindness in checking the correctness of both pictures and texts.

I should also like to express appreciation for the generous aid and advice given me by the following: Dr. Robert A. Nordyke, now of the Straub Clinic, Honolulu, Hawaii, for his aid in planning the illustration of the use of radio isotopes in tests of absorption (Plate 22, Section XI); Dr. Robert J. Matthews of Van Nuys, California, for demonstrating to me the test for occult blood in the stool (Plate 24, Section XI); and Dr. Paul K. McKissock of Veterans Administration Center, Los Angeles, California, for his advice in connection with the sketch of reversal of an intestinal loop (Plates 1 and 2, Section XI).

For the Plates in Sections IX and X, dealing with the blood vessels of the abdominal wall and of the intestine, Dr. Michels and I were helped a great deal by Paul Kornblith, a medical student at Jefferson Medical College, and by Dr. Padmanabhan Siddharth of Madras Medical College, India, presently a teaching fellow at the Daniel Baugh Institute of Anatomy.

Throughout this project there has been to me one source of encouragement and stimulation, one fountainhead of counsel and advice, my very dear friend, the editor of these volumes, Dr. Ernst Oppenheimer, to whom I shall be forever grateful. I cannot here recount the multitudinous ways in which he has helped. Suffice it to say that his devotion to the work, his confidence in me, and his tireless attention to organization and detail have been an inspiration.

**Frank H. Netter, MD**

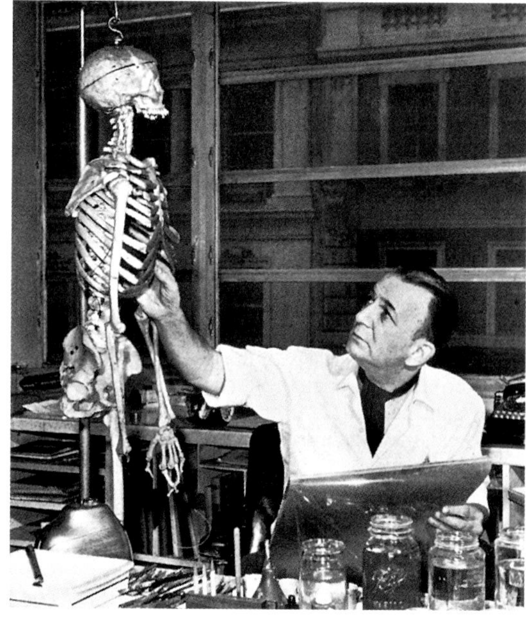

# CONTRIBUTORS


## EDITOR-IN-CHIEF

**James C. Reynolds, MD**
Professor of Clinical Medicine
Co-director, Neurogastroenterology and Motility Program
Division of Gastroenterology and Hepatology
Department of Medicine
Perelman School of Medicine at the University of Pennsylvania
Philadelphia, Pennsylvania
PLATES 1.11–1.26

## SENIOR ASSOCIATE EDITOR

**Peter J. Ward, PhD**
Professor of Anatomy
Department of Biomedical Sciences
West Virginia School of Osteopathic Medicine
Lewisburg, West Virginia
PLATES 1.1–1.10, 2.1–2.7, 3.1–3.19

## ASSOCIATE EDITORS

**Suzanne Rose, MD, MSEd**
Professor of Medicine
Senior Vice Dean for Medical Education
Perelman School of Medicine at the University of Pennsylvania
Philadelphia, Pennsylvania
PLATES 3.20–3.100

**Missale Solomon, MD**
Gastroenterologist
GastroHealth Maryland
Catonsville, Maryland
PLATES 2.8–2.83

**Christopher Steele, MD, MPH**
Assistant Professor of Medicine
University of Connecticut School of Medicine
Farmington, Connecticut
PLATES 3.20–3.100

## CONTRIBUTORS

**Roopjeet K. Bath, MBBS**
Assistant Professor of Medicine
Division of Gastroenterology
University of Connecticut School of Medicine
Farmington, Connecticut
PLATES 3.35–3.36, 3.63

**Kevin Dieckhaus, MD**
Professor of Medicine
Division of Infectious Diseases
University of Connecticut School of Medicine
Farmington, Connecticut
PLATES 3.46–3.62

**Eric Girard, MD**
Assistant Professor of Surgery
University of Connecticut School of Medicine
Farmington, Connecticut
PLATES 3.30–3.34, 3.37–3.45, 3.73–3.76, 3.89, 3.92–3.96

**John Harrison, PhD**
Associate Professor
Division of Craniofacial Sciences
University of Connecticut School of Medicine
Farmington, Connecticut
PLATES 3.24–3.29

**Christina E. Metcalf, MD**
Division Director, Breast Surgery
Associate Professor of Surgery
University of Connecticut School of Medicine
Trinity Health of New England Medical Group
Comprehensive Women's Health Center
St. Francis Hospital
Hartford, Connecticut
PLATES 3.30–3.34, 3.37–3.45, 3.73–3.76, 3.89, 3.92–3.96

**Rishabh Sachdev, MD**
Assistant Professor of Medicine
Division of Gastroenterology
University of Connecticut School of Medicine
Farmington, Connecticut
PLATES 3.97–3.100

**Haleh Vaziri, MD**
Associate Professor of Medicine
Division of Gastroenterology
University of Connecticut School of Medicine
Farmington, Connecticut
PLATES 3.22, 3.65–3.72, 3.90–3.91

**Haresh Visweshwar, MD, MS**
Assistant Professor of Medicine
University of Connecticut School of Medicine
Farmington, Connecticut
PLATES 3.20–3.21, 3.23, 3.64, 3.77–3.88

# CONTRIBUTORS TO THE SECOND EDITION

We would like to acknowledge the work of the previous edition contributors.

**Eva Alsheik, MD**

**Rosemarie Arena, MD**

**Reena V. Chokshi, MD**

**Kevin D. Dieckhaus, MD, FIDSA**

**Faripour Forouhar, MD**

**John R. Harrison, PhD**

**Marco Molina, MD**

**Neilanjan Nandi, MD**

**Ajish Pillai, MD**

**Christopher Steele, MD, MPH, MS**

**Christina E. Stevenson, MD, FACS**

**Savanna Thor, MD**

**Haleh Vaziri, MD**

**Tobias Zuchelli, MD**

# CONTENTS OF THE COMPLETE VOLUME 9—DIGESTIVE SYSTEM: THREE-PART SET




**ISBN: 978-0-323-88130-2**





**ISBN: 978-0-323-88131-9**





**ISBN: 978-0-323-88090-9**

# CONTENTS

SECTION 1

# OVERVIEW OF LOWER DIGESTIVE TRACT

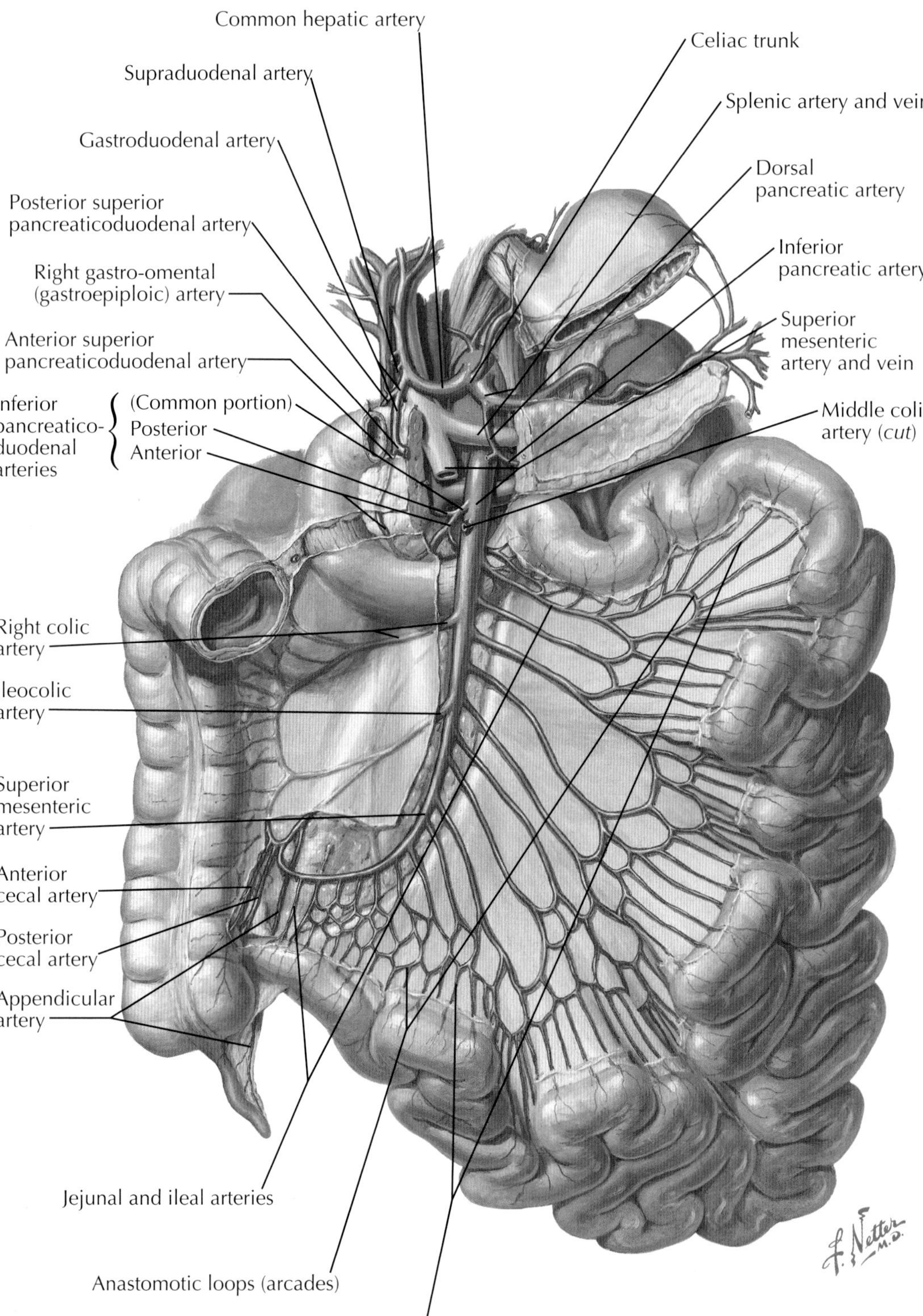


## Blood Supply of Small and Large Intestines

The blood supply to the small and large intestines is extremely variable and unpredictable. The variations concerning the origin, course, anastomoses, and distribution of the intestinal vessels are so frequent and so significant that conventional textbook descriptions are inadequate and, in many respects, even misleading. Because of this variability, surgeons should have an intimate acquaintance with the entire spectrum of the gut's arterial supply to avoid operative errors, such as devascularization of intestinal sections, which might inadvertently induce necrosis and lead to rupture and peritonitis. This section illustrates the most typical branching patterns of the vessels associated with the small and large intestines. In the later sections devoted to each organ, the complex variations that may be encountered are considered.

The digestive tract within the abdominal cavity receives nearly all of its blood supply from three unpaired branches of the abdominal aorta. The foregut organs (distal esophagus, stomach, liver, gallbladder, spleen, pancreas, and proximal duodenum) are supplied by the *celiac trunk,* a large artery that leaves the abdominal aorta shortly after passing through the diaphragm. The small and large intestines receive their blood supply from the other two unpaired vessels of the aorta, the superior mesenteric and inferior mesenteric arteries.

The superior mesenteric artery (SMA) arises from the anterior wall of the abdominal aorta immediately inferior to the celiac trunk. It supplies the midgut organs (distal duodenum, part of the pancreas, jejunum, ileum, cecum, vermiform appendix, ascending colon, and transverse colon) before forming anastomoses with the inferior mesenteric artery. One of the first arteries to arise from the SMA is the *middle colic artery,* which supplies the most distal midgut structure, the transverse colon. The position of the transverse colon is a remnant of the rotation and extreme elongation of the embryonic gut tube that occurs as it reaches its mature state. This artery will be described again as it anastomoses with the blood supply to the ascending colon.

Another proximal branch of the SMA is the *inferior pancreaticoduodenal artery.* It splits into an anterior branch and a posterior branch that sandwich the inferior aspect of the head of the pancreas. These vessels, as their name implies, also supply the distal duodenum as it transitions to become the jejunum. The anterior and posterior branches of the inferior pancreaticoduodenal artery anastomose with two adjacent branches of the celiac trunk, the anterior and posterior branches of the *superior pancreaticoduodenal artery.* The inferior pancreaticoduodenal artery also forms an anastomosis with the next branch off of the SMA that supplies the jejunum.

The next branches from the SMA are 15 to 18 intestinal branches that are either *jejunal arteries* or *ileal arteries.* These exit the left side of the SMA and travel within the intestinal mesentery until they reach the jejunum and ileum. The point at which these vessels become covered by the two peritoneal folds that become the small intestine's mesentery is termed the *root of the mesentery.* As these vessels approach the small intestine, they interconnect to form a series of loops, or *arterial arcades.* These arcades ensure redundancy in the blood supply to the small intestine so that an interruption in one region will not cause ischemia of the nearby intestine. The arterial arcades give off *straight arteries* (vasa recta) that actually reach the gut tube. Although there is no clear transition between the jejunum and ileum, the

## Blood Supply of Small and Large Intestines (Continued)

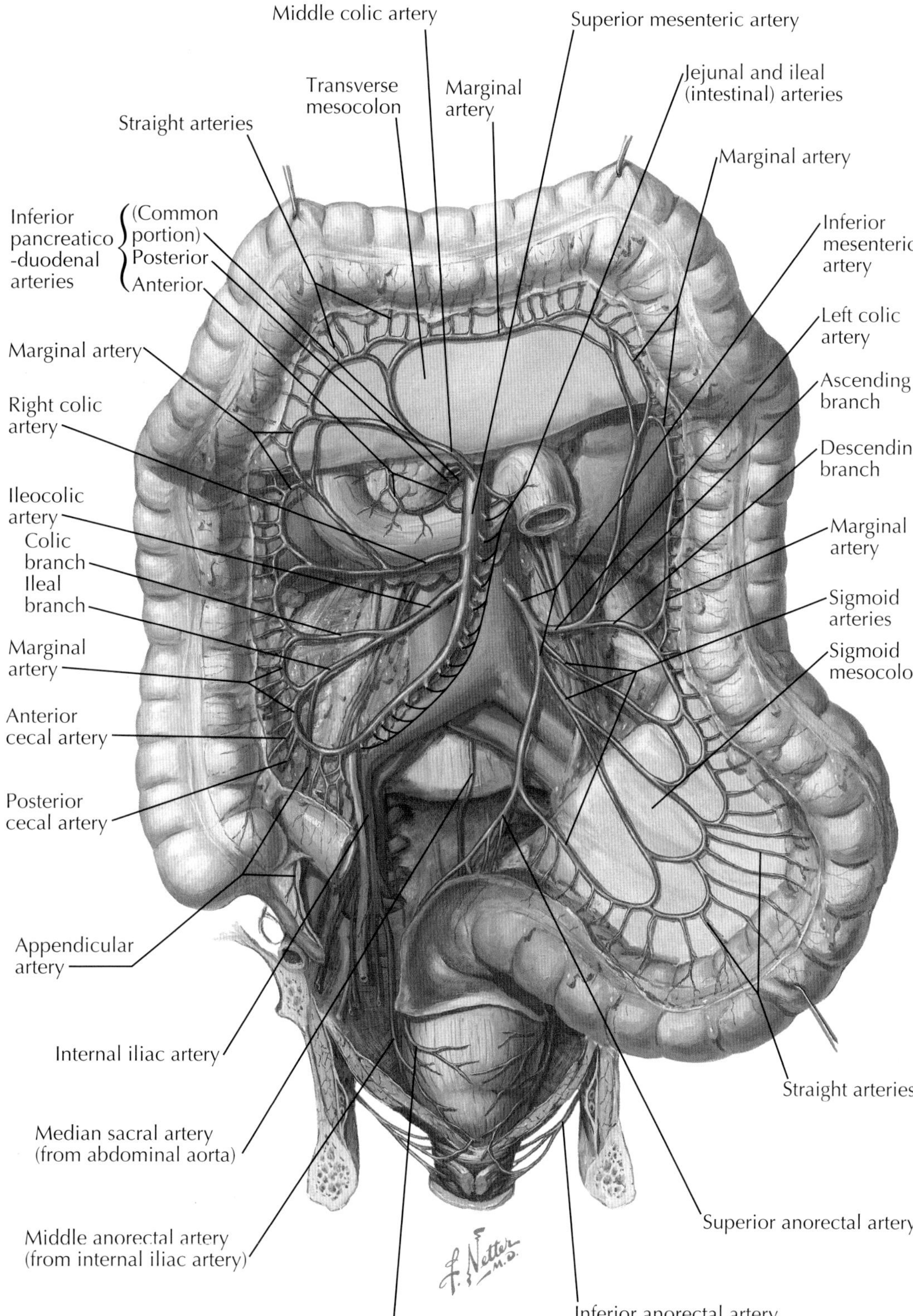


appearance of the arterial arcades and straight arteries can assist in differentiating one from the other. The jejunum tends to have simple arcades with one loop between adjacent jejunal arteries and fairly elongated straight arteries. In contrast, the ileum has more complex arcades with two or more loops and relatively short straight arteries that reach the ileum.

Exiting the right side of the SMA are the ileocolic and right colic arteries. The *ileocolic artery* travels inferiorly and to the right, branching into an *ileal branch* and a *colic branch*. The ileal branch anastomoses with the arterial arcades of the ileal artery, supplying the terminal ileum. The ileal branch also typically gives off the important *appendicular artery*, which travels posterior to the ileal arterial arcades, through the mesoappendix, and finally to the vermiform appendix itself. In the vicinity of the appendicular artery, the ileal branch of the ileocolic artery gives off an *anterior cecal artery* and a *posterior cecal artery*, which supply blood to their respective sides of the cecum. The *right colic artery* exits the SMA superior to the ileocolic artery and travels transversely toward the ascending colon. It forms significant anastomoses with the colic branch of the ileocolic and middle colic arteries. The anastomosis occurs primarily through a large artery, the *marginal artery* (of Drummond), which parallels the entire large colon and receives blood from the ileocolic, right colic, middle colic, left colic, and sigmoid arteries. The marginal artery is a vessel that allows blood to reach the entire length of the colon even if one of the feeder arteries is compromised. From the marginal artery, blood reaches the colon itself via the vasa recta.

The *inferior mesenteric artery* is the last of the three unpaired vessels that supply the digestive tract. It arises from the left anterior aspect of the abdominal aorta approximately 3 to 5 cm above the bifurcation of the right and left common iliac arteries. It quickly gives off several branches: the left colic, sigmoid, and superior rectal arteries. The *left colic artery* travels transversely to the left, giving off an *ascending branch* that travels toward the left colic flexure to anastomose with branches of the middle colic artery. The rest of the left colic artery contributes blood primarily to the descending colon via the marginal artery and straight arteries. The *sigmoid arteries* are a series of three to four arteries branching off of the inferior mesenteric artery that travel within the *sigmoid mesocolon* to reach the sigmoid colon. The branches of the sigmoid artery form interconnecting arterial arcades before giving off straight arteries that enter the sigmoid colon itself. Typically, the marginal artery does not continue as a distinct structure into the sigmoid mesocolon.

The final direct branch of the inferior mesenteric artery is the *superior anorectal artery*. It communicates with the sigmoid arterial arcades and may also supply some distinct branches to the sigmoid colon, termed the *rectosigmoid arteries*. The sigmoid mesocolon disappears as the sigmoid colon transitions to become the rectum, which is retroperitoneal. As this transition occurs, the superior anorectal artery bifurcates into two lateral anorectal arteries that parallel the rectal wall and supply blood to the organ. These branches of the superior anorectal artery anastomose with the *middle anorectal artery*, a branch of the internal iliac artery, and to a lesser degree, the *inferior anorectal artery*, a branch of the internal pudendal artery.

Veins of Small Intestine

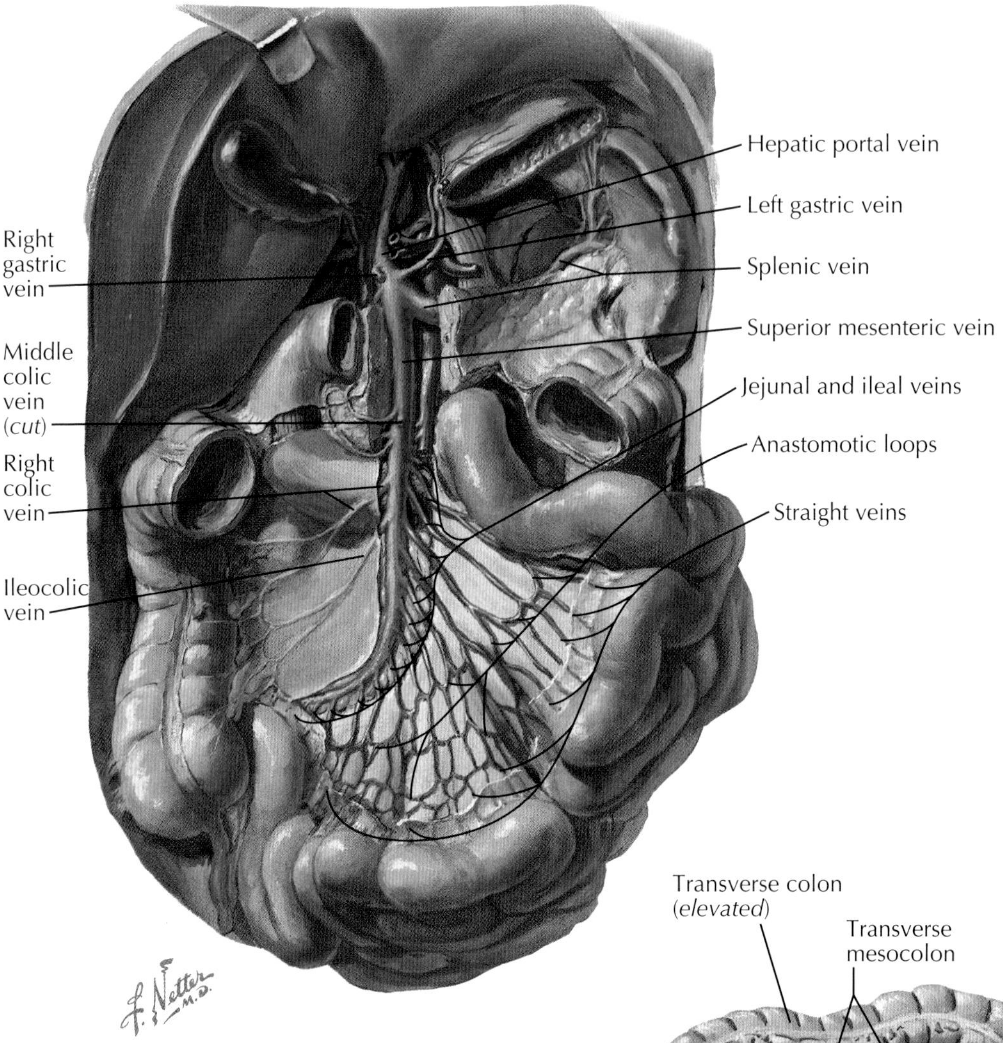

Hepatic portal vein
Left gastric vein
Splenic vein
Superior mesenteric vein
Jejunal and ileal veins
Anastomotic loops
Straight veins
Right gastric vein
Middle colic vein (*cut*)
Right colic vein
Ileocolic vein

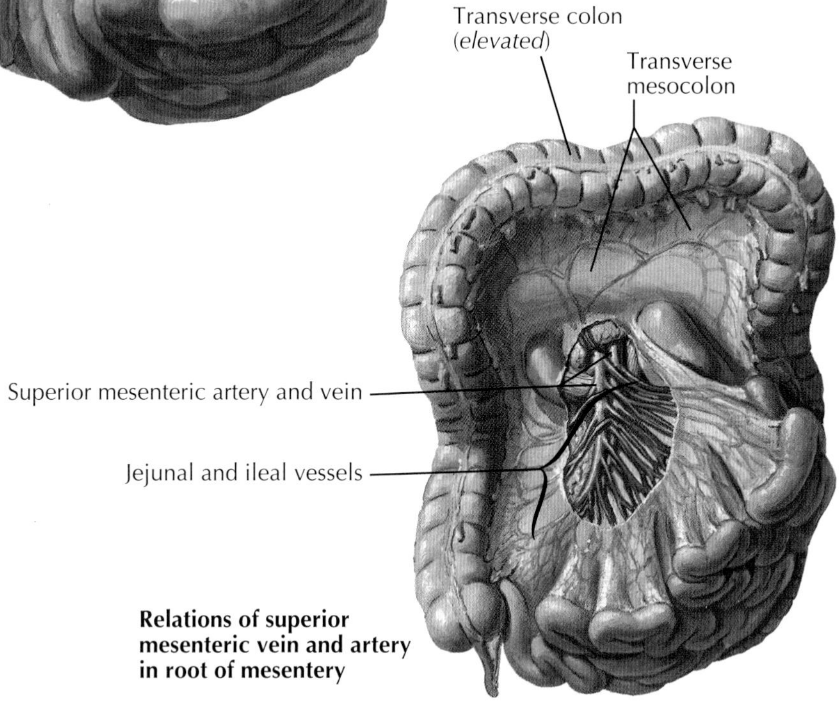

Transverse colon (*elevated*)
Transverse mesocolon
Superior mesenteric artery and vein
Jejunal and ileal vessels

**Relations of superior mesenteric vein and artery in root of mesentery**

## Venous Drainage of Small and Large Intestines

The veins that drain blood from the small and large intestines largely parallel the arteries that supply each organ and share the same names. However, because the veins eventually drain to the hepatic portal vein and liver, there are some notable departures from the arterial scheme. The *superior mesenteric vein* drains the midgut organs and receives blood from the *inferior pancreaticoduodenal, jejunal, ileal, ileocolic,* and *right* and *middle colic veins.* These veins run parallel to the concordantly named arteries as they leave the SMA, although blood is flowing in the opposite direction. Because of its position near the superior mesenteric vein and the fact that there is no celiac vein, the *right gastroomental vein* drains to the right side of the superior mesenteric vein shortly before the latter drains into the hepatic portal vein. The artery of the same name is a branch of the gastroduodenal artery, which branches from the common hepatic artery and celiac trunk.

The *jejunal* and *ileal veins* conform in number and appearance of their arcades and straight arteries with those of their respective arteries. Lying, as a rule, to the right of the arteries, the veins from the small intestine extend from the duodenojejunal junction close to the ileocecal junction, where the *anterior* and *posterior cecal veins* and the *appendicular veins* unite to form the *ileocolic vein.* The first or first two jejunal veins frequently receive, either via a common trunk or as a separate vessel, an *inferior pancreaticoduodenal vein* running alongside the corresponding arteries. The venous drainage of the first part of the jejunum is often not into the superior mesenteric vein but rather into either the anterior or posterior pancreaticoduodenal vein. These venous pancreaticoduodenal arcades are fashioned in the same way as the arcades of the corresponding arteries. The posterior pancreaticoduodenal vein, lying over the artery, is covered by a thin layer of connective tissue, composed of remnants of the fetal dorsal mesoduodenum, which may be readily seen during surgery when the duodenum and the head of the pancreas are mobilized.

Around the head of the pancreas, two venous arcades are formed (similar to the situation with the arteries), one anteriorly by the *anterior superior* and *anterior inferior pancreaticoduodenal veins* and the other posteriorly by the *posterior superior* and *posterior inferior pancreaticoduodenal veins.* Both inferior pancreaticoduodenal veins empty predominantly into the first and second jejunal veins (70%) or into the superior mesenteric vein (30%), either separately or via a common trunk. Deviating from the arterial arrangement, the posterior superior pancreaticoduodenal vein joins the portal vein directly behind the head of the pancreas, its entry point lying shortly ahead of that of the left gastric vein. The anterior superior pancreaticoduodenal vein joins the *right gastroepiploic vein,* which, after passing behind the first part of the duodenum, enters into the superior mesenteric vein at the pancreatic notch, shortly before the latter empties into the hepatic portal vein formed by the union of the superior mesenteric and splenic veins.

Starting in the region of the terminal ileum, the superior mesenteric vein first follows an oblique course and then a straight superior course, lying to the right of and somewhat anterior to the accompanying artery. In this way, both vessels describe a curve with the convexity to the left. Both also cross anterior to the third portion of the duodenum, a fact worth remembering in cases of

## Venous Drainage of Small and Large Intestines (Continued)

duodenal obstruction due to compression by the vessels, perhaps caused by the excessive weight of a neoplastic growth or weakness of the anterior abdominal wall.

The *inferior mesenteric vein* starts as a continuation of the superior rectal vein, which brings blood from the rectum and superior part of the anal canal. During its upward course, it receives venous blood from the *rectosigmoid, sigmoid,* and *left colic veins,* which drain the sigmoid colon and descending colon. All these tributaries follow the corresponding arteries closely, lying mostly to their left. Their anastomosing and arcade formations are the same as those described for the respective arteries. However, the main trunk of the inferior mesenteric artery lies to the right, where it branches from the abdominal aorta. Instead of paralleling it, the inferior mesenteric vein continues superiorly after it receives blood from the left colic and upper sigmoid veins, separating from the artery. The vein ascends anterior to the left psoas muscles, just to the left of the fourth portion of the duodenum. It continues behind the body of the pancreas to enter most frequently (in 38% of observed cases) the *splenic vein.* The splenic vein, in turn, combines with the superior mesenteric vein (at times 3–3.5 cm from the union of the inferior mesenteric and splenic veins). Sometimes (29%), the inferior mesenteric vein enters the superior mesenteric vein, and at other times (32%), it joins the superior mesenteric vein and the splenic vein at their junction. In a few instances, a second inferior mesenteric vein may exist.

The splenic vein emerges from the hilus of the spleen as several fan-like veins that converge into a single large vessel. It has an average length of 15 cm and is never, unlike its accompanying artery, tortuous or coiled. It demonstrates a great number of different divisional patterns, which may include the short gastric veins and a superior polar splenic vein.

The *portal vein* and, especially, the variations of its tributaries are extremely important when considering a portocaval shunt for redirecting the portal blood flow to relieve or ameliorate the consequences of portal hypertension. It seems, therefore, appropriate to discuss in this volume variations that particularly involve the venous drainage of the intestine in which the superior or inferior mesenteric veins participate. The *superior pancreaticoduodenal vein* is sometimes (38%) only a single vessel but more frequently (50%) is duplicated, with one branch terminating in the portal vein and the other in the superior mesenteric vein. The *right and left gastroomental veins,* corresponding to arteries of the same name, which are branches to the celiac arterial trunk, drain to the superior mesenteric vein (sometimes portal vein) and the splenic vein, respectively. The *left gastric vein,* also corresponding to an artery branching from the celiac trunk, can join the rest of the portal circulation at the superior aspect of the union of the splenic and superior mesenteric veins but has been found to join the portal vein directly in some instances as well as the splenic vein distal to the just-mentioned junction. The *right gastric vein,* which is usually a small vein, typically terminates in the portal vein within 3 cm of its division into right and left branches, but it may also enter the base of the superior mesenteric vein or, far less frequently, the proximal segment of the right gastroomental vein or the inferior pancreaticoduodenal vein.

The veins serving the rectum and anal canal are the unpaired *superior anorectal veins* as well as the *right* and *left middle anorectal veins* and the *right* and *left inferior*

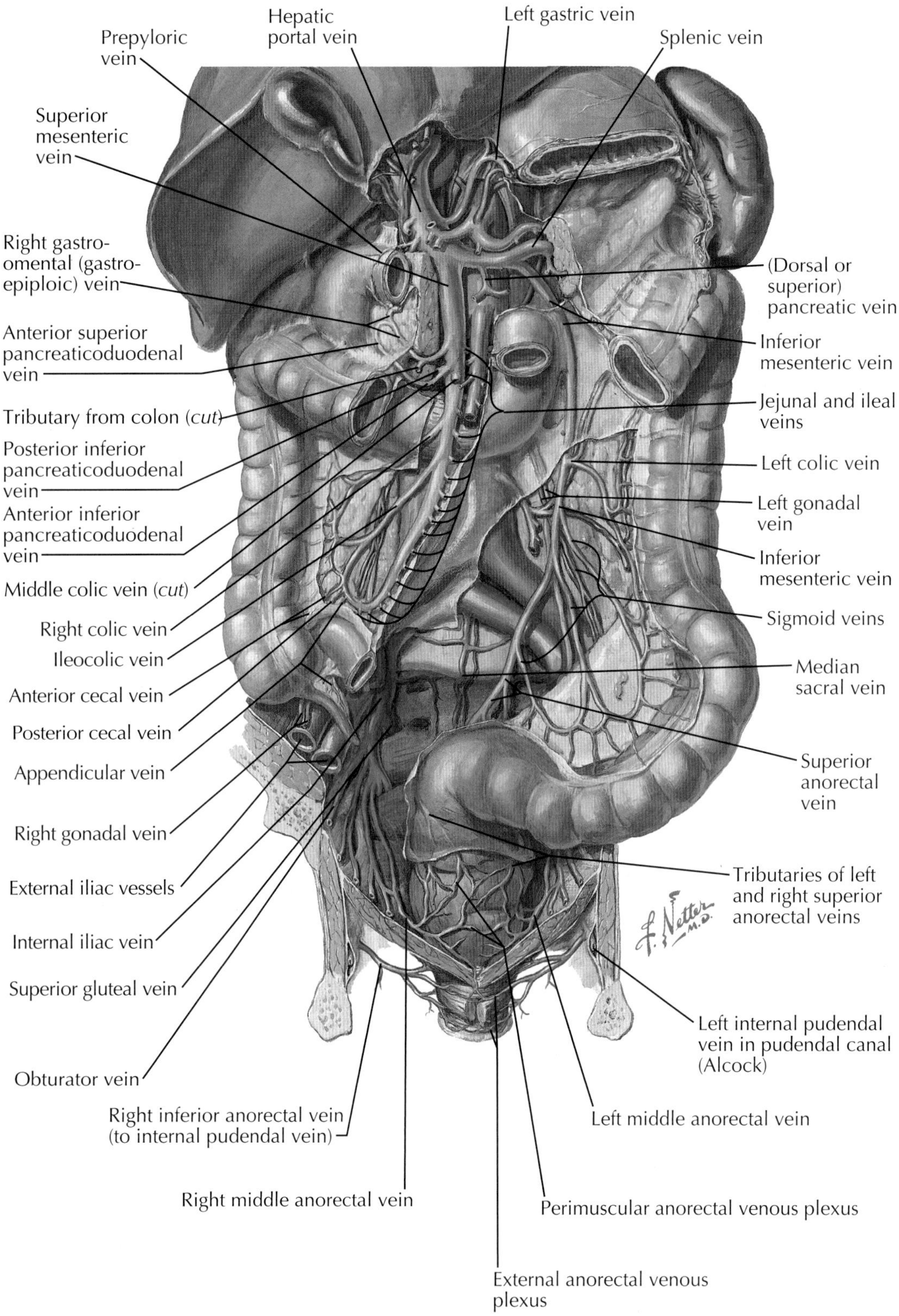

## Venous Drainage of Small and Large Intestines (Continued)

*anorectal veins.* These vessels follow the same course as the arteries of the same name, but they return the blood into two different systems. The superior anorectal vein drains blood into the portal system via the inferior mesenteric vein, whereas the middle anorectal veins drain into the *internal iliac vein* and then the *common iliac veins* before entering the inferior vena cava. Blood in the inferior anorectal veins follows a similar course, first draining to the *internal pudendal vein* before entering the internal iliac veins.

The blood draining into the anorectal veins begin in three venous plexuses situated in the walls of the anorectal canal. The lowest of these plexuses, the *external anorectal plexus,* lies in the perianal space, in the subcutaneous tissue surrounding the lower anal canal near the external opening of the anus. The *internal anorectal plexus* is located in the submucosal space of the rectum superior to the pectinate line. These two plexuses are sometimes collectively referred to as the *submucosal plexus* or the *superior* and *inferior submucosal plexuses.* The third venous plexus surrounds the muscular wall of the rectum below its peritoneal reflection and is called the *perimuscular anorectal plexus,* although some authors refer to it as the external anorectal plexus, a term that leads to confusion with the first of the three plexuses described above. The perimuscular anorectal plexus withdraws blood chiefly from the muscular wall of the rectum and evacuates the upper portion into the superior anorectal vein, although the chief route of drainage of the perimuscular plexus is to the middle anorectal veins.

The internal and external anorectal plexuses serve the mucosal, submucosal, and perianal tissues. The internal plexus encompasses the rectal circumference completely, but the greatest aggregation of small and large veins is in the rectal columns (of Morgagni). Dilation of the internal anorectal plexus results in internal hemorrhoids, and dilation of the external anorectal plexus or thrombosis of its vessels results in external hemorrhoids. The internal and external anorectal plexuses are separated by the internal anal sphincter as well as the dense tissue of the pecten, but they communicate with each other by slender vessels that increase in size and number with age and are also more voluminous in the presence of hemorrhoids.

These connections between the external and internal anorectal plexuses as well as the perimuscular plexuses constitute anastomoses between the inferior and superior anorectal veins and between the caval and portal venous systems. The significance of this situation is enhanced by the fact that the inferior and middle anorectal veins and their collecting vessels, the internal pudendal veins, have valves. In contrast, the superior anorectal vein is devoid of such valves, so that when the pressure in the portal vein rises, perhaps owing to portal hypertension, the circulation in the superior anorectal vein may reverse and portal blood may traverse the anorectal plexuses and be carried away by the middle and inferior rectal veins. This shunts portal blood via the internal iliac vein to the caval system. When this collateral venous circulation develops, the increased blood volume and pressure in the vessels dilate them to the extent that internal and/or external hemorrhoids may result.

In the absence of portal hypertension, spasms of the anal sphincter may also cause external hemorrhoids, because they may shut off the outflow of blood to the inferior anorectal veins. Internal hemorrhoids, on the other hand, may develop when alterations (dilation as well as constriction) occur within the apertures of the rectal wall through which branches of the internal anorectal plexus pass.

### Veins of Rectum and Anal Canal: Female

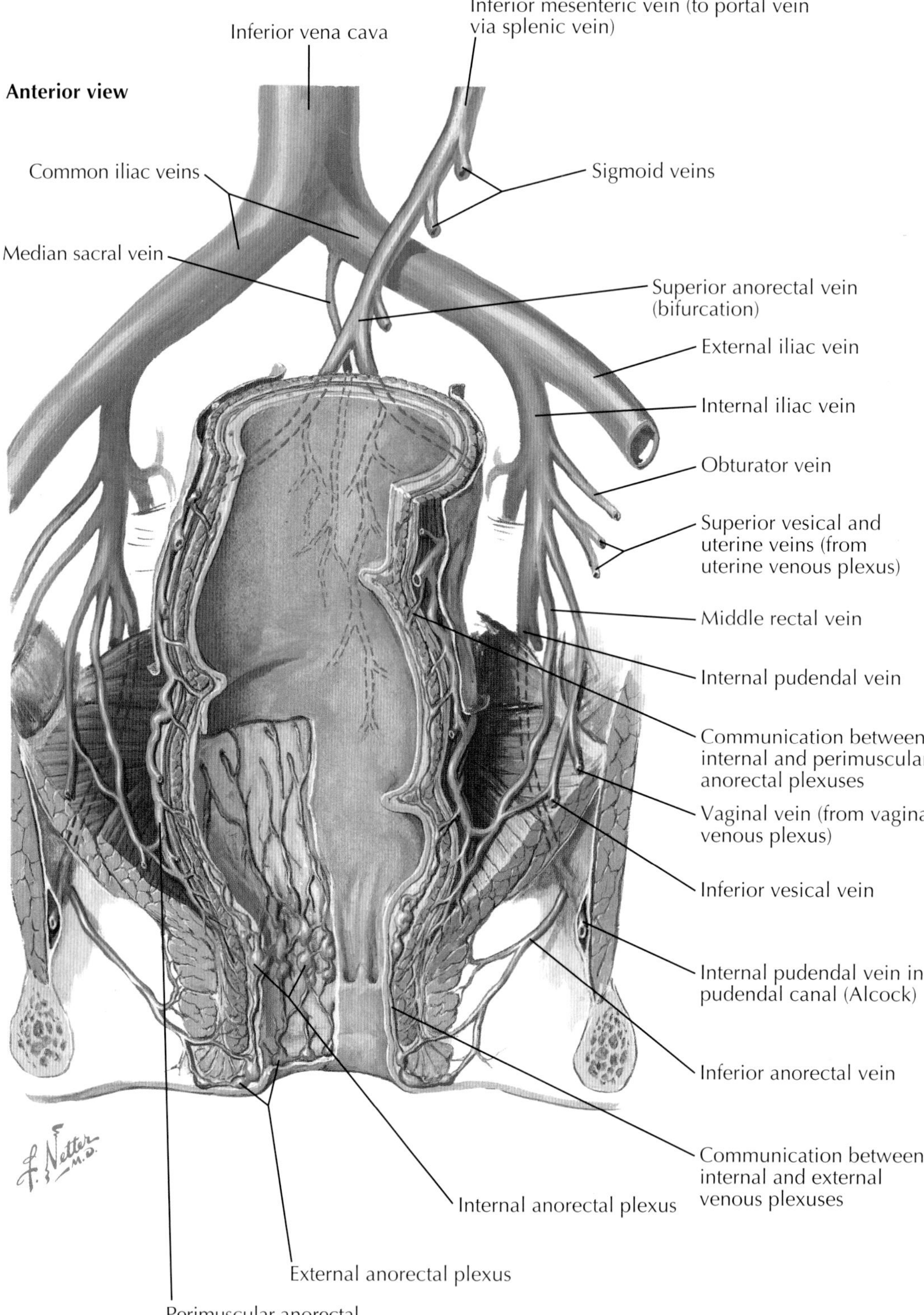

## Innervation of Small and Large Intestines

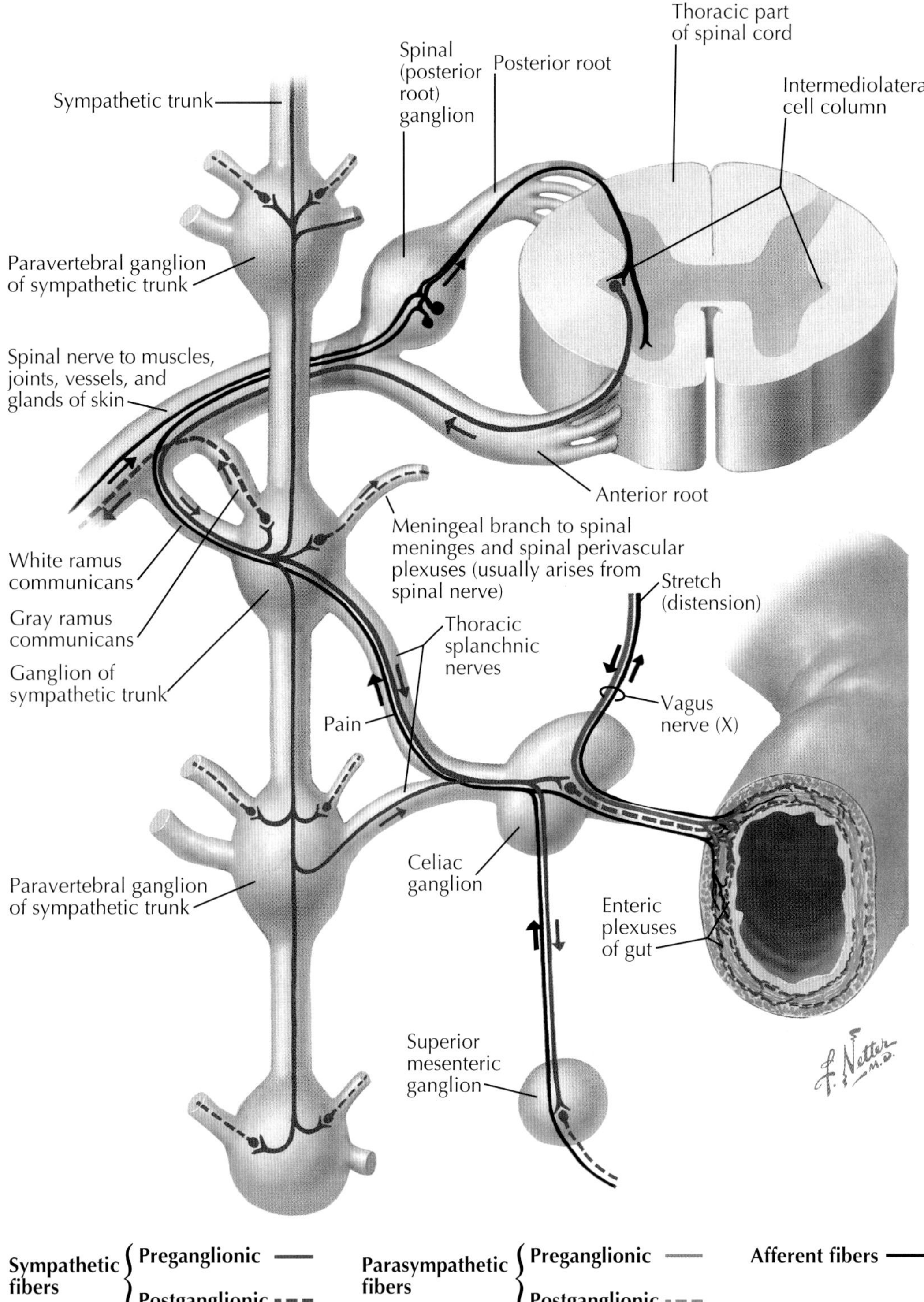


The nerves supplying the small and large intestines (and their vessels) contain both visceromotor (sympathetic and parasympathetic efferent) fibers and viscerosensory (afferent) fibers. Although nerve cells scattered through the entire alimentary tract and locally produced hormones can maintain some degree of intrinsic intestinal activity, it is the activities of the visceromotor and viscerosensory nerves that markedly affect the activity or quiescence of the intestines. Generally, increased sympathetic activity will constrict the blood supply to the intestines and decrease their activity. In contrast, increased parasympathetic activity will increase the rate of peristalsis and glandular secretion. Viscerosensory responses to either painful or nonpainful stimuli prompt the central nervous system (CNS) to modulate visceromotor activity.

Although the visceromotor and viscerosensory systems operate as complex, continuous-feedback loops, the *hypothalamus* can be considered as a source and terminus of pathways concerned with visceral activities. The hypothalamus is a small region of the CNS located superior to the pituitary gland and anteroinferior to the thalamic nuclei. It is primarily concerned with regulating the body's homeostatic drives by adjusting body temperature, appetite, and blood flow as well as the level of aggression. It has extensive cortical connections with the premotor areas of the frontal cortex, cingulate gyrus, and orbital surfaces of the frontal lobes. It sends axons to many structures; for our purposes, the most important are the reticular formation, dorsal motor nucleus of the vagus, and specific regions of the thoracic, lumbar, and sacral levels of the spinal cord. The nuclei of the reticular formation also project to the dorsal motor nucleus of the vagus and spinal cord, and these are the distinct locations where visceromotor (both parasympathetic and sympathetic) impulses to the organs are generated. The similarities between the two systems are discussed below, and their differences are discussed in subsequent plates.

Visceromotor activity occurs along a two-neuron chain. The preganglionic nerve cell body is always found in the CNS, and it projects an axon to reach a second nerve cell body somewhere in the body. The preganglionic axon synapses with this postganglionic cell, which projects another axon to reach the target structures that are actually being innervated, such as smooth muscle and glands.

Preganglionic sympathetic nerve cell bodies are located in the gray matter of the spinal cord in an area between the anterior and posterior horns, the *intermediolateral column* (nucleus), which stretches from the first thoracic segment of the spinal cord inferiorly to the second or third lumbar segment of the spinal cord. The preganglionic sympathetic nerve cells that specifically innervate the small and large intestines arise, respectively, from segments T8–T10 and T10–L2/L3 of the intermediolateral column. The preganglionic sympathetic neurons from each segment of the intermediolateral column send their axons to exit the spinal cord via the *anterior rootlets,* which coalesce to form an *anterior root* from each segment. The anterior roots, and the preganglionic sympathetic axons within them, join posterior roots to form the *spinal nerve,* which traverses the intervertebral foramen. The spinal nerve splits to form posterior rami to innervate somatic structures of the back, and anterior rami that innervate somatic structures of the trunk and limbs. The preganglionic sympathetic axons travel briefly into the anterior rami before leaving as a separate structure, the *white rami communicans,* which connects to a nearby longitudinal string of nerve cell bodies, the *sympathetic chain* (sympathetic trunk and paravertebral ganglia). The preganglionic sympathetic axons that innervate the sweat glands, arrector pili, and precapillary sphincters of the somatic body will synapse with cells in each of these sympathetic chain ganglia; however, the preganglionic sympathetic axons that innervate abdominal organs, such as the small and large intestines, pass through these ganglia without synapsing. These axons leave the medial aspect of the sympathetic chain ganglia as *thoracic, lumbar,* or *sacral splanchnic nerves.* Although there is considerable variation in the exact branching pattern, generally the preganglionic sympathetic axons of T5–T9 combine to form *greater thoracic splanchnic nerves* on each side. Similarly, the T10 and T11 contributions fuse to form the *lesser thoracic splanchnic nerve* and the T12 axons form the *least thoracic splanchnic nerve.* These thoracic splanchnic nerves travel medially and inferiorly on each side of the thoracic vertebral bodies before passing posterior to the diaphragm and entering the abdomen to reach postganglionic ganglia. The *lumbar splanchnic* and *sacral splanchnic nerves* leave the sympathetic chain ganglia in the lumbar and sacral regions but do not merge; instead, they each travel medially to reach their ganglia.

## Innervation of Small and Large Intestines (Continued)

The targets for all of these splanchnic nerves are the *prevertebral ganglia* that lie anterior to the abdominal aorta and vertebral column. Each of these ganglia is a collection of postganglionic sympathetic nerve cell bodies that will send their axons to the target tissues of the abdominal organs. The members of this group are the *celiac, aorticorenal, superior mesenteric,* and *inferior mesenteric ganglia.* There are additional postganglionic sympathetic nerve cell bodies scattered throughout the *intermesenteric plexus* (located between the superior and inferior mesenteric ganglia) as well as the *superior hypogastric* and *inferior hypogastric plexuses,* located within the pelvis. The celiac ganglion gives off postganglionic sympathetic axons that contribute to the *celiac plexus,* which innervates the foregut organs (distal esophagus, stomach, proximal duodenum, parts of the pancreas, spleen, liver, and gallbladder). Similarly, the aorticorenal ganglia on the right and left contribute postganglionic sympathetic nerves to the *aorticorenal plexus,* supplying targets in the suprarenal gland, kidney, proximal ureters, and gonads. The superior mesenteric and inferior mesenteric ganglia contribute postganglionic sympathetic axons to the *superior* and *inferior mesenteric plexuses,* which supply the midgut (distal duodenum, part of the pancreas, jejunum, ileum, cecum, appendix, ascending colon, and transverse colon) and hindgut (descending colon, sigmoid colon, and rectum), respectively. The *intermesenteric plexus* connects the superior and inferior mesenteric ganglia and is composed of visceral afferent axons passing between the two as well as lumbar splanchnic nerves contributing preganglionic sympathetic axons to the abdominal organs. Postganglionic sympathetic nerve cells may be found within the intermesenteric plexus. Extending inferiorly from the inferior mesenteric ganglion is the *superior hypogastric plexus.* It is similar to the intermesenteric plexus but also carries a large number of preganglionic parasympathetic axons. The superior hypogastric plexus extends inferiorly and splits into two bundles, the *right* and *left hypogastric nerves,* which pass into the true pelvis and terminate as the *left* and *right inferior hypogastric plexuses.* The inferior hypogastric plexuses consist of preganglionic sympathetic axons from the sacral splanchnic nerves, postganglionic sympathetic nerve cell bodies, preganglionic parasympathetic axons, and viscerosensory axons. They wrap around the pelvic organs and may be referred to as having subplexuses such as the *rectal, vesical, prostatic, vaginal,* and *uterine plexuses.*

Although there is variation in their targets, the sympathetic splanchnic nerves tend to follow a certain pattern. The greater thoracic splanchnic nerves contribute preganglionic sympathetic axons to synapse with postganglionic nerve cells in the celiac and superior mesenteric ganglia. Thus they innervate foregut and midgut organs. The lesser thoracic splanchnic nerves contribute preganglionic sympathetic axons to synapse with postganglionic nerve cells in the aorticorenal and superior mesenteric ganglia. Therefore they innervate midgut structures, gonadal structures, and structures associated with the kidneys. The least thoracic splanchnic nerves contribute preganglionic sympathetic axons to the superior mesenteric ganglion, also innervating midgut organs. The lumbar splanchnic nerves contribute to the superior mesenteric and inferior mesenteric ganglia as well as the intermesenteric and superior hypogastric plexuses. Thus the lumbar splanchnic nerves innervate midgut and hindgut organs and may contribute to the innervation of other pelvic organs. The preganglionic sympathetic axons in the sacral splanchnic nerves exit the sympathetic chain ganglia and enter the inferior hypogastric plexus on each side. They may synapse with postganglionic nerve cells within it or ascend to the superior hypogastric plexus and synapse there. The inferior hypogastric plexuses supply postganglionic sympathetic axons to the distal rectum and other pelvic organs.

In regard to parasympathetic efferent activity, descending fibers arising from the anterior region of the hypothalamus synapse with cells in the *dorsal vagal motor nuclei* in the medulla oblongata and also with cells in the *second to fourth sacral segments* of the spinal cord. The dorsal vagal motor nucleus contributes preganglionic parasympathetic axons to the *left* and *right vagus nerves,* which leave the jugular foramen to innervate thoracic and abdominopelvic organs. Activity of the vagus nerve in the thorax is not part of this discussion other than to mention that the left and right vagus nerves are closely associated with the esophagus and interweave to produce the *anterior* and *posterior vagal trunks,* which pierce the diaphragm alongside the esophagus to enter the abdomen. The anterior vagal trunk travels on the anterior aspect of the stomach, across the *hepatogastric ligament,* to innervate some of the liver and gallbladder. When each vagal trunk reaches the target organ, it synapses with postganglionic parasympathetic nerve cell bodies located within its wall. The posterior vagal trunk moves further posteriorly from the esophagus to run into the nearby celiac

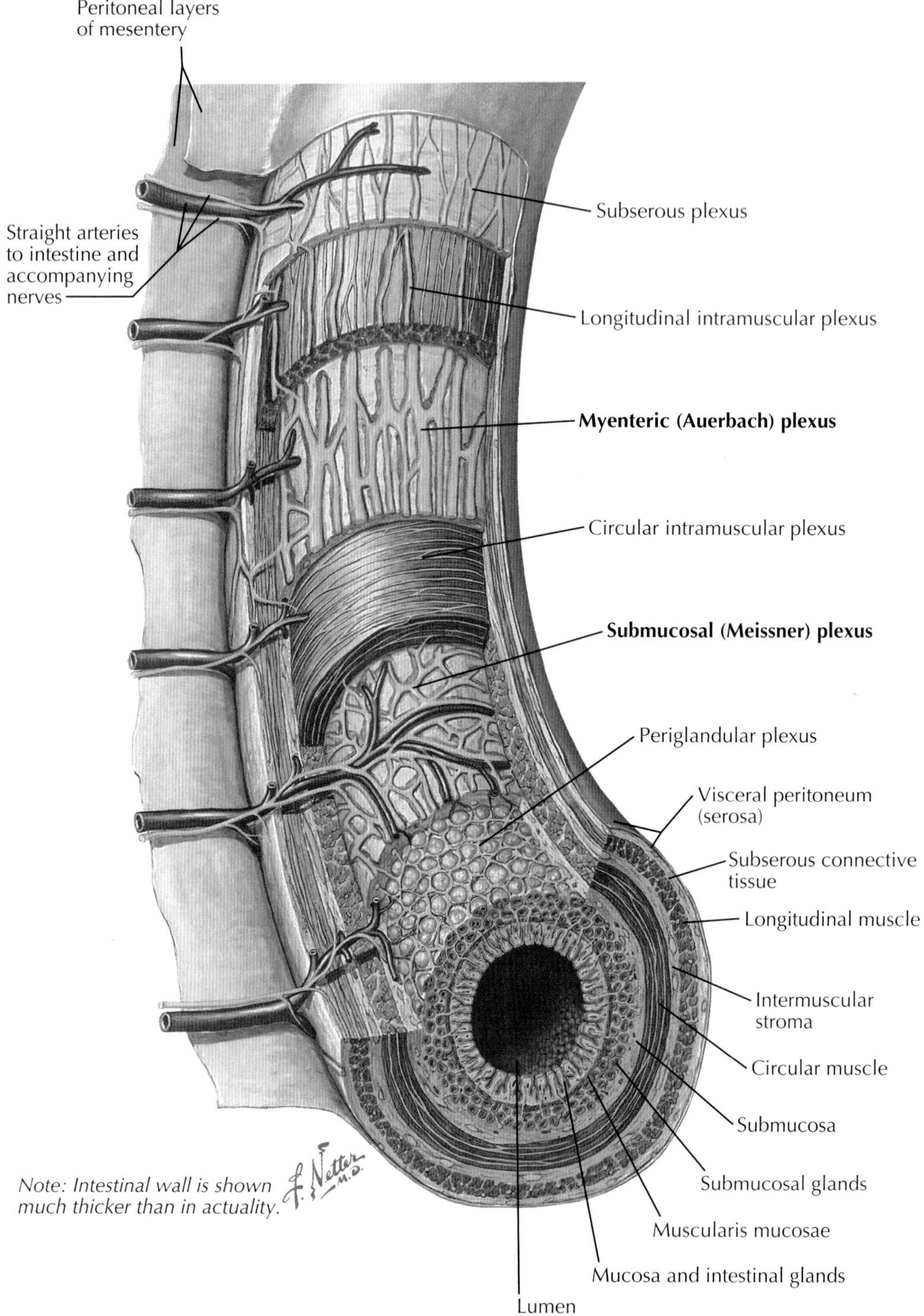

Autonomic Innervation of Small and Large Intestines: Schema

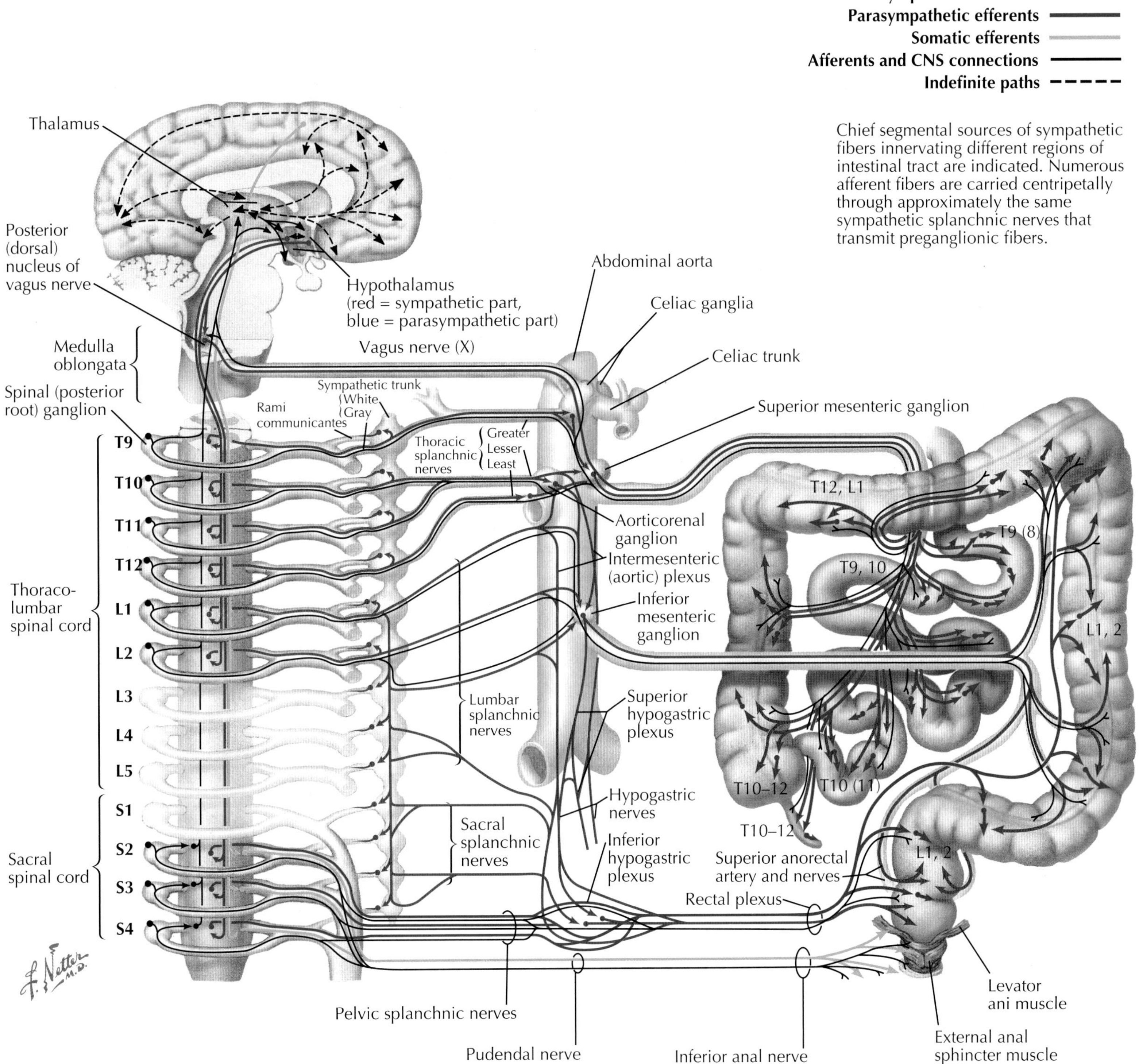


## Innervation of Small and Large Intestines (Continued)

ganglion. In contrast to the preganglionic sympathetic axons entering the celiac ganglion, the preganglionic parasympathetic axons do not synapse there but instead pass through the ganglion to enter the *celiac plexus*. From there, these axons, alongside the postganglionic sympathetic axons from the celiac ganglion and viscerosensory axons, travel along branches of the celiac trunk to reach the foregut organs. Once the celiac plexus reaches the foregut organs, the preganglionic parasympathetic axons within it synapse with postganglionic parasympathetic nerve cells within the wall of each organ.

Preganglionic parasympathetic axons from the posterior vagal trunk also pass inferiorly to reach the aorticorenal and superior mesenteric ganglia. As before, the preganglionic parasympathetic axons do not synapse in these ganglia but instead join the aorticorenal and superior mesenteric plexuses, which follow the arteries from the aorta to reach each of the target organs. In the case of the intestines, preganglionic parasympathetic axons from the posterior vagal trunk pass through the superior mesenteric ganglion to join postganglionic sympathetic and viscerosensory axons within the *superior mesenteric plexus*. The superior mesenteric plexus follows the branching of the SMA along its course through the mesentery and can be subdivided into plexuses named for each artery: *inferior pancreaticoduodenal, middle colic, jejunal, ileal, ileocolic, appendicular,* and *right colic plexuses,* which innervate the regions supplied by each vessel. The preganglionic parasympathetic axons synapse with a series of postganglionic parasympathetic nerve cell bodies that are scattered throughout the walls of the organs. These nerve cells make up the *enteric nervous system.*

## INNERVATION OF SMALL AND LARGE INTESTINES (Continued)

The vagus nerve supplies preganglionic parasympathetic axons that innervate structures of the thorax, foregut, and midgut, but the hindgut and other pelvic organs receive preganglionic parasympathetic axons from nerve cell bodies located within the sacral spinal cord. These cells project axons through the anterior rootlets, anterior roots, spinal nerves, and anterior rami of levels S2–S4. Once the anterior rami have exited the anterior sacral foramina, the preganglionic parasympathetic axons leave as *pelvic splanchnic nerves* and join the nearby right and left inferior hypogastric plexuses. Some of these axons form synapses in minute ganglia located near, or in the wall of, the pelvic structures (distal colon, rectum, bladder, and external and internal genital organs), to which they carry the impulses for visceromotor activity, vasodilation, and glandular secretion. These preganglionic parasympathetic axons may travel within the inferior hypogastric plexuses to synapse with postganglionic nerve cells in the pelvic organs and distal rectum. They may also ascend through the right and left hypogastric nerves to reach the superior hypogastric plexus and then the inferior mesenteric ganglion. Preganglionic parasympathetic axons pass through the inferior mesenteric ganglion without synapsing and join the *inferior mesenteric plexus* alongside postganglionic sympathetic axons and visceral afferent axons. The inferior mesenteric plexus follows the branches of the inferior mesenteric artery, branching into *left colic, sigmoid,* and *superior anorectal plexuses,* corresponding to the artery that carries the axons. The preganglionic parasympathetic axons synapse with a series of postganglionic parasympathetic nerve cell bodies that are scattered throughout the walls of the organs. These nerve cells form the enteric nervous system, and the axons of these ganglionic cells become the *postganglionic parasympathetic axons,* which, together with the postganglionic sympathetic axons in the plexus, innervate the smooth muscle of the intestinal wall, the vessels supplying the intestines, and the intestinal glands.

The enteric nervous system stretches the entire length of the alimentary tract from the esophagus to the rectum. This plexus consists of small groups of nerve cells interconnected by networks of fibers, and it is subdivided into myenteric (Auerbach) and submucosal (Meissner) plexuses. The *myenteric plexus* is found between the longitudinal and circular layers of the muscularis externa. Each main plexus, or primary plexus, gives off fibers that form finer secondary plexuses and even finer tertiary plexuses, which ramify both within and between the adjacent layers of muscle. Some fibers from the longitudinal intramuscular plexus enter the subserous tissue and constitute a rarefied subserous plexus. The *submucosal plexus* is located at the interface of the submucosal and muscularis externa layers. It is also subdivided into superficial and deep parts. Fibers from the deep part enter the mucosa, where they form delicate periglandular plexuses. The name of each subdivision of the enteric nervous system describes its location and histologic appearance. These distinctions are somewhat arbitrary, because all parts of the enteric nervous system are interconnected and form an exceedingly complex, self-regulating network. Sympathetic input to the enteric nervous system tends to restrict blood flow and slow the activity of the alimentary tract. Conversely, parasympathetic input tends to increase smooth muscle contraction and peristalsis as well as glandular secretion into the tract.

### AUTONOMIC INNERVATION OF SMALL INTESTINE

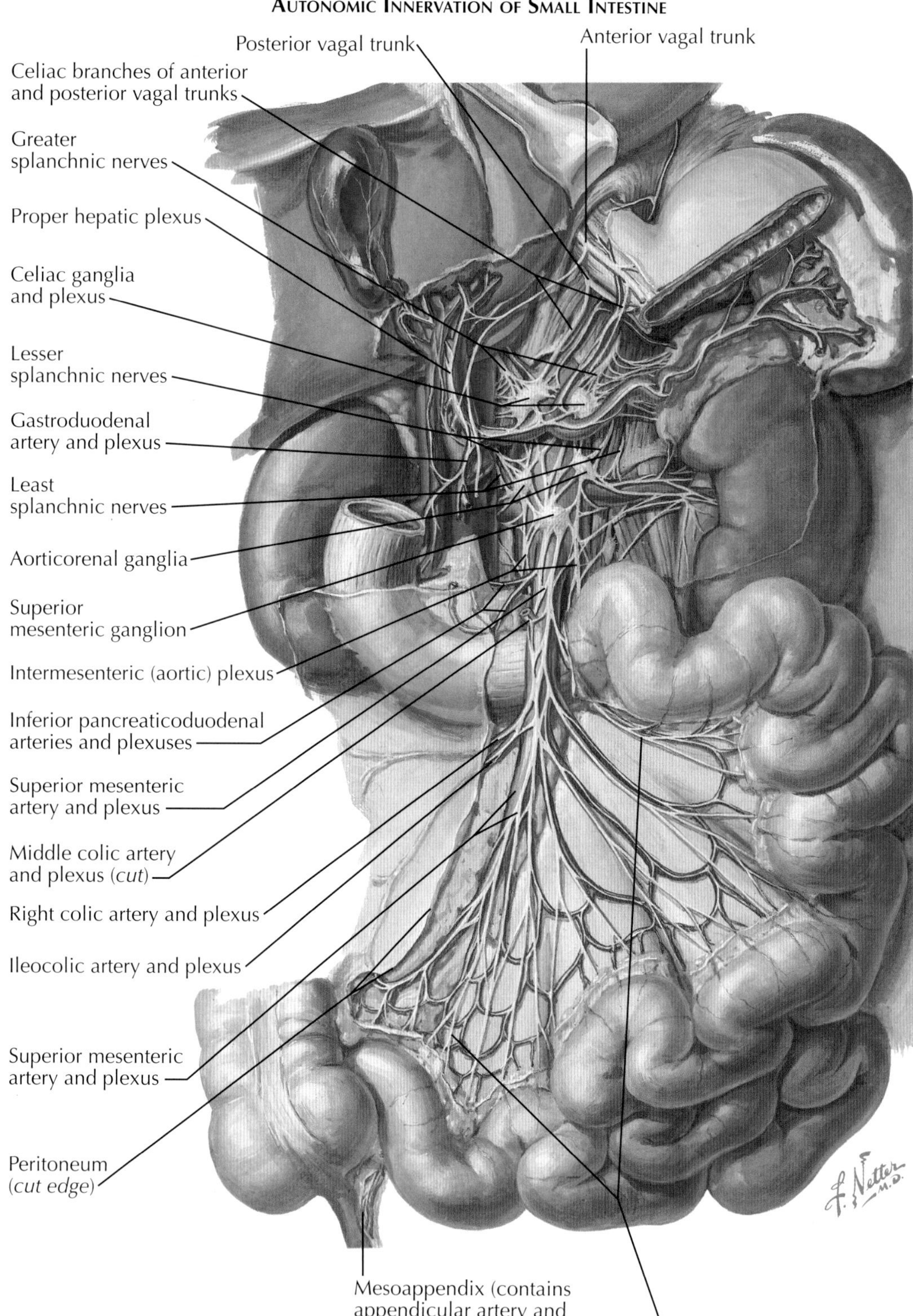


Viscerosensory activity related to the small and large intestines falls into two broad categories, visceral pain and normal visceral reflexive stimuli. The intestines are insensitive to ordinary tactile, painful, and thermal stimuli, although they respond to tension, ischemia, and chemical irritations with visceral pain. The free nerve endings of visceral pain axons extend from the intestines and join the plexus related to their blood supply in a retrograde fashion. For example, visceral pain from the jejunum would be carried back to the CNS by axons traveling along the jejunal plexus and the superior mesenteric plexus. Thereafter, visceral pain fibers travel in a retrograde fashion along the sympathetic innervation of the target organ. So in the case of visceral pain from the jejunum, after the axon has exited the superior mesenteric plexus, it continues along the lesser or least thoracic splanchnic nerves and through the sympathetic chain ganglia, white rami communicans, anterior ramus, and spinal nerve. At this time, being afferent, the axon travels along the posterior root to reach the spinal cord. Before reaching the spinal cord, the axon encounters (but does not synapse within) its nerve cell body. The nerve cell bodies of these viscerosensory axons are located in the spinal (posterior root) ganglia. Because these nerve cells are pseudounipolar, their axons extend from the target tissue to reach

## Innervation of Small and Large Intestines (Continued)

the cell body but also proximally to reach the posterior gray horn of the spinal cord.

Nonpainful, reflexive stimuli from the small and large intestines travel in a retrograde manner along the parasympathetic innervation of each organ. For this reason, a stimulus can follow two pathways. Foregut and midgut organs receive their preganglionic parasympathetic innervation via the vagus nerves; therefore reflexive visceral afferents from these organs contribute to the vagus nerves as they ascend to reach the brainstem and then project to the inferior aspect of the solitary nucleus. There are so many visceral afferents that they constitute the bulk of each vagus nerve. The pseudounipolar cell bodies for these axons are located in the *inferior vagal ganglion,* which is near the point where each vagus nerve exits from the jugular foramen. Hindgut organs do not receive parasympathetic input from the vagus nerves but rather from the pelvic splanchnic nerves. So in this case, reflexive afferent inputs from the hindgut project along the inferior mesenteric plexus, to the superior hypogastric plexus, right and left hypogastric nerves, right and left inferior hypogastric plexuses, pelvic splanchnic nerves, anterior rami of S2–S4, spinal nerves of S2–S4, posterior rami of S2–S4, and, finally, sacral spinal cord. As before, the cell bodies of these afferent axons are located in the spinal (posterior root) ganglia of S2–S4, and their smaller, proximal extensions project to the posterior horn of the sacral spinal cord.

An exception to this pattern occurs in abdominopelvic organs that are entirely covered by the peritoneum. In these organs (distal rectum, inferior aspect of the bladder, inferior aspect of the uterus, cervix, prostate, and seminal vesicles), both visceral pain and normal reflexive stimuli follow the parasympathetic pathways back to the sacral spinal cord. Once in the spinal cord, the exact course followed by visceral afferent pathways within the CNS is very complex.

There is evidence that these pathways behave in a fashion similar to that of the somatic pathways. Some of the visceral axons that enter the cord through the posterior roots form synapses with cells of the posterior horn near their level of entry, and the impulses are conveyed superiorly through tracts that lie near, or are commingled with, the anterolateral system. Other fibers ascend in the posterior white columns and may relay at higher levels in the brainstem. Some of these afferent visceral fibers, as well as the nonpainful reflexive inputs to the solitary nucleus, may pass with somatic fibers to the *thalamus* and be relayed onward to the postcentral gyrus. Other fibers form synapses in the *hypothalamus,* from whence fibers project to the premotor areas of the frontal cortex, the orbital surfaces, and the cingulate gyrus. In actuality, many of these hypothalamocortical connections are via relays in the anterior and medial nuclei of the thalamus. Possibly, the hypothalamus plays the same role in visceral afferent pathways as does the thalamus in their somatic counterparts. (To indicate the fact that the hypothalamocortical and the corticohypothalamic connections follow similar routes, the lines representing these pathways have arrows on both ends.)

Finally, the innervation of the anorectal transitional region combines features of the autonomic innervation of the rectum and the somatic innervation of the anus and perineum. This area develops from the anal pit, an invagination of the skin and surrounding mesoderm that meets the developing hindgut, forming a continuous tube as the membrane between the two regions ruptures. The two regions retain their distinct epithelium, innervation, and blood supply, transitioning in the region of the pecten. The portions of the rectum that are covered by peritoneum are innervated by postganglionic sympathetic axons from the inferior mesenteric ganglia and plexus as well as preganglionic parasympathetic axons that will synapse on postganglionic nerve cells in the wall of the rectum, the myenteric and submucosal plexuses. These plexuses supply the involuntary smooth muscles of the rectum and the internal anal sphincter. They dwindle as one progresses inferiorly through the anal region and are entirely absent below the intersphincteric groove (white line of Hilton) within the anal canal. The voluntary external anal sphincter is innervated mainly by somatomotor branches of the *inferior anal nerves,* branches of the pudendal nerve. These same nerves also convey the somatosensory axons from this region of the anal canal. Therefore below the pecten this innervation resembles that of the perineal skin and is very sensitive to tactile, painful, and thermal stimuli, whereas the upper part of the anal canal is almost insensitive to such stimuli but responds readily to alterations in tension or ischemia. From a practical point of view, this neuroanatomic situation explains why an anal fissure is so painful and why, in injections for internal hemorrhoids, the puncture is scarcely felt if the needle is inserted through the mucosa.

### Autonomic Innervation of Large Intestine

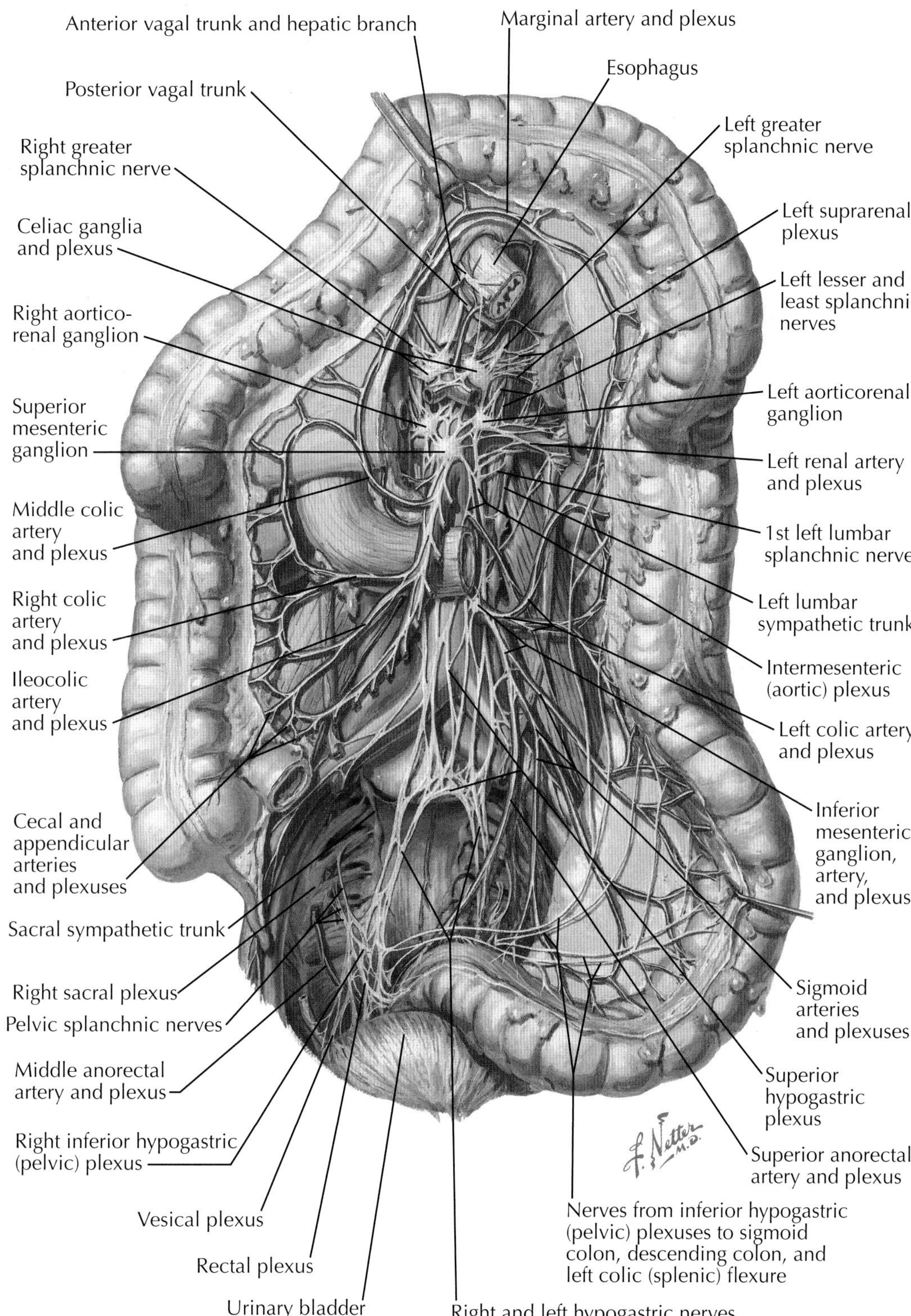

## SECRETORY, DIGESTIVE, AND ABSORPTIVE FUNCTIONS OF SMALL AND LARGE INTESTINES

The purpose of the complex enzymatic reactions to which foodstuffs are exposed within the intestinal lumen is to prepare nutrients for transfer into and assimilation within the organism. The lumen of the digestive system, which is the space encompassed by the wall of the digestive tube, belongs, fundamentally speaking, to the outside world, and the processes by which the products of digestion enter and pass through the intestinal wall into the circulation are called *secretion* and *absorption*, respectively. The mucosa of the small intestine throughout its length is lined by cells involved with both secretion and absorption: mucus-secreting cells, neuroendocrine cells, and immune active cells. The incredible efficiency of intestinal function is emphasized by the fact that of the approximately 8 L of fluid that enters the small intestine, only 100 to 200 mL is excreted from the rectum, for an efficiency rate in excess of 98%. In disease states, the large and small intestines absorb even more fluid, sometimes exceeding 25 L per day. Alternatively, in secretory disorders and infection, the volume of diarrhea lost may rapidly pose a life-threatening risk of dehydration, with the loss of many liters of fluids and their accompanying electrolytes.

### SECRETION

The secretory product of the duodenal glands is an alkaline, pale-yellow, viscous fluid, rich in bicarbonates and also containing mucus. Its primary function is protecting the proximal duodenum against the corrosive action of the acidic gastric contents entering the intestine. Whereas there is an increasing relative absorption to secretion as nutrients pass into the jejunum and ileum, secretion persists from epithelial cells, goblet cells, and submucosal glands. The resulting luminal contents, or *succus entericus,* are constantly being mixed with mucus, bile, and digestive enzyme–laden pancreatic juice. The intestinal secretion contains a wide variety of digestive enzymes, namely, peptidases, nucleases, nucleosidases, phosphatase, lipase, maltase, sucrase, and lactase. Brush-border enterokinase is essential in activating the cascade of proenzymes secreted by the pancreas, including the cascades of trypsinogen to trypsin and chymotrypsinogen to chymotrypsin. The fact that digestion can proceed even in patients who have undergone total pancreatectomy indicates that the brush-border and secreted digestive intestinal enzymes are important. Motility of the small intestine is activated by parasympathetic nerves, enteric nerves, and a host of enteric hormones acting both locally (paraendocrine hormones) and through the systemic circulation (most notably, cholecystokinin and secretin). These neurologic and hormonal reflexes are stimulated by the presence of acids and nutrients and by distension of the stomach and small intestine. These processes are slowed when nutrients, especially fats and essential amino acids, reach the distal small bowel. There they activate the so-called *ileal brake* by means of neural mechanisms and release of hormones, including peptide YY and glucagon-like peptide-1. Throughout the digestive process, mucus is being secreted from the intestinal crypts and epithelial cells on the villi to ensure adequate lubrication and protection of the surface epithelial cells.

Mucus is also secreted by colonic epithelium when it has been stimulated mechanically or chemically. The epithelium also secretes an alkaline-rich fluid high in potassium, which is exchanged for sodium as the fecal stream is solidified through dehydration processes.

DIGESTION OF PROTEIN

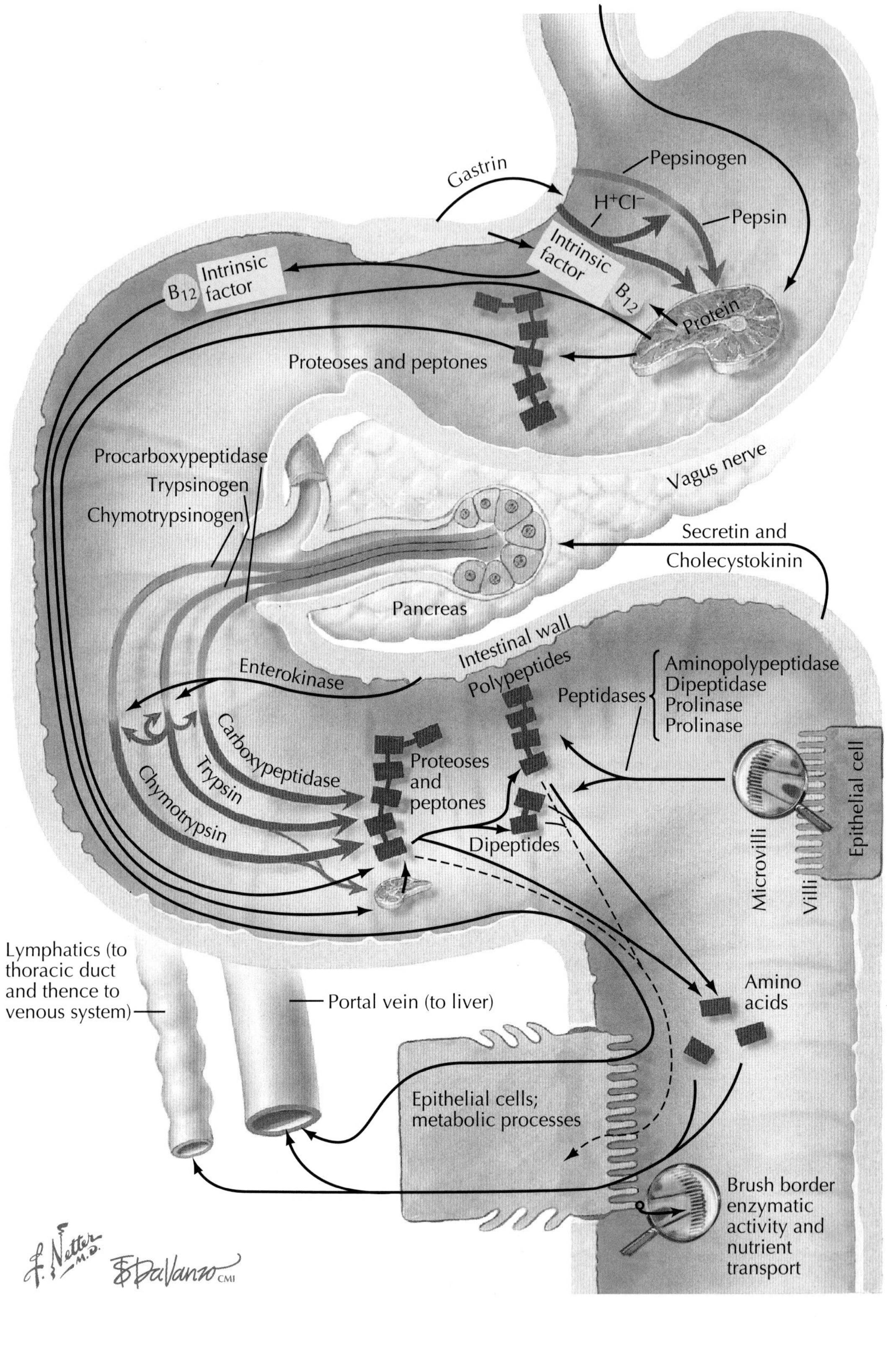

# Secretory, Digestive, and Absorptive Functions of Small and Large Intestines (Continued)

## DIGESTION

The normal diet includes a variety of macronutrients composed of carbohydrates, nucleic acids, and proteins that are soluble in water and of fats, which are not. It also contains minerals, vitamins, and other micronutrients. Each requires specific, distinct pathways for digestion in preparation for absorption.

The digestion of proteins is carried out by gastric peptidases, an array of brush-border enzymes, and enzymes secreted by the pancreas. The primary gastric peptidase is pepsin, but chymosin is also active in an acidic environment. Chief cells secrete an inactive substance, pepsinogen, which is activated by acid in the stomach to become pepsin. Pancreatic juices contain a rich supply of proteins that make up over 20 isoforms of 12 distinct enzymes and cofactors, most of which are proteases. All proteases are secreted as inactive proenzymes (zymogens), as are phospholipase and colipase. The proteolytic actions of each protein-splitting enzyme have a highly specific effect. Each attacks only certain linkages of the protein molecule or of the degradation products resulting from the preceding effects of one or more catalytically active compounds. According to their functions, they are typically grouped as either exopeptidases or endopeptidases. Trypsinogen is activated by the brush-border enzyme enterokinase to become its active form, trypsin, which in turn activates other enzymes. Trypsin, chymotrypsin, carboxypeptidase, and the intestinal aminopeptidases act only on polypeptides or peptides containing a free amino group. The dipeptidases act only on dipeptides. As the peptide is digested within the lumen, it diffuses to the epithelial surface, where a number of membrane-bound peptidases continue the digestive process. This cascade of proteolytic effects breaks down the original protein until it has been fragmented into its elementary components, the 26 amino acids, dipeptides, or tripeptides, in preparation for absorption.

For the *digestion of nucleoproteins,* the pancreas supplies nucleases, ribonuclease, deoxyribonuclease, and other substances that specifically hydrolyze nucleosides: pentose or deoxypentose is conjugated to purines and pyrimidine bases. Intestinal secretion also provides nucleases and, particularly, phosphatases, which split nucleotides (phosphoric esters of nucleosides) into their components.

Dietary carbohydrates may consist of monosaccharides such as glucose and fructose, disaccharides such as lactose and sucrose, or polysaccharides. The processes involved in the *digestion of carbohydrates* are therefore primarily concerned with the enzymatic cleavage of polysaccharides and oligosaccharides into monosaccharides. Polysaccharides include starch, glycogen, and fibers such as cellulose, gums, and pectins. In human nutrition, the most important carbohydrate is *starch,* which is a polysaccharide occurring as an energy reservoir in plants, particularly cereals, grains, roots, and tubers. The counterpart in animals is glycogen, another polysaccharide ingested with meat and liver. In both starch and glycogen, a large number of hexoses (monosaccharides) are linked together, forming either a straight chain or a branched chain of molecules. The linkage between these molecules varies, and to open them, the organism is equipped with a variety of specifically active enzymes.

DIGESTION OF CARBOHYDRATES

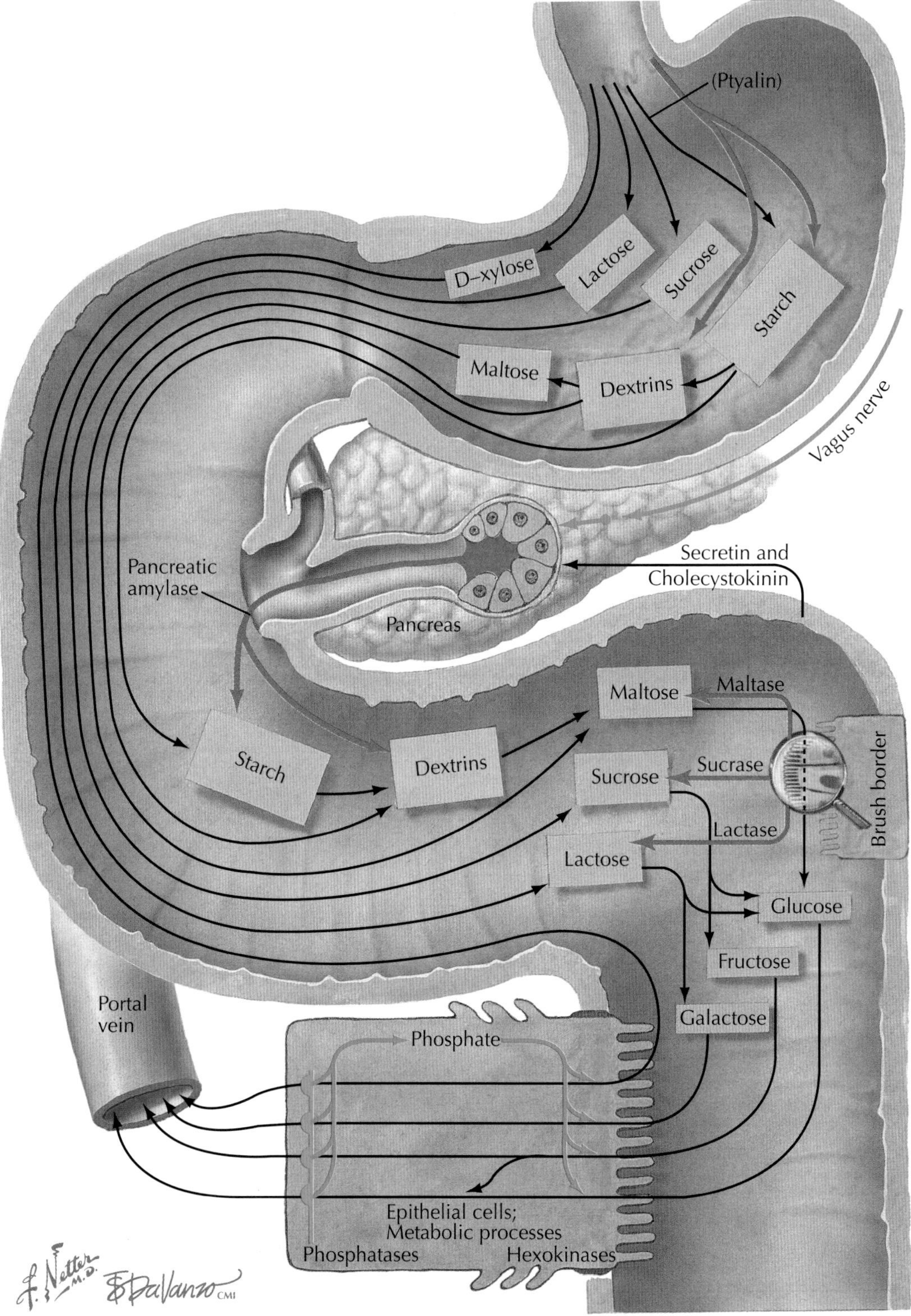

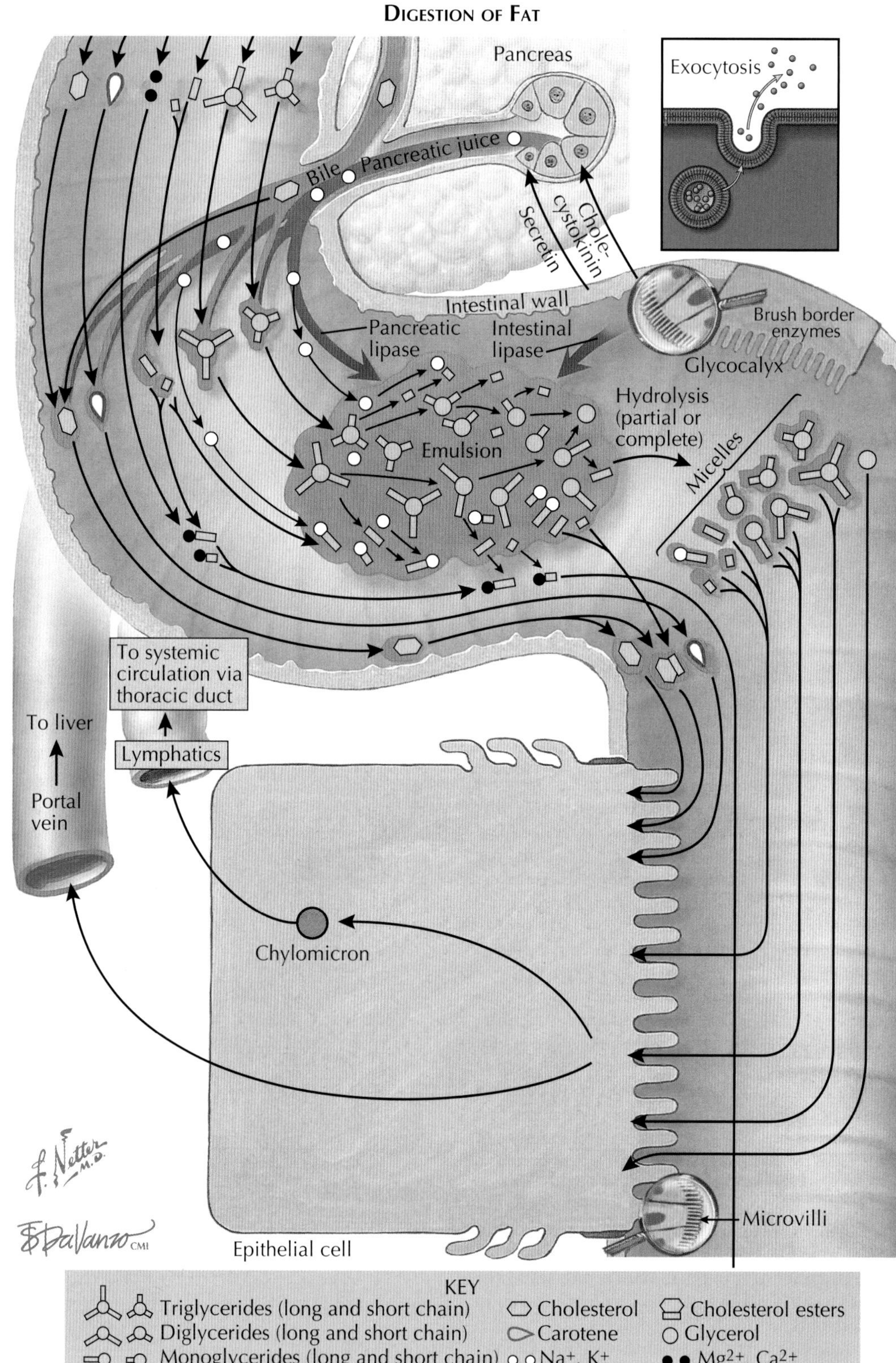


## SECRETORY, DIGESTIVE, AND ABSORPTIVE FUNCTIONS OF SMALL AND LARGE INTESTINES (Continued)

Starch-splitting enzymes called *amylases* are secreted by the pancreas and, to a lesser extent, by the salivary glands. The digestion of carbohydrates begins in the mouth with the action of salivary amylase. Because salivary amylase is inactivated by gastric acid in the stomach, the actions of the enzyme mainly affect the outer portions of the food mass. Once it reaches the stomach and the gastric acid has penetrated the food mass, digestion of carbohydrates slows or stops until the food mass reaches the duodenum. In the duodenum, carbohydrates are acted on by the more effective enzymes α-amylase and β-amylase, which are synthesized in the pancreas and then secreted in their active forms. The action of the amylases yields the disaccharide *maltose* and a polysaccharide fragment called *dextrin,* which cannot be further digested by amylase. Therefore except during the period of infancy, when the secretory activity of the pancreas has not yet fully developed, the degradation of starch into the disaccharide *maltose* and the monosaccharide *glucose* is completed in the lower part of the duodenum and in the jejunum and ileum. The splitting of maltose into two molecules of glucose is catalyzed by *maltase,* an enzyme formed by the intestinal glands. Disaccharides are primarily digested by intestinal brush-border enzymes such as *sucrose-isomaltase,* which converts sucrose (common table sugar) into a molecule of glucose and a molecule of fructose, and *lactase-phlorizin hydrolase,* which converts lactase (milk sugar) into glucose and *galactose.* Other brush-border disaccharidases include glucoamylase and trehalase. The end products, therefore, are simple monosaccharides, which the intestinal epithelial cell is prepared to absorb.

In humans, cellulose is indigestible, because humans, in contrast to some animals, lack enzymes capable of attacking the specific bonds of cellulose. The enzymes derived from the bacterial flora of the human colonic microbiota can act on cellulose and on the undigested starch reaching the distal gut. This action of the microbiota produces increased osmotically active substances that attract fluid into the lumen and produce gas through fermentation. Both result in distension that increases colonic motility; when this distension is excessive, it can lead to discomfort interpreted as "gas" and to increased flatulence and bloating.

Lipids include a variety of heterogeneous molecules often described as fats. The term includes triglycerides, phospholipids, cholesterol, steroids, and fat-soluble vitamins. From the dietary point of view, the triglycerides are of major importance due to their high-energy value. Triglycerides, whether of plant origin (unsaturated) or animal origin (mostly saturated), are esters of glycerol and fatty acids. The esters are named *triglycerides* because the three alcoholic hydroxyl groups of glycerol are bound in an ester linkage to the carboxyl group (the group that determines the acid character) of either saturated or unsaturated organic acids, such as palmitic, stearic, oleic, or linoleic acid. The term *neutral fat* has also been used to describe these important nutrients because no acidic group is free. In an aqueous milieu, fats align with their hydrophobic groups adjacent to each other and their polar groups facing the surrounding water. This arrangement creates bilayers or micelles. Nonpolar lipids accumulate in the inner portions of these micelles. Further digestion of fats requires access to these molecules within the micelle. Bile salts and the coenzyme colipase are essential factors that facilitate this access. Triglycerides are *digested*

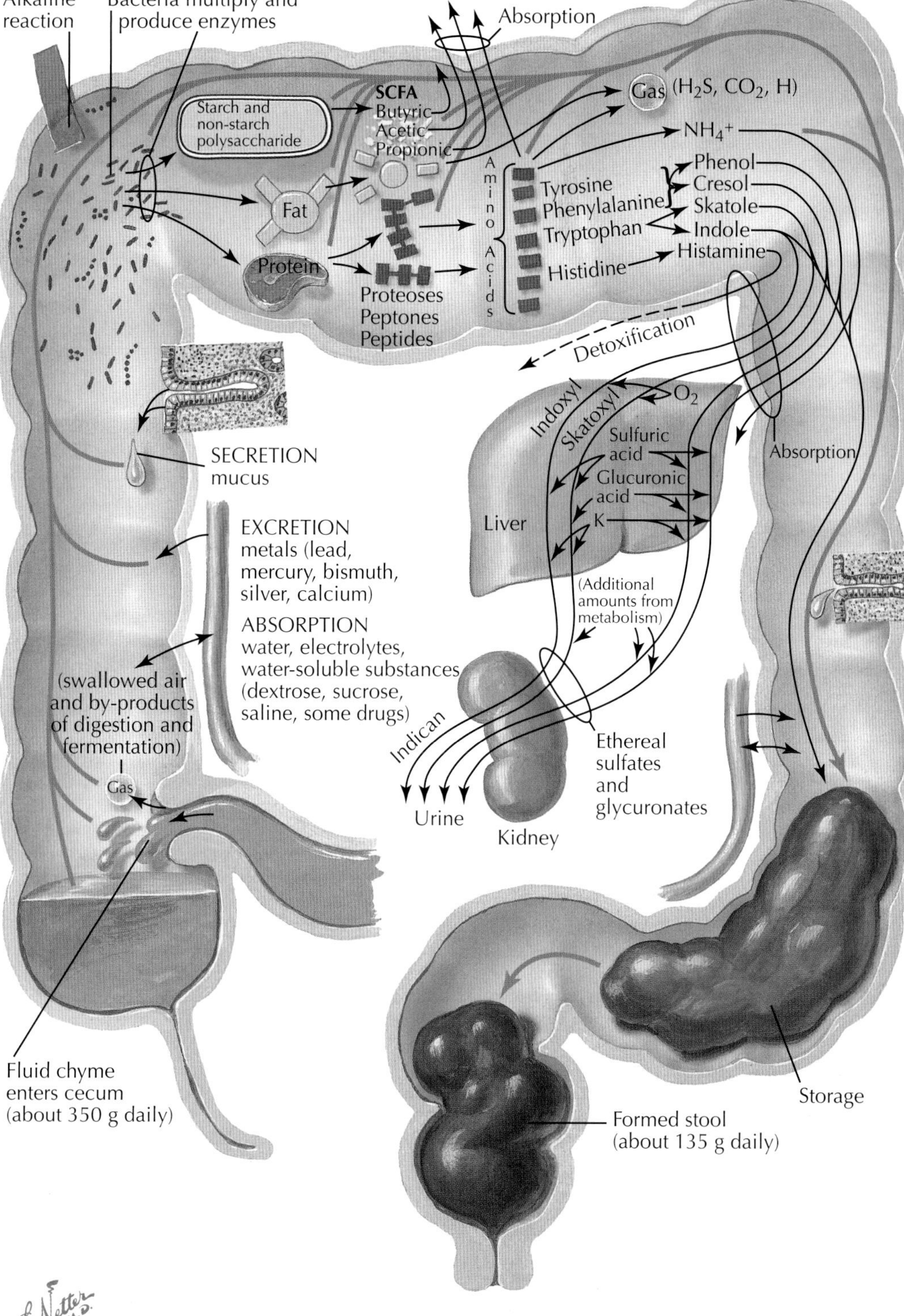


## Secretory, Digestive, and Absorptive Functions of Small and Large Intestines (Continued)

by hydrolyzation of the ester linkage, yielding the components of the esters, namely, *glycerol* and the various *fatty acids.* The splitting of fat occurs in stages, meaning that the *triglycerides* lose first one of their three acid molecules, leaving a *diglyceride* (i.e., a glycerol ester containing only two acids), and this, in turn, is hydrolyzed to a *monoglyceride,* which possesses only one acid molecule.

The hydrolysis of triglycerides and phospholipids is accomplished by *lipases* and *phospholipases,* respectively, that are secreted by the salivary glands, stomach, pancreas, and intestinal glands. A limited amount of fat is digested in the stomach by a lingual lipase originating in saliva and the gastric lipase originating from the chief cells in the stomach. The gastric lipase can function in an acidic environment, in contrast to other lipases, which act in a nearly neutral environment. In most adults, this gastric lipase is of limited significance, but it is important in patients with pancreatic insufficiency; it is also important in infants, in whom it is capable of hydrolyzing the highly emulsified fat of milk. The pancreas is the major source of bicarbonate, which serves to neutralize gastric acidity, and of lipase activity. It also is the source of colipase, which plays an important role as a cofactor at the interface of water, bile salt, and lipid by enhancing lipolysis. The phospholipids undergo hydrolysis into their component parts by secretions of a proenzyme from the pancreas that is activated by trypsin to produce phospholipase A. This hydrolysis produces glycerol, fatty acids, phosphate, and the special compound characteristic of the particular phospholipid (choline, serine, inositol, or ethanolamine). In contrast to the enzymes involved in protein and carbohydrate digestion, which act with a high degree of specificity on certain compounds or chemically well-defined groups or bonds, the action of lipases of animal or plant origin is far less specific.

In the lower duodenum, fat is mixed with bile and dispersed into a fine emulsion. The components of bile responsible for this action are the bile acids, mostly glycocholic acid and taurocholic acid, which act as detergents. The result of the emulsification of fat in the aqueous medium of the intestinal chyme is an enormous increase of the surface area of the fat particles, facilitating the hydrolytic action of the pancreatic and intestinal lipases. The fatty acids, whether ingested with food or arising as split products of fat hydrolysis, combine in the intestine with bile salts and cations, forming soluble soaps with sodium and potassium and insoluble soaps with calcium and magnesium. Bile is important for the emulsification of ingested water-insoluble or less-soluble fats in the digestion mixture. Insoluble soaps, the monoglycerides, are "ferried" through the lumen to the cellular barrier with complexes of colipase and bile acids. The soluble alkali soaps aid in the emulsification of fat and the stabilization of emulsified lipids by the same principle that makes soap useful in the household for cleansing and detergent effects.

Much of ingested cholesterol is not esterified in the lumen, although some hydrolysis occurs through the action of cholesterol esterase. Instead, cholesterol can be taken up intact through specific facilitated transport. Other lipids, such as vitamin A (and its provitamin, carotene), vitamins E and K, and other steroids, including vitamin D, are not broken down within the intestine.

## ABSORPTION

The absorption of nearly all nutrients is achieved by the small intestinal cells of the duodenal, jejunal, and ileal epithelia. The small, but important, amount of nutrient absorption and the significant amount of water and electrolyte absorption that take place in the colon are described at the end of this section. Selective absorption also occurs across the oral and gastric epithelia. The epithelial lining of the small intestine is preeminently and specifically equipped for its function by its length and its large surface area. The surface area of the intestinal tube is increased by the presence of luminal folds, villi, and, most importantly, microvilli. Small intestinal folds are arrayed in a special circular design perpendicular to the axis of the lumen, which enhances the turbulent flow of the luminal contents, known as the *plicae circulares.* Villi further increase the surface area 15- to 30-fold, and microvilli increase the surface area an additional 20- to 40-fold.

Ions are transported across the epithelium by ion channels and ion exchangers and by cotransporters that facilitate diffusion, osmosis, and solvent drag. Other complex molecular transport mechanisms involve specific receptor-mediated transport proteins and other active transport mechanisms. The presence of transport proteins on the apical surface and the tight junctions between cells permit movement of fluid as the epithelium actively transports substances against a concentration gradient. Ion-specific channel proteins permit the movement of hydrophilic ions through the hydrophobic bilayer of the cell membrane along concentration gradients (facilitated diffusion). These ion channels are also "gated," so that they permit transport only for a brief period in which the channel is open; then the gate closes.

Water crosses the intestinal wall in both directions, depending on hydraulic and osmotic forces based on the osmolality of luminal contents and the location within the small intestine. This occurs across the cell membrane and between cells in the paracellular channels that are exquisitely regulated by tight junctions and their regulatory and contractile proteins. Aquaporin water channels are less common in the gut than in the renal tubules. If the aqueous phase of the intestinal contents is hypotonic, water moves from the lumen through the cells and between the cells through paracellular spaces into the blood. Alternatively, if the luminal content is hypertonic, water will be transferred from the blood into the lumen. As solutes enter the wall, an obligatory transport of water from the lumen occurs to keep the solution within the tube isosmotic.

Most minerals, such as the salts composed of sodium, potassium, and chloride ions, move with the water across channels, but, in addition, specific ion pumps, exchangers, and cotransport mechanisms exist to bring needed ions into the epithelial cells and then into the circulation, often against a steep concentration gradient. Active transport by ion pumps requires energy expenditure through the hydrolysis of adenosine triphosphate. Carrier proteins can couple electrolyte transport with specific nutrients, including glucose and amino acids. For example, the cotransport of each molecule of glucose brings two molecules of sodium into the epithelial cell. Chloride is transported into the lumen by means of the chloride channel on the apical cell membrane, primarily the cystic fibrosis transmembrane conductance regulator. It is absorbed across tight junctions and via exchange proteins with bicarbonate.

Calcium must be solubilized before it can be absorbed through acidification in the stomach or at the brush-border surface by the action of the $Na^+$-$H^+$ exchanger. Absorption through channels or by carriers is tightly regulated through vitamin D–mediated processes. Once in the lumen, it is bound by a calcium-binding protein, calbindin-D9k.

Like calcium, magnesium is absorbed by both passive and active processes, primarily in the duodenum and upper jejunum. Magnesium absorption is much less efficient than is calcium absorption; this accounts for the efficacy of its salts to function as osmotic laxatives.

Males absorb 1 mg of iron daily; 2 mg of iron daily is absorbed by menstruating females, again primarily through the duodenum. Ferric iron must be solubilized to ferrous iron to be absorbed. This occurs through the effect of gastric acid, ascorbic acid, or brush-border reductases. The divalent brush-border transporter carries this essential nutrient into the cell, where it is oxidized by heme-oxidase before being transported out of the cell. Its absorption is tightly regulated by the hepatic synthesis of the peptide hepcidin, based on the needs of the body.

The concentration of bile in the intestine diminishes as the chyme enters the distal intestine. Effective active transport of bile acids by the distal ileum is necessary to maintain healthy concentrations of these complex molecules. Malabsorption will lead to bile salt diarrhea.

The products of protein digestion formed by the combination of gastric, pancreatic, and brush-border peptidases result in dipeptides or tripeptides and *amino acids* that can diffuse to the cell membrane surface. There they are brought into the cell by more than a dozen specific sodium-coupled transport mechanisms. The rate of absorption for various amino acids is different, and quantitatively most may be absorbed as dipeptides and tripeptides. Once in the enterocyte, all are degraded further to isolated amino acids. Although some amino acids entering the cells are synthesized within them, most are transported by the basolateral membrane directly into the circulation. Under special circumstances, intact protein molecules may be absorbed through specialized channels and the process of pinocytosis associated with M cells as part of the gut immune regulatory system.

*Carbohydrates* are absorbed almost exclusively in the form of monosaccharides, that is, as hexoses (glucose, fructose, and galactose) or pentoses (ribose and deoxyribose). Monosaccharides are absorbed via specific sodium-coupled cotransport proteins that recognize only the D isomer of the molecule. Galactose is more rapidly absorbed than is glucose. Fructose is absorbed via facilitated transport down a concentration gradient via its own specific transport protein, GLUT5. Within fairly wide limits, the rate of hexose transfer is independent of the intraluminal concentration. The presence of enzymes (hexokinases) catalyzing the conversion of hexoses to hexose phosphates in the intestinal mucosa and the reduction of glucose and galactose absorption can occur when the hexokinases are inhibited by phlorizin. The picture of the absorption of pentoses is still less clear. The transfer of xylose, used now as an indicator of the efficiency of intestinal absorption, may involve diffusion or phosphorylation, or both.

Lipolysis hydrolyzes fats to diglycerides, then monoglycerides, and then completely hydrolyzed fat components, glycerol, and fatty acids that enter the cell through a specific transport mechanism, including fatty acid translocase CD36. Once absorbed, the split products are transported in the cell by fatty acid–binding proteins to the endoplasmic reticulum, where they are resynthesized back to triglycerides. Other lipids are added, including apolipoproteins, in the Golgi apparatus, and the product is packaged into secretory granules. These leave the cell by exocytosis as chylomicrons, moving into the lymphatics to the rest of the body. Some lipids exit the cell in very-low-density lipoproteins. Other lipids and some phospholipids may be further degraded, leave the cell, and enter the portal system. Similarly, cholesterol is transported into the cell by specific transport proteins located on the apical brush borders. It is processed within the cell and exits in chylomicrons or very-low-density lipoproteins.

The absorption of other lipids, cholesterol, phosphatides, and fat-soluble vitamins is intimately related to the mechanisms of fat absorption. Although some *cholesterol* may be esterified in the lumen, most is transported into the cell through receptor-mediated transport. Free cholesterol and the cholesterol esters leave the intestinal cells by way of the lymph stream. The absorption of the hydrolytic products of phospholipid digestion (see above) follows the line indicated for fat absorption.

Vitamin A is a water-insoluble lipid derived from dietary carotenoid. The vitamin is actually made up of a family of biologically active retinoids. These retinoids are esterified to long-chain fatty acids that are hydrolyzed by pancreatic enzymes. Absorption occurs via passive, noncarrier-mediated transport into the cell, where the vitamin is further oxidized and eventually bound to retinol-binding protein for distribution to the rest of the body. Active vitamin D is the result of a complex series of steps, including actions in the kidney, liver, and skin. Although the skin can synthesize vitamin D under adequate exposure to sunlight, in more northern climates, absorption of the inactive unesterified sterol precursors vitamin $D_3$ (cholecalciferol) and $D_2$ (ergocalciferol) is important for their nutrient value. After absorption by the enterocyte, they are exported in chylomicrons to the circulation, where they become bound to transport proteins. In the liver, they are metabolized to 25-hydroxyvitamin D and then to 1,25-dihdroxyvitamin $D_3$ by the kidney.

The mechanisms involved in the absorption of the water-soluble vitamins (thiamine, riboflavin, nicotinic acid, pyridoxine, pantothenic acid, ascorbic acid, and cyanocobalamin [vitamin $B_{12}$]) involve vitamin-specific, complex, receptor-mediated mechanisms after partial intraluminal metabolism. As discussed elsewhere, vitamin $B_{12}$ is absorbed by complex interactions of two binding proteins. The salivary glands secrete a pH-dependent binding protein (R protein) known as *haptocorrin* that protects the vitamin from intragastric digestion. Once the complex reaches the duodenum, proteolysis releases haptocorrin, permitting the intrinsic factor secreted by the gastric parietal cells to bind $B_{12}$ and facilitate its protection until absorbed in the distal ileum. The intrinsic factor–vitamin $B_{12}$ complex is bound to the cubam receptor on ileal epithelium. There the complex is actively absorbed by endocytosis into the ileum.

Unlike other important nutrients and vitamins, vitamin K is primarily derived from synthetic actions of the microbiota and is absorbed by the colonic epithelium. Although malabsorption of most fat-soluble vitamins is due to a deficiency of pancreatic enzymes or bile salts, vitamin K deficiency more commonly results from inadequate nutrition and the deleterious effects of antibiotics on the microbiota.

As mentioned, the role of the colon in absorbing nutrients to be used by the rest of the body is negligible. Colonic epithelial cells, however, are able to absorb short-chain fatty acids that are a major source of energy for the epithelial cells. Effective absorption of fluid and electrolytes by the colon is important and serves to limit the loss of fluid in the stool by nearly a liter under normal circumstances and by more when small intestinal fluid delivery to the colon increases during disease states. It also limits the volume of fluid loss and the inconvenience of frequent defecations.

**Causes of Gastrointestinal Hemorrhage**

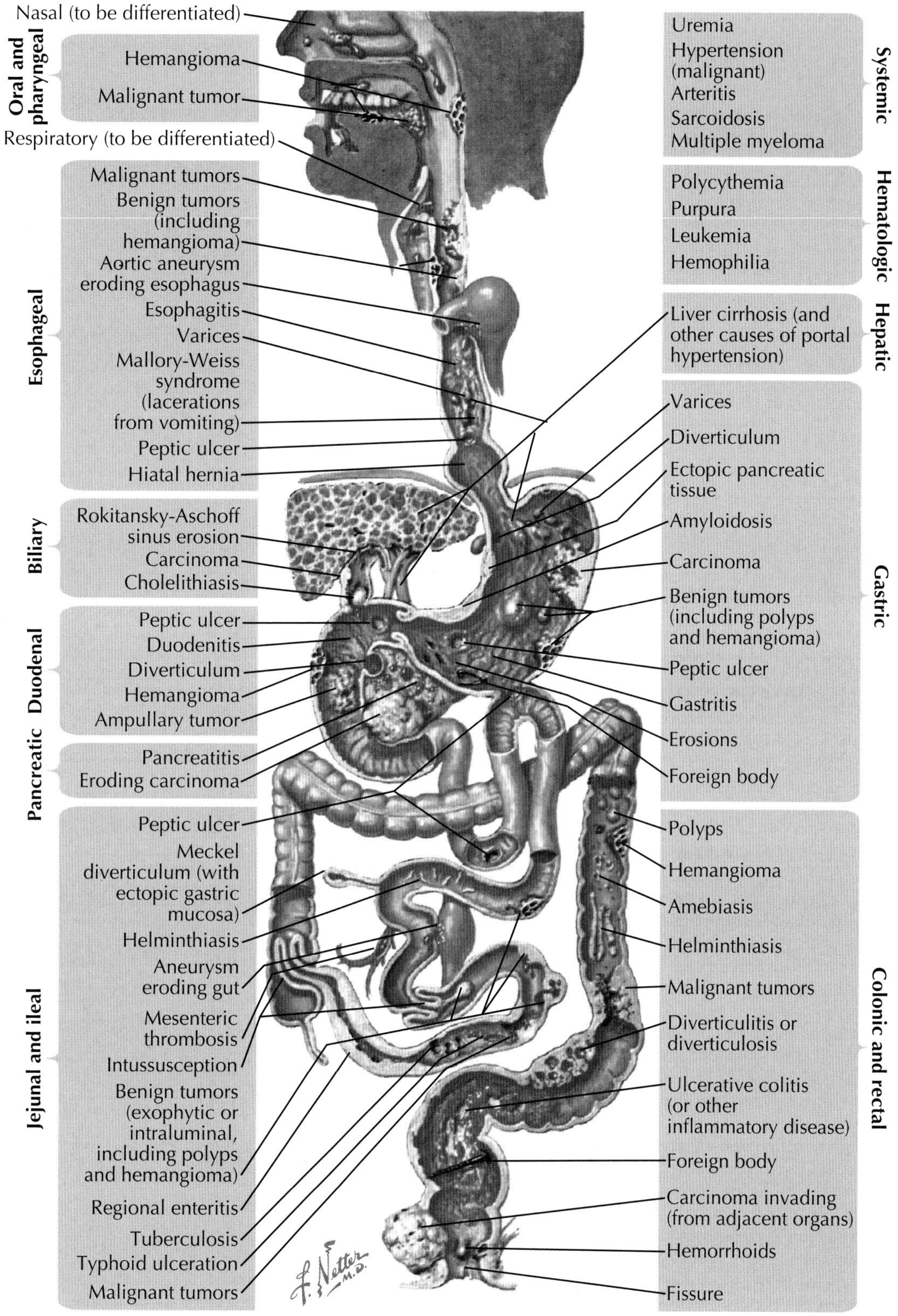

## Overview of Gastrointestinal Hemorrhage

Many gastrointestinal disorders manifest themselves by bleeding. Intestinal bleeding may present as bright-red blood, suggesting gross lower bleeding (hematochezia), passage of black stool (melena), or other findings of bleeding but no change in stool color (occult bleeding). When no cause of bleeding can be detected with the usual examinations, obscure gastrointestinal bleeding is occurring.

More severe hemorrhages reveal themselves by the appearance of visible blood in the stool, where it may be intermingled with the fecal material as bright-red blood (*hematochezia*) or appear as bloody diarrhea. Hematochezia in small volumes is almost always caused by a colonic lesion. In contrast, passage of large volumes of red blood or bloody stools may be caused by intestinal disorders or upper gastrointestinal hemorrhage, in which case it signifies massive bleeding. It is often noted that the most common etiology of hemodynamically significant lower GI bleeding is an upper GI source originating above the ligament of Treitz. Lesions causing upper gastrointestinal bleeding can accurately be detected in more than 95% of cases by upper endoscopy. Upper endoscopy is a procedure of shorter duration than colonoscopy, does not require bowel preparation, and often detects lesions that can be easily treated by a wide variety of effective devices. If upper endoscopy is negative, attention should be directed to the colon as the most likely source and to the small intestine only if thorough evaluations of both the upper digestive tract and colon are negative.

Distinguishing upper bleeding from lower bleeding is often challenging, even for experts. Bleeding that is at first thought to originate in the colon will later be determined to be from an upper source in 15% of patients. An upper digestive organ source is confirmed in patients with hematemesis, blood in a nasogastric lavage, or blood seen endoscopically. An upper source should be pursued before proceeding with colonoscopy whenever bleeding is brisk and hemodynamically significant, there is melena, there is known or suspected liver disease, the patient has been taking nonsteroidal antiinflammatory drugs, or there are known upper pathologic findings. Lower gastrointestinal bleeding is less likely if the blood urea nitrogen–to-creatinine ratio is higher than 25 and very unlikely if the ratio is higher than 50.

Substantial bleeding may also present as black stool, known as *melena*. The black color indicates that blood has been exposed to the digestive activity of intestinal secretions, and therefore, as a rule, it is a sign that the bleeding originates from a lesion in the gut above the cecum. Rarely, however, melena may occur with lesions located as low as the left colon. Because colonoscopy will detect a source of bleeding in the colon in less than 5% of patients with melena who have had a negative

Management of Gastrointestinal Hemorrhage

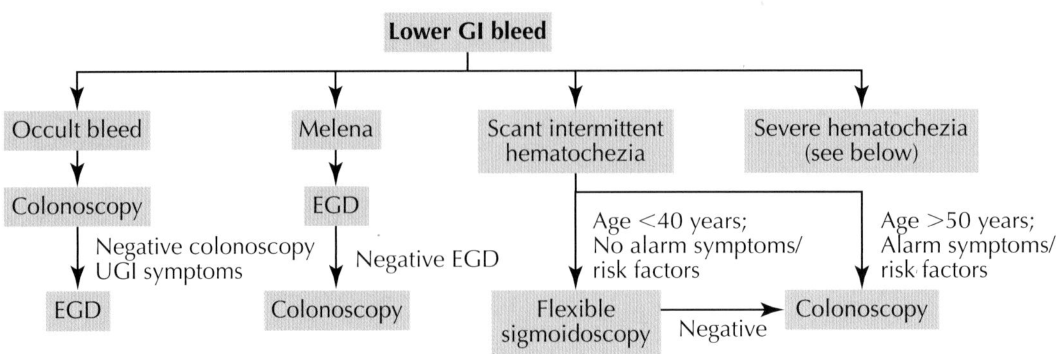


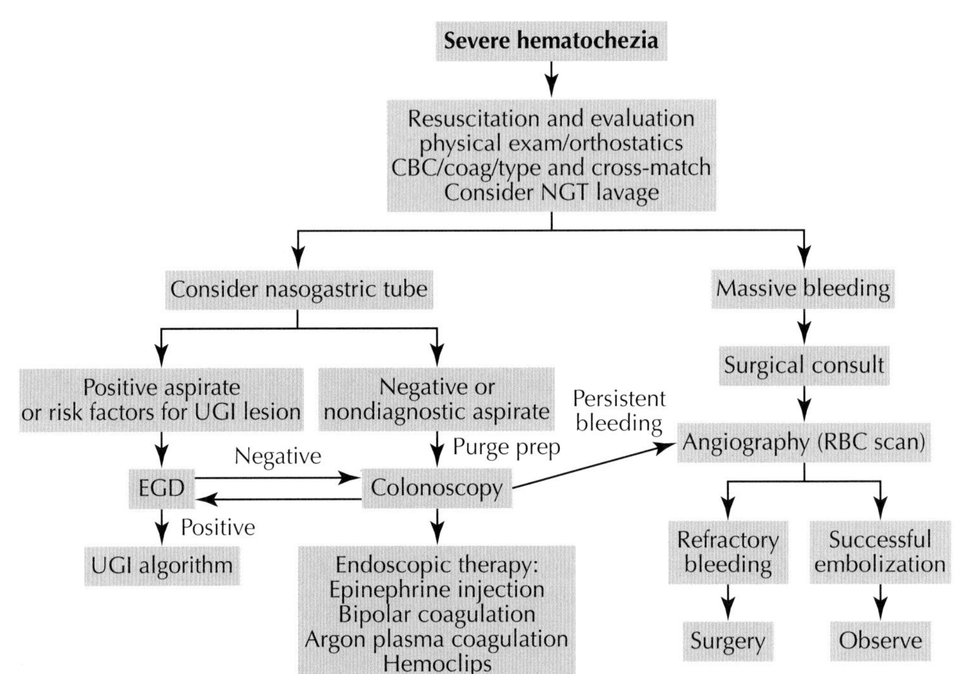


EGD = Esophagogastroduodenoscopy; CBC = complete blood count; Coag = coagulation; RBC = red blood cell; UGI = upper gastrointestinal; NGT = nasogastric tube.
*From ASGE Standards of Practice Committee, Pasha SF, Shergill A, Acosta RD, et al. The role of endoscopy in the patient with lower GI bleeding. Gastrointestinal Endoscopy, 2014;79(6):875–888.*

## Overview of Gastrointestinal Hemorrhage (Continued)

endoscopic examination, it is imperative that a thorough upper examination be performed first in all patients with melena as well as in those with overt bleeding.

The loss of blood from the intestines may be so minimal that, in the absence of other symptoms, it may escape attention until microcytic anemia is seen as the first sign of a gastrointestinal disorder. Because bleeding is often the only sign of serious pathologic situations in the digestive tract, it is important to include an evaluation for fecal "occult" blood at the slightest suspicion of a lesion in the gut.

To avoid pitfalls, remember that neither stool color nor the presence of blood on fecal occult blood testing is conclusive evidence that a lesion is present in the digestive system. The stool may be discolored for reasons other than the presence of blood. The stool is often gray or black in patients taking iron or bismuth preparations. It may be reddish when the patient has eaten beets or other red substances if transit is rapid, as occurs with severe diarrhea. Likewise it is important to appreciate that bleeding originating in the *oral* or *pharyngeal cavity* or from *hemorrhagic lesions in the respiratory tract* can be detected in the feces. Vaginal bleeding may also be mistaken for rectal bleeding. More commonly, false-positive testing for occult blood occurs in patients eating red meat. Such false-positive results can be avoided if testing is performed with immune techniques that accurately detect only human hemoglobin.

Before proceeding with definitive testing and possible treatment with endoscopic techniques, the airway, breathing, and circulatory status of the patient must be promptly assessed and secured (ABCs of emergency care). The history should focus on potential causes, the volume of blood lost, the presence of any signs or symptoms of coagulopathy (including use of nonsteroidal antiinflammatory drugs), and the presence of comorbidities. Correcting any of these existing problems must be the foremost priority during the first 24 hours after the patient is admitted to the hospital. Laboratory testing, including a complete metabolic panel, complete blood count, and coagulation studies, should be sent for stat analysis. Blood should be drawn for blood typing and, when appropriate, for cross-matching. Only when the patient is hemodynamically stable and any ongoing concurrent illnesses have been addressed and optimized should the bowel be thoroughly prepped for an urgent colonoscopic examination.

The source of lower gastrointestinal bleeding can be accurately detected in most patients by colonoscopy. In a select clinical setting, particularly when the patient has recently had a normal colonoscopy and describes low-volume hematochezia, a sigmoidoscopy may be all that is needed. It is particularly useful to perform sigmoidoscopy when the patient is actively experiencing bleeding. Hemorrhoids missed by flexible endoscopic techniques may be more accurately detected with rigid proctoscopy. When upper endoscopy and colonoscopy fail to identify a source, balloon-assisted enteroscopy can reach most, if not all, of the jejunum and ileum. Sources of bleeding can often be treated using these endoscopic techniques. The use of other techniques to detect bleeding sources, including capsule enteroscopy, nuclear scans, angiography, and cross-sectional imaging techniques, is described in Plates 1.15, 1.16, and 2.13.

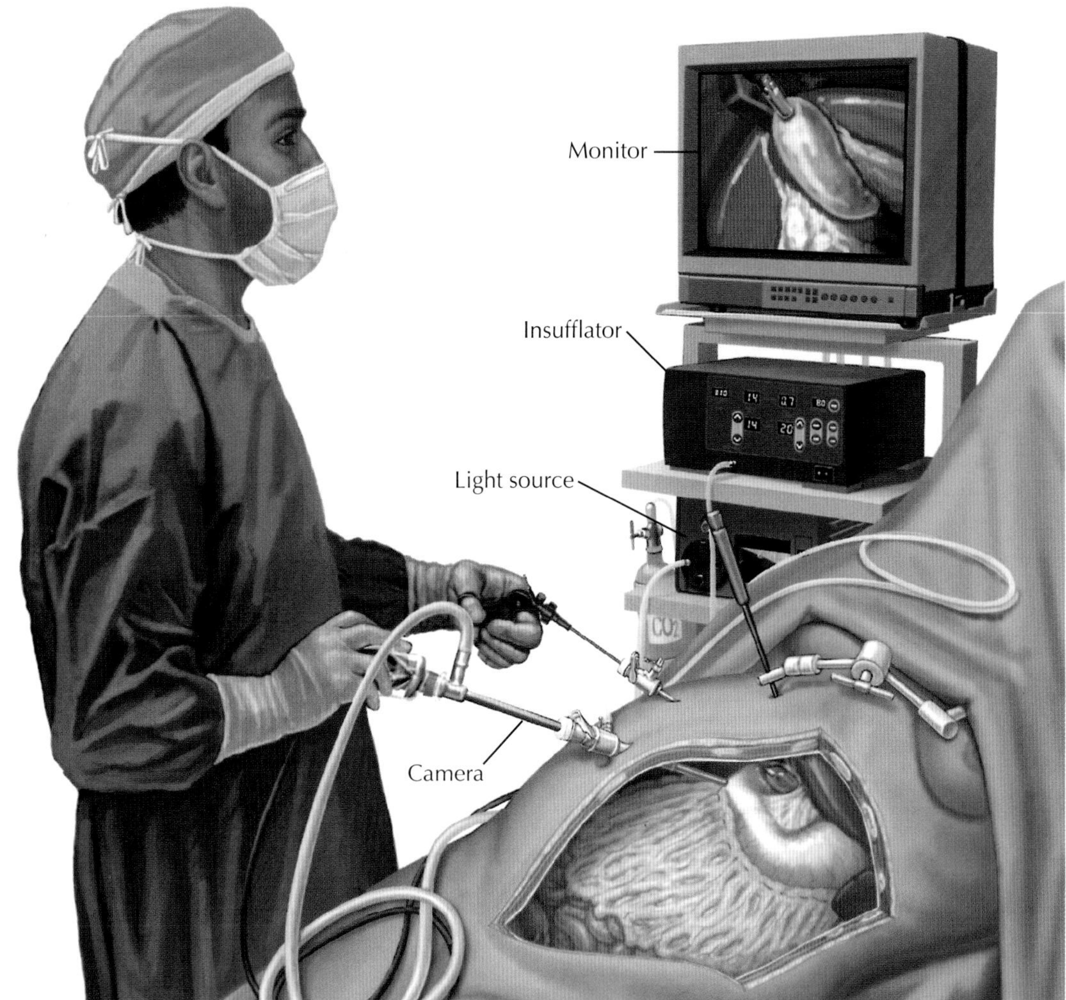


## Laparoscopic Peritoneoscopy

Laparoscopic peritoneoscopy is the direct inspection of the peritoneal cavity and its contents by means of an endoscopic instrument introduced through the abdominal wall. Laparoscopic surgery has revolutionized the field of surgery and has gradually been replacing many conventional surgical procedures. The procedure is used in gastroenterologic, general surgical, and gynecologic disorders in which a positive diagnosis cannot be established by simpler methods. Its value lies in the fact that it can frequently supply information that otherwise would be obtained only by exploratory laparotomy. In addition to being a surgical method, it is particularly valuable as a diagnostic tool for visualizing and obtaining biopsies from peritoneal surfaces, the liver, the omentum, and the small bowel as well as the pelvic organs. Intraabdominal adhesions, peritoneal carcinomatosis or tuberculosis, ascites, or hemorrhage can readily be recognized and sampled via a laparoscope. In malignant disease, laparoscopy is useful for staging.

The examination is carried out in an operating room using all aseptic precautions, as would be expected with open laparotomy. Laparoscopy requires lifting of the abdominal wall from the abdominal organs. The method used by most surgeons is the creation of a pneumoperitoneum by insufflation with carbon dioxide into the peritoneal cavity through a needle or cannula. An alternative to pneumoperitoneum is an abdominal lift device that can be placed through a 10- to 12-mm trocar at the umbilicus. These devices have the advantage of creating little physiologic derangement, but they are bulky and do not allow as much working room as a pneumoperitoneum does.

The first step in the procedure is to establish abdominal access. This is achieved by two methods. The first, closed technique allows the surgeon to place a specialized, spring-loaded Veress needle into the abdominal cavity without damaging the underlying organs. The umbilicus is usually selected as the preferred point of access because, in this location, the abdominal wall is thin, even in patients with obesity. The abdomen is then inflated with carbon dioxide gas.

The other method is the open (Hasson) technique. With this technique, the surgeon makes a small incision just below the umbilicus and, under direct vision, locates the abdominal fascia. A small incision is made through the fascia and underlying peritoneum. A finger is placed in the abdomen to make certain that bowel is not adherent before insufflation is begun. This technique is preferable for patients who have undergone previous operations that may have caused the small bowel to be adherent to the undersurface of the abdominal wound.

The usual site of initial insufflation is the umbilicus; the primary trocar/laparoscope port is placed at the same site. The locations of multiple other ports are chosen to triangulate the camera and the instruments around a focal point within the abdomen, thereby maintaining optimal access for manipulation of the instruments. Certain areas, such as areas of scarring from prior operations (because of the likelihood of adhesions), the upper right quadrant (because of the round ligament), and the midline of the rectus abdominis muscle (because of the course of epigastric vessels), should be avoided. Alternative access techniques for laparoscopic surgery include single-incision surgery, single-port access, and natural orifice transluminal endoscopic surgery. In single-incision surgery, a single incision is made, usually at the umbilicus, rather than multiple incisions for multiple ports. In natural orifice transluminal endoscopic surgery, a multichannel endoscopic technique is used to reach the peritoneal cavity through the mouth, stomach, vagina, or rectum. This technique is a truly "scarless" operation with minimal pain. Turning the patient on the right side may help expose the spleen, and applying the Trendelenburg position causes the pelvic organs to become visible.

Laparoscopic peritoneoscopy has proved its value in diagnosing peritoneal tuberculosis and abdominal malignant diseases and determining whether they are operable, in diagnosing hepatobiliary diseases, in identifying obscure abdominal masses, and in diagnosing diseases involving the pelvic organs. The risks of laparoscopy are few but include accidental injury such as air embolism, hemorrhage from a ruptured blood vessel, perforation of a hollow viscus, pneumothorax, and pneumomediastinum. Laceration of the inferior epigastric artery has been reported. Most complications can be avoided with a perfect technique and a proper selection of patients. Absolute contraindications to the procedure include hemodynamic or respiratory instability, serious heart and lung diseases, and diaphragmatic defects. It is sometimes necessary to exclude from examination patients with extensive operative scars.

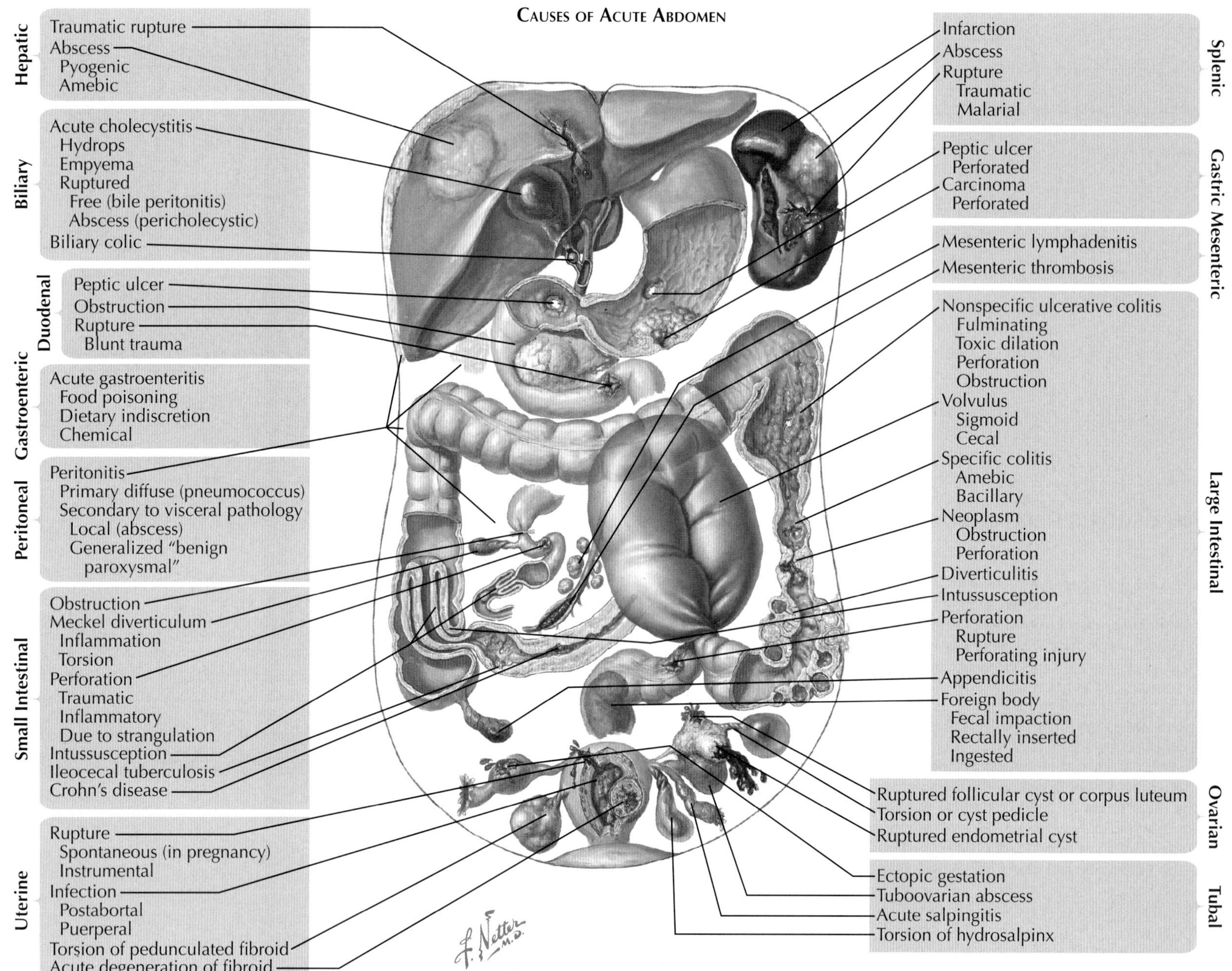


## The "Acute Abdomen"

An acute abdominal condition should be described as *acute abdomen* when a patient complains of abdominal pain that persists for more than a few hours and is associated with tenderness or other evidence of an inflammatory reaction or a visceral dysfunction. The diagnosis of the cause of acute abdominal conditions remains one of the most challenging problems in medicine. Many pathologic processes, both intraabdominal and extraabdominal, may result in an acute abdomen. An accurate history, thorough physical examination, and proper laboratory examinations help make the broad differential diagnosis of causes.

Pain in the right upper quadrant may originate from cardiac, pulmonary, GI, and renal conditions. Evidence of cardiac failure may implicate the heart; a pleuritic type of pain, cough, sputum, and auscultatory findings over the right lower lobe point may implicate disease above the diaphragm. A prodromal period of nausea and anorexia, followed by pain, jaundice, and enlargement of the liver, suggests hepatitis, which must be differentiated from acute cholecystitis, which presents with colicky pain and a tender, globular mass in the right upper quadrant. Urinalysis showing red and/or white blood cells will suggest pyelonephritis or renal stone, whereas glycosuria and ketonuria may be the first positive evidence that the pain is a clinical facet of diabetic acidosis. Unquestionably, the most difficult area in which to make a diagnosis is the right lower quadrant in females. Although persistent pain in this region should be considered a sign of appendicitis until proved otherwise, keep in mind that a twisted, ruptured, or bleeding ovarian cyst, a pelvic inflammatory process, or a twisted pedunculated fibroid may cause identical symptoms. The situation is simplified only by the fact that surgery is indicated for all these lesions, provided that systemic and renal diseases have been excluded. With pain and tenderness on the left side, a tumor or diverticulitis must enter into the differential diagnosis. Intestinal obstruction, whatever its cause, may start its clinical appearance with the signs and symptoms of acute abdomen. A patient with an abdominal scar from previous surgery who complains of cramps and vomiting must be assumed to have intestinal obstruction until proved otherwise.

Although the location of pain usually fixes the site of a disease process, pain may be felt at a distance from the pathologic process. During a careful physical examination in which the maximal area of tenderness is being assessed, guarding or rebound tenderness may accurately disclose the site of disease; the imprecise nature of nociception localizing in all viscera can be humbling to even the best clinician. Appendicitis frequently

ACUTE ABDOMEN: THORACIC, RETROPERITONEAL, SYSTEMIC, ABDOMINAL WALL

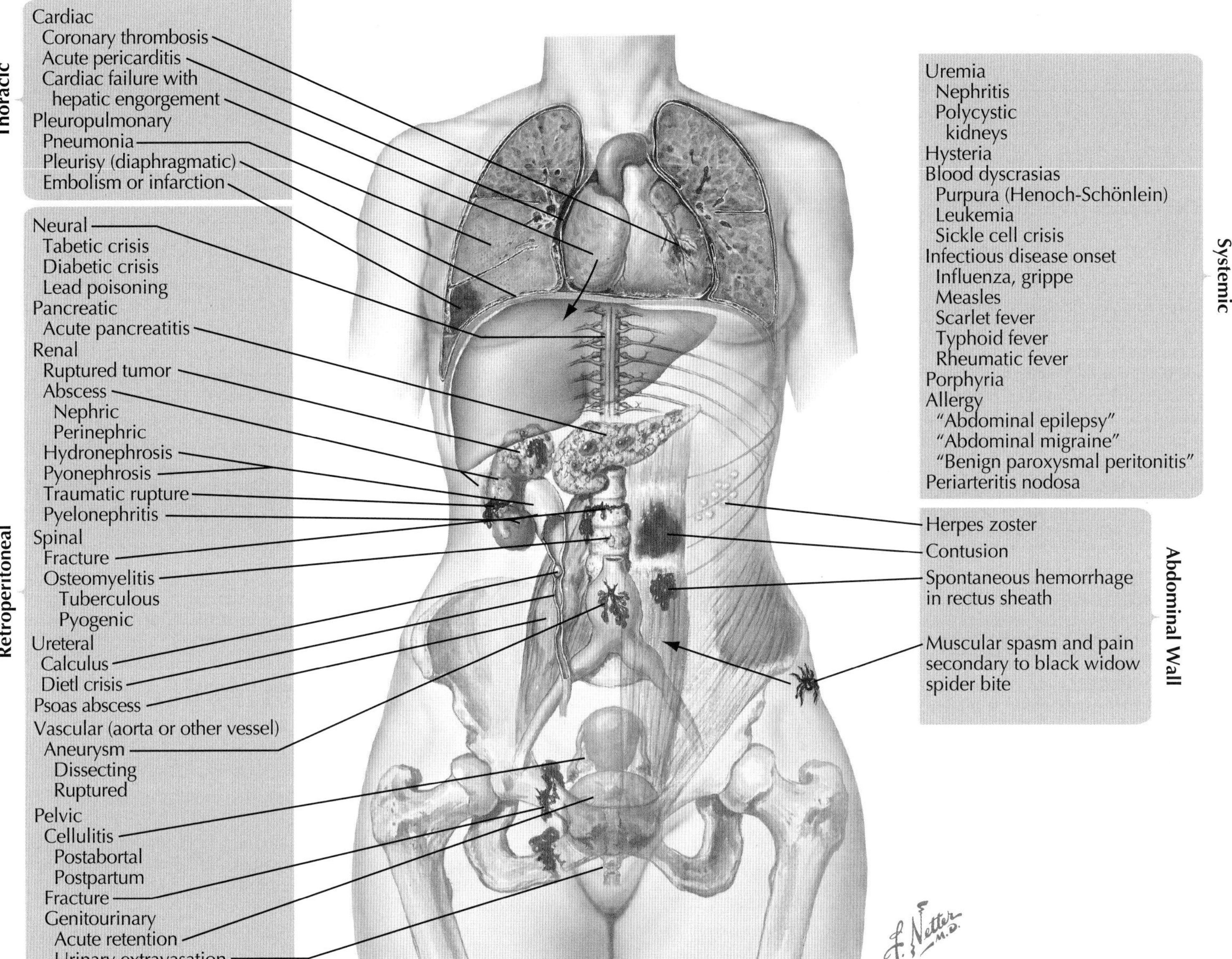


## THE "ACUTE ABDOMEN" (Continued)

begins with epigastric or periumbilical pain before localizing to the right lower quadrant, a site often referred to as the McBurney's point. Although acute cholecystitis is most commonly identified in the right upper quadrant and will result in a positive Murphy sign, it commonly presents with epigastric pain or pain in other quadrants, the periumbilical area, or the right shoulder. Similarly, perforated peptic ulcer and pancreatitis may manifest themselves with lower abdominal pain, particularly if there has been extravasation of inflammatory exudate down the pericolonic gutters. Rebound tenderness, the most significant if not truly pathognomonic sign of peritoneal inflammation, is almost always an indication of the need for surgical intervention. The exception to this rule is a peritoneal reaction that can be shown to be due to a systemic disease (e.g., systemic lupus erythematosus or sickle cell crisis).

With any doubt about the abdominal diagnosis, upright and supine views of the abdomen and an upright chest radiograph should be obtained immediately. The latter will exclude or ascertain the presence of pneumonia, pulmonary infarction, congestive heart failure, pericardial effusion, or fractured ribs, all of which can present with the clinical picture of an acute abdomen. On the abdominal or chest film, free air under the diaphragm usually indicates a perforated viscus and, thus, the need for urgent surgical intervention. Opaque calculi may be visible and lead to a diagnosis of cholecystitis, chronic pancreatitis, renal lithiasis, or even gallstone ileus. In cases of injury manifesting paralytic ileus, radiographic examination may disclose fracture of a vertebra or the pelvis. Localized ileus (the *sentinel loop*) may be seen in pancreatitis, appendicitis, or mesenteric infarction. Volvulus of the sigmoid or cecum presents with a characteristic appearance on radiography. In most cases, emergency computed tomography (CT) scanning of the abdomen and pelvis will reveal the diagnosis. Until perforation has been definitively ruled out, liquid-soluble contrast should be used rather than ingestion of barium.

Examining the abdominal fluid at the time of laparoscopy or in an emergency setting with a peritoneal tap performed with a fine needle may yield considerable information. Clear fluid is obtained in the presence of an early peritoneal response to an inflammatory process. The process has progressed if leukocytes and bacteria are found in a turbid fluid. Sanguineous fluid with a positive amylase reaction points to acute hemorrhagic pancreatitis, whereas a frankly bloody fluid must be attributed to trauma, a ruptured spleen or liver, mesenteric vascular occlusion, a ruptured or twisted and infarcted ovarian cyst, or ectopic pregnancy.

## Overview of Digestive Tract Obstructions

Any organic or functional condition that primarily or indirectly impedes the normal propulsion of luminal contents from the esophagus to the anus could be considered a partial or complete obstruction. In the newborn, a variety of congenital anomalies (esophageal, intestinal, anal atresias, colonic malrotation, volvulus of the midgut, meconium ileus, aganglionic megacolon) resulting in obstruction are illustrated here. Other causes of mechanical interference of intestinal function in early infancy include incarceration in an internal or external (inguinal) hernia, congenital peritoneal bands, intestinal duplications, volvulus due to mesenteric cysts, and annular pancreas, although the latter may not become clinically manifested until the patient is an adult or an aged adult.

Esophageal diseases that interfere with the normal passage of fluids and solids are illustrated in the uppermost row of the illustration on the next page. Esophageal strictures can be iatrogenic from endoscopic procedures, irradiation, medications, or surgery; vascular; neoplastic; or, most commonly, gastroesophageal reflux. Congenital or acquired webs and rings, particularly Schatzki rings, are common, easily treatable causes of esophageal obstruction. Fundoplications performed to treat reflux and repair an esophageal hernia will, by design, reduce the size of the lumen at the gastroesophageal junction and hence produce a functional stricture. Creating a surgical narrowing that is snug but not excessively tight (so that it causes a functional or mechanical obstruction) is the essence of a successful surgical intervention. Extraluminal pressure on the esophagus by a tumor mass, goiter, aberrant or enlarged arteries, or visceral abnormalities in the neck or mediastinum will lead to the same results.

Functional or mechanical impairment of gastric emptying is common. Gastroparesis implies a functional delay, but this diagnosis should only be made when intrinsic and extrinsic causes of mechanical obstruction, metabolic causes, and medication-related causes have been excluded. Gastroparesis is commonly seen in patients with hypothyroidism, amyloidosis, or connective tissue disease; after surgery; and as a complication of diabetes. Gastroparesis can be difficult to distinguish clinically from partial gastric obstruction because both present with early satiety, nausea, vomiting, bloating, distension, and, if prolonged, weight loss. Habitual intake of excessive indigestible material that accumulates in the stomach—such as hair (trichobezoar), fruit or vegetable fibers (phytobezoar), undissolved medications (pharmacobezoar), and even plastic materials—can result in chronic partial gastric obstruction. Initially these materials may persist as accumulations of loose semisolids, but with time, they will be compressed by gastric contractions into a solid ball that can add to the impaired emptying. Intrinsic benign mechanical occlusion occurs most commonly from antral, prepyloric, or pyloric peptic ulcer. Surgery, irradiation, ingestion of caustic substances, and benign neoplasms such as large epithelial polyps, leiomyomas, or gastrointestinal stromal tumors commonly also lead to partial gastric obstructions. Intrinsic or extrinsic malignant neoplasms are all too common mechanical causes of gastric outlet obstruction.

Obstruction of the duodenum is most commonly due to peptic ulcer disease. As with other severe complications of peptic ulcer, peptic strictures should raise concern for the presence of a gastrinoma *(Zollinger-Ellison syndrome)*. Extraluminal compression may occur, as in *superior mesenteric artery syndrome,* in which the SMA can cause mechanical obstruction of the duodenum. Similarly, the duodenum can be occluded by a local extension of a carcinoma of the head of the pancreas, colon, or upper pole of the left kidney that puts pressure on or invades the duodenum. Other extrinsic neoplastic causes of duodenal obstruction include lymphadenopathy in the small bowel mesentery or extension of cancer into the transverse mesocolon.

Small intestinal obstruction typically leads to periumbilical pain, bloating, and, eventually, vomiting of feculent liquids. Of the wide variety of conditions that can lead to obstruction of the small intestine, the most common in adults are adhesions after previous surgery. The small bowel may develop strictures after radiation therapy, typically delivered to adjacent gynecologic organs or in the treatment of lymphoma. In children and adults, the presence of an incarcerated loop of small bowel in a hernia should be considered as a potential cause that will require urgent surgical attention before ischemic injury ensues. Hernias are described, based on their location, as inguinal, femoral, diaphragmatic, paraesophageal, incisional, umbilical, ventral, or internal, including spigelian hernia. Incarceration of a hernia resulting from entrapment of a loop of small intestine in a congenital, traumatic, or surgical ring is a surgical emergency. The small intestine can also be obstructed by large intraluminal objects, including ingested foreign bodies, bezoars, or a large biliary calculus, or as a consequence of an accumulation of parasitic worms. Mechanical obstruction of the small intestine may also be produced by intussusception, which will be found to be secondary to a mucosal lesion in a frequency that increases with the patient's age. Varying degrees of small bowel obstruction may be the result of segmental fibrotic stricture formation in patients with Crohn's disease, most commonly in the ileum and jejunum. Small bowel loops may become stenotic as the result of healing after localized infarction sustained in hernial incarceration or mesenteric vascular occlusion. Primary neoplasms of the small intestine, although rare, should always be considered in the differential diagnosis and include carcinomas, neuroendocrine tumors, gastrointestinal stromal tumors, leiomyosarcomas, and lymphomas. Finally, iatrogenic intestinal obstruction may occur on occasion, including anastomotic stenosis, torsion or angulation, or antiperistaltic anastomosis of intestinal loops, or as the result of other faulty surgical techniques. Common extrinsic causes of intestinal obstruction other than postoperative adhesions include congenital peritoneal bands, metastatic tumor implants, Meckel diverticulum, and adhesive peritonitis (tuberculosis, *Mycobacterium avium-intracellulare,* or other foreign body granulomas).

Nonmechanical impairment of intestinal motor function has been descriptively termed *reflex, adynamic,* or *paralytic ileus.* The continued use of this last term is unfortunate. Although it is used widely to describe functional intestinal motility, it almost never is restricted to the ileum alone and, in fact, is often used indiscriminately when both the small bowel and large bowel are dysfunctional. The term *ileus* should not be used to describe impaired motility isolated to the colon. The patient typically presents with failure to pass flatus, abdominal distension, a "silent abdomen," and the radiographic findings of dilation of the small and/or large intestine with accumulation of fecal material, fluids, and excess gas.

Ileus can be a complication of various conditions that can lead to delayed intestinal transit, including metabolic disorders, metastatic neoplasms, vascular or inflammatory disorders, and infectious mesenteritis. Other causes include CNS lesions, spinal disorders, postoperative complications, or complications after pancreatitis, peritonitis, penetrating or blunt trauma, or extensive rib fractures. Other clinical conditions in which ileus has been said to occur as a "reflex" phenomenon include renal or biliary colic, pneumonia, torsion infarction of an ovarian cyst, coronary thrombosis, and retroperitoneal hemorrhage (incident to fracture of the spine or pelvis, a dissecting aortic aneurysm, urinary extravasation, or rupture of the kidney). Causes of constipation are described elsewhere.

So-called *paralytic* or *adynamic ileus* occurs commonly in the setting of purulent peritonitis (due to a perforated appendix, perforated hollow viscus, pelvic inflammatory disease, leakage or dehiscence of an intestinal suture line, wound evisceration, and other problems). Ileus may follow the intraperitoneal extravasation of gastric or duodenal contents (perforated peptic ulcer), pancreatic juice (acute hemorrhagic pancreatitis), bile (perforated gallbladder, bile leakage from the liver or bile ducts), and blood (postoperative hemorrhage, rupture of the liver or spleen, ectopic gestation, or "chocolate" cyst of the ovary).

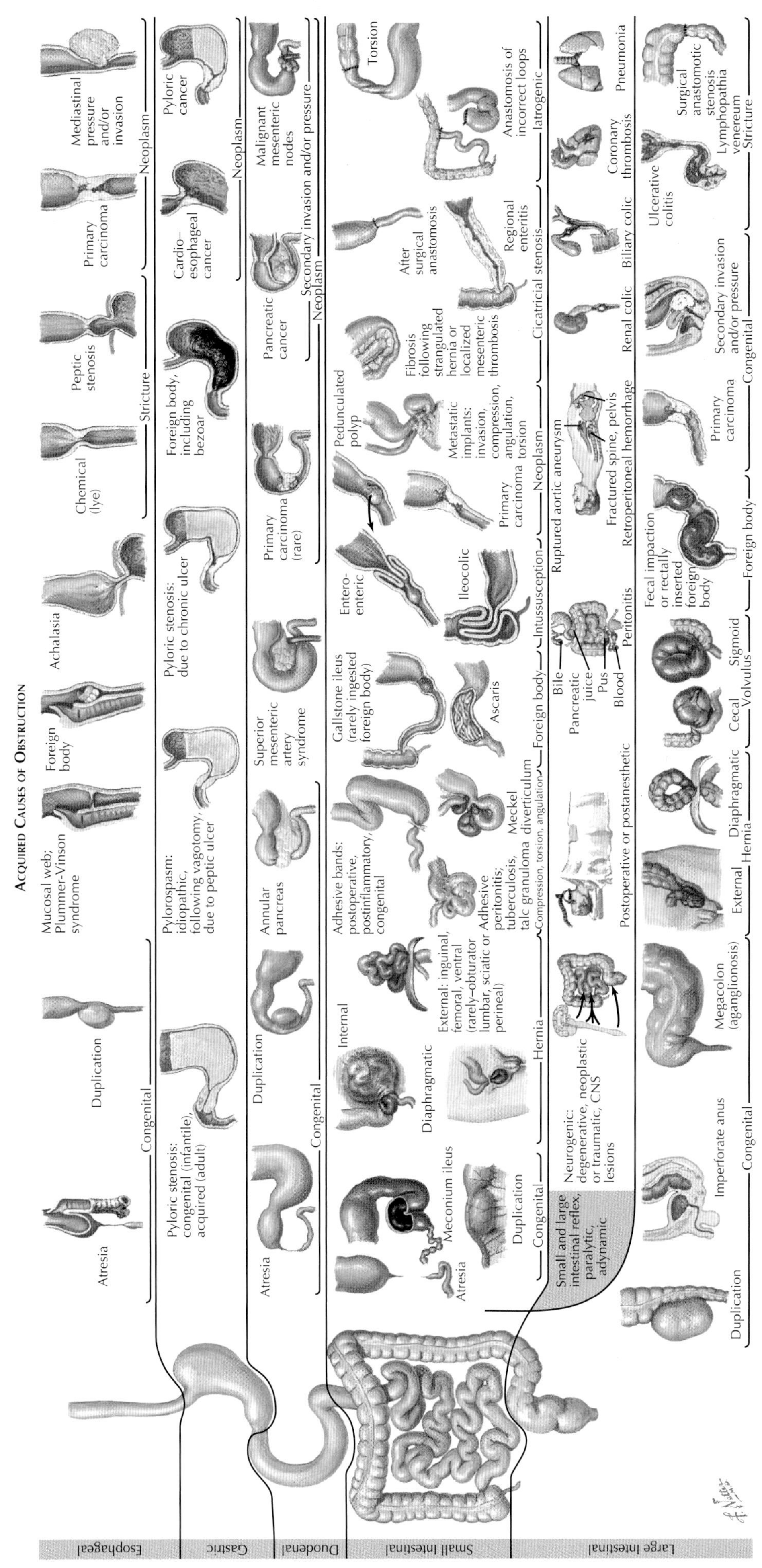
Acquired Causes of Obstruction
Esophageal
Atresia
Duplication
Congenital
Mucosal web; Plummer-Vinson syndrome
Foreign body
Achalasia
Chemical (lye)
Peptic stenosis
Stricture
Primary carcinoma
Mediastinal pressure and/or invasion
Neoplasm
Gastric
Pyloric stenosis: congenital (infantile), acquired (adult)
Congenital
Pylorospasm: idiopathic, following vagotomy, due to peptic ulcer
Pyloric stenosis: due to chronic ulcer
Foreign body, including bezoar
Cardio-esophageal cancer
Pyloric cancer
Neoplasm
Duodenal
Atresia
Duplication
Congenital
Annular pancreas
Superior mesenteric artery syndrome
Primary carcinoma (rare)
Pancreatic cancer
Neoplasm
Malignant mesenteric nodes
Secondary invasion and/or pressure
Small Intestinal
Atresia
Meconium ileus
Duplication
Congenital
Diaphragmatic
Internal
External: inguinal, femoral, ventral (rarely–obturator lumbar, sciatic or perineal)
Hernia
Adhesive bands: postoperative, postinflammatory, congenital
Adhesive peritonitis; tuberculosis, talc granuloma
Meckel diverticulum
Compression, torsion, angulation
Gallstone ileus (rarely ingested foreign body)
Ascaris
Foreign body
Entero-enteric
Ileocolic
Intussusception
Primary carcinoma
Pedunculated polyp
Metastatic implants: invasion, compression, angulation, torsion
Neoplasm
Fibrosis following strangulated hernia or localized mesenteric thrombosis
After surgical anastomosis
Regional enteritis
Cicatricial stenosis
Torsion
Anastomosis of incorrect loops
Iatrogenic
Small and large intestinal reflex, paralytic, adynamic
Neurogenic: degenerative, neoplastic or traumatic, CNS lesions
Postoperative or postanesthetic
Bile
Pancreatic juice
Pus
Blood
Peritonitis
Ruptured aortic aneurysm
Fractured spine, pelvis
Retroperitoneal hemorrhage
Renal colic
Biliary colic
Coronary thrombosis
Pneumonia
Large Intestinal
Duplication
Imperforate anus
Megacolon (aganglionosis)
Congenital
External
Diaphragmatic
Hernia
Cecal
Sigmoid
Volvulus
Fecal impaction or rectally inserted foreign body
Foreign body
Primary carcinoma
Secondary invasion and/or pressure
Congenital
Ulcerative colitis
Surgical anastomotic stenosis
Lymphopathia venereum
Stricture

## Acute Peritonitis

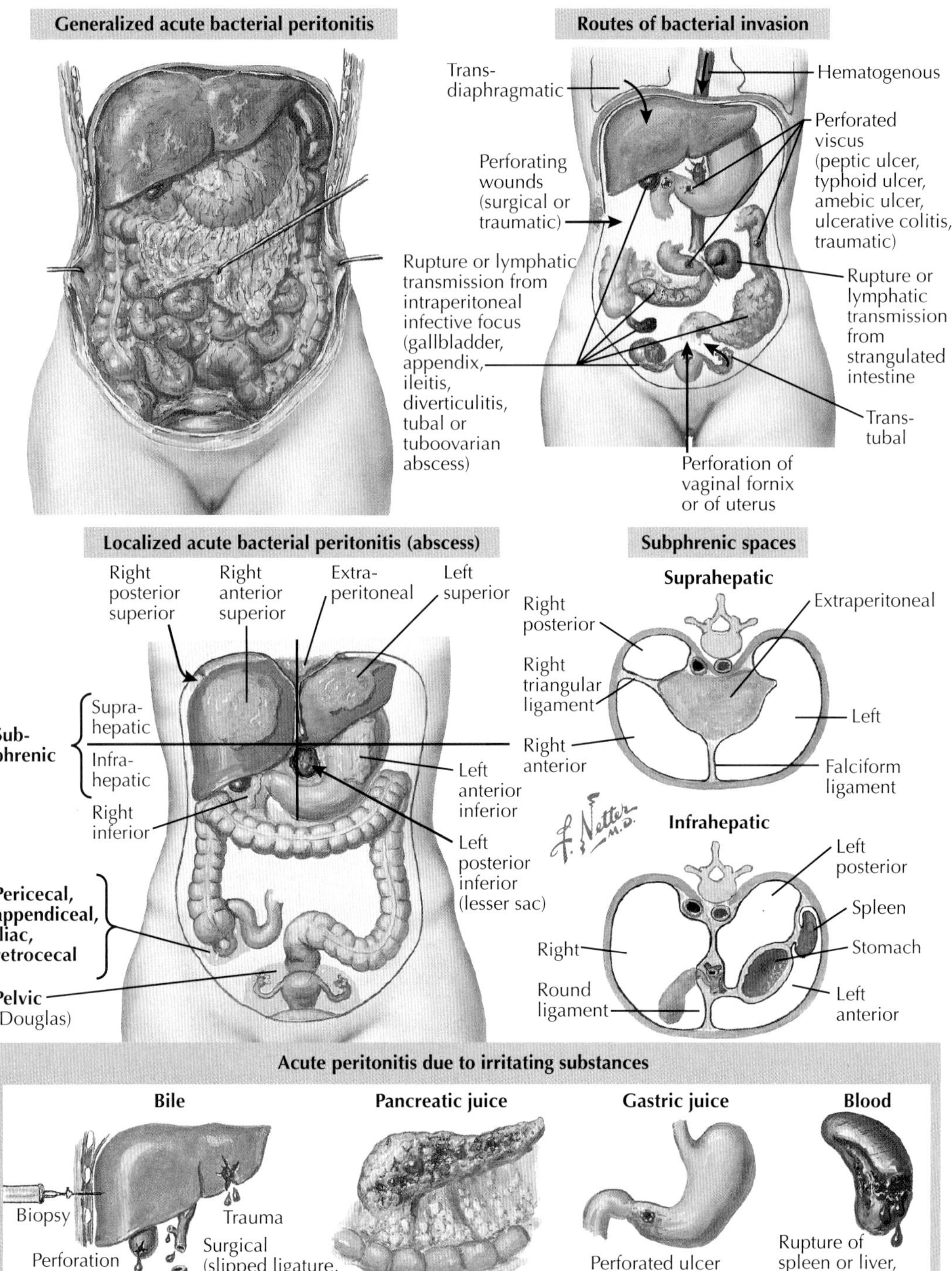


Acute infectious peritonitis results from chemical injury, autoimmune inflammation, or infection from a variety of microorganisms. The latter reach the peritoneum (1) from the exterior by *penetrating wounds* of the abdominal wall (trauma, surgery), (2) from an infectious process in an abdominal organ *via the lymphatics* or ostia of the *fallopian tubes,* (3) by *rupture of a viscus,* (4) from a distant organ *via the bloodstream,* or (5) spontaneously without a bowel injury. Rupture of a viscus can result from a wide variety of inflammatory, vascular, or malignant injuries of the bowel. Spontaneous infections result from bacterial translocation across the mucosa and into adjacent fluid, most commonly ascites or dialysis fluid. Infections involve a variety of species of pathogenic microorganisms, including *Escherichia coli,* streptococci, enterococci, staphylococci, diphtheroids, *Clostridium* species, *Klebsiella,* and pneumococci. When peritonitis results from bowel perforation, there is invariably more than one species involved. Identification of the organisms provides clues as to the source of the infection. When multiple gram-negative or anaerobic species are involved that are typical of the intestinal flora, they are a consequence of bowel injury. In contrast, when the organism is atypical for gut flora, such as gonococci, streptococci, or staphylococci, the source is extraintestinal. Gonococcal peritonitis occurs almost exclusively in females as a complication of gonorrheal salpingitis; it is usually confined to the pelvis. A form of gonococcal peritonitis localized in the upper right abdominal quadrant is characterized by the appearance of thin fibrin bands (violin strings) between the anterior surface of the liver, the diaphragm, and the anterior abdominal wall and, clinically, by severe acute pain in this region *(Fitz-Hugh–Curtis syndrome).* Pneumococcal peritonitis may develop as a complication of a pneumococcal infection elsewhere in the body (e.g., pneumonia, empyema, otitis), but it may occur also as a primary disease; as such, it is observed mostly in female children between the ages of 3 and 7 years, and it is believed that the pneumococci reach the peritoneum from the genital tract through the fallopian tubes.

The course of peritonitis is determined by the quality and quantity both of the injurious agents and of the body's defenses. The infection may remain localized and walled in by the adhesion of adjacent structures, or it may spread and become *generalized.* The pathologic changes are those seen in inflammation of any serous membrane; the peritoneum becomes congested and, owing to the deposition of fibrin, loses its normal sheen. The exudate is serous during the earliest stages but later becomes purulent. The inflammatory process may reach the blood vessels in the mesentery, where thrombosis may develop and develop gangrene in a part of the bowel. *Localized peritonitis* in the form of an abscess may occur at the primary point of infection or at some distance from it. The most common causes of localized abdominal abscess include those that arise from perforated appendix, diverticulitis, and ruptured cholecystitis. Pelvic abscesses may also result from appendicitis, although they are more commonly due to gynecologic infections. The most important form of localized peritonitis is, however, the *subphrenic abscess* characterized by the collection of pus in one of the subphrenic spaces. The pus usually originates in the upper abdomen, but it may also come from the right iliac fossa or even the pelvis. The most common causes of a subphrenic abscess are *gastric* or *duodenal perforation, appendicitis,* and *hepatobiliary infections.*

Acute peritonitis may result from the entrance of *irritating substances* into the peritoneal cavity. *Bile* may escape from an injury to the intrahepatic or extrahepatic biliary system sustained during trauma or surgical procedures or caused by rupture. Irritating quantities of *blood* enter the cavity usually from a rupture of the spleen, uterine tube (in a tubal pregnancy), liver, or other structures. Pancreatic *enzymes* reach the peritoneum in the course of acute hemorrhagic pancreatitis, whereas the entrance of gastric juice results from gastric or duodenal perforation.

The typical symptoms of generalized peritonitis are abdominal pain, rigidity of the abdominal musculature, and vomiting; in the early stages, hyperperistalsis may develop, but as the process extends, paralysis of the intestinal tract sets in. Both the temperature and pulse rate are elevated. The blood picture usually shows leukocytosis. If peritonitis is due to perforation of a hollow viscus, the presence of free air or fluid may be elicited on examination or shown on radiographic imaging. If the infection is virulent and the body's defenses are poor, the disease is particularly severe and often rapidly fatal.

## CHRONIC PERITONITIS

*Tuberculous peritonitis* can occur at any age but is seen more commonly in young adults and children, patients undergoing dialysis, or patients who are immunocompromised such as those with acquired immunodeficiency syndrome. It is practically always secondary to some other focus in the body, the most frequent sources of infection being tuberculous lesions in the bowel, mesenteric glands, and fallopian tubes. In the course of general miliary tuberculosis, the tuberculous peritonitis may occur as an acute infection; much more commonly, however, it appears as a chronic condition that manifests itself in one of two main forms: (1) exudative or moist and (2) plastic or dry. In the first variety, the exudation is marked and the abdominal cavity becomes filled with a thin ascitic fluid; *numerous tubercles,* about the size of a pinhead or larger, appear *on the peritoneal surfaces.* In the second variety, the exudate is dense and rich in fibrin, formation of adhesions occurs most readily, and the viscera become matted together; the peritoneum is studded with tubercles, which, however, may be covered by deposits of fibrin; and the omentum is often greatly thickened and rolled up. Caseous necrosis of tuberculous lesions may lead to formation of fistulous tracts. The two varieties may occur together, giving rise to the so-called encysted or encapsulated form characterized by loculated collections of fluid encysted by the *dense adhesions.*

Tuberculous peritonitis may have a sudden or an insidious onset. The most common clinical manifestations are diffuse or localized abdominal pain of variable intensity and abdominal distension due to ascites; in the dry form, however, the effusion may be small and difficult to demonstrate by physical examination. Fever is common but is typically intermittent and of low grade. Other symptoms include nausea and vomiting, constipation or diarrhea, and, of course, general constitutional symptoms that usually accompany a tuberculous infection. Physical examination of the abdomen may reveal signs of fluid, a diffuse or localized tenderness, and, eventually, intraabdominal masses. Ascitic fluid obtained by paracentesis may be clear, cloudy, lemon-yellow, or bloody, and, in the case of erosion of the mesenteric lymphatic system, chylous. Its cellular analysis shows, in the very early stages, the predominance of polymorphonuclear neutrophils, which are gradually replaced by lymphocytes and monocytes. Tubercle bacilli may eventually be isolated from the ascitic fluid by culture or QuantiFERON. Exposure to tuberculosis can be assessed with skin testing or the interferon gamma release assay. Neither test is very sensitive in the setting of intestinal or peritoneal disease. The most definitive procedure for diagnosis of peritoneal tuberculosis is laparoscopic peritoneoscopic biopsy of a tubercle.

*Chronic granulomatous peritonitis* grossly resembling that caused by tuberculosis may occur in a number of other diseases. *Mycobacterium avium-intracellulare* infection is a mycobacterial disease that can mimic tuberculosis in every way; it occurs most commonly in patients who are immunocompromised. *South American blastomycosis* and *coccidioidomycosis* (caused by *Paracoccidioides brasiliensis* and *Coccidioides immitis,* respectively), actinomycosis, syphilis, and tularemia occasionally involve the peritoneum and produce granulomatous lesions. *Foreign substances,* such as talcum, liquid petrolatum, radiographic contrast media, and others, introduced into the peritoneal cavity during operations or diagnostic procedures (e.g., hysterosalpingography) as well as extruded gastrointestinal contents left in the abdominal cavity after operations, and contents of ruptured dermoid and other cysts, may all cause a chronic inflammatory reaction, with formation of adhesions and foreign body granulomas. A similar reaction may be produced by *Enterobius vermicularis* and *ova of Schistosoma* that may, by erratic migration, reach the peritoneum.

Fibrous bands and adhesions may form in the peritoneal cavity as a late result of acute peritonitis or a result of localized chronic peritonitis (perivisceritis) occurring over the site of an ulcerative or inflammatory lesion in the stomach, intestine, gallbladder, liver, or genital organs. Fibrinous perihepatitis and perisplenitis may accompany liver cirrhosis and other conditions with persistent ascites.

Serositis may mimic bacterial peritonitis. This most commonly is due to systemic lupus erythematosus and related forms of vasculitis. Less commonly, noninfectious peritonitis may be due to familial Mediterranean fever or porphyria. A rare form of polyserositis characterized by intense fibrosis with hyalinization of the peritoneum and other serous membranes, particularly the pericardium and pleura, is known as *Pick* or *Concato disease.*

CHRONIC PERITONITIS

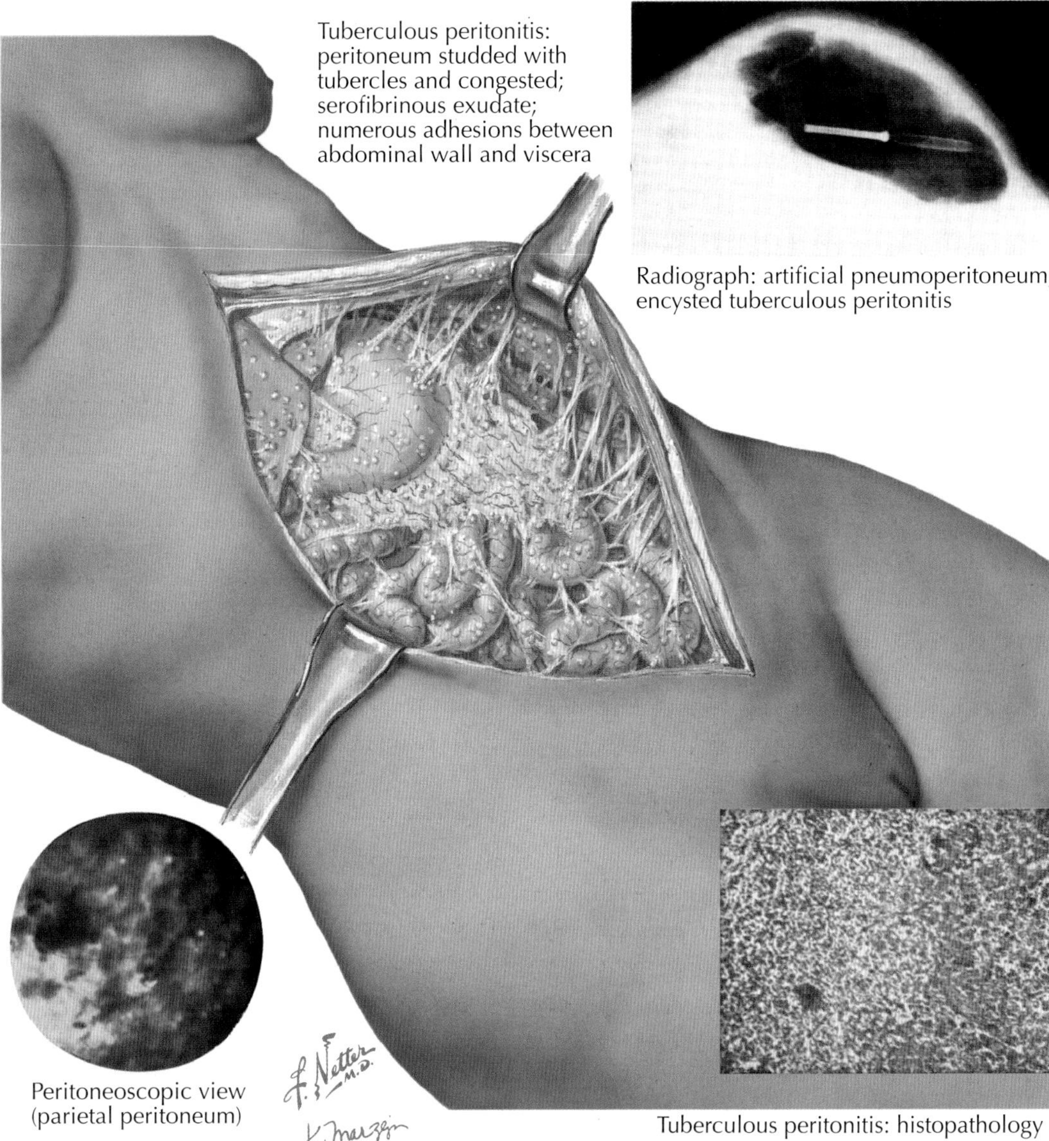


**Granulomatous peritonitis due to causes other than tuberculous**

Foreign body granuloma

South American blastomycosis: granuloma containing *Paracoccidioides brasiliensis*

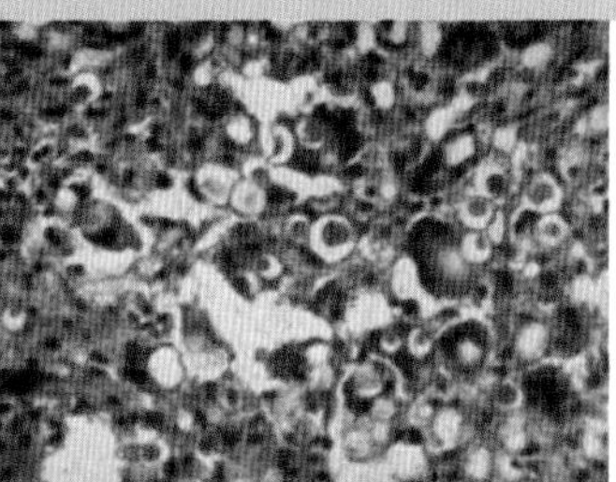

Schistosomiasis: granuloma (late stage) containing ova of *Schistosoma mansoni*

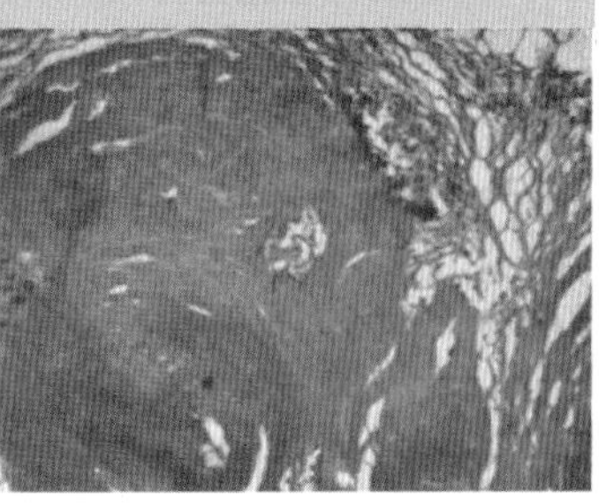

## Cancer of Peritoneum

Primary malignant tumors of the peritoneum (mesotheliomas or endotheliomas) are rare, but secondary malignant tumors are relatively common. Tumor cell spread into the peritoneum occurs by direct extension, hematogenous spread, or lymphatic spread. Once the peritoneum has been invaded, dissemination of malignant cells throughout the peritoneal cavity and implantation diffusely throughout the peritoneal surfaces can occur rapidly. Epithelial primary carcinomas commonly metastasize to the peritoneum (e.g., adenocarcinomas of the stomach, intestine, ovaries, and, less commonly, lung and breast). Melanomas also frequently metastasize to the digestive system, including the mesentery. Malignant neoplasms of the retroperitoneal connective, nervous, or muscular tissue, as well as sarcomas and teratomas, although rare, invade the peritoneum or become metastasized within it.

Mesothelioma, the most common primary tumor, is a rare, aggressive tumor arising from mesothelial cells within the serosal lining of the peritoneum, pleura, and pericardium. Although the cause is unclear, there is a strong association with asbestos exposure. Peritoneal mesothelioma is classified as either benign-borderline (multicystic or well-differentiated papillary) mesothelioma or diffuse peritoneal (epithelial, sarcomatoid, or biphasic) mesothelioma.

Normally, peritoneal stromal tissue is a rich source of growth factor and chemokines. Infiltration of malignant cells often increases exudative secretions and occludes the lymphatics. Accumulation of excess fluid in the peritoneum *(malignant ascites)* may be serous, serofibrinous, hemorrhagic, or chylous from malignant fatty degeneration. Chylous pleural effusions, in contrast, are caused by damage to the thoracic duct or its main tributaries.

Peritoneal metastases have various morphologic findings, with the gross pattern dependent on the histology of the primary tumor, manner of spread, and intensity and type of peritoneal reaction. Most common are *nodules* scattered over the omentum, mesentery tissue, and visceral and parietal peritoneum; smaller nodules, measuring a few millimeters in diameter, are semitranslucent, whereas larger ones are opaque, white, yellowish white, gray, or reddish. When surface growth exceeds growth in depth, *plaque-like masses* develop, which vary in size and usually have a waxy appearance. Such lesions may be difficult to detect by even the most accurate cross-sectional imaging. Necrotic changes can produce ulcer-like depressions and most commonly occur with metastases from ovarian papillary serous cystadenoma. In the *adhesive form,* extensive adhesions may develop in the peritoneal cavity due to organized fibrin bands produced by dense exudate, the confluence of adjacent implants, or tumor infiltration from one organ to another. Gastric carcinoma is prone to produce metastases; many experts recommend peritoneal fluid cytologic analysis before attempting extensive surgical resection. When more advanced, such metastases may merge into a mass that can lead to fistula formation or obstruction. Other types of peritoneal metastases appear as pedunculated nodules or as small sessile or pedunculated cysts. The cause is usually papillary serous cystadenocarcinoma or cystic ovarian tumors. Metastases of appendicular adenocarcinoma or of ovarian pseudomucinous cystadenocarcinoma on the peritoneal surfaces may produce *pseudomyxoma peritonei,* in which a large quantity of gelatinous material accumulates in the peritoneal cavity. Rupture of a nonmalignant mucocele of the appendix with fistula formation may also lead to accumulation of mucus in the peritoneal cavity.

Most frequent sites of primary tumor

1. Ovary
2. Stomach
3. Intestine

Less frequently other abdominal organs; rarely lung, breast, or other organs

Adenocarcinoma of appendix (malignant mucocele) and pseudomucinous carcinoma of ovary may give rise to pseudomyxoma peritonei

Ascitic fluid cytology in peritoneal carcinomatosis: tumor cells, mesothelial cells, and lymphocytes (Leishman stain)

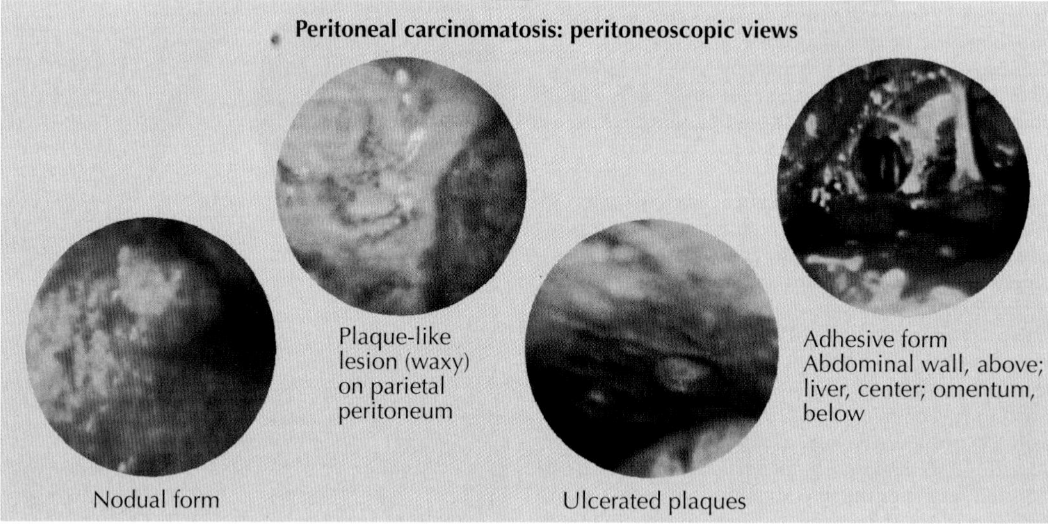


The symptoms of peritoneal carcinomatosis are chiefly abdominal distension due to ascites and abdominal pain but may include weight loss, anorexia, fever, and diarrhea. Physical examination reveals signs of fluid and, eventually, palpable masses. The differential diagnosis should consider all chronic peritoneal conditions. The initial diagnostic procedure is paracentesis for analysis of fluid, including the cell count, Gram-stained smear and culture, acid-fast bacilli stain and culture, cytologic studies, and chemistry testing. Malignant ascites is typically exudative with a low albumen gradient. Cytologic demonstration of *tumor cells in ascitic fluid* is also diagnostic. False-positive results may occur because reactive mesothelial cells can simulate carcinoma. Immunohistochemistry can also establish the diagnosis. CT scanning and magnetic resonance imaging may show mesenteric thickening, peritoneal studding, a tumor mass, and ascites, although advanced disease may present without radiologic evidence. When the diagnosis remains unclear, *peritoneoscopy* by laparoscopy permits visualization of peritoneal deposits, cytologic assessment, and/or biopsy.

There is no staging system for primary peritoneal mesothelioma, although one has been proposed. The expected median survival time for peritoneal carcinomatosis is 1 to 2 years. Local invasion of the liver, abdominal wall, diaphragm, retroperitoneum, GI tract, and bladder commonly occurs. Treatment involves a multidisciplinary approach, combining cytoreductive surgery, chemotherapy, hyperthermic perioperative intraperitoneal therapy, and irradiation. Surgical intervention can be palliative for debulking, particularly when intestinal obstruction is present.

## Abdominal Wounds: Blast Injuries

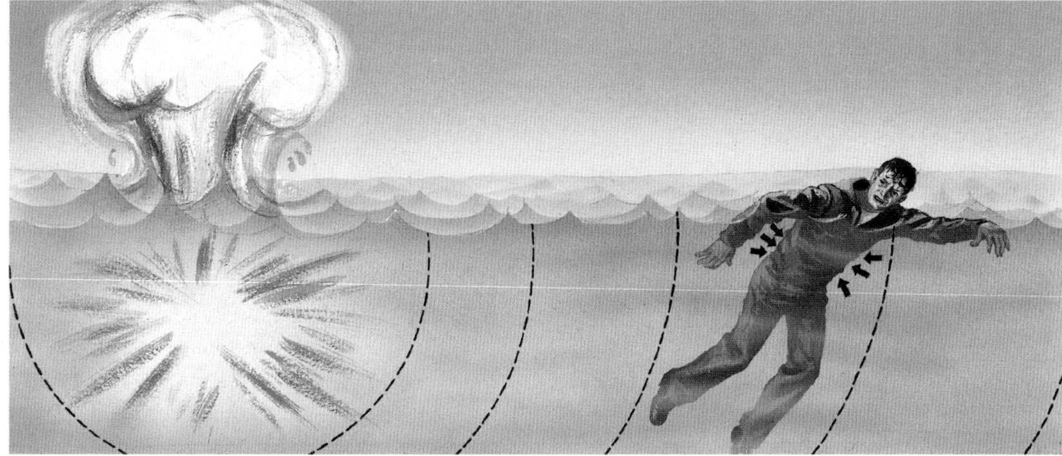

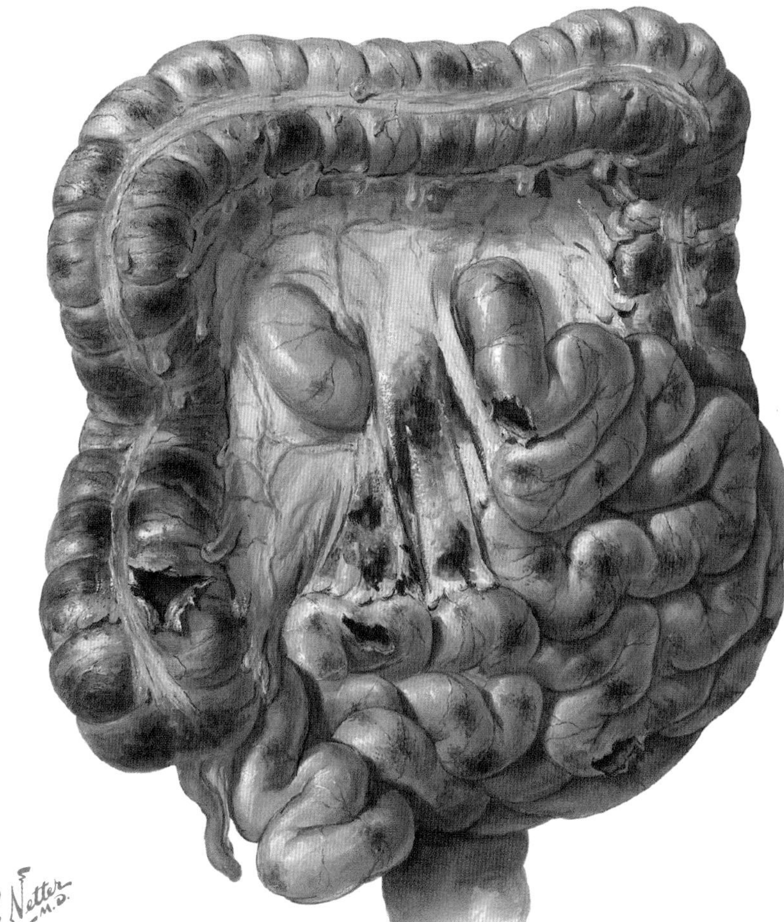


Abdominal wounds and blunt trauma are common acute injuries encountered in emergency settings. The depth and severity of a penetrating wound cannot be determined by history or physical examination alone. After stabilizing the airway, breathing, and circulation, emergency cross-sectional imaging is essential as the operating room is being prepared and surgical expertise recruited. Broad-spectrum intravenous antibiotics should be hung on admission as the patient is prepped for operation. If extensive intraabdominal bleeding is occurring, laparotomy should be done as early as possible. Exploration must be thorough, and all perforations must be closed. Diversion of the fecal stream is often advised when there has been peritoneal soiling. In extensive damage, resection is necessary. In addition to customary preoperative and postoperative measures, oxygen, continuous gastroduodenal suction, multiple drains, and broad-spectrum antibiotic therapy are essential.

Blunt and immersion or "underwater" blast injuries of the abdomen are challenging. Blast-related injuries occur from one of four mechanisms. Primary blast injuries are caused when the blast wave propagates from the detonation center through the victim, causing damage to predominantly air-filled organs; the small intestine is the visceral organ most commonly injured. Effects of the blast wave are far more pronounced than in a closed space because instead of dissipating, the wave may be enhanced as it reflects and reverberates off surfaces. In immersion or "underwater" injury, underwater explosions produce waves; the soft abdominal organs and, to some extent, intrathoracic organs experience the most damage. The severity of the impact or size of the charge, distance from the explosion, amount of gas in the hollow viscera, and, perhaps, position and degree of submersion influence the extent and type of injury. Tertiary blast injuries occur when a victim is physically displaced or crushed by forceful air movement, a motor vehicle collision, or a structural collapse. Quaternary injuries include burns and inhalation injury.

Intestinal tract injuries from blunt trauma or blasts consist primarily of intramural hemorrhages and perforations. The former are mostly multiple and petechial and involve the submucosal and subperitoneal layers of the small intestine, especially the lower ileum and cecum; therefore the severity of the injury may be underestimated on examination of the peritoneal surface. The stomach, esophagus, colon, mesentery, and omentum may also be injured. Injuries vary widely in size and shape. Larger lesions can occur in the colon and, if massive, may lead to gangrene of the bowel. Bleeding also occurs in the loose areolar retroperitoneal tissue. Perforations or tears are less frequent and are more likely to involve the small intestine. They are circular or linear, with everted edges and a blown-out appearance. Generalized or localized peritonitis often appears later. Alternatively, there may be signs of frank perforation at the outset.

Coincident with the explosion, the patient experiences a shock-like sensation, a gripping pain, a temporary paralyzing numbness of abdomen and legs, testicular pain, or an urge to urinate or defecate. Severe, sharp, and stabbing or colicky abdominal pain soon develops. Severe nausea, hematemesis, bloody diarrhea, and diffuse abdominal tenderness may develop. Rigidity appears in cases with perforation, along with physical findings of peritoneal irritation, including guarding and severe rebound tenderness, which can become pronounced and usually portend the presence of free air in the peritoneal cavity. Symptoms may subside relatively rapidly in the absence of perforation or pancreatitis. Evidence of blast injury to the lung may be present. Cautious observation is essential because intraabdominal hematomas can lead to perforation as late as 2 weeks after injury.

The prognosis depends on the extent of visceral injury; mortality rates in cases without intestinal perforation are probably not above 10%, whereas in cases with intestinal perforation, mortality rates can be over 25%. Early deaths are due to shock and late deaths to peritonitis. Associated injury of the lungs increases the gravity of the condition. If there are clinical or radiographic signs of perforation, laparotomy should be performed as early as possible.

When it is fairly certain that no perforation has occurred, treatment is conservative and like that of other nonpenetrating abdominal injuries. Resuscitative measures must be instituted early, but plasma and blood transfusions should be administered cautiously in cases of lung injury. For the same reason, delivering effective general anesthesia is challenging. Prognosis depends on the extent of visceral injury, the time to intervention, and the presence of associated injuries to other organs. Late deaths due to peritonitis or delayed bleeding have occurred.

## PHYSIOLOGY OF GASTROENTERIC STOMAS

**Gastrojejunostomy (patent pylorus)**

Preferential emptying may be by way of patent pylorus

Gastric irritation, nausea and vomiting

Entry of duodenal content into stomach

Gastric juice may act on susceptible jejunum

Irritation, ulcer

**Gastrojejunostomy (stenotic pylorus)**

Stenotic pylorus

Stasis in antrum

Hypersecretion

Gastric acid acts on jejunum, predisposing to ulcer

Long afferent loop

Decreases neutralizing effects of duodenal secretions, increases susceptibility to ulcer, decreases hormonal effects

Stoma too small

Delayed gastric emptying

Stoma too large

Jejunal distension

Dumping syndrome

**Ileotransversostomy with resection**

Loss of storage capacity

Loss of absorptive capacity

Increased bulk and irritating property of colonic content

Loss of portion of colon

Loss of ileocecal sphincter

Unregulated entry of ileal content into colon

Loss of terminal ileum

Loss of absorptive capacity

Loss of storage capacity

Increased fluidity of colonic content

Diarrhea

**Ileotransversostomy in continuity (bypass)**

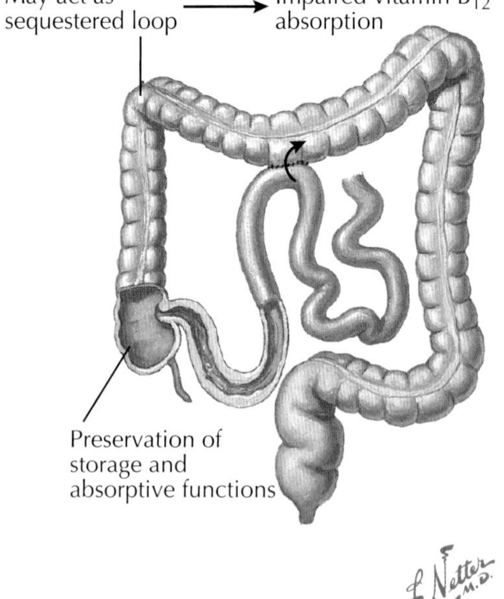


F. Netter M.D.

Creation of a well-constructed ostomy by a highly skilled surgeon at the site of an anastomosis or as a cutaneous stoma that preserves normal digestive functions can result in an excellent quality of life for a patient undergoing resection of portions of the digestive system. Technical risks associated with the creation of any stoma include anastomotic leak, dehiscence, and stricture. The size of the anastomosis varies with the organs involved and the desired outcome of the procedure, but it is important to note that although stricture-related closure is always a risk, larger stomas are not always better. Cutaneous ostomies have an additional risk of prolapse, bleeding, and peristomal ulceration. Evaluation of ostomy function and anatomy may require skilled radiologic assessment with barium studies, CT studies, or endoscopy, or a combination of these studies. Endoscopic evaluation also provides the potential for therapeutic interventions to correct stomal problems, including dilation and placement of self-expanding stents.

Esophagogastrostomy is one of the most challenging of surgical anastomoses. The position of the distal esophagus is significantly influenced by the posture of the patient, and a foreshortened esophagus is prone to dehiscence from the anastomosis if the stomach is not freed adequately from its position in the abdomen to be pulled high enough into the chest. The gastric portion of the anastomosis is prone to ischemia and dehiscence if an adequate blood supply is not provided as the surgeon frees up the stomach and pulls it into the chest. Leakage of the ostomy has a particularly high risk of becoming a life-threatening complication when it occurs in the mediastinum, where it will be adjacent to the vital structures of the trachea, lungs, aorta, and heart. For this reason, esophagogastrostomies are typically safer if adequate resection of the gastroesophageal junction can be performed and still permits a low anastomosis or if the stomach is pulled through the mediastinum or retrosternally and anastomosed in the neck where any leak can be easily addressed.

Gastrojejunostomy is one of the most common surgical ostomies. In previous years, gastrojejunostomy was most commonly performed to treat recurrent peptic ulcer disease. Since the advent of effective medical therapy for peptic ulcer disease, partial gastrectomy with gastrojejunostomy is rarely needed. In fact, even when the patient has a bleeding duodenal ulcer resistant to endoscopic treatment, an ostomy is rarely created because of the risk of performing this complex surgical procedure in the setting of a surgical emergency procedure. Instead, oversewing of the ulcer with or without a selective vagotomy is the procedure of choice. This surgery is followed by treatment of *Helicobacter pylori* and/or education as to the risk of using nonsteroidal antiinflammatory drugs. Gastrojejunostomies are more commonly performed after subtotal gastrectomy for gastric cancer, after gastric outlet obstruction from peptic ulcer–related stricture or extrinsic tumor, or as part of an obesity bypass procedure.

Subtotal gastrectomy and anastomosis of the proximal stomach to the jejunum eliminates or severely impairs several important functions of the stomach and proximal duodenum, resulting in severe impairment of normal digestive functions. The benefit of the adaptive capacitance of the fundus and gastric body, as well as receptive relaxation of the stomach, is lost when a subtotal gastrectomy is performed. Although this is one of the goals of obesity bypass surgery, it can contribute significantly to further weight loss in a patient recovering from gastric cancer surgery. The size of the residual stomach is therefore an important influence on the size of a meal that the patient can tolerate after partial gastrectomy.

With resection of the distal stomach, gastric peristalsis can no longer triturate food into particles smaller than 4 mm (which it had easily been able to do for most foods). If food is swallowed with minimal mastication, the residual stomach is prone to develop bezoars unless the anastomosis is large. When distal gastrectomy leads to loss of the pylorus, indiscriminate gastric emptying develops. Loss of the sieving function of the pylorus permits solid material to enter the jejunum. Larger materials have much less surface area on which digestive enzymes can act to reduce them to basic molecules for absorption. Loss of the regulatory functions of the

## PHYSIOLOGY OF GASTROENTERIC STOMAS (Continued)

pylorus and duodenum also results in adverse effects from rapid emptying of liquid gastric contents. A common complication of gastrojejunostomy is the development of a peptic ulcer distal to the anastomosis. This occurs for three reasons: (1) there is rapid emptying of gastric fluids with high concentrations of acid; (2) the jejunal mucosa is more susceptible to injury by gastric juice than is the duodenal mucosa; and (3) alkaline bile juice refluxing into the stomach can increase acid secretion. Emptying of the gastric contents directly into the jejunum, besides predisposing to jejunal ulcer, as mentioned above, may also lead to the postprandial syndrome of abdominal distress, sweating, weakness, and syncope resulting from jejunal distension known as the *dumping syndrome.* A host of other complications are well documented from the loss of hormonal and neural regulation of digestion by the duodenum. Positioning of the gastrojejunostomy below the point at which the proximal duodenum remains connected to the sphincter of Oddi also has associated risks; this results in a blind loop and multiple related complications described as *afferent* and *efferent loop syndromes.* The general recommendation is to limit the length of the afferent jejunal loop.

*Ileocolostomy* is needed after resection of the terminal ileum and portions of the colon. Functional changes after ileocolostomy are determined by the length of ileum removed, the underlying disease, and the degree to which colonic contents reflux into the small intestine. Extensive resections of the colon can result in a diminished storage capacity of the colon, with acceleration of colonic passage time, diminished absorption of fluid, and corresponding reduction in consistency of the fecal residues. Resection of the ileum can result in impaired vitamin $B_{12}$ absorption, decreased bile salt absorption leading to choleretic diarrhea, and loss of important ileal mucosal hormones responsible for regulation of small intestinal transit, known as the *ileal brake.*

When an ileocolostomy is performed for ileitis, the operation may consist of a side-to-side anastomosis in continuity or a resection with an end-to-end or end-to-side ileocolic anastomosis. The anastomosis in continuity preserves some function in the bypassed small intestine and colon, depending on the extent of the disease and the site of the anastomosis.

Permanent *ileostomy* is sometimes necessary for extensive Crohn disease or ulcerative colitis. Ileoanal anastomosis is preferred for severe ulcerative colitis and colonic polyposis syndromes but is not recommended for Crohn's disease. If the ostomy is too narrow or strictured, a dilation may develop adjacent to the stoma. Other complications from a stoma include excess fluid losses resulting from extensive small bowel resection or underlying enteritis, vigorous peristaltic contractions that may produce a "noisy" ileostomy, and leakage around the ostomy that may lead to irritation of the peristomal skin. Satisfactory appliances and adhesive materials and education and care of the patient by a team of experts, including an expert ostomy nurse, are needed for a good outcome.

*Colostomy* is usually performed for neoplasms of the sigmoid colon or diverticulitis. Unlike ileal fluids that are always liquid, distal colonic contents may become inspissated. In this case the colostomy must be irrigated regularly to evacuate the fecal content mechanically. Keeping the fecal contents semiliquified is preferred.

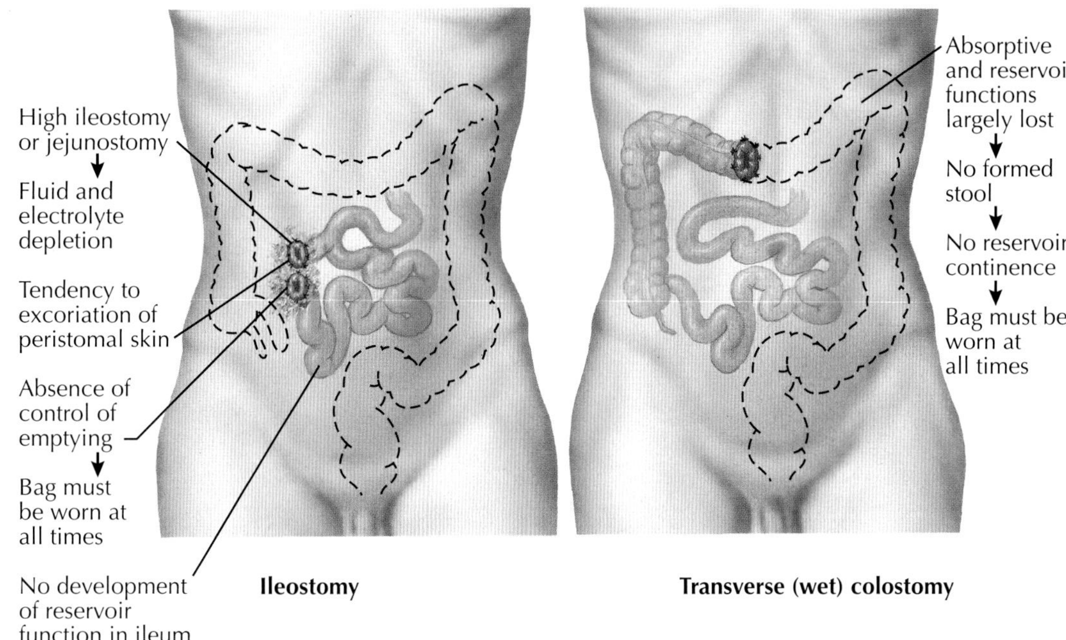


**Ileostomy** **Transverse (wet) colostomy**

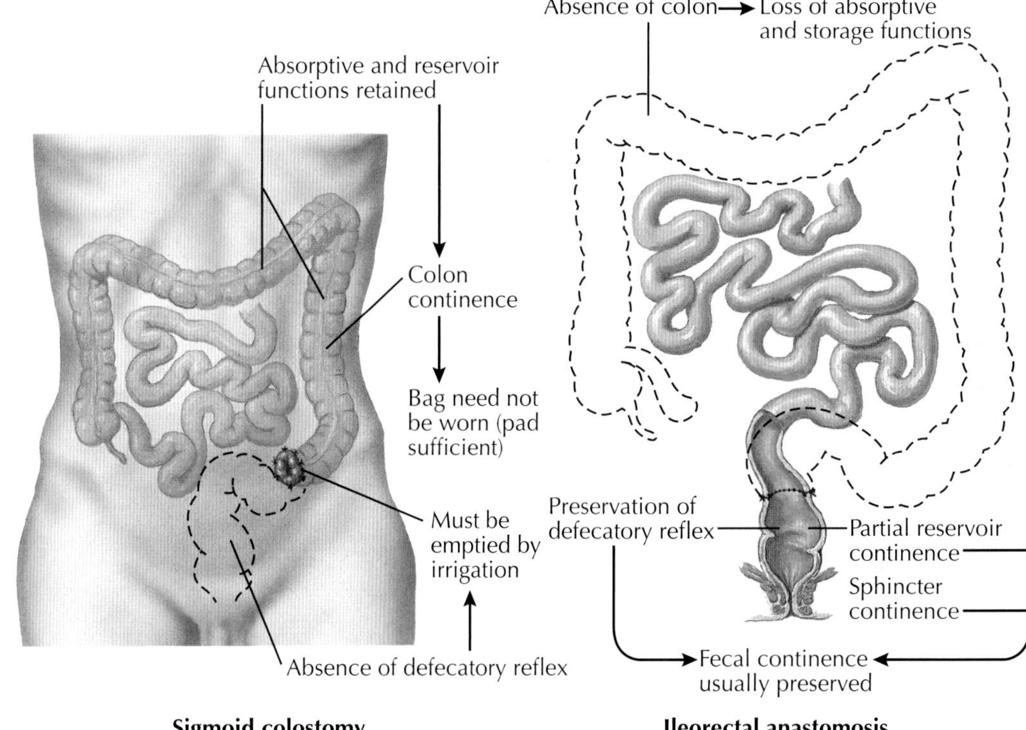


**Sigmoid colostomy** **Ileorectal anastomosis**

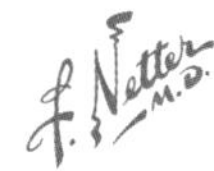

Anastomosis of the ileum to the anus (ileoanal anastomosis) is the procedure of choice for total colectomy, including ulcerative colitis and diffuse polyposis of the colon. The aim of the procedure is to permit controlled defecation through the natural orifice by preserving the anal sphincters. Reducing fluid volumes presented to the rectum is achieved by creating a J-shaped ileal pouch. Immediately after surgery, the patient must deal with a high frequency of bowel movements. Diarrhea typically decreases over time to four to seven bowel movements daily, one or two of which will be at night. Leaving a sleeve of rectum to create an ileorectal anastomosis should be avoided because it will continue to provide a risk for recurrent colitis or cancer, depending on the initial indication for total colectomy. Fecal incontinence is a common complication, particularly during sleep, when volitional control of the sphincter is diminished. Inflammation of the J-pouch may result in pouchitis.

# SMALL BOWEL

## Development of Small Intestine

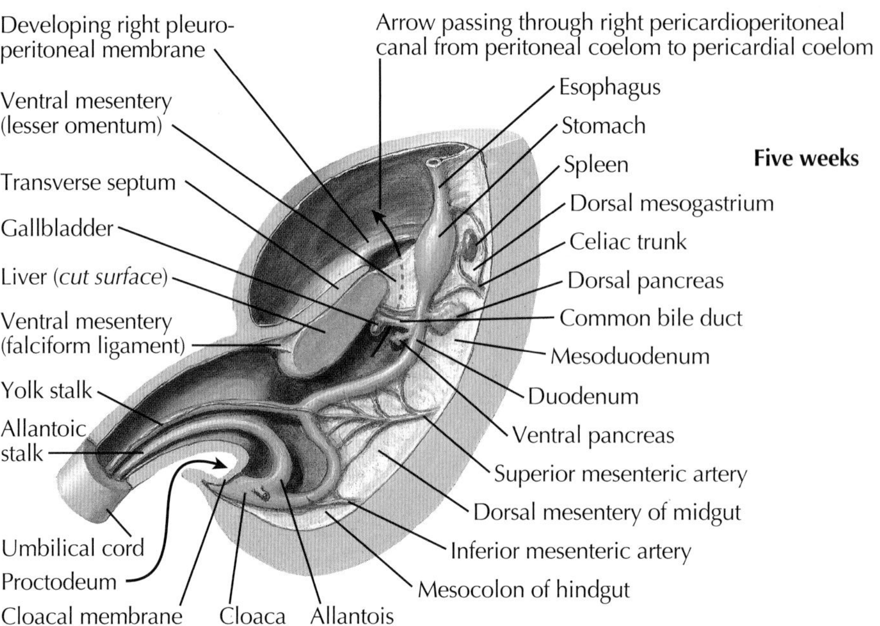


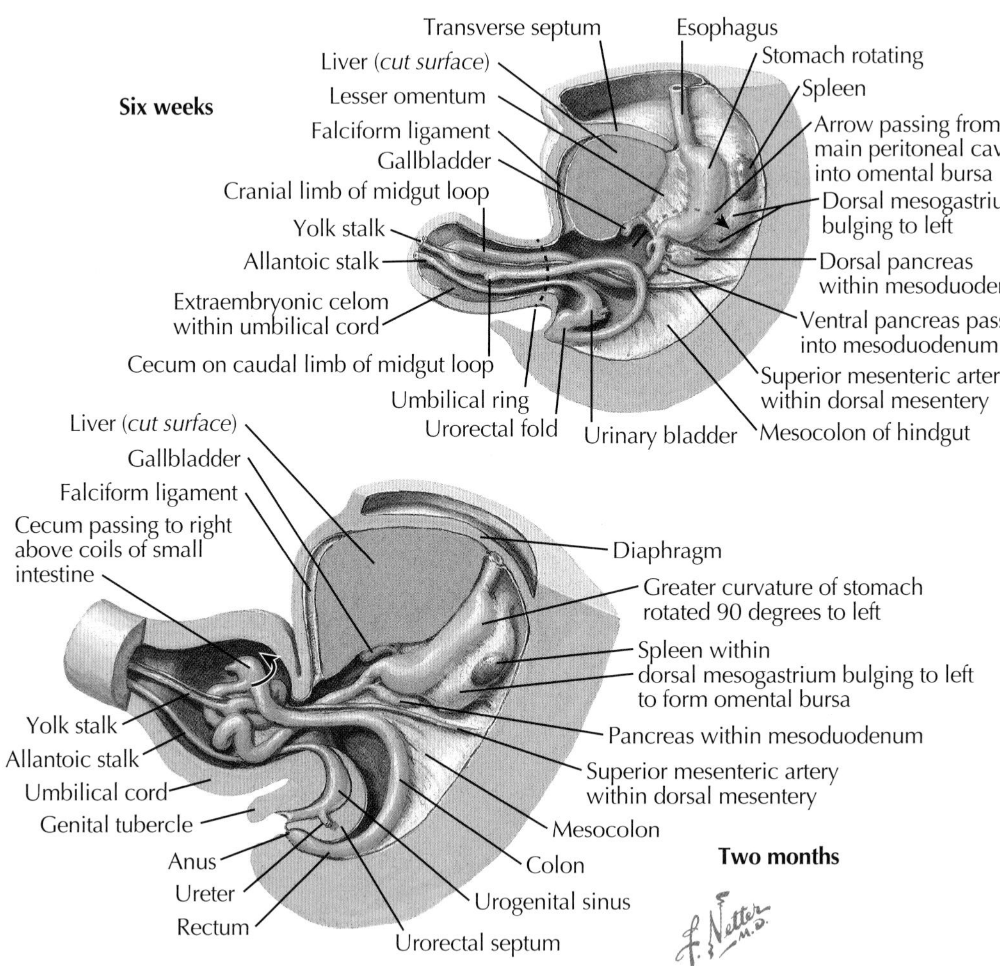


The small intestine includes the duodenum, jejunum, and ileum. During development of the gastrointestinal (GI) system, the duodenum comes from the distal portion of the foregut, whereas the jejunum and ileum come entirely from the midgut. The duodenum moves to the right of the midline as the stomach rotates and shifts to the left side of the abdomen during weeks 4 to 6 of fetal life. As development proceeds, the common bile duct moves to the posterior side of the gut tube as the stomach rotates and the liver enlarges. One aspect of duodenal development that is clinically important is that during weeks 5 and 6, the epithelial lining of the duodenum, derived from the endoderm, proliferates to the point that it completely blocks its own lumen. However, the lumen of the duodenum typically recanalizes so that the fetus can begin swallowing amniotic fluid. If the lumen of the duodenum does not recanalize or opens incompletely, *duodenal atresia* or *stenosis* will occur. As a region of gut that links the foregut and midgut, the duodenum is supplied by branches of both the celiac and superior mesenteric arteries. The descending and horizontal portions of the duodenum are the regions where this anastomosis occurs, and these are also the regions in which atresia or stenosis is most likely to manifest.

The jejunum and ileum are, in their entirety, midgut structures and are supplied by branches of the superior mesenteric artery (SMA). As it elongates, a loop of midgut herniates into the umbilical cord, with the SMA extending between the loop's proximal limb (cranial) and distal limb (caudal). The vitelline duct extends off the apex of the loop, connecting the midgut temporarily to the secondary yolk sac. The proximal limb of the midgut loop will become the jejunum and ileum, and the distal limb will become the terminal ileum, cecum, appendix, ascending colon, and transverse colon. Although it may sound as though the proximal and caudal portions are unbalanced, the jejunum and ileum elongate tremendously, creating many loops within the umbilicus. While in the umbilicus, the midgut rotates 90 degrees in a clockwise motion (when viewed from the perspective of the embryo) and also elongates. This rotation moves the proximal limb to the right and the distal limb to the left side of the cord. During the 10th week, the midgut begins to return to the abdominal cavity, which has grown more expansive as the relative size of the liver and kidneys decreases. As the loop of midgut finishes returning to the abdomen in the 11th week, it undergoes a further 180-degree rotation around the SMA, with the proximal limb moving to the left side of the body (where most of the jejunum will be found) and the distal limb moving to the right side of the body (where the distal ileum, cecum, appendix, and ascending colon are typically found). During this process, the ileum loses its connection to the vitelline duct, unless it remains as a blind pouch (*ileal* or *Meckel diverticulum*).

The dorsal mesentery of the duodenum lays back and fuses with the parietal peritoneum of the posterior body wall to become secondarily retroperitoneal. The jejunum and ileum retain the mesentery; it allows these intramesenteric organs a degree of freedom within the abdominal cavity. Because the stomach and the proximal jejunum have a mesentery, the first and fourth portions of the duodenum may have a small section of mesentery. The morphologic changes of the midgut during development are largely complete at this time, apart from expansion as the individual grows during childhood and adolescence. The development of the large intestine, the colon, is covered in the next section.

## Topography and Relations of Small Bowel

The small intestine consists of a retroperitoneal portion, the duodenum, and a mesenteric portion made up of the coils of the *jejunum* and *ileum*. The total length of the mesenteric portion of the small intestine varies considerably. The average for adults is roughly 5 m. The proximal jejunum forms approximately two-fifths of the mesenteric portion, and the ileum forms the remaining three-fifths. The jejunum commences at the *duodenojejunal flexure* on the left side of the second lumbar vertebra or, occasionally, somewhat more cranially. The ileum terminates when it joins the cecum in the right iliac fossa. Although the division between the jejunum and ileum is not grossly visible (the appearance of the arteries and histologic structure can be used to distinguish the two regions), the coils of the jejunum tend to be on the superior left side of the abdomen and those of the ileum on the inferior right side.

The duodenojejunal flexure is situated at the superiormost end of the region covered by the mesentery of the transverse colon. It may sometimes be partially concealed by the parietal line of attachment of the transverse mesocolon. From the duodenojejunal flexure to the ileocolic junction, the line of attachment of this mesentery runs obliquely from superior left to inferior right, passing across the lumbar portion of the spine, aorta, inferior vena cava, right psoas major, and right ureter. The mesentery is formed by two layers of peritoneum that reflect off the posterior body wall and become continuous as they cover the intestinal surface. The space between the two layers of peritoneum is filled with connective tissue and adipose cells, the quantity of the latter varying greatly from one individual to another. Sandwiched between the two layers of peritoneum and embedded in this tissue are blood and lymph vessels running between the intestine and the posterior abdominal wall as well as nerves and mesenteric lymph nodes. The mesentery is only about 15 to 20 cm in length as it attaches to the body wall, compared with several meters (corresponding to the length of the intestine) along its intestinal attachment, so the mesentery can be conceptualized as fanning outward as it approaches the intestines. The existence of the mesentery affords the intestinal coils a wide range of movement.

The various *portions of the large intestine* form a horseshoe-shaped frame enclosing the coils of the small intestine. This frame may be overlapped anteriorly by the coils of the small intestine, particularly the descending colon on the left side. Similarly, depending on their filling and on their relationship with the pelvic organs, the coils of the small intestine may extend inferiorly into the true pelvis or, if the pelvic organs are greatly distended (e.g., in pregnancy), may be displaced superiorly.

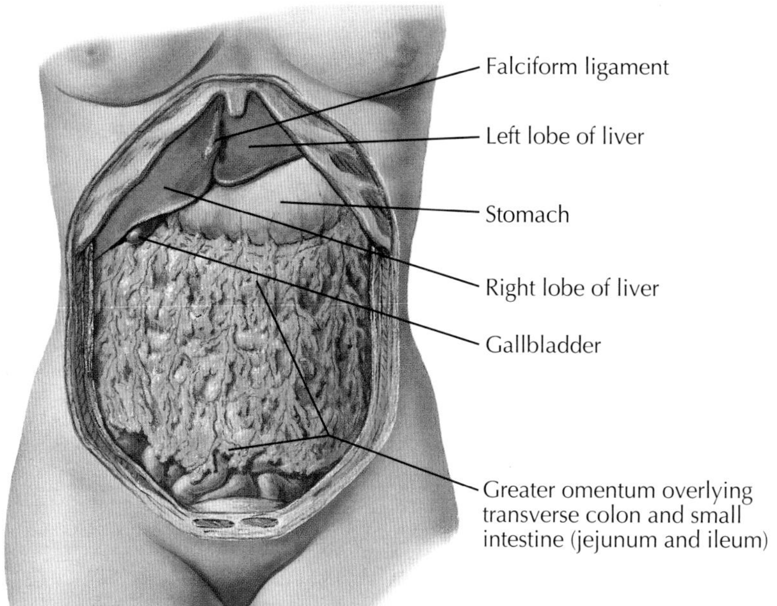


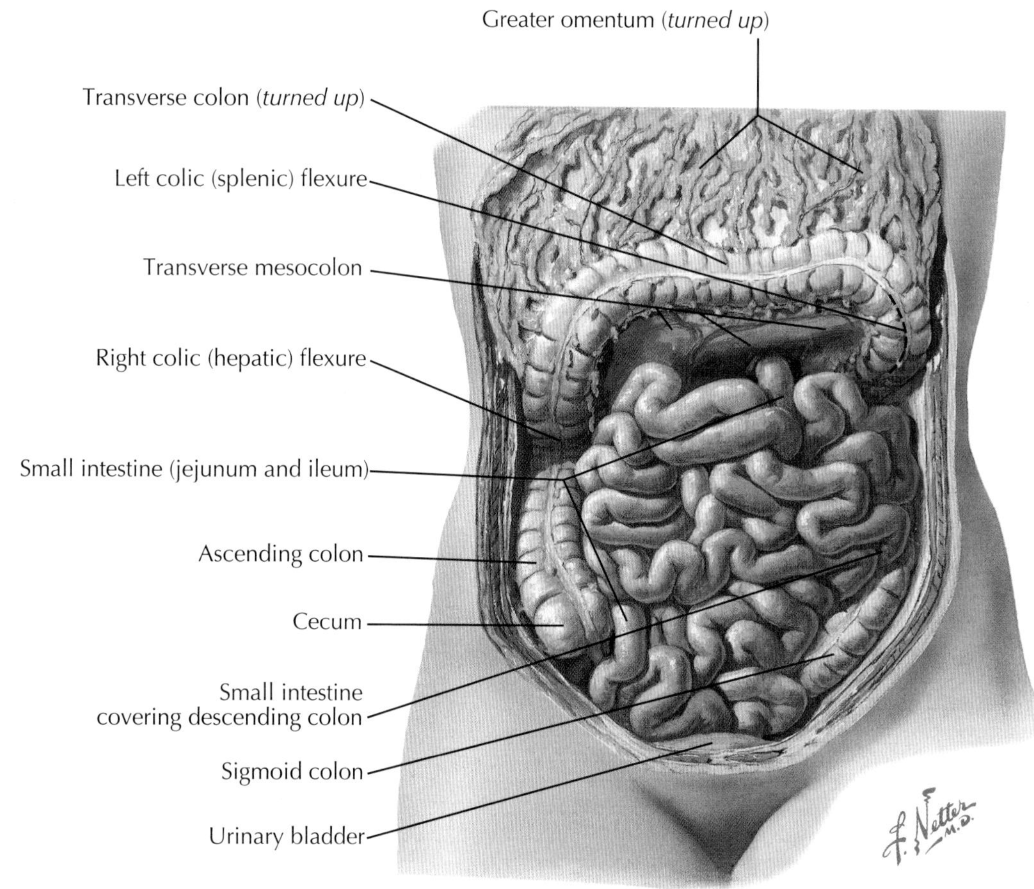


Greatly varying in shape and highly mobile, the *greater omentum* hangs down apron-like from the greater curvature of the stomach and spreads between the anterior abdominal wall and the coils of the small intestine. This large sheet of connective tissue, adipose tissue, and outer coating of the peritoneum frequently obscures the small intestines but can often be reflected, so that its free end is lifted superiorly. However, it also may form adhesions to the anterior and lateral abdominal wall that make it difficult to reflect.

Because it is suspended from the body wall by a mesentery, the small intestine is capable of considerable movement, and its individual coils vary greatly in position. This is true between individuals and even in the same subject at different times, depending on the state of intestinal filling and peristalsis and the position of the body. The only portion that, in line with its progressively shortened mesentery, has a more or less constant position is the terminal ileum, which passes to the right, across the right psoas major muscle, to the site of the ileocolic junction.

## Structure of Small Intestine

The freely mobile portion of the small intestine, which is attached to the mesentery, extends from the duodenojejunal flexure to the ileocolic orifice, where the small intestine joins the large intestine. This portion of the small intestine consists of the jejunum and the ileum. They run imperceptibly into each other, the transition being marked by a gradual change in the diameter of the lumen and by several structural alterations.

The walls of the jejunum and ileum are virtually identical in structure but have slight modifications that make them histologically distinct. Like the rest of the GI tract, the jejunum and the ileum have four layers: the *mucosa, submucosa, muscularis externa,* and *serosa.* The innermost layer, the mucosa, is thickly plicated by macroscopically visible *circular folds (plicae circulares, Kerckring folds).* These folds vary in height, projecting into the lumen by 3 to 10 mm. Some of these plicae extend all the way around the internal circumference, some of them extend only halfway or two-thirds of the way around the circle, and still others spiral around the circle twice or even more times. The circular folds projecting into the lumen slow down the progression of the luminal contents to a slight degree, but their most important function is to increase the absorptive surface area of the intestinal lumen. The visible increase in surface area created by the circular folds is mirrored on the microscopic level by tiny finger-like projections, *intestinal villi.*

In fact, the entire mucosal surface of the small intestine, over and between the circular folds, is covered with intestinal villi, projections that are 0.5 to 1.5 mm long (just barely visible to the naked eye). The mass of these villi (estimated at 4 million altogether in the jejunum and ileum) accounts for the velvety appearance of the mucosa. They are somewhat longer and broader in the jejunum than they are in the ileum. The valleys or indentations between the villi form nonramified pits, each of which harbors tubular structures, the *intestinal glands* (crypts of Lieberkühn). The entire inner surface of the small intestine, including the villi, is covered by a single layer of epithelial cells, the majority of which are *enterocytes,* highly prismatic columnar cells with a surface covered by *microvilli,* microscopic projections from these cells' apical surfaces. Between these columnar cells are interspersed other types of cells, such as *goblet cells, Paneth cells,* and *enteroendocrine cells.* The goblet cells secrete an alkaline, mucous fluid that coats the whole mucosa. Most goblet cells are found lining the crypts or along the lower parts of the villi, but a considerable number of them are located near the apex of the villi, where they seem to be squeezed between neighboring enterocytes. The Paneth cells are found almost exclusively near the base of the intestinal glands. They are easily identified histologically due to the eosinophilic granules they contain. Paneth cells are primarily involved in moderating the normal bacterial flora of the small intestine. They do so by secreting the antimicrobial enzyme lysozyme as well as α-defensins. They are able to phagocytose bacteria and other invaders within the intestinal lumen. Last, the enteroendocrine cells (argentaffin cells, yellow cells, cells of Schmidt or of Kulchitsky) contain basal-staining granules with a high affinity for silver and chromium. These cells are typically found at the bottom of intestinal glands but can migrate upward. They regulate the activity of the digestive system by releasing hormones such as cholecystokinin (stimulates secretion of the gallbladder and pancreas and inhibits gastric emptying), secretin (stimulates pancreatic secretion and inhibits gastric secretion), motilin (stimulates peristalsis), and gastric inhibitory peptide (stimulates insulin secretion and inhibits gastric secretion) into the bloodstream. Enteroendocrine cells in the small intestine may also secrete somatostatin (inhibits release of gastrin and gastric secretion) and histamine (stimulates gastric secretion from parietal cells) in a paracrine fashion, affecting nearby tissues. Lymphocytes, eosinophils, neutrophils, macrophages, mast cells, and plasma cells are also sometimes seen in the epithelial lining of the small intestine, but these have generally migrated from the underlying layer of the mucosa, the lamina propria.

The *lamina propria* lies deep to the epithelial surface of the mucosa, but it extends into both the circular folds

**Mucosa and Musculature of Duodenum**

**Jejunum**

Mesentery
Anastomotic loop (arcade) of jejunal arteries
Straight arteries
Serosa (visceral peritoneum)
Longitudinal muscle layer
Circular muscle layer
Submucosa
Mucosa
Solitary lymphoid nodule
Circular folds (valves of Kerckring)
F. Netter M.D.

**Ileum**

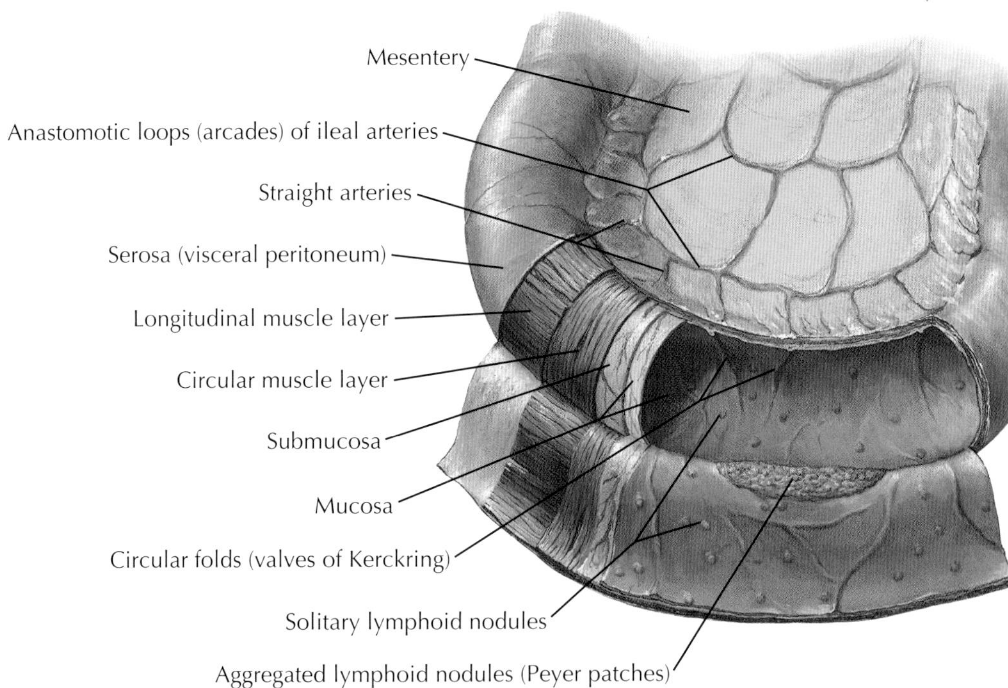

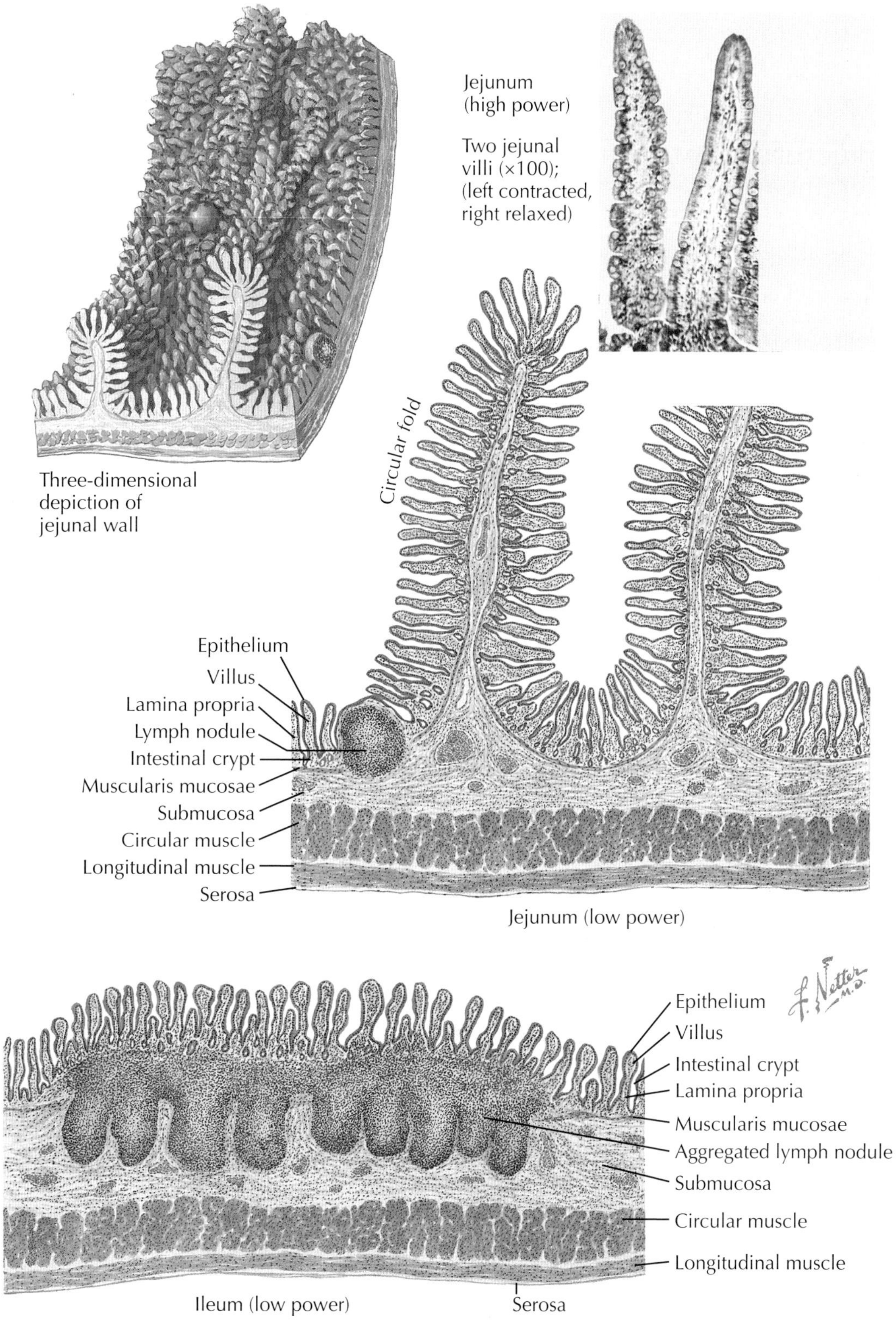

## STRUCTURE OF SMALL INTESTINE (Continued)

and intestinal villi, forming the core of each villus. This diffuse reticular connective tissue allows for the easy diffusion of nutrients and gases to and from the epithelial lining of the intestine. The lamina propria frequently assumes a lymphatic character owing to the large number of lymphocytes that migrate through it. The lamina propria also contains thin fibers of smooth muscle that radiate from the muscularis mucosae upward to the tips of the villi. When these fibers are relaxed, the villi have a smooth surface, whereas they become jagged or indented when the fibers contract. These muscular fibrils are assumed to act as motors that maintain the pumping function of the villi. At the core of each villus is a lymphatic vessel, the *central lacteal,* which transports fat-soluble substances and lymph to the cisterna chyli and from there to the venous circulation. The *muscularis mucosae,* which separates the lamina propria from the submucosa, is composed of two thin layers of smooth muscle, which keep the movable mucosal layer in place. The outer longitudinal layer is thinner than the inner circular layer, from which the muscular fibers in the core of the villi, mentioned above, emanate.

The *submucosa* is a relatively stout layer that is deep to the mucosa. It is made up of type I collagen bundles forming dense, irregular connective tissue. By altering the angles of its meshes, this submucosal network is able to adapt itself to changes in the diameter and length of the intestinal lumen. The submucosa contains a rich network of arteries, veins, and lymphatics that supply the submucosa and overlying mucosal structures. It also has a substantial network of viscerosensory and visceromotor axons; preganglionic parasympathetic axons terminating in the submucosa synapse on the *submucosal plexus (Meissner plexus),* a collection of ganglia (nerve cells) scattered throughout the small and large intestines that contribute to the enteric nervous system.

The *muscularis externa* is a large and powerful two-layered coat of smooth muscle that covers the submucosa. The thick inner circular layer and the thinner outer longitudinal layer are connected by convoluted transitional fascicles in the area where they border on each other. Between the two layers is a network of viscerosensory and visceromotor axons. As in the submucosa, preganglionic parasympathetic axons synapse with the *myenteric plexus (Auerbach plexus),* which are the ganglia located between the two layers of smooth muscle. The myenteric plexus and submucosal plexuses are major components of the enteric nervous system. The muscularis externa is responsible for creating the powerful movements of peristalsis that move intestinal contents progressively down the lumen, or in retrograde motion during vomiting.

Lining the outside surface of the small intestines is the final layer, the *serosa* (visceral peritoneum). This layer is composed of mesothelial cells on the surface that are connected to the muscularis externa by a thin layer of loose connective tissue. The mesothelial cells release fluid that lubricates the external surface of the small intestine and helps to prevent irritation and adhesions between the intestines and other peritoneal structures. The serosa covers the entire circumference of the small intestines, except for a narrow strip where the mesentery anchors the intestines to the posterior body wall.

Although very similar in many ways, the jejunum and ileum differ in several respects. The lumen of the ileum is narrower and the diameter of the total wall is thinner than that of the jejunum. The average diameter of the jejunum measures 3 to 3.5 cm and that of the ileum is 2.5 cm or less. Due to this difference, the contents of the intestine are more visible through the wall of the ileum than the jejunum. Because of this, in the operative view, the jejunum typically has a whitish-red hue, whereas the ileum takes on a darker appearance. The circular folds within the lumen vary in frequency and height, as do the villi. They decrease in height and number as the small intestine approaches the cecum, and in the distal ileum the folds appear only sporadically.

SMALL INTESTINE MICROSCOPIC STRUCTURE

## Structure of Small Intestine (Continued)

In the jejunum, lymphatic tissue is encountered only in the form of *solitary lymphoid nodules* that appear as pinhead-sized elevations on the surface of the mucosa. They become more numerous and more pronounced near the large intestine. Within the ileum, such nodules are very pronounced, forming *aggregated lymphoid nodules (Peyer patches)*. They are invariably situated opposite the attachment of the mesentery and are generally of an elongated oval or ellipsoid shape, their longest diameter always coinciding with the longitudinal axis of the intestinal lumen. Their average width is 1 to 1.5 cm and they vary in length from 2 cm up to 10 or 12 cm or, occasionally, even more. They differ in number from one individual to another, the average total fluctuating from 20 to 30. Another difference between the jejunum and ileum concerns the fat content of their mesenteries. In the adult, the mesentery of the ileum contains more fatty tissue and appears to be thicker than that of the jejunum. The blood vessels that supply each region also have different appearances, which are described in Plates 1.1 and 1.2.

The principal task of the GI tract is to supply the body with its caloric requirements and metabolic material. The structures of the entire GI tract, from the mouth to the large intestine, are optimized to accomplish this task. It is within the small intestines, especially the jejunum and ileum, where the majority of absorption occurs through the enterocytes that coat the inner surface of the small intestine. These epithelial cells, together with the villi they cover, should properly be considered *the* organ of absorption. The surface area available for absorption is maximized in several ways. The circular folds of the small intestine (including the epithelial cells, lamina propria, muscularis mucosae, and submucosal layers) increase the surface area grossly. The villi that project from the lumen and circular folds further increase the surface area available for absorption. Finally, the apical surfaces of the enterocytes themselves have a brush-like border, which is actually composed of microvilli extending from each enterocyte into the lumen. It has been calculated that each epithelial cell is provided with about 1000 microvilli, which increase the cellular surface approximately 24 times. The microvilli seem to vary only a little in size (average length, 1 μm; width, 0.07 μm) and have a core of actin microfilaments extending down their length to attach to a network of fibrils, the *terminal web*, at the apical edges of the cells. Contraction or relaxation of this web can widen or narrow the space between adjacent villi.

At some time after the ingestion of a meal containing fat, fine lipid droplets can be observed in the intermicrovillous spaces; slightly later, the droplets appear in the area of the terminal web, where they accumulate in minute vesicles that owe their existence to a *pinocytotic activity*, probably of the intermicrovillous plasma membrane. The droplets then can be found in the main body of the epithelial cell, where they coalesce to form larger units in vesicles or cisternae, which are connected with each other by intracellular tubules. The fat droplets pass toward the lateral cell surfaces. From the intercellular spaces, the droplets traverse the basement membrane and the interstitial spaces of the lamina propria to enter the central lacteals of the villi. The lacteals carry fats and fluid proximally via lymphatic channels that ultimately drain to the cisterna chyli, thoracic duct, and, finally, the left subclavian vein. For this reason, fat-soluble substances can bypass the liver, which receives other substances absorbed from the lumen that are transported to it via blood in the hepatic portal vein.

The nucleus of the enterocytes is typically located in its basal region, near the Golgi apparatus. Mitochondria and other organelles of the cell body show no particular or specific features. To maintain a separation between the lumen of the intestines (which is technically outside the body) and the extracellular space within the body, the apical region of enterocytes and other cells of the intestinal epithelium are bound to each other by junctional complexes in the vicinity of the terminal web. The enterocytes are anchored to the underlying connective tissue of the lamina propria by tight junctions. This allows the enterocytes to be selective about the substances that are released into the lamina propria and, thereafter, the bloodstream.

### Epithelium of Small Intestine

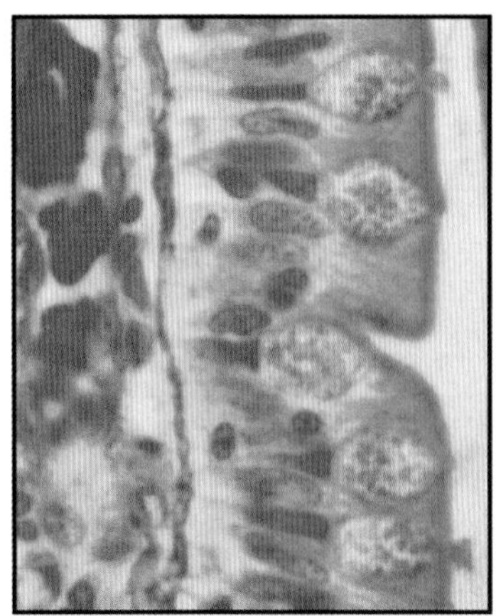
Goblet cells and striated border of human jejunal villus (azan stain, ×650)

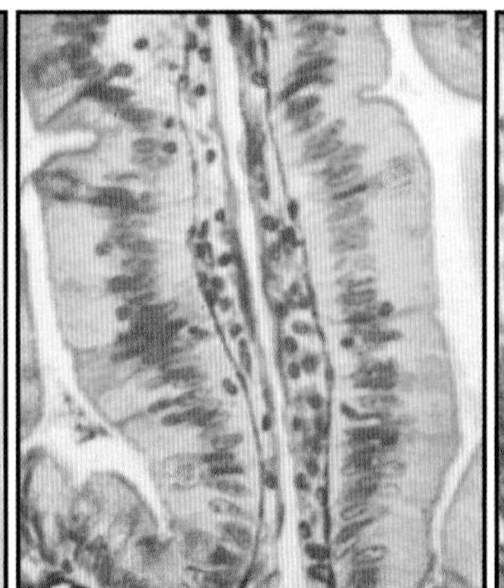
Central lacteal (chyliferous vessel) in human jejunal villus (azan stain, ×325)

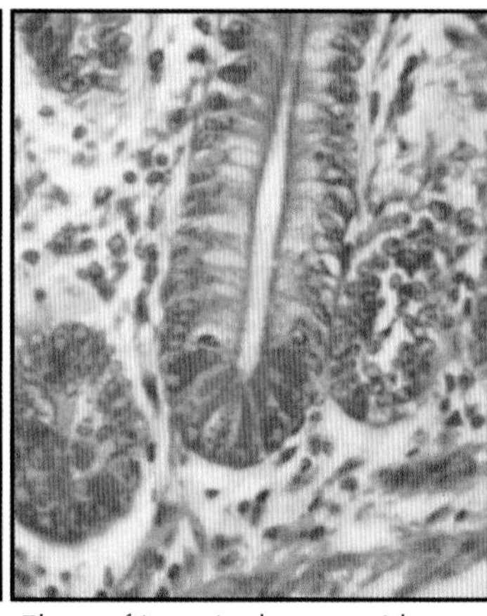
Floor of intestinal crypt with granulated, oxyphilic cells of Paneth (hematoxylin-eosin, ×325)

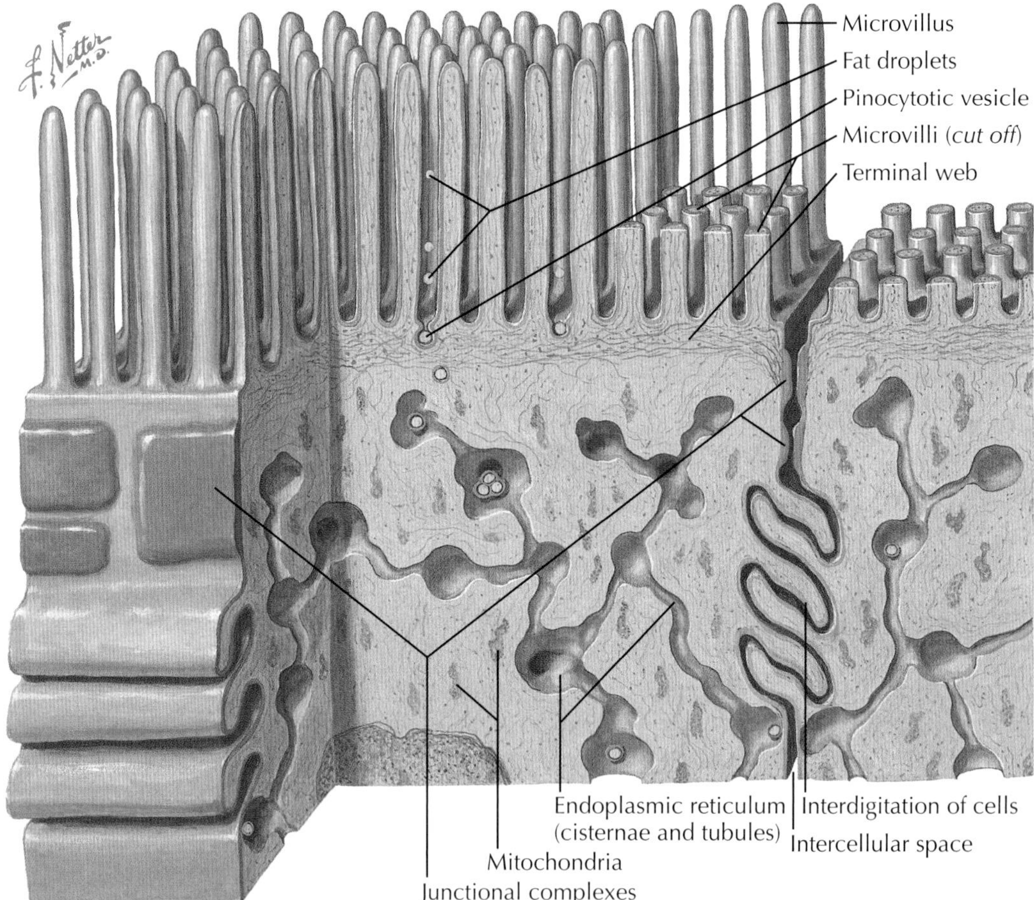

Three-dimensional schema of striated border of intestinal epithelial cells (based on ultramicroscopic studies)

## Blood Supply of Small Intestine

For the typical pattern of arterial branching of the small intestines, refer to Plates 1.1 and 1.2. This section describes common variations concerning the origin, course, anastomoses, and distribution of the vessels supplying the small intestine. These variations are so frequent that conventional textbook descriptions are inadequate for anyone attempting procedures in the area. Typically, the SMA supplies almost all of the small intestine aside from the proximal duodenum, which receives blood from the *supraduodenal* and *superior pancreaticoduodenal arteries.* These arteries are branches of the *gastroduodenal artery,* a branch of the *common hepatic artery,* which is itself a branch of the *celiac trunk.*

The distance between the celiac trunk and the SMA varies from 1 to 23 mm but is typically between 1 and 6 mm. These major vessels branch from the abdominal aorta; in rare cases, the vessels form a single massive vessel, a *celiacomesenteric trunk* (A), that gives off the common hepatic, splenic, left gastric, and superior mesenteric arteries. However, in some cases of celiacomesenteric trunk the left gastric artery is a small separate branch arising directly from the abdominal aorta. A far more frequently encountered variation (0.4%–6% of the population) of these vessels is a *hepatomesenteric trunk.* This occurs when the SMA fuses with the common hepatic, right hepatic, or left hepatic artery (B, C, D, and E). If the hepatomesenteric trunk includes the common hepatic artery, there will also be a *gastrosplenic trunk* giving rise to the splenic and left gastric arteries (B). If the hepatomesenteric trunk gives rise to a right hepatic artery (C) or an accessory right hepatic artery (D and E), there will be either an incomplete celiac trunk or a complete celiac trunk contributing the remaining hepatic vessels (C and D). The cystic artery may arise from either the right hepatic artery or accessory right hepatic artery (C, D, and E).

Variations that are even less frequent have been described. A *splenomesenteric trunk* develops when the superior mesenteric and splenic arteries arise from a common trunk (F). In such cases, there will be a separate *hepatogastric trunk* branching into common hepatic and left gastric arteries. If the superior mesenteric, splenic, and common hepatic arteries come from a common trunk of the abdominal aorta (G), the result is a *hepatosplenomesenteric trunk,* with a separate left gastric artery arising from the aorta or from the left inferior phrenic artery, creating a *gastrophrenic trunk.* Occasionally, the right *gastroomental artery* may branch from the SMA (H) instead of taking its normal departure from the gastroduodenal artery.

The first jejunal branch of superior mesenteric origin may be very large (6 mm in diameter), but in many instances, it is very small (1–2 mm) and forms anastomoses with the inferior pancreaticoduodenal artery or has a common origin with it. The distribution, as well as the caliber, of all the following intestinal branches of the SMA varies considerably, and smaller branches may alternate without any general rule or order. An odd situation may be faced during gastric resection, when the right gastroomental artery and the first jejunal branch arise from a common pancreaticoduodenal trunk coming from the SMA. Closer to the small intestine itself, small (4- to 6-cm) segments may be vascularized by straight arteries derived from a separate anterior and posterior arcade, each serving the anterior and posterior surface of the same region of the gut. Although numerous other examples of variations concerning the origin and communication of the first jejunal branches could be enumerated, those cited seem sufficient to justify the requirement of a careful inspection of these vessels while operating in this region.

Common origin of celiac trunk and superior mesenteric artery.

Celiacomesenteric trunk

A

Replaced hepatic artery takes origin from superior mesenteric (note inferior pancreaticoduodenal artery from 1st jejunal).

Splenogastric trunk

Hepatomesenteric trunk

B

Replaced right hepatic artery takes origin from superior mesenteric; inferior pancreaticoduodenal and 1st jejunal arteries from replaced right hepatic.

Incomplete celiac trunk

Hepatomesenteric trunk

C

Accessory right hepatic artery takes origin from superior mesenteric; inferior pancreaticoduodenal arteries from accessory right hepatic; 1st jejunal artery from anterior inferior pancreaticoduodenal.

Complete celiac trunk

Hepatomesenteric trunk (Note accessory left gastric artery from left hepatic.)

D

Accessory right hepatic artery takes origin from superior mesenteric.

Complete celiac trunk

Hepatomesenteric trunk

E

Splenic artery takes origin from superior mesenteric (note replaced left hepatic artery from left gastric).

Hepatogastric trunk

Splenomesenteric trunk

F

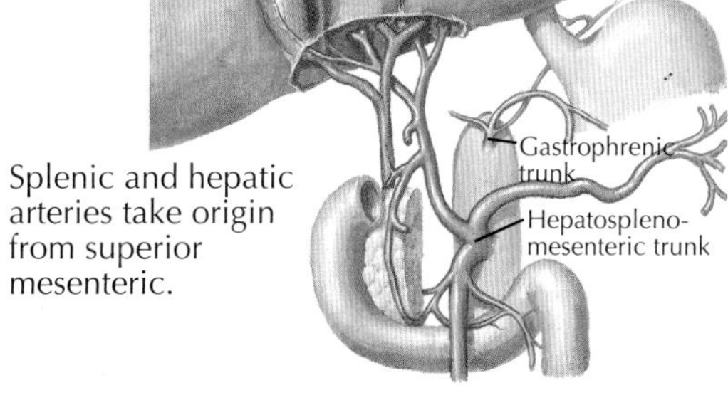

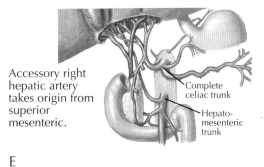


Splenic and hepatic arteries take origin from superior mesenteric.

G

Right gastroepiploic (gastroomental) artery takes origin from superior mesenteric (note accessory left hepatic artery from left gastric).

H

F. Netter M.D.

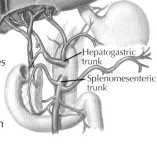

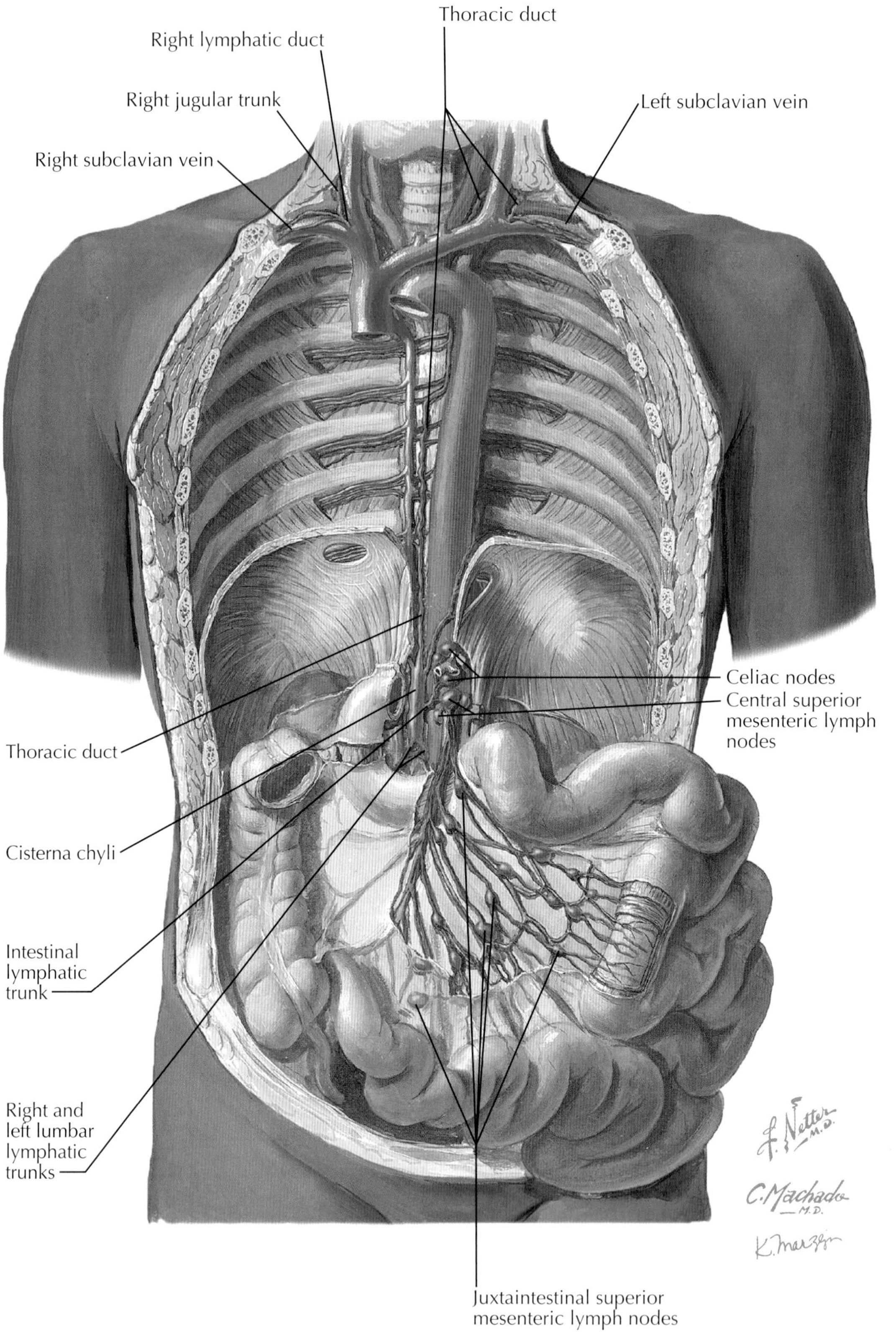

## Lymph Drainage of Small Intestine

The lymph vessels of the small intestine begin with the *central lacteals of the villi.* At the base of the villi, each central lacteal joins with lymph capillaries, draining the nearby intestinal crypts. These lymph capillaries form a fine network within the lamina propria, in which the first lymphatic valves are already encountered. Many minute branches emerge from this network, penetrating through the muscularis mucosae into the submucosa, which hosts a sizable network of lymphatic vessels. The vessels of this network have conspicuous valves that prevent retrograde motion of the lymphatic fluid once it is inside the vessels. Progressively larger lymph vessels, receiving additional lymph from the layers of the muscularis mucosae and from the serosa and subserosa, pass toward the attachment of the mesentery to the small intestine. Within the mesentery, the lymph vessels travel alongside arteries and veins. These larger lymph vessels have been referred to as *chyliferous vessels* or *lacteals* because they transport emulsified fat absorbed from the intestines and appear as milky-white threads after the ingestion of fat-containing food. Lymph fluid traveling through these vessels encounters several *juxtaintestinal* (within the mesentery, alongside the intestines) *superior mesenteric lymph nodes,* which number some 100 to 200 and constitute the largest aggregate of lymph nodes in the body. They increase in number and size toward the root of the mesentery, where larger lymphatic branches are situated, which lead into the *central superior mesenteric nodes* in the area where the SMA arises from the aorta.

The proximal duodenum and nearby pancreas receive blood from branches of the celiac trunk; its distal sections are supplied by the SMA; and lymphatic drainage from the duodenum can pass to either celiac or superior mesenteric lymph nodes. Lymphatic fluid from the duodenum and the nearby pancreatic head travels to lymph nodes lying inferior, superior, and posterior to the head of the pancreas. The inferior nodes are the already-encountered central superior mesenteric nodes. The superior group of lymph nodes is known as the *subpyloric* and *right suprapancreatic nodes,* and the posterior group is known as the *retropancreatic nodes.* Lymphatic fluid from the latter two groups of nodes drains parallel to branches of the celiac trunk to reach the celiac lymph nodes.

From the superior mesenteric nodes and the celiac nodes, lymphatic fluid passes through the short intestinal or GI lymph trunk, which is sometimes divided into several smaller parallel trunks, and enters the *cisterna chyli,* a sac-like expansion at the beginning of the *thoracic duct.* The cisterna chyli also receives much of the lymphatic fluid drained from the lower limbs, pelvic organs, and hindgut organs. From the cisterna chyli, lymph drains superiorly through the thoracic duct. This large lymphatic vessel has prominent valves in its wall and is found in the posterior mediastinum between the aorta and esophagus. It ascends and travels posterior to the arch of the aorta to ultimately drain the lymphatic fluid into the venous system at the left subclavian vein near its junction with the left internal jugular vein.

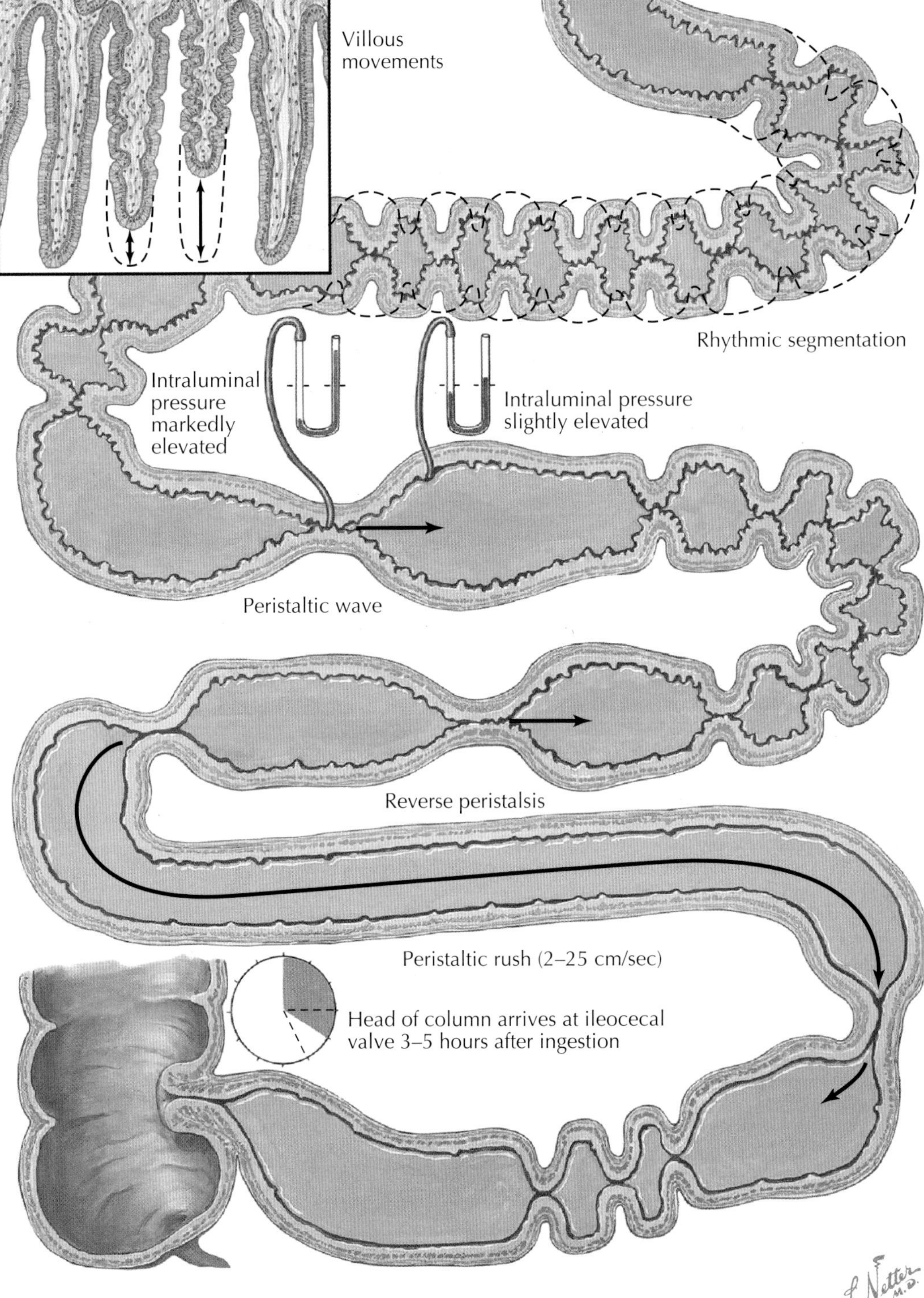


## Motility of Small Intestine

The primary function of the small bowel is absorption of nutrients. The motor activity or the *motility* of the small bowel supports this function by facilitating the mixing of chyme with digestive enzymes and other intestinal fluid and creating a to-and-fro movement of the chyme that allows adequate contact time with the intestinal mucosa. The digestive status (i.e., the fasting or fed state) is a key component of small bowel motility. During fasting, a wave of electrical activity, termed the *migratory motor complex* (MMC), originates in the gastric antrum and duodenum, and migrates distally in a recurring pattern, every 90 to 120 minutes, until it is interrupted by feeding. In addition to facilitating the transport of indigestible substances and sloughed cells from the stomach to the colon, the MMC also sweeps bacteria from the small intestine to the large intestine and inhibits the reflux of colonic bacteria to the terminal ileum. This complex is often termed the "intestinal housekeeper" and can be divided into four phases.

Phase 1 of the MMC lasts 5 to 20 minutes and is characterized by a prolonged period of quiescence. Phase 2 lasts 10 to 40 minutes and is defined by an increased frequency of random (irregular) contractions. Phase 3 lasts 3 to 6 minutes and is characterized by bursts of rhythmic high-amplitude contractions and is also the most active, albeit short, phase. Phase 4 is a transitional period between phases 3 and 1 with rapid decrease in contractions. In the duodenum, phase 3 contractions have a frequency of 1 to 12 contractions per minute and last for at least 3 minutes with the velocity progressively decreasing from the proximal duodenum to the distal jejunum. Alterations in the MMC have been implicated in the pathophysiology of small intestinal bacterial overgrowth, irritable bowel syndrome, functional dyspepsia, gastroparesis, Chagas disease, and intestinal pseudoobstruction.

The control of the MMC is complex, and it appears to be influenced by the extrinsic and intrinsic nervous system. Smooth muscle cells of the GI tract undergo periodic depolarization of their membrane potential. These are called *slow waves,* and they are generated by the interstitial cells of Cajal, which act as pacemakers and produce spontaneous electrical slow waves with a frequency of 12 per minute in the duodenum and 10 per minute in the ileum. A contraction is achieved when a slow wave occurs at the same time that an excitatory neurotransmitter is released from a motor neuron of the enteric nervous system.

Studies suggest a humoral control of MMC activity because phase 3 of the MMC with an antral origin can be induced through intravenous (IV) administration of motilin and erythromycin, whereas administration of serotonin or somatostatin induces phase 3 activity with duodenal origin. The role of the vagus nerve in control of the MMC seems to be restricted to the stomach, as vagotomy abolishes the motor activity in the stomach but leaves the periodic activity in the small bowel intact.

The fed state, or the postprandial phase, is defined as the time between ingestion of a meal with sufficient caloric content until the return of phase 3 of the MMC. When nutrients enter the small bowel, transit is initially rapid, and chyme is distributed throughout the bowel.

## Motility of Small Intestine (Continued)

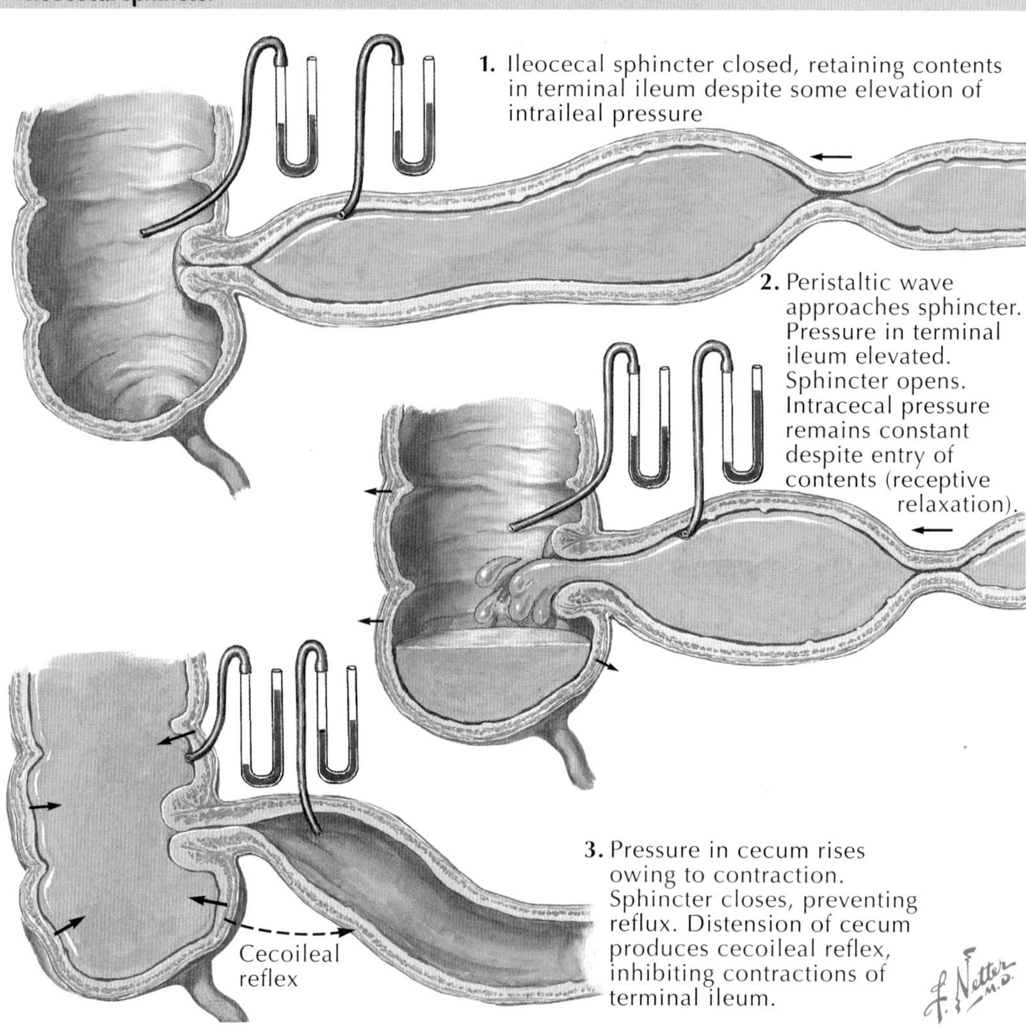

GRADIENT AND ILEOCECAL SPHINCTER
Gradient
A
A1
B1
B
A
B1
A1
B
Ileocecal sphincter
1. Ileocecal sphincter closed, retaining contents in terminal ileum despite some elevation of intraileal pressure
2. Peristaltic wave approaches sphincter. Pressure in terminal ileum elevated. Sphincter opens. Intracecal pressure remains constant despite entry of contents (receptive relaxation).
3. Pressure in cecum rises owing to contraction. Sphincter closes, preventing reflux. Distension of cecum produces cecoileal reflex, inhibiting contractions of terminal ileum.
Cecoileal reflex


During digestion, transit slows down to promote absorption by increasing contact time of the chyme with the small intestinal lining. Pressure waves after a meal are similar to those occurring during the MCC but propagate half the distance of phase 3 pressure waves on average. Most postprandial pressure waves propel the contents less than 2 cm and mainly serve to mix and grind the chyme. Flow rates during this period are highly variable and rely on caloric content and the nature of the meal. In addition, the enteric nerves, hormonal function, and level of paracrine mediators, including gastrin, cholecystokinin, neurotensin, peptide YY, pancreatic polypeptide, and motilin, play a role.

The stationary pressure waves of the postprandial period favor absorption, as does phase 1 of the MMC. The stationary pressure waves work in two ways: (1) by stirring intestinal contents and (2) by providing propulsive pressure waves to spread and expose the chyme to a larger absorptive surface. This type of activity is also referred to as *rhythmic segmentation.* Intestinal peristalsis is generated by the contraction of the muscularis propria, made up of outer longitudinal and inner circular layers, forming a continuous tube that lengthens, shortens, twists, and constricts so that the enclosed contents are constantly agitated and propelled. A meal generally traverses the small bowel in approximately 5 hours, a period that is shortened by the intake of another meal.

The *ileocecal valve* is a distinct feature of the small bowel that plays an important role in peristalsis. It is located at the end of the ileum, wedged into the wall of the colon, and operates independently of the ileum and the colon. The ileocecal junction functions as a true sphincter and regulates the flow of material from the ileum to the cecum as well as preventing its retrograde passage. The sphincter remains contracted at rest, which allows prolonged contact of intestinal contents with the terminal ileal mucosa favoring maximal intestinal absorption. The sphincter opens when a peristaltic wave, passing along the terminal ileum, builds up enough pressure to overcome the resistance of the sphincter. Relaxation of the ileocecal sphincter is stimulated by gastrin released upon ingestion of a meal or gastric distension and the *gastroileal reflex.* The cecum at first manifests receptive relaxation. Increasing pressure in the cecum, either by overdistension or by a peristaltic contraction, causes a reflex contraction of the sphincter, preventing overfilling of the cecum and cecoileal reflux.

Motility studies (manometry) and transit studies are used to investigate small bowel motor function. Small bowel or antroduodenal manometry study is conducted via a nasoenteral catheter that measures intraluminal pressure induced by smooth muscle contractions. Transit studies include hydrogen breath testing, small bowel scintigraphy, and wireless motility capsule testing. The wireless motility capsule measures the transit time, pressure, pH, and temperature from the mouth to the anus. It correlates well with scintigraphy. Patients can resume normal daily activities while data are being collected by the capsule. It also eliminates radiation exposure and provides a complete transit profile of the GI tract.

## GASTROINTESTINAL HORMONES

The epithelium of the GI tract contains multiple cell types, including specialized cells termed *enteroendocrine cells* that number less than 1% of the cell population and yet form the largest endocrine system of the body. Enteroendocrine cells synthesize, store, and release chemical transmitters that are involved in GI motility, secretion, and absorption and in regulation of appetite. These transmitters are predominantly small polypeptides that are also found in the enteric nervous system and the central nervous system (CNS). There are more than 30 gut peptide hormone genes identified, which express more than 100 bioactive peptides. They are grouped into "families" according to their primary structure. In this section, the pancreatic polypeptide family and somatostatin will be discussed.

The pancreatic polypeptide family of peptides include peptide YY, pancreatic polypeptide, and neuropeptide Y. Despite sharing structural similarities and the same 36 amino acid lengths, the gut peptides vary in their biologic functions and locations. Peptide YY, neuropeptide Y, and pancreatic polypeptide bind to a family of G protein–linked receptors (called *Y receptors*). At present, five receptor subtypes have been identified.

*Peptide YY* is a gut peptide secreted from L cells in the ileum and H cells in the colon in response to an oral nutrient load. Peptide YY levels start to rise within 15 minutes of any caloric ingestion, long before the nutrients themselves reach the distal gut, implying that other neural or hormonal mechanisms are involved in its release. The actions of peptide YY are largely inhibitory. It inhibits GI motility, pancreatic and gastric secretion, and chloride secretion, causing a delay in intestinal transit, or the so-called *ileal brake*. This allows for a longer contact time between nutrients and the small intestine. Peptide YY is also believed to be involved in the regulation of food intake and satiety, acting mainly via the $Y_2$ receptors in the hypothalamus.

*Pancreatic polypeptide* is secreted by specialized pancreatic islet cells and inhibits gallbladder contraction and pancreatic exocrine secretion. It may influence food intake, energy metabolism, and the expression of gastric ghrelin and hypothalamic peptides. *Neuropeptide Y* is a neurotransmitter predominantly found in sympathetic neurons and is the most potent known stimulant of food intake.

*Somatostatin* was originally identified as a growth hormone inhibiting factor. Since its discovery, it has been identified in various organs of the body and throughout the GI tract, possessing a broad inhibitory action in the gut. Somatostatin is secreted by the D cells of the stomach and duodenum and the δ cells of the islets of Langerhans of the pancreas. Its secretion is stimulated by the presence of glucose, amino acids, and glucagon-like peptide-1. In the stomach, somatostatin regulates acid secretion by directly inhibiting gastrin release and indirectly inhibiting release of histamine and reducing secretion of pepsinogen. It inhibits cholecystokinin, profoundly inhibits secretion of pancreatic enzymes and bicarbonate along with glucagon and insulin secretion, and reduces bile flow. Somatostatin also reduces splanchnic blood flow and has inhibitory effects on intestinal transport of nutrients and fluid and tissue growth and proliferation. The effects of somatostatin on intestinal motility are similarly inhibitory with the exception of stimulating the MMC, probably through its effects on motilin.

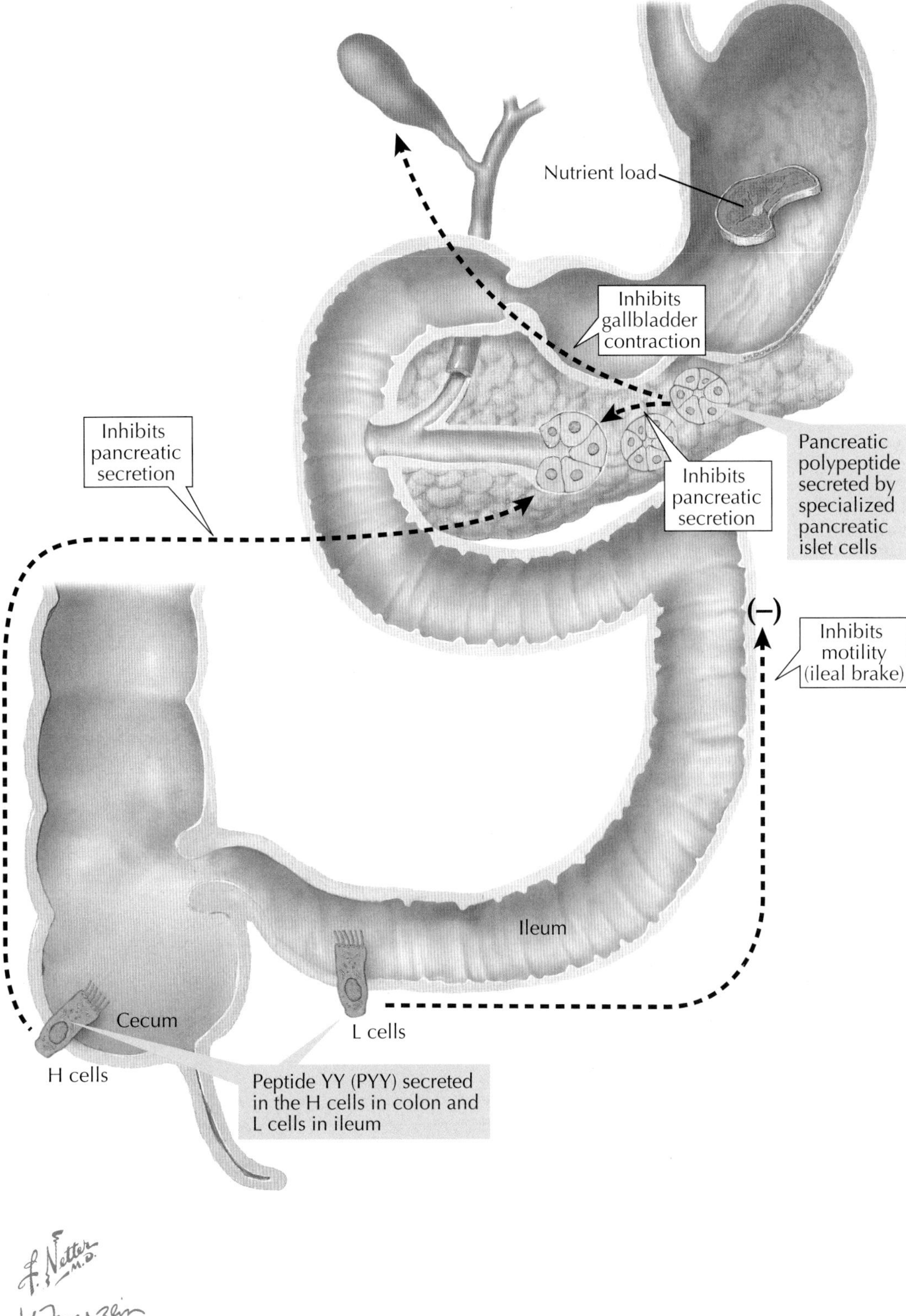


These varied physiologic effects of somatostatin have enabled its use for multiple diagnostic and pharmacologic purposes, and the development of synthetic long-acting analogs has circumvented the very short half-life of the native compound. The presence of abundant somatostatin receptors in several endocrine tumors has made it possible to use radiolabeled somatostatin analogs, such as octreotide, to localize even small tumors throughout the body. The effect on reducing splanchnic blood flow and portal venous pressure has led to somatostatin analogs being used in variceal bleeding and other forms of GI bleeding. The inhibitory effect on hormonal secretion and cell proliferation on many endocrine cells render somatostatin a logical candidate for the management of neuroendocrine tumors that express somatostatin receptors, including acromegaly, carcinoid tumors, and islet cell tumors (including gastrinomas). Somatostatin analogs can also be useful as an antidiarrheal in certain high-output states as well as for closing pancreatic fistulas. Long-term use of these agents can lead to certain side effects, particularly cholelithiasis and impaired glucose tolerance, and patients need to be monitored closely.

# Pathophysiology of Small Intestine

The most important functions of the small intestine are digestion and absorption of nutrients. These are achieved by an interaction between a healthy small bowel motility and GI hormones. Clinically recognizable disturbances of small bowel function arise mainly from alterations in the motor activities and/or interference with digestion and absorption.

## ABDOMINAL PAIN

Abdominal pain is a common manifestation of several processes involving the small intestine. The pain is often located in the midabdomen (periumbilical region) but can also be diffuse across the abdomen. Progressive small bowel distension with or without obstruction causes colicky pain in the early stages, which later becomes constant. Bacteria such as *Yersinia* and *Salmonella* or Crohn's disease (CD) have an affinity to the terminal ileum, causing enteritis that manifests with severe pain and tenderness in the right lower quadrant, often mimicking acute appendicitis. Severe postprandial pain that incites fear of eating *(sitophobia)* is suggestive of mesenteric ischemia, especially when it is accompanied by weight loss in a patient with atherosclerosis. Luminal small bowel lesions can cause episodic periumbilical abdominal pain due to intermittent intussusception or persistent, unrelenting pain with luminal blockage and local advancement by a malignant mass.

## NAUSEA AND VOMITING

Distension or irritation of the small bowel tends to provoke nausea and vomiting. Because the second portion of the duodenum is most sensitive in this respect, it has been termed the "organ of nausea." Small intestinal obstruction from any source invariably causes vomiting. Luminal examples include blockage by tumors, intussusception, or strictures from CD. Extrinsic processes such as adhesions as a result of radiation, strangulation by an internal hernia, or impingement by vascular structures as in SMA syndrome all present with varying degrees of vomiting. Enteric infections with viruses such as norovirus or bacteria such as *Staphylococcus aureus* often cause vomiting by elaborating enterotoxins that cause visceral irritation and induction of ileus.

## DIARRHEA

Acute profuse watery diarrhea is often infectious in etiology and resolves within 2 to 4 weeks. Chronic diarrhea that lasts more than 4 weeks has a broad differential diagnosis and includes secretory causes such as ingestion of drugs or toxins, neuroendocrine tumors, and bile acid malabsorption (choleric diarrhea). Diarrhea accompanied by weight loss is common in bowel resection or mucosal diseases such as inflammatory bowel disease (Crohn's ileitis), celiac disease (gluten-sensitive enteropathy), and primary intestinal lymphangiectasia. Infectious diseases can also directly target the small bowel, as in Whipple disease, *Mycobacterium avium-intracellulare* infection, and giardiasis.

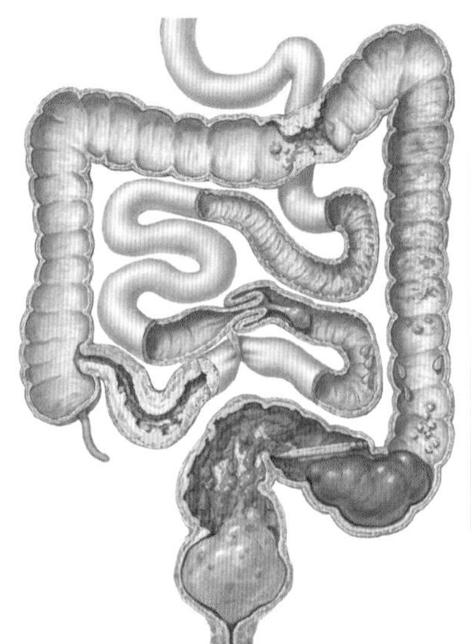

**Diarrhea**

| Infectious | Mechanical |
|---|---|
| Giardiasis | Small bowel tumors |
| Whipple disease | Intussusception |
| Bacterial enteritis | Adhesions |
| Viral enteritis | Hernias |
| Tropical sprue | Metastatic disease |
| Tuberculosis | |
| **Malabsorptive** | **Miscellaneous** |
| Celiac disease | Eosinophilic gastroenteritis |
| Carbohydrate malabsorption | Small intestinal bacterial overgrowth |
| Lactose malabsorption | Crohn's enteritis |
| Lymphangiectasia | Ischemia |
| | Connective tissue disease |

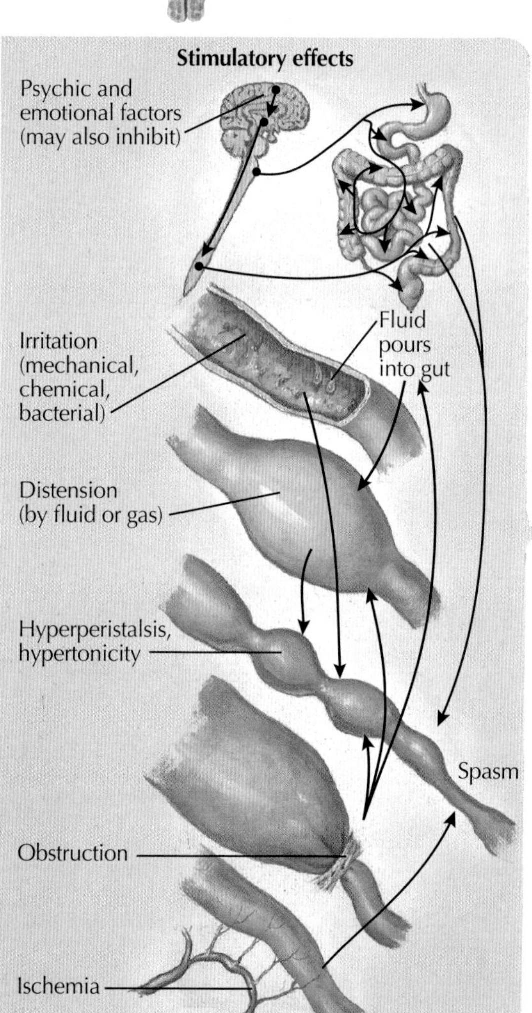


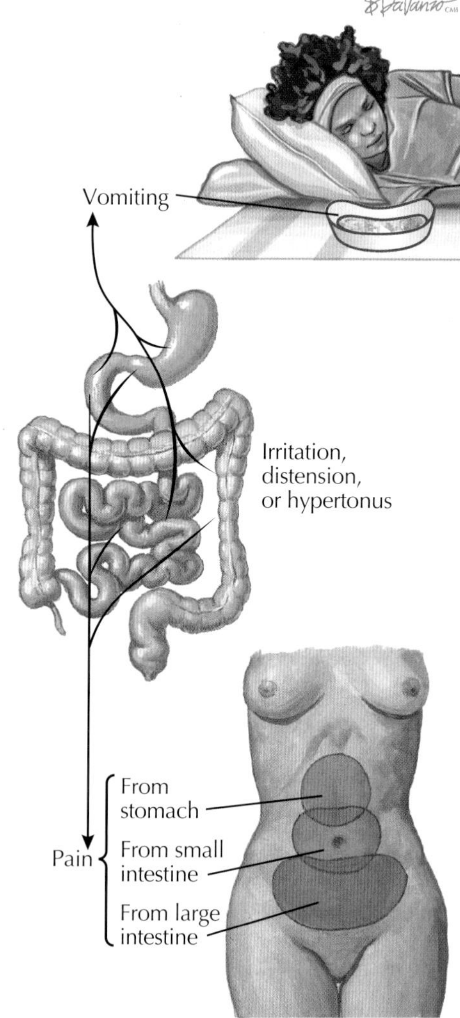


## DYSMOTILITY

Disordered small bowel motility, or *dysmotility*, can be an inherited defect as part of a familial visceral myopathy or neuropathy. It can also be caused by systemic disease or infection, or it can be a paraneoplastic syndrome. In some cases, no etiology is evident, and the process is deemed idiopathic. Mild forms of intestinal dysmotility may be asymptomatic. Symptomatic disease can range from mild discomfort to chronic intestinal pseudoobstruction.

## BLOATING

Bloating is a ubiquitous complaint that can indicate pathologies in the upper and lower GI as well as pancreatic and even pelvic diseases. It is described as a sensation of abdominal fullness with or without obvious abdominal distension. Small bowel pathologies often lead to bloating by excessive gas accumulation in the intestine. Carbohydrate malabsorption, particularly that of lactose, is a common cause as well as small intestinal bacterial overgrowth. Many patients with bloating, however, often have no clearly identifiable abnormality.

## Tests for Small Bowel Function

### TESTS OF INTESTINAL MOTILITY

*Small bowel manometry,* also called *antroduodenal manometry,* is a procedure that assesses small bowel motility. It involves placing a long tube with pressure sensors into the small intestine past the stomach. These sensors are able to measure intraluminal pressure induced by smooth muscle contractions. The test generally takes 6 hours, with the patient fasting during the first 4 hours; the patient then eats a standard meal, and a postprandial recording is made during the next 2 hours.

The *wireless motility capsule system* or *SmartPill Motility Monitoring system* is a useful diagnostic tool that can be used to assess gut transit time. The system consists of a wireless ingestible motility capsule that the patient swallows and a portable data receiver that is worn by the patient for acquiring and transmitting data, which is then downloaded and analyzed. It senses pH, temperature, and pressure, and the data can be reviewed in real time or after study completion. The small bowel transit time is the time interval between capsule entry into the duodenum and its entry into the cecum. Delayed small intestinal transit is determined when transit times exceed 6 hours (normal range 2–6 hours), based on 95% cutoff values from control studies.

*Small bowel scintigraphy* provides valuable physiologic and quantitative information and allows the assessment of the orocecal transit time. The test involves ingestion of either a liquid or solid material labeled with indium-111 or technetium-99m after which sequential scans are obtained over several hours. The small bowel transit time can be calculated as the time for 10% or 50% of the activity to arrive at the terminal ileum or cecum after correcting for gastric emptying. A hepatobiliary iminodiacetic acid (HIDA) scan, which is a test used to evaluate the biliary system, can give a more specific measure of duodenocecal transit time by avoiding the influence of gastric emptying. This can be calculated using a technetium-99m HIDA IV tracer, which is taken up by the liver and excreted in the bile directly into the duodenum. However, there is limited published information regarding this technique.

### TESTS OF ABSORPTION

Nutrient absorption occurs primarily in the small intestine, and, consequently, disorders of the small intestine commonly cause malabsorption. The gold standard test of fat malabsorption (steatorrhea) is the quantitative 72-hour fecal fat determination, which requires stool collection for 3 to 5 days while the patient consumes a high-fat diet (usually 100 g/day). Stool fat analysis is performed via the traditional van de Kamer method. An alternative, less cumbersome method, near-infrared reflectance analysis, exists but is not widely available. The latter has excellent correlation with the van de Kamer method and allows for simultaneous measurement of fecal fat, nitrogen, and carbohydrates in a single sample. Daily fecal fat excretion in healthy individuals is usually less than 6 g/day, but values up to 14 g/day can be seen with diarrhea. Qualitative tests that can be performed on a spot sample of stool are also available and include the Sudan III stain test and the acid steatocrit test. If properly performed, these tests can detect more than 90% of patients with clinically significant steatorrhea; however, they have not replaced the 72-hour stool collection.

Carbohydrate absorption can be assessed by a blood test such as the lactose tolerance test, where blood glucose levels are monitored after oral administration of a 50-g test dose of lactose or by breath tests. Breath tests are based on the fact that unabsorbed carbohydrates reaching the colon are fermented by the colonic microflora, leading to an increase in gases, specifically hydrogen, carbon dioxide, and methane, that can then be measured in the breath. Specific forms of carbohydrate malabsorption (e.g., lactose, fructose, sucrose, sorbitol, and others) can be diagnosed with these tests. The D-xylose test is a measure of the absorptive capacity of the proximal small bowel. The test is performed by measuring D-xylose levels in venous blood and urine after oral administration of a 25-g dose of D-xylose. Low blood and urinary levels

Wireless Motility Capsule

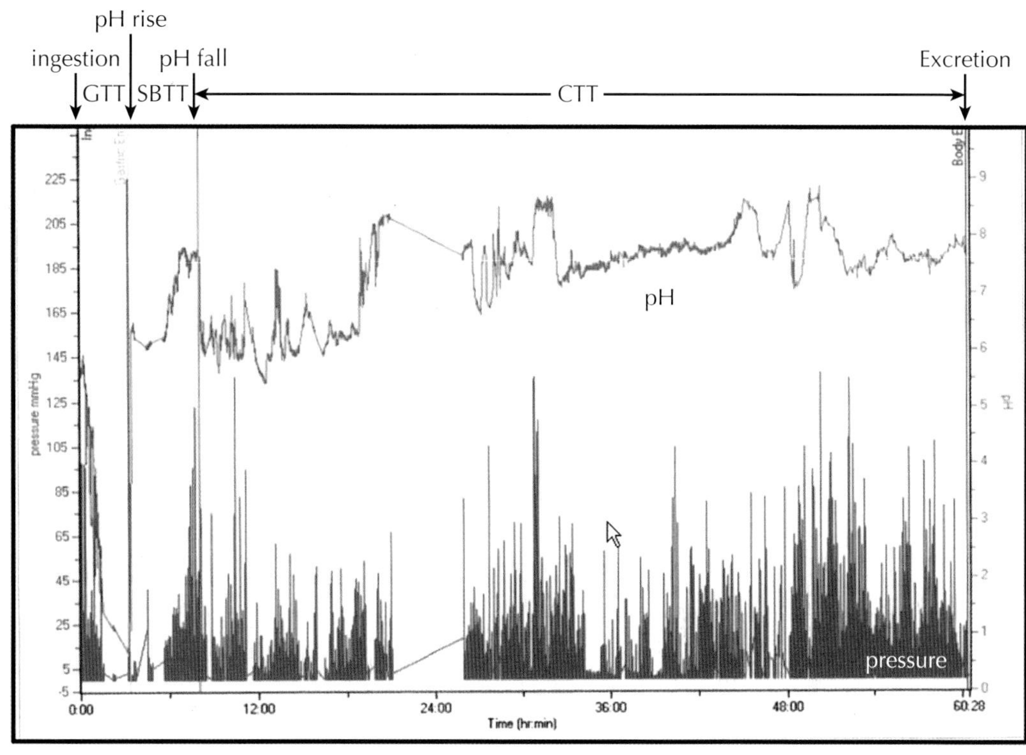


GTT = gastric transit time; SBTT = small bowel transit time; CTT = colonic transit time; WGTT = whole gut transit time.

**Barium small bowel series**

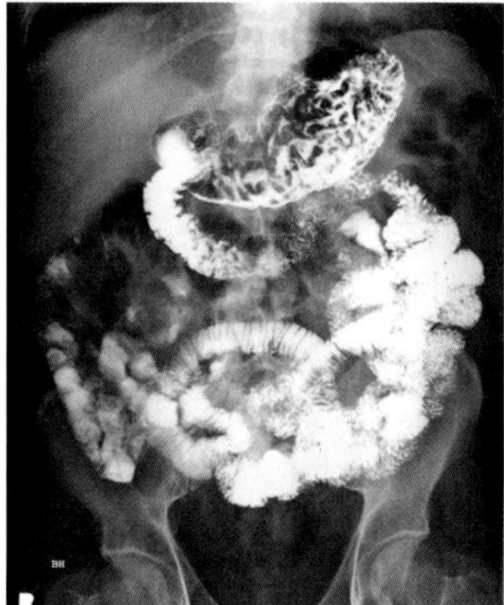


Normal small bowel series

**CT enterography**

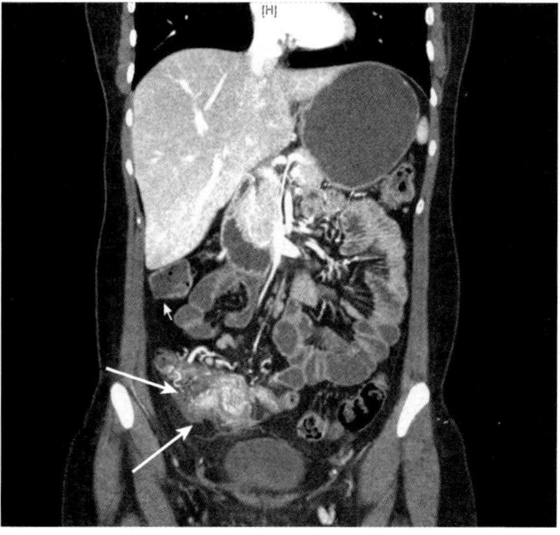

Mucosal enhancement and wall thickening with surrounding inflammatory changes and tethering involving the terminal ileum and cecum consistent with acute Crohn's disease flare

# Tests for Small Bowel Function (Continued)

suggest mucosal malabsorptive disease such as celiac disease. However exocrine pancreatic insufficiency would show normal levels because pancreatic enzymes are not required for the absorption of D-xylose.

The classic test for quantifying protein malabsorption is the measurement of fecal nitrogen content in a quantitatively collected stool specimen. However, this is rarely used. Enteral protein loss can be established by determining the clearance of alpha-1 antitrypsin from plasma. Alpha-1 antitrypsin is a protein synthesized in the liver and has a molecular weight similar to that of albumin. It is neither actively secreted nor absorbed in the intestine and resists proteolysis; therefore it is excreted in the stool while still intact. A blood sample and a 24-hour stool collection are required to measure alpha-1 antitrypsin clearance. The presence of an elevated alpha-1 antitrypsin level above the normal values is diagnostic. Test limitations include the presence of diarrhea, which can interfere with the test, and the inability to distinguish between a gastric and an intestinal source of the protein. If the former is suspected, then the test should be performed while the patient is receiving antisecretory therapy.

## Capsule Endoscopy

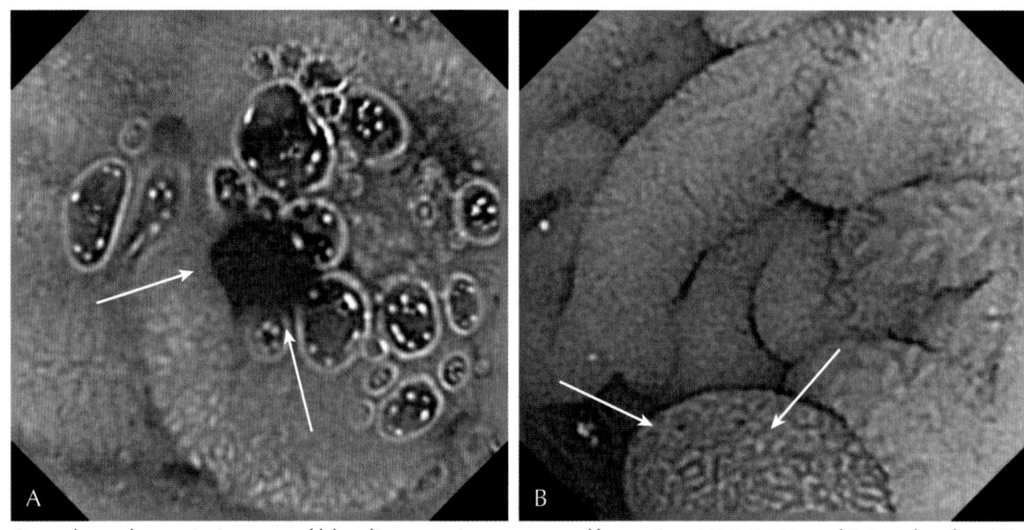

Capsule endoscopic images of bleeding arteriovenous malformation (AVM) **(A)** and jejunal polyp **(B)**.

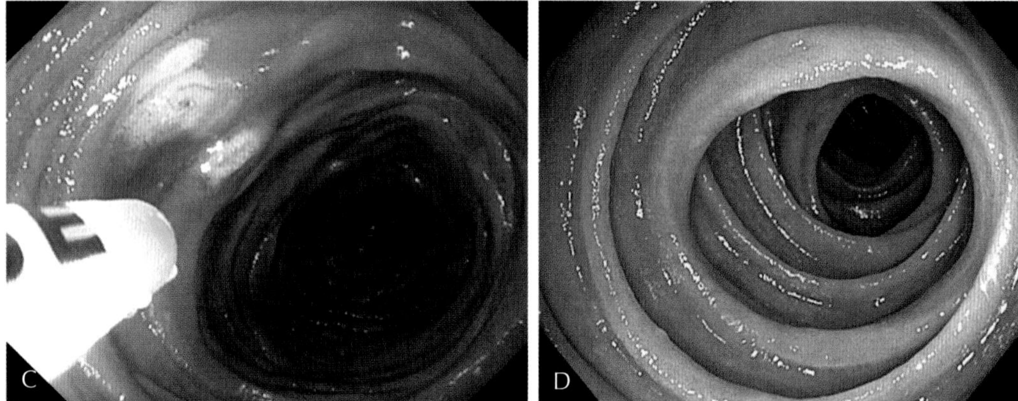

Enteroscopic images of postablation of a bleeding AVM **(C)** and normal jejunum **(D)**.

### RADIOLOGIC TESTS

Plain abdominal radiography is usually the first-line imaging study obtained when intestinal obstruction is suspected. Typical findings include dilated bowel loops with or without air-fluid levels. Thickened small bowel walls can sometimes be demonstrated on plain radiographs although contrast is usually necessary to enhance the luminal processes. Barium examination of the small bowel allows good mucosal detail and can provide useful information on luminal irregularities or narrowing as seen in CD. Small intestinal diverticula, fistulae, and mural or intraluminal filling defects can also be visualized with these studies. Small bowel barium studies can be performed via two methods. In a *small bowel follow-through,* the patient drinks a barium suspension and films are taken every 20 to 30 minutes until the barium reaches the terminal ileum. A *small bowel enteroclysis* requires nasojejunal intubation with a 10-Fr catheter and infusion of barium suspension to achieve optimal small bowel distension. Spot films of the small bowel with compression views to separate small bowel loops and visualize the terminal ileum are taken. Conventional computed tomography (CT) scans of the abdomen and pelvis lack the mucosal detail of small bowel barium studies but can identify small bowel wall thickening and associated extraluminal diseases such as fat wrapping, fistulae, abscess formation, lymphadenopathy, or local and metastatic tumor spread from small bowel neoplasms. CT enterography and CT enteroclysis permit viewing of enhanced bowel wall and mucosal abnormalities and combine luminal imaging with an examination of extraintestinal space. These tests use large volumes (1500–2000 mL) of enteral contrasts. A positive enteral contrast agent can be used without an IV contrast agent, or a neutral enteral contrast agent can be used with an IV contrast agent. Limitations of CT enterography include the the high volume of enteral contrast material that is not tolerated by all patients and the high radiation dose involved. Magnetic resonance imaging (MRI) offers excellent soft tissue resolution with no ionizing radiation, making it a very attractive choice for imaging the small bowel, especially in inflammatory bowel disease. Similar to other enterographic studies, adequate bowel distension can be achieved with oral administration of the contrast or via infusion of the contrast through a nasojejunal tube (enteroclysis).

### ENDOSCOPIC TESTS

*Esophagogastroduodenoscopy* (EGD) is the first-line endoscopic procedure performed for most upper GI disorders. It involves insertion of a fiberoptic endoscope through the mouth past the esophagus and stomach and into the duodenum. *Push enteroscopy* requires a longer endoscope that can reach the jejunum. *Device-assisted enteroscopy using single-balloon* or *double-balloon enteroscopy* allows for more extensive examination of the small bowel with a potential for therapeutic intervention. A flexible overtube with a balloon and a pump controller allows deep advancement of the endoscope by using a push-and-pull method with inflation and deflation of the balloon and telescoping of the intestine onto the overtube. Although these techniques are arduous and time-consuming, examination of the entire small bowel is possible with their use. *Intraoperative enteroscopy* is often necessary in cases of obscure GI bleeding where endoscopic evaluation is performed through enterotomies created during laparotomy. *Video capsule endoscopy* is a safe and noninvasive wireless endoscopic technique that allows examination of the entire small bowel. The procedure usually requires a modified bowel preparation after which the video capsule, measuring approximately 11 by 26 mm, is swallowed with water and obtains approximately 50,000 images over 8 continuous hours, at a rate of 2 to 4 images per second. After ingestion, the capsule travels past the stomach, small bowel, and colon and is eliminated via the stool after 24 to 36 hours or longer depending on the patient's bowel transit. The images are transmitted to and stored within a portable recording device worn by the patient for the 8-hour period. At the end of the procedure, the images are downloaded from the recording device and viewed at a computer workstation, although newer generations of the device do allow real-time viewing. For patients who are not able to swallow the capsule or those with known gastroparesis, the capsule can be deployed directly into the duodenum via an EGD. Video capsule endoscopy is useful for evaluating obscure GI bleeding in adults and can identify small bowel CD or small bowel tumors, and it has been shown to be superior to small bowel follow-through in detecting mucosal lesions. One disadvantage of a video capsule endoscopy is the potential for it to become impacted or lodged, and the test should not be used in individuals with known or suspected stricture to avoid additional endoscopic or surgical procedure to retrieve it.

# Congenital Intestinal Obstruction: Intestinal Atresia, Malrotation of Colon, Volvulus of Midgut

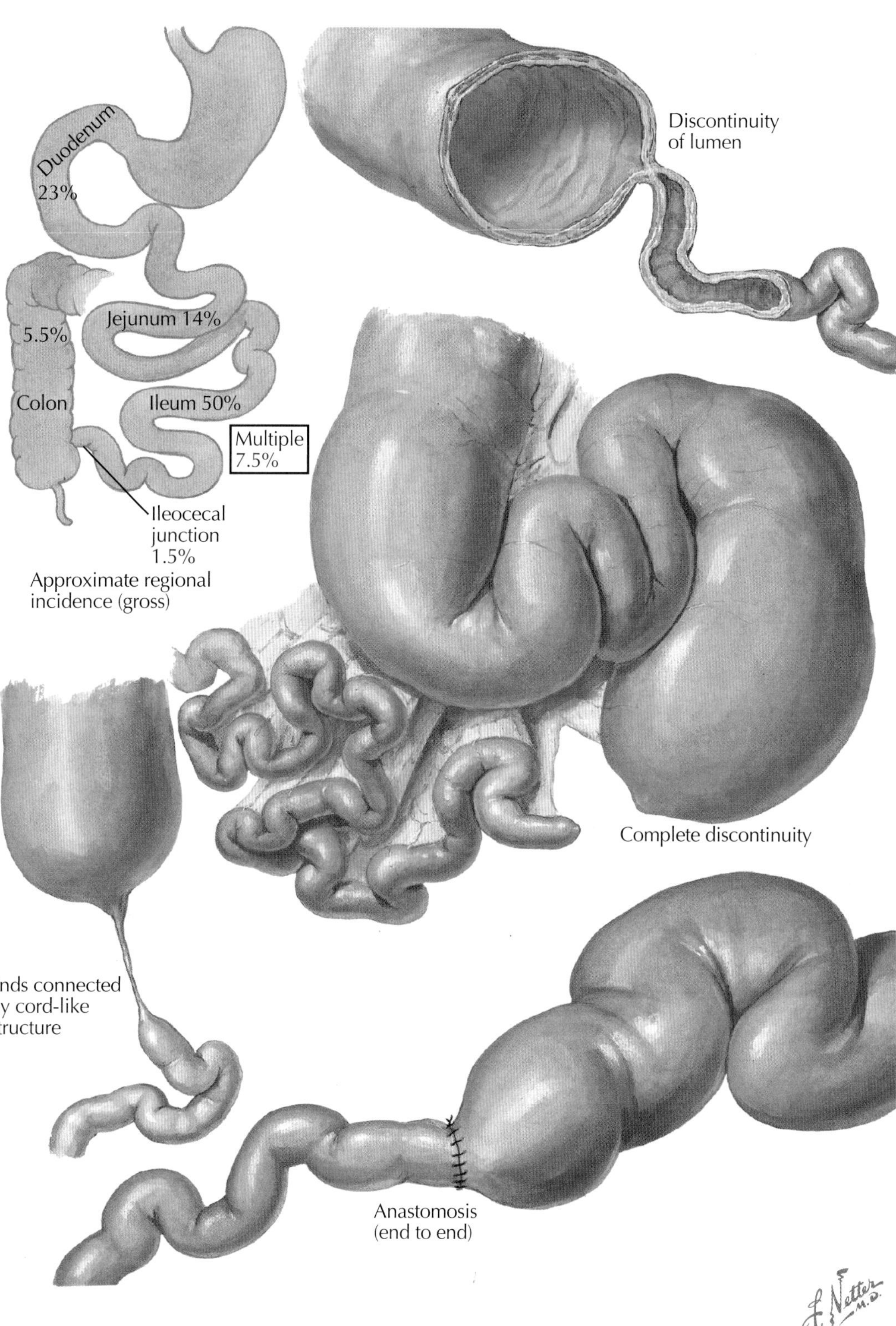


Congenital intestinal obstruction occurs in approximately 1 out of 2000 live births, caused by a variety of congenital anomalies, and prompt diagnosis and treatment can be lifesaving. The causes of such intestinal obstructions include atresia of the esophagus, diaphragmatic hernia, annular pancreas, malrotation of the colon with volvulus of the midgut, peritoneal bands mostly compressing the duodenum, internal or mesentericoparietal herniations, meconium ileus (MI), aganglionic megacolon, imperforate anus, and *atresia* or *congenital stenosis* of the bowel.

*Atresia* refers to the complete congenital obstruction of the lumen of a hollow viscus, whereas *stenosis* refers to luminal narrowing of varying degrees. The most common site of intestinal atresia is the small bowel, particularly the jejunum, with the colon least affected. Intestinal atresia results from an interruption in the normal development of the GI tract, usually during the second and third months of fetal life. In the proximal small bowel, this is often caused by failure of the intestine to recanalize. As the intestine changes from a solid structure to a hollow tube, one or more septa may persist, leaving a diaphragm of tissue with only a minute opening as stenosis. In the middle and distal small bowel, atresia often results from vascular disruption, leading to ischemic necrosis of the fetal intestine. Because the fetal bowel is sterile, the necrotic tissue is resorbed, leaving blind proximal and distal ends, often with a gap in the mesentery.

Intestinal atresia can be classified into four types based on the anatomic arrangement. In type 1, there is occlusion of the lumen by a diaphragm composed of mucosa and submucosa with an otherwise intact bowel wall and mesentery and no discontinuity. In type 2, the proximal and distal atretic segments are connected by a short band with bowel (but not mesentery) discontinuity evident. In type 3, there is complete discontinuity of the bowel and mesentery, whereas type 4 can have multiple atretic segments with a combination of types 2 and 3.

The diagnosis of intestinal atresia or stenosis can be made with prenatal ultrasonography (US). Findings that suggest intestinal atresia on US include bowel dilation or ascites. Prenatal diagnosis allows the infant to get prompt treatment shortly after birth, thus avoiding the complications associated with intestinal obstruction.

Postnatally, the diagnosis of intestinal atresia or stenosis should be suspected in newborns who develop abdominal distension, vomiting, or an abdominal mass with or without obstipation. However, the timing of these signs is variable and depends on the location of the obstruction as well as its nature, whether it is a stenosis or an atresia. Plain abdominal radiographs are indicated in any newborn suspected to have intestinal obstruction. The presence of persisting bile-stained vomitus in the absence of meconium stools for more than 4 hours is often a common initial finding in proximal obstruction. A double-bubble sign on plain radiograph (dilated stomach and proximal duodenum) with no distal gas strongly suggests duodenal atresia. If an enema is indicated, it should be a diagnostic *barium* enema, unless MI is suspected, in which case water-soluble diatrizoate (Gastrografin) should be used. It may be necessary to aspirate air from the stomach because it might distort or obscure the pattern of gas distribution in the small bowel. Alternatively, if gas is absent in a more proximal small bowel obstruction, insufflation of a small (20 mL) volume of gas into the stomach may be necessary. Differentiation between the shadows of the small and large intestines on a radiograph is often difficult in neonates because the circular folds of jejunum and colonic haustrations are often underdeveloped. For this reason, the point of obstruction in an infant is commonly assumed to be lower than it actually is. Total absence of air in the abdomen is indicative of esophageal atresia

# Congenital Intestinal Obstruction: Intestinal Atresia, Malrotation of Colon, Volvulus of Midgut (Continued)

without tracheoesophageal communication. In general, obstructive lesions in the alimentary canal are marked by air distension above and complete absence of air below the point of obstruction.

The management of intestinal atresia is primarily surgical and depends on the location of the obstruction. In all cases, the mandatory principle is to preserve as much of the small intestine as possible. In cases with a long atretic portion, the lack of an adequate absorptive surface can interfere with maintenance of nutrition postoperatively. Preoperative care includes decompression of the proximal segment via the placement of a nasoenteric tube, cessation of feedings, and fluid and electrolyte resuscitation.

Surgery can be performed laparoscopically, but the possibility of multiple atresias should always be entertained and properly evaluated preoperatively. The prognosis of intestinal atresia is very good. Most deaths occur in infants who are premature or have associated anomalies.

*Volvulus* is the term generally used to indicate the torsion and/or coiling of an organ at its attachment, which, in the specific case of the intestines, is the mesentery. It may occur at all ages when, for one reason or another, an intestinal segment becomes longer and the mesentery narrower. In the newborn, *volvulus of the midgut,* which leads to serious intestinal obstruction, is a complication of a *malrotation of the colon.* Normally, around week 10 of fetal life, the ileocecal area rotates in a counterclockwise direction, bringing the cecum into the right lower abdominal quadrant and permitting the mesentery of the ascending colon to be fixed posteriorly and laterally to the parietal peritoneum. Genetic mutations that disrupt signaling result in the arrest of this process. With the mesenteric attachment of duodenojejunal junction and mid transverse colon missing, a long mass of intestine remains suspended between the two points of fixation. Such malrotation can lead to a volvulus producing not only intestinal obstruction but also occlusion of the superior mesenteric vessels. Alternatively, the cecum may be held in this abnormal position in the right upper quadrant by adventitious *peritoneal bands* and be fixed to the liver, parietal peritoneum, or posterior abdominal wall in such a way as to compress the duodenum. Peritoneal bands, not associated with malrotation of the colon, may occasionally cause obstruction of the duodenum and rarely of other parts of the small bowel.

*Volvulus of the midgut* presents with symptoms and signs consistent with intestinal obstruction, including vomiting, abdominal pain, GI bleeding, and shock. The radiographic appearance is consistent with dilated loops proximally and decompressed segments distal to the obstruction. Residual air bubbles, however, may be observed distal to the obstruction due to air that has moved down before the onset of the volvulus. Any patient suspected to have volvulus of the midgut should be rapidly resuscitated and taken to emergent surgery. The volvulus occurs clockwise and should therefore be untwisted counterclockwise, recalling the phrase "turning back the hands of time." Then the Ladd's procedure should be undertaken, which is the standard corrective measure for intestinal malrotation. This procedure consists of division of peritoneal (Ladd's) bands that traverse the posterior abdomen, appendectomy, and functional positioning of the intestine with or without fixation.

*Internal hernia* (paraduodenal or duodenojejunal) may also be responsible for intestinal obstruction in infants. A loop of bowel may become incarcerated, or even strangulated, by entering a congenital defect in the mesentery or by passing between adventitious bands of peritoneum. The herniation is generally diagnosed either by exclusion or on the operating table. The obvious procedure is to reduce any existing hernia and repair the defect or divide any obstructing adventitious bands.

Malrotation of Colon and Volvulus of Midgut

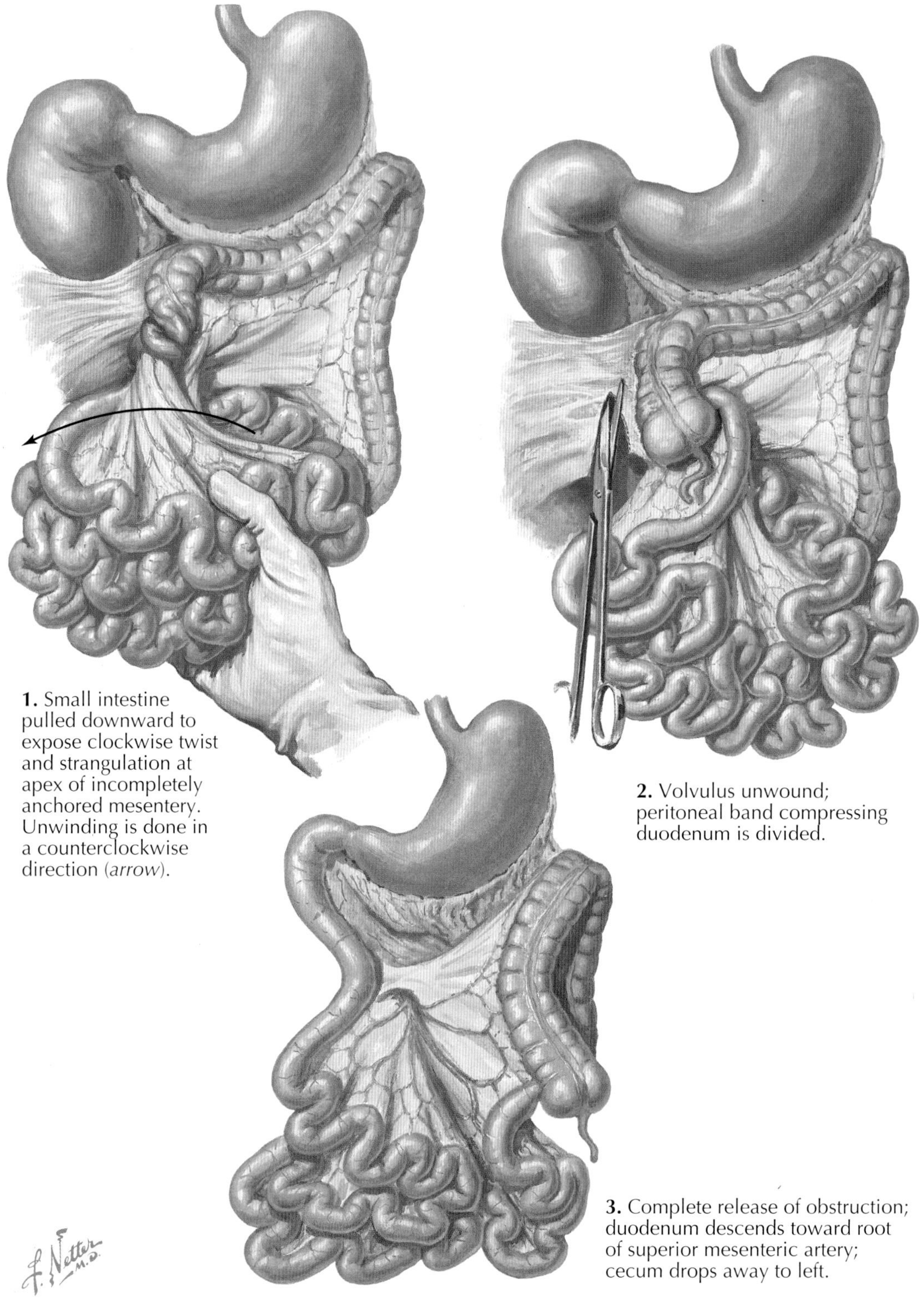

**1.** Small intestine pulled downward to expose clockwise twist and strangulation at apex of incompletely anchored mesentery. Unwinding is done in a counterclockwise direction (*arrow*).

**2.** Volvulus unwound; peritoneal band compressing duodenum is divided.

**3.** Complete release of obstruction; duodenum descends toward root of superior mesenteric artery; cecum drops away to left.

F. Netter M.D.

## Congenital Intestinal Obstruction: Meconium Ileus

*Meconium ileus* (MI) is a condition where thick, inspissated meconium causes impaction of the ileum, leading to intestinal obstruction. It develops almost exclusively in infants born with cystic fibrosis (CF) and has an incidence of 10%. CF is a lethal autosomal recessive disorder caused by mutation of the cystic fibrosis transmembrane conductance regulator (CFTR) protein. CFTR mutation primarily interferes with chloride transport in various acinar structures, including the intestinal, bronchial, and pancreatic glands. Pancreatic damage can occur in utero, and two-thirds of affected infants have severe pancreatic insufficiency at birth.

Meconium is the newborn's feces made up of cells and intestinal secretions that normally passes in the first few hours and days after birth. In patients with CF, the meconium becomes thick and tenacious, adhering to the intestinal mucosa. Progressively, it can cause complete obstruction, with an empty, collapsed segment distally and a dilated segment proximally. The *ileum frequently resembles a strand of beads,* as the bowel wall conforms to the contour of the *aggregations of meconium,* which is gray in color and of a dried, putty-like consistency. Just proximal to the occlusion, the *bowel is slightly larger* in caliber, and the meconium sticking to the wall is less firm and more greenish but still viscous enough to prevent peristaltic propulsion.

MI is classified into two forms (simple MI and complex MI) based on the presence of complications. MI is considered simple if there is no associated complication and complex if complicated by perforation, peritonitis, atresia, or volvulus. Typical radiographic findings in MI are described as varying degrees of proximal bowel distension, ranging from loops that appear smaller than normal to some that are enormously ballooned. This is in marked contrast to intestinal obstruction from atresia, stenosis, or aganglionic megacolon, where the whole segment proximal to the obstruction is distended to the same extent. The inspissated meconium is seen on radiography as a radiopaque mass, with a mottled appearance due to air bubbles that have been forced into it. It is important to remember, however, that inspissated meconium may also be visualized in aganglionic megacolon (see Plate 3.30) and that both conditions, MI and aganglionic megacolon, may exist without any evidence of fecal shadows on radiographic examination. Flecks of calcium, either scattered throughout the abdomen or attached to the bowel wall, are an ominous sign, suggesting *meconium peritonitis* caused by rupture of the intestine in utero.

The management of MI depends on the degree of obstruction and the presence of complications. Patients with simple MI can be treated nonoperatively by methods that help disimpact the inspissated mucus. In this approach, hyperosmolar enema using a water-soluble contrast such as diatrizoate (Gastrografin), or *N*-acetylcysteine (Mucomyst) can be infused transanally via a catheter into the dilated portion of the ileum. This procedure should be performed by an experienced team, and the use of fluoroscopy is recommended. These agents help dissolve the impacted meconium by pulling fluid from the bowel wall into the intestinal lumen; therefore these infants are at risk of fluid and electrolyte abnormalities, and expectant and adequate resuscitation is mandatory. This approach is successful in up to 40% of cases and can be followed for several days provided no complications occur. In those who do not respond to conservative therapy or with complex MI, surgical intervention should be performed. Operative irrigation can be attempted using the same agents delivered through a purse-string suture. Alternatively, the distended terminal ileum should be resected with the meconium pellets flushed from the distal small bowel. An end ileostomy is created, with the distal bowel brought up as a mucous fistula or sewn to the side of the ileum. Reanastomosis can be carried out at a later time after appropriate deflation of the dilated proximal bowel and institution of pancreatic enzyme replacement therapy. *Distal intestinal obstructive syndrome* (DIOS) is a similar phenomenon that occurs later in life and is more commonly seen in patients with CF who have a history of MI as an infant.

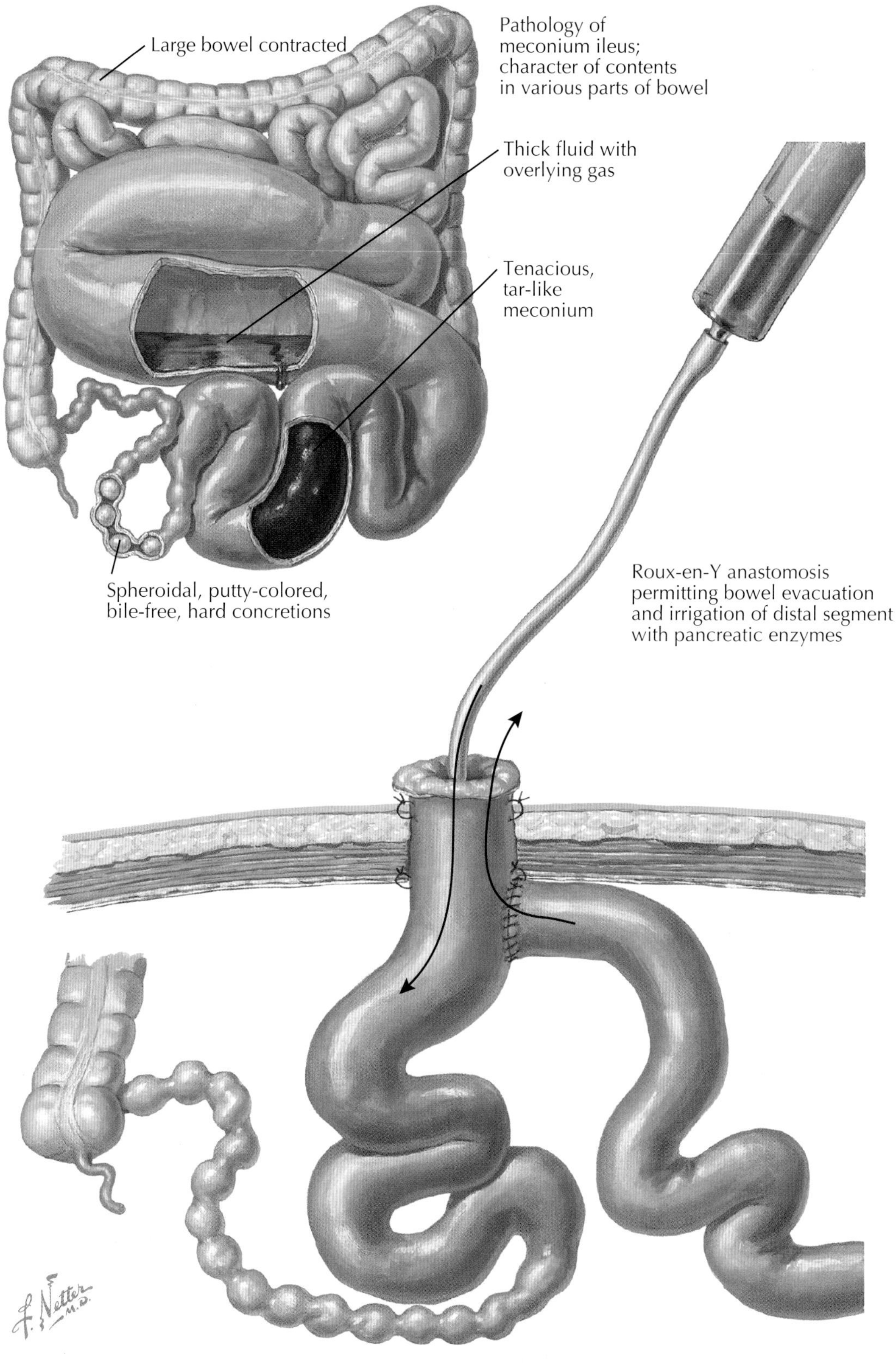

Sites of Diaphragmatic Hernias and Herniation of Abdominal Viscera

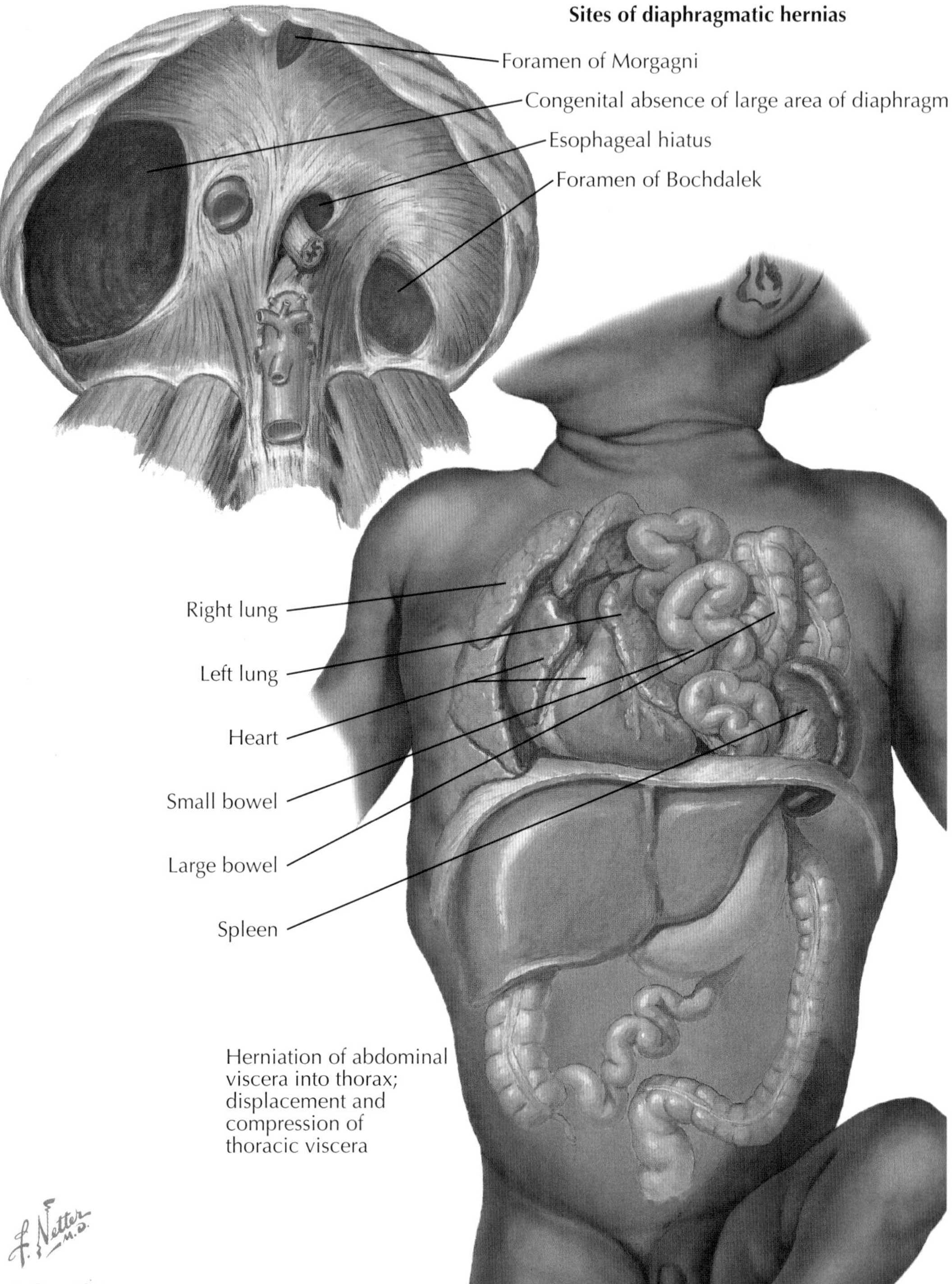


## Diaphragmatic Hernia

Congenital diaphragmatic hernia is a developmental birth defect resulting in discontinuity of the diaphragm that allows herniation of abdominal viscera into the thoracic cavity. It is present in 1 in 3000 live births and has the potential for high neonatal morbidity and mortality.

The most usual site of a congenital diaphragmatic hernia is the foramen of Bochdalek in the posterolateral portion. Herniation most often occurs in the left side and usually involves the stomach and the bowels. Right-sided hernias are rare and may contain the liver. Less common hernias occur at the esophageal hiatus and at the foramen of Morgagni in the retrosternal portion of the diaphragm. Herniation through these latter defects usually does not produce severe respiratory distress. *Diaphragmatic eventration* must be distinguished from diaphragmatic herniation. The former refers to elevation of a portion of the diaphragm that is thin and membranous due to incomplete muscularization. The diaphragm in this case forms a sac that covers abdominal contents displaced into the thorax. In rare cases, the diaphragm may completely or partially fail to develop *(diaphragmatic* or *hemidiaphragmatic agenesis).* Failure of normal closure of the pleuroperitoneal folds during the 4th to 10th weeks after fertilization appears to be the initial step in formation of these hernias. Genetic or environmental factors are believed to trigger disruption of mesenchymal cell differentiation during formation of the diaphragm. However, clear understanding of the etiology remains unclear.

Most cases of congenital diaphragmatic hernia are diagnosed prenatally on routine US screening at approximately 24 weeks of gestation. Visualization of a chest mass with or without mediastinal shift is suggestive of a diaphragmatic hernia. Fetal MRI can confirm the finding and estimate lung volumes as well as identify associated anomalies, which frequently occur with diaphragmatic hernias and fetal echocardiogram, and genetic studies should concurrently be performed. In utero therapy is investigational at this time and involves fetal tracheal occlusion, which averts pulmonary hypoplasia and pulmonary hypertension by increasing transpulmonic pressure. The birth should take place at a tertiary care center via vaginal delivery induced at term.

Although routine prenatal US examination can identify most congenital diaphragmatic hernias, the diagnosis may not be made until after delivery. The characteristic signs include a barrel-shaped chest with a left-sided respiratory lag (if the hernia is on the left, as it is in most instances) and a small and frequently scaphoid abdomen. The heart is displaced to the right, often to an extreme degree. Breathing sounds are absent over the left chest and are heard only over the upper right thorax portion, where they are harsh in character. Gas fills the herniated bowel usually only later, so that the percussion sounds over the chest are not necessarily tympanitic directly after birth. Auscultatory findings, suggestive of peristaltic movements in the chest, may be present but are not reliable. Some

THORACIC APPROACH TO REPAIR OF DIAPHRAGMATIC HERNIA

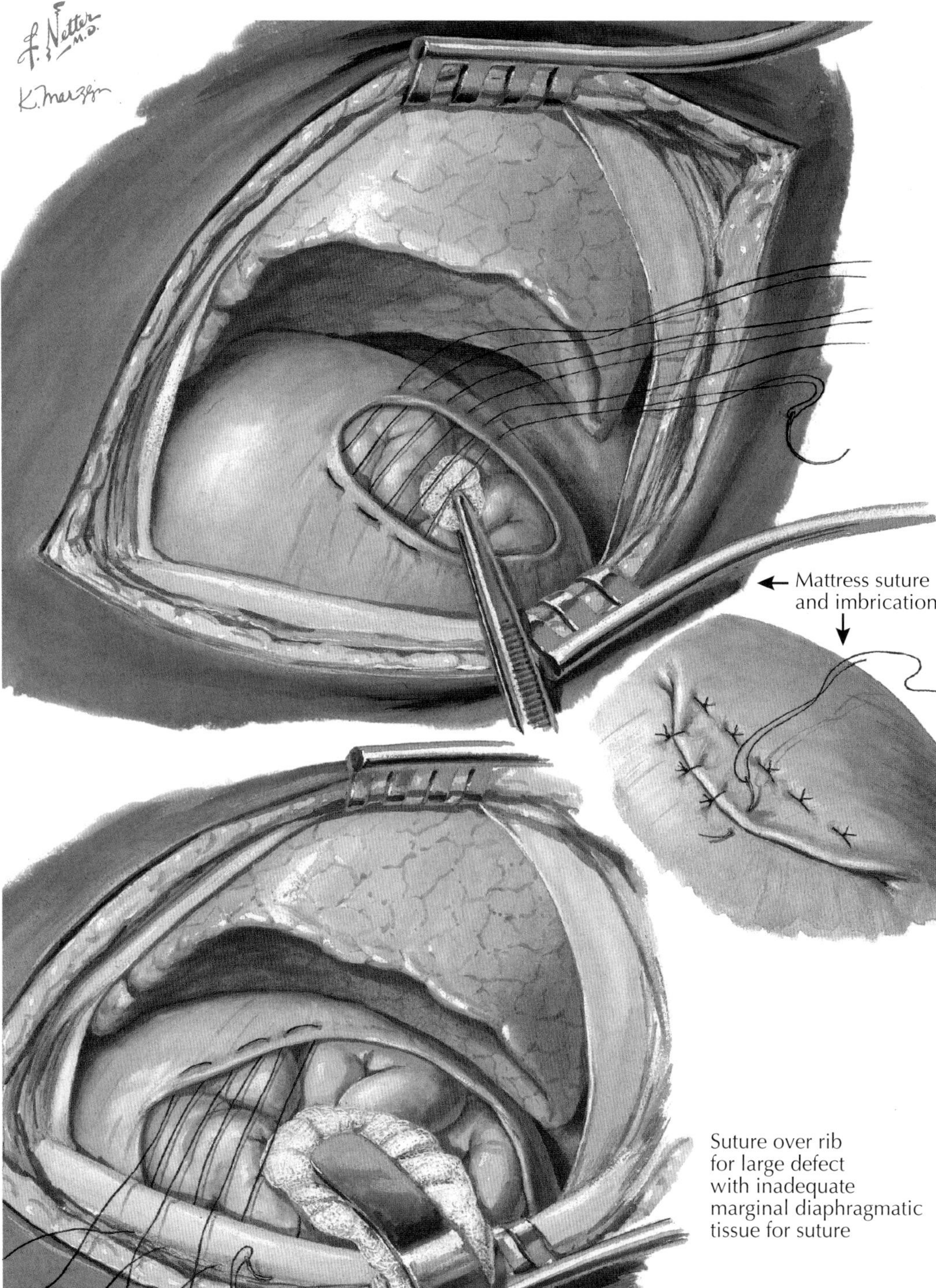


## DIAPHRAGMATIC HERNIA (Continued)

infants, able to compensate for the presence of abdominal viscera in the chest, exhibit signs and symptoms only when the gas-filled intestines cause a greater mediastinal shift. Although the diagnosis can be made on physical findings alone, chest radiograph confirms the clinical impression, except when the severity of the infant's respiratory distress does not allow time for such a procedure.

Once the diagnosis of a diaphragmatic hernia is made, treatment encompasses preoperative medical management followed by surgical repair. Aggressive preoperative medical management has improved survival rates to well over 90% and involves ventilatory support after immediate endotracheal intubation. Use of extracorporeal membrane oxygenation should be employed for infants who do not respond to conventional ventilatory support. Echocardiography is performed to evaluate pulmonary hypertension and identify underlying cardiac anomalies. The circulatory system is maintained by administration of fluids and inotropic agents. To avoid additional distension of the abdominal viscera, nasogastric tube placement before anesthesia is recommended. Premature infants with respiratory distress syndrome should receive surfactant therapy.

In the past, surgical repair of these types of hernias was considered an emergency and infants underwent surgery shortly after birth. It is now accepted that emergent surgery is not necessary, and the timing of surgery has shifted to delaying surgical repair until the patient has been stabilized. Infants requiring minimal support with no evidence of pulmonary compromise can undergo surgical repair within 72 hours. In infants with some degree of pulmonary hypoplasia and reversible pulmonary hypertension, surgery should be delayed until pulmonary compliance improves and pulmonary hypertension is reversed.

Surgical repair of the diaphragmatic hernia can be performed via an abdominal or a transthoracic approach using either open or minimally invasive techniques.

The repair of the diaphragmatic defect may be accomplished by primary closure; however, larger defects often need a synthetic patch repair to allow a tension-free closure. The abdominal cavity may also be too small and underdeveloped to accommodate the intestine and permit closure of the abdominal wall muscle and fascial layers. In such cases, a temporary abdominal wall silo or mobilization of abdominal wall skin flaps may be necessary to allow for gradual visceral reduction and concomitant abdominal cavity expansion, so that a staged closure of the abdominal wall is possible.

Complications after repair can be seen immediately after surgery with persistent pulmonary hypertension or can occur late with chronic respiratory disease, recurrent hernia, patch infection, spinal or chest wall abnormalities, and gastroesophageal reflux.

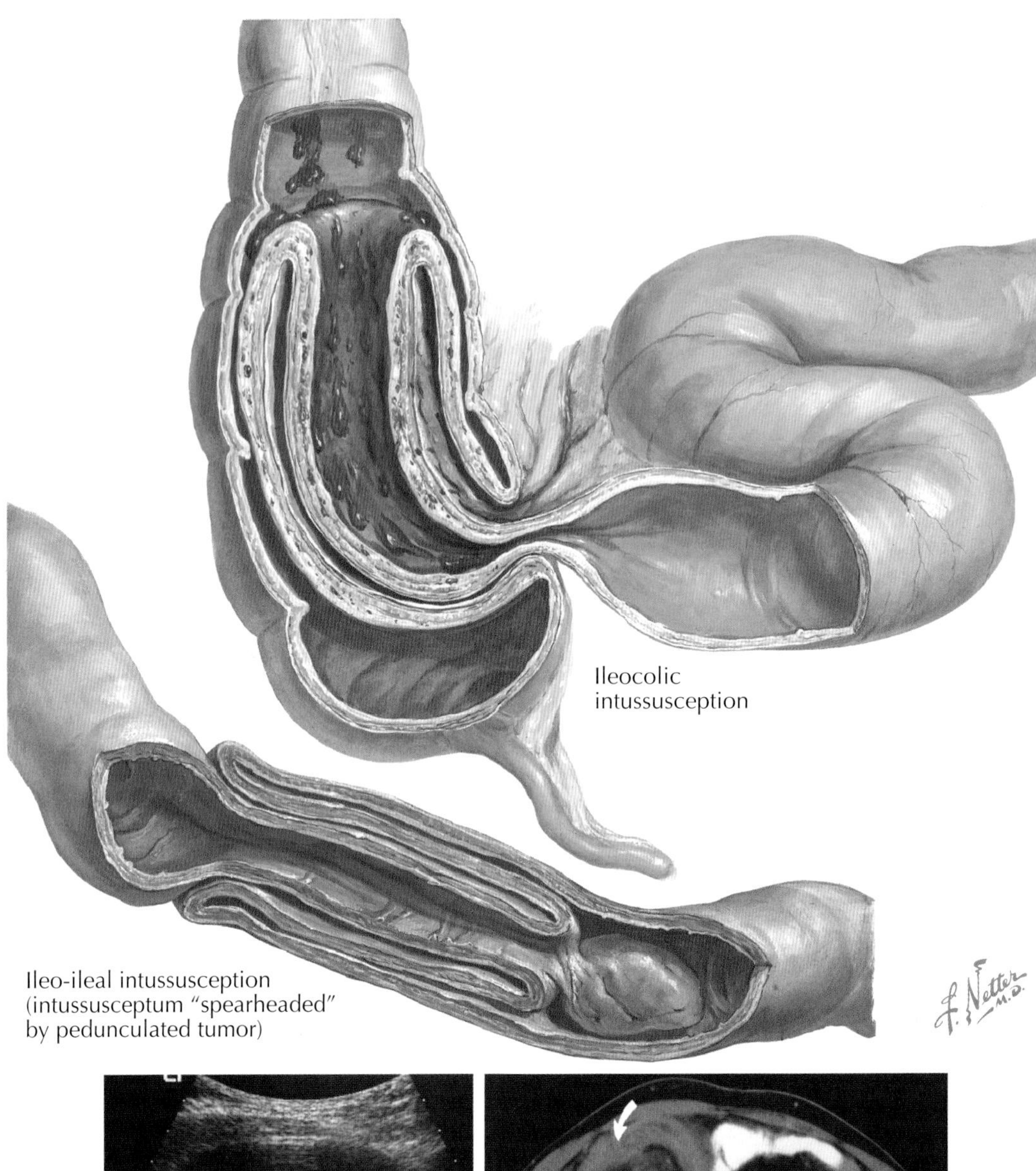


Ileocolic lymphoma leading to ileocolic intussusception. **(A)** Ultrasound image of the right iliac fossa showing the "pseudotumor" or "kidney" sign. The ileum can be seen centrally (*arrow*), surrounded by mesenteric fat that is hyperechoic, all within the thickened ascending colon. **(B)** CT showing oral contrast medium in the ileal lumen, the surrounding mesenteric fat accompanying the intussusceptum, and the thickened ascending colon, which is the intussuscipiens (*arrow*). *(From Grant LA, Griffin, N. Grainger & Allison's Diagnostic Radiology Essentials. Elsevier; 2013.)*

## INTUSSUSCEPTION

Intussusception occurs when a proximal segment of the bowel telescopes into an adjacent distal segment. It is one of the most common abdominal emergencies in children but is rare in adults. Intussusception commonly occurs near the ileocecal junction, where the intussusceptum telescopes into the intussuscipiens, dragging the associated mesentery with it. This leads to the development of venous and lymphatic congestion with resulting intestinal edema, which can ultimately lead to ischemia, perforation, and peritonitis. Rarely, the proximal bowel is drawn into the lumen of the distal bowel *(retrograde intussusception);* this phenomenon is seen in roux-en-Y gastric bypass surgery. The majority of cases in children are idiopathic, although evidence points to a preceding viral infection triggering the intussusception in some of these cases. On the other hand, adults usually have a distinct underlying pathologic lead point, which can be malignant in half of cases. Intermittent abdominal pain is the most common presentation in both children and adults. Symptoms progress over time and are accompanied by nausea and vomiting. In children, a sausage-shaped abdominal mass may be felt in the right side of the abdomen accompanied by the "currant jelly" stool mixed with blood and mucus.

An intussusception is sometimes discovered incidentally during an imaging study performed for other reasons or for nonspecific symptoms. If these intussusceptions are short and if the patient has few symptoms, intervention may not be required.

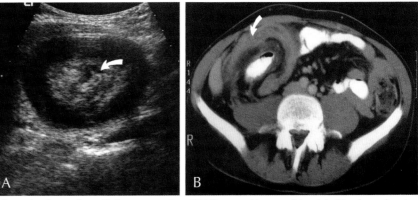

US is the method of choice for detecting intussusception in children and can demonstrate layers within the intestine *(target sign)*. Plain abdominal radiographs are less sensitive and are used to exclude other causes and confirm the presence of small bowel obstruction. In adults, contrast-enhanced CT scanning of the abdomen and pelvis is the investigation of choice and may also reveal a target sign.

The treatment approach differs in pediatric and adult populations. In stable children with no signs of bowel perforation, nonoperative reduction using either hydrostatic or pneumatic enema is preferred to surgery. With this approach, the recurrence rate reaches 10%. In adults, surgical resection of the involved segment is recommended with pathologic evaluation to rule out underlying malignant disease.

## OMPHALOCELE

An *omphalocele,* or *exomphalos,* is a midline abdominal wall defect at the base of the umbilical cord that is covered only by a membrane of amnion and peritoneum; it often contains bowel and occasionally the spleen and liver. When the defect is less than 4 cm, it is termed a *hernia of the umbilical cord,* whereas a defect greater than 5 cm or one containing >75% of the liver is termed a *giant omphalocele.* It results from the persistence of the physiologic midgut herniation beyond the 12th postmenstrual week. Associated abnormalities occur in 30% to 70% of infants and include chromosomal abnormalities (e.g., trisomy 13, 18, 21), congenital heart disease, Beckwith-Wiedemann syndrome, and prune belly syndrome. The diagnosis of an omphalocele can usually be made by inspection, but if the omphalocele is small, it may appear to be a normal part of the umbilical cord. The major differential diagnosis to consider is gastroschisis. *Gastroschisis* is a defect in the abdominal wall that usually occurs to the right of the normal insertion area of the umbilical cord and is believed to arise at the site of involution of the right umbilical vein. The absence of a membranous sac with free-floating loops of bowel distinguishes gastroschisis from omphalocele. In cases with in utero rupture of the membranous sac of the omphalocele, other clues such as the location of the liver and site of the cord insertion should be sought.

When omphalocele is identified prenatally, fetal genetic studies, including amniocentesis and fetal echocardiography, should be offered because of the high risk of aneuploidy and other congenital and genetic disorders. Fetal growth should subsequently be monitored closely. Precluding other obstetric indications, spontaneous labor and delivery should be allowed to occur. However, referral to a tertiary care center is highly recommended.

In the delivery room, neonatal management involves stabilizing the airway and covering the defect with saline-soaked gauze dressings or submerging the entire content in a sterile "bowel bag." Peripheral IV access should be established, and an orogastric tube should be inserted to decompress the stomach. The primary goal of surgery is to return the viscera into the abdominal cavity and close the defect. Small defects (<2 cm) can generally be managed by primary direct closure, whereas medium to large defects require a staged repair or the "paint and wait" approach. The latter has become a more frequently employed strategy for giant omphaloceles. Reepithelialization of the sac is promoted by daily application of a sclerosing solution, commonly silver sulfadiazine cream or povidone iodine solution, over the exposed sac surface with a supportive gauze wrap until cicatrization is completed and delayed closure is achieved.

A staged repair aims to create a protective extraabdominal extension of the peritoneal cavity (termed a *silo*), allowing gradual reduction of the viscera and gradual abdominal wall expansion. This is achieved by using two parallel sheets of reinforced silastic sheeting sutured to the fascial edges or a preformed one-piece silo with a collapsible ring at its base for ease of insertion. A prosthetic patch repair bridges the fascial gap with a synthetic material (e.g., polytetrafluoroethylene), and the skin is closed over the patch. The silo is progressively compressed to invert the amniotic sac. Care is taken not to exceed a pressure of 20 cm of water and to avoid impaired venous return. The contents gradually return into the abdominal cavity, bringing the edges of the linea alba together by stretching the abdominal wall muscles over 5 to 7 days, after which the silo is removed, the amnion is left inverted, and the defect is primarily closed.

Management of an omphalocele may be complicated by rupture of the omphalocele sac either in utero or during delivery. The frequency of multiple congenital anomalies in these infants must also be borne in mind, especially intestinal obstruction caused by anomalies of rotation and fixation of the colon. If intestinal obstruction is suspected based on signs or radiologic findings, then the proper corrective intraabdominal procedure must be undertaken before the closure is completed.

The survival rate for infants with small omphaloceles is excellent (>90%). Infants with large omphaloceles have increased morbidity and mortality related to wound infection, dehiscence, or associated anomalies.

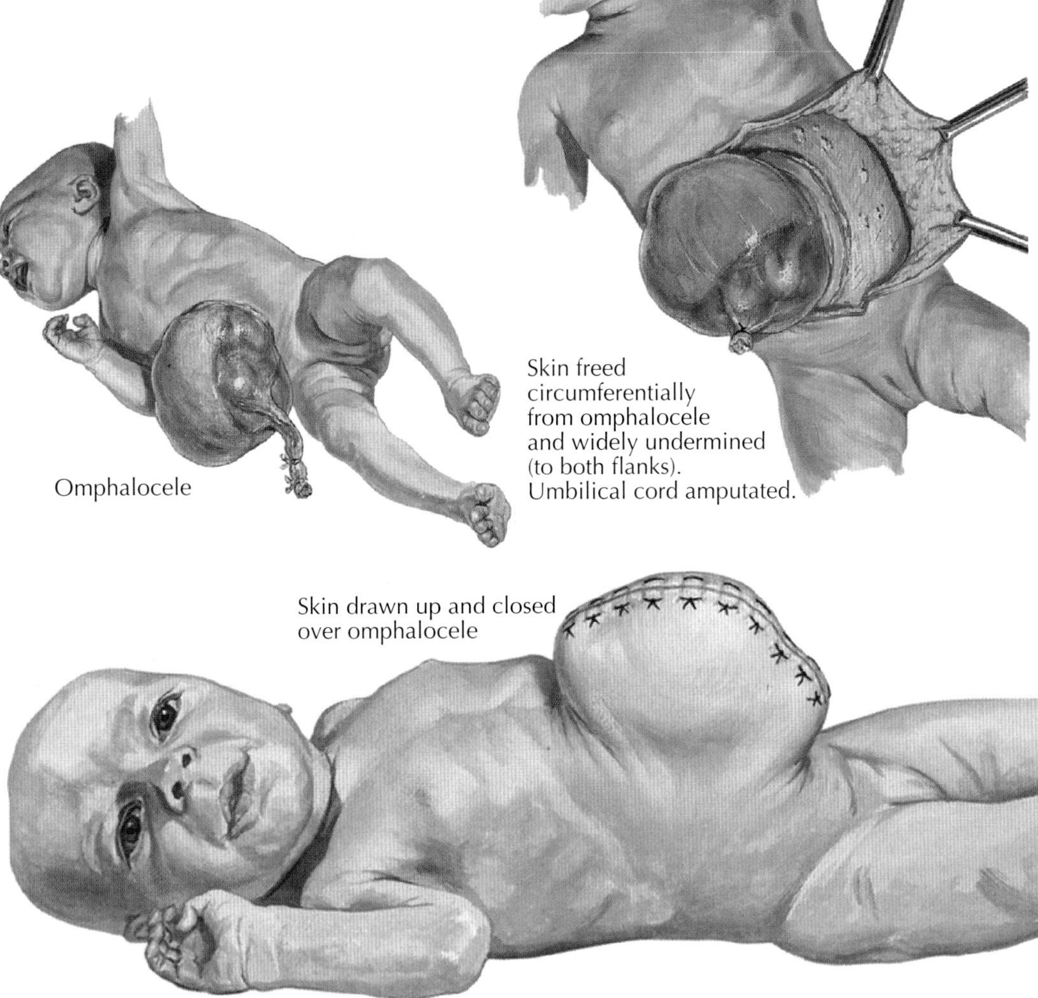

Omphalocele
Skin freed circumferentially from omphalocele and widely undermined (to both flanks). Umbilical cord amputated.
Skin drawn up and closed over omphalocele


Direct closure (small omphalocele)

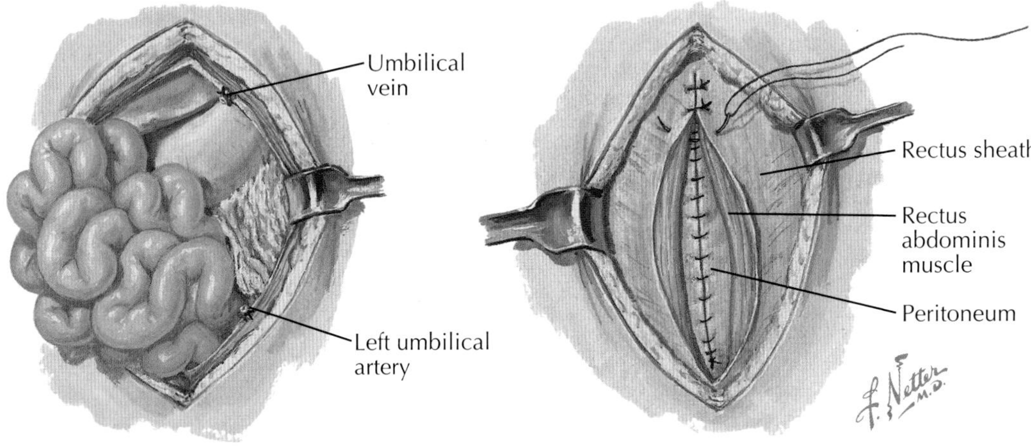


Sac and adjoining rim of skin cut away; umbilical arteries and vein ligated

Layers of abdominal wall dissected out and sutured serially

## Duplications of Alimentary Tract

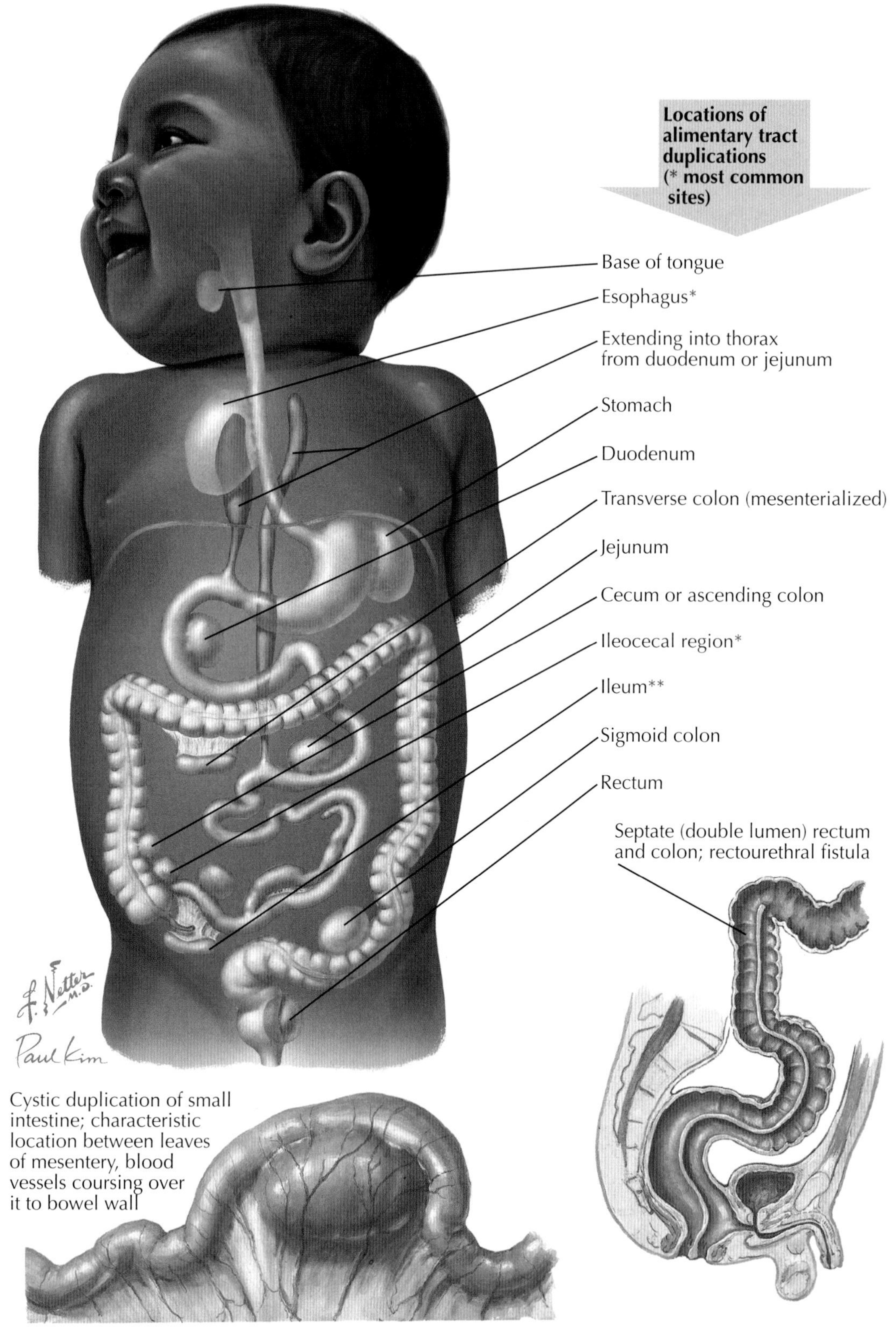

Duplications of the alimentary canal, sometimes referred to as *mesenteric cysts, giant diverticula,* or *enteric cysts,* are rare congenital malformations that develop during fetal life. These spherical or tubular structures may be single or multiple and possess all the layers of that part of the alimentary tract to which they are intimately attached, including the muscular coat. This is in distinction to diverticula, which lack a muscular coat. GI duplication cysts may or may not communicate with the adjacent lumen of the GI tract.

Most intestinal duplications are diagnosed in newborn infants and children, but some remain asymptomatic until adulthood. With the routine use of prenatal US, however, many are being diagnosed in utero. Associated anomalies are present in one-third of cases and involve the spine and GI tract.

They arise from defective embryogenesis, but no unifying explanation exists to describe all possible combinations of duplications, locations, and associated anomalies; however, several theories have been proposed. Failure of recanalization can explain duplications located in the GI tract, which passes through a "solid" stage with temporary occlusion of the lumen around the fifth week of life. Intrauterine vascular accidents can explain duplication cysts associated with atresia. Incomplete twinning can explain duplications of the hindgut associated with genitourinary malformations.

Duplications can occur in all parts of the alimentary canal, from the *tongue* to the *rectum,* with the majority located in the jejunoileal area. Small intestinal duplications are typically located on the mesenteric border and share a blood supply with the adjacent intestine.

The walls of the two structures (i.e., of the intestine and its corresponding duplication) are not sharply separated but have muscular fibers in common; hence it is often difficult to remove the duplicated segment without damaging the blood supply or the wall of the contiguous intestine.

Intestinal duplications may remain asymptomatic, and the diagnosis may be made incidentally by physical examination or during a radiologic or endoscopic procedure. Symptoms, when present, depend on the location and size of the duplication, with dysphagia (esophageal) or abdominal pain and vomiting (intestine) being common presentations. Ectopic gastric mucosa is present in 24% of intestinal duplications, potentially leading to penetrating ulcers and severe GI bleeding. Rarely, these cysts can serve as the lead point to intussusception or get superinfected. In adults, malignant diseases (commonly adenocarcinoma) arising from alimentary tract duplications have been reported and are often advanced at diagnosis.

The diagnosis is confirmed radiologically, with the choice of imaging largely dictated by the site of the duplication, clinical urgency, and the potential for associated anomalies. Abdominal sonography is invaluable for intraabdominal duplications and typically shows a cystic structure situated next to the intestine with a "double wall" sign (a hyperechoic inner layer produced by the mucosa and a relatively hypoechoic outer layer produced by smooth muscle). The presence of peristalsis is also a helpful sign. When ectopic gastric mucosa is suspected, $^{99m}$Tc pertechnetate scintigraphy should be performed to confirm the finding. MRI and CT cross-sectional imaging are particularly useful for thoracic and pelvic duplications. Contrast studies and endoscopy may provide additional information in selected duplications.

The definitive management of intestinal duplications is surgical resection, which is indicated even if the cysts are asymptomatic because the potential complications can be grave. Complete excision of the duplication in continuity with the adjacent bowel is preferred whenever possible. If complete excision is not feasible or the patient is unable to tolerate the surgery, then the cyst may be excised or "shelled out" and the mucosa stripped. Additionally, a simple exteriorization by the Mikulicz technique can be performed, with the final repair postponed to a later date. Minimally invasive surgery (thoracoscopic or laparoscopic) is favored when possible and has a low rate of postoperative pain and better aesthetics. Endoscopic resection of duodenal duplications has been reported, but the long-term outcome has not been documented.

Locations of alimentary tract duplications (* most common sites)

Base of tongue
Esophagus*
Extending into thorax from duodenum or jejunum
Stomach
Duodenum
Transverse colon (mesenterialized)
Jejunum
Cecum or ascending colon
Ileocecal region*
Ileum**
Sigmoid colon
Rectum

Septate (double lumen) rectum and colon; rectourethral fistula

Cystic duplication of small intestine; characteristic location between leaves of mesentery, blood vessels coursing over it to bowel wall

F. Netter M.D.
Paul Kim

# Meckel Diverticulum and Other Remnants of the Omphalomesenteric Duct

*Meckel diverticulum* is the most frequent congenital anomaly of the GI tract. It is an outpouching of the GI tract that forms due to a failure of the omphalomesenteric (vitelline) duct to disappear between the 5th and 10th weeks of gestation. Meckel diverticulum has classically been described by the rule of twos. It is prevalent in approximately 2% of the population, is usually located within 2 feet of the ileocecal valve, and measures approximately 2 inches in length. It is two times as prevalent in males as in females, with approximately 2% of patients developing a complication, usually within the first 2 years of life. This diverticulum is always attached to the antimesenteric side of the ileal wall with a funnel shape and wide neck resembling that of a finger of a glove. In reality, the length varies from 1 to 10 cm with width ranging from 1 to 4 cm in diameter. The artery supplying the diverticulum, the *vitelline artery,* is a branch of the SMA, which crosses over the ileal wall along the diverticulum to its tip.

Meckel diverticulum is a "true" diverticulum involving all the layers of the small bowel (the mucosal, muscular, and serosal layers), in contrast to an acquired intestinal diverticulum, in which the mucosa and submucosa herniate through the muscle layer, covered only by serosa. The mucosal lining of a Meckel diverticulum corresponds to that of the ileum, but occasionally islands of heterotopic (jejunal, duodenal, or gastric) mucosa or nodules of pancreatic tissue may be present, giving rise to serious complications (see below).

In the majority of individuals with Meckel diverticulum, the rest of the former vitelline duct becomes completely obliterated. In up to 15% of cases, a *nonpatent fibrous cord* may remain, attaching the blind end of the *diverticulum to the umbilical site of the abdominal wall* or to another intestinal loop. Rarely a *solid fibrous cord without development of a diverticulum* persists, resulting in fixation of an ileal loop to the umbilicus. All these can predispose to intestinal obstruction and strangulation of bowel loops.

In rare instances, the entire patent vitelline duct persists and leads to an *umbilicointestinal fistula,* which becomes obvious soon after birth. The umbilical cord in such cases is usually thicker than normal at its base, and once the umbilical stump has regressed and sloughed off, a reddish mass with a small central opening is noted at the umbilicus. The fistula may leak depending on the duct caliber and changes in the abdominal pressure.

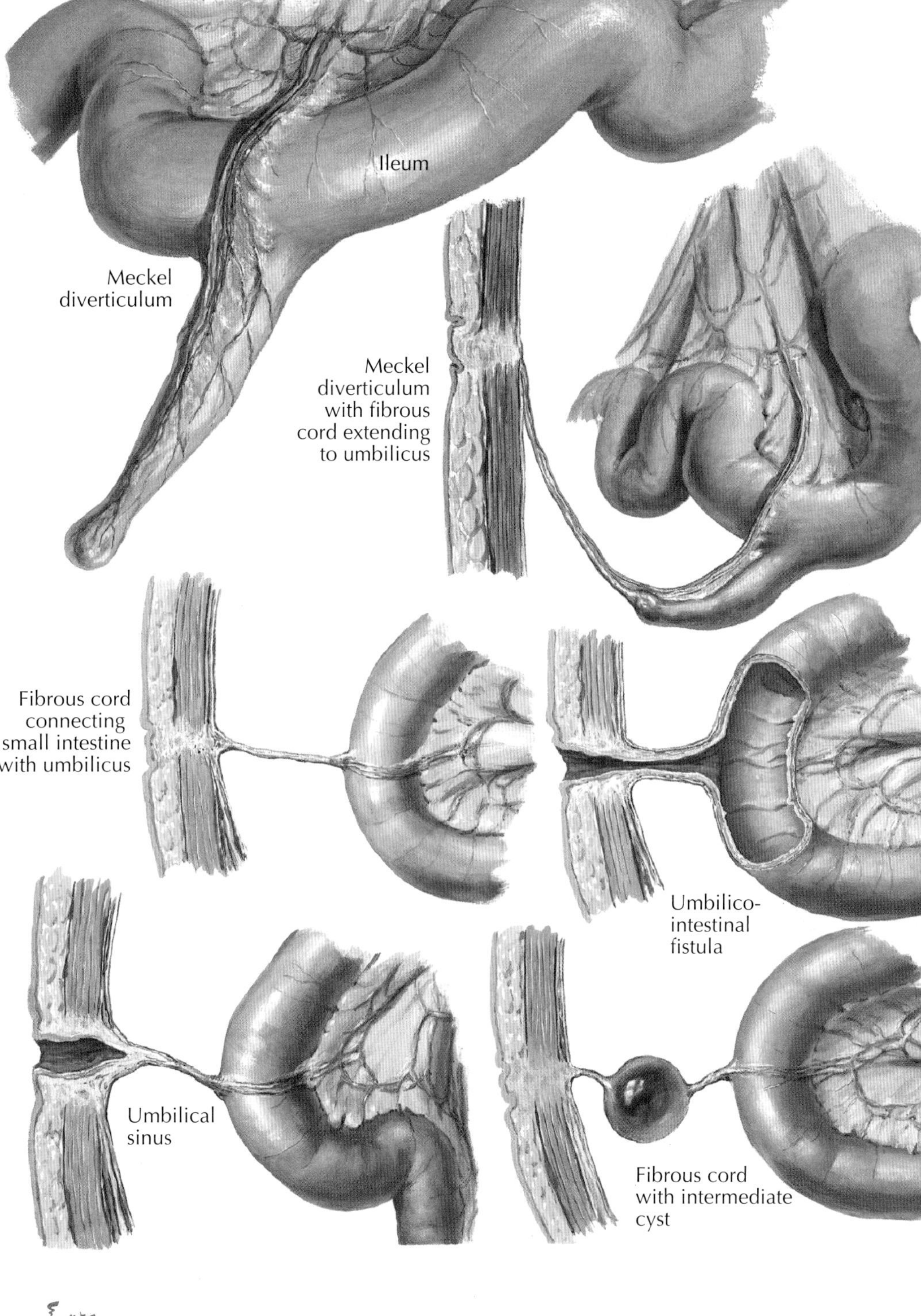


The discharge can vary from scant intermittent mucus to profuse continuous enteric contents. In such cases, an umbilical polyp frequently forms at the external opening of the fistula. Even larger caliber fistula can allow the prolapse of the ileum, which protrudes as a dark-red, sausage-like mass.

Another anatomic variant of a vitelline duct remnant is an *umbilical sinus.* In these cases, the vitelline duct may remain open only at its outer portion, resulting in a *sinus* rather than a fistula. In such instances, the proximal part of the duct closer to the ileum is usually transformed into a fibrous cord attached on one end to the sinus and on the other to the ileum. Finally, the vitelline duct may undergo *fibrosis* on the *outer and inner end* leaving the central portion patent as a *cyst* (enterocyst), which later in life may give rise to symptoms.

Meckel diverticula, as well as the other variants of vitelline duct remnants, often remain silent and are

COMPLICATIONS OF MECKEL DIVERTICULUM AND VITELLINE DUCT REMNANTS

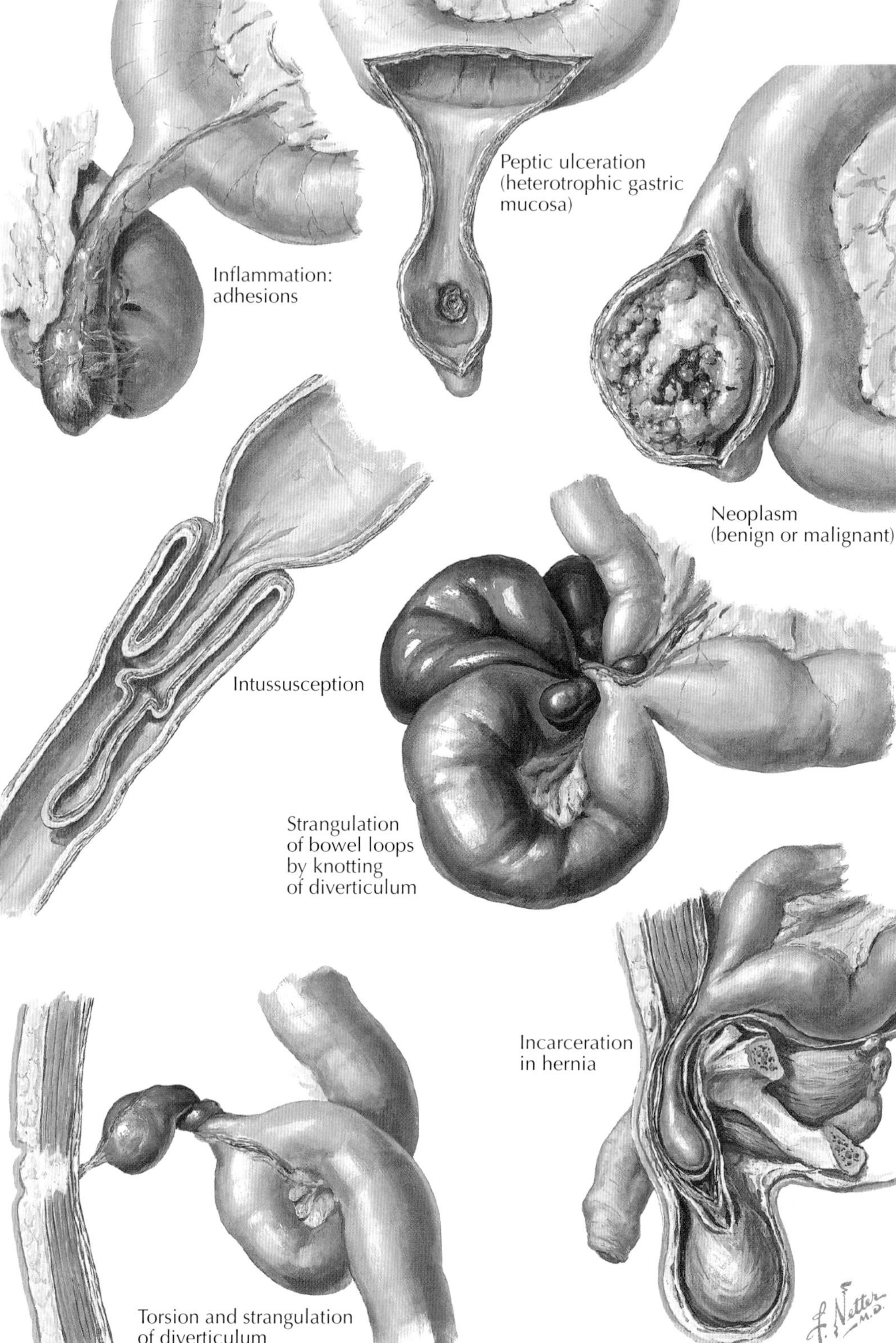


## MECKEL DIVERTICULUM AND OTHER REMNANTS OF THE OMPHALOMESENTERIC DUCT (Continued)

only discovered incidentally by imaging or during abdominal exploration for an unrelated pathology. Symptomatic presentation usually follows one of four clinical syndromes (i.e., peptic ulceration, intestinal obstruction, acute inflammation, and tumors).

GI bleeding can occur as a result of peptic ulceration caused by heterotopic gastric mucosa in the lining of a diverticulum, which is present in over 20% of patients with Meckel diverticulum. The ulcer is located adjacent to or distal to the diverticulum and presents with an acute and massive hemorrhage or with chronic, insidious bleeding. The diagnosis should be suspected in children who develop painless rectal bleeding or in younger adults who present with obscure GI bleeding. The gastric mucosa, even when ectopic, is able to concentrate and secrete $^{99m}$Tc-labeled pertechnetate and forms the basis of the Meckel scan, which can help localize ectopic gastric mucosa in symptomatic Meckel diverticulum. Mesenteric arteriography may be useful in patients with brisk bleeding. Wireless capsule endoscopy and device-assisted enteroscopy can identify the diverticulum and exclude other etiologies of GI bleeding. If the source of the bleeding is not identified with these diagnostic tests or in a patient with massive hemorrhage and hemodynamic instability, then abdominal exploration becomes necessary.

Meckel diverticulum can lead to intestinal obstruction through various pathways. Intussusception occurs when the diverticulum serves as the lead point of ileal or ileocolonic intussusception. A remnant fibrous cord or band attached to the diverticulum can lead to volvulus, and torsion of the diverticulum alone could cause intestinal obstruction. In rare instances, Meckel diverticulum can herniate into a groin (inguinal or femoral) or abdominal wall (umbilical), hernia leading to strangulation *(Littre hernia).*

Meckel diverticulitis can develop when enteroliths or inspissated food particles or infection lead to increased intraluminal pressure that causes erosion of the diverticular wall. This evolves into inflammation and focal necrosis, which can result in perforation and peritonitis. Symptoms and signs of Meckel diverticulitis are often indistinguishable from acute appendicitis, with sudden onset colicky pain that initiates around the umbilicus and shifts to the right lower quadrant with accompanying tenderness, nausea, vomiting, and fever. CT of the abdomen and pelvis is the imaging of choice based on these symptoms; however, the diagnosis is made upon exploratory laparotomy.

*Benign tumors* (myoma, lipoma, adenoma, and neurogenic neoplasm) and malignant lesions (adenocarcinoma, sarcoma, and carcinoid) can develop in a Meckel diverticulum. These can be identified incidentally or cause intestinal obstruction, perforation, or GI bleeding.

Management of a Meckel diverticulum mainly depends on the clinical presentation. Symptomatic Meckel diverticulum should be resected with either diverticulectomy or segmental intestinal resection and primary anastomosis. This can be achieved via open or laparoscopic approach with the latter favored when feasible. The decision to resect the diverticulum in patients who are asymptomatic remains controversial. Adults younger than 50 years of age with a diverticulum longer than 2 cm or one with a fibrous band or palpable abnormality are at increased risk of developing complications, and elective resection should be considered.

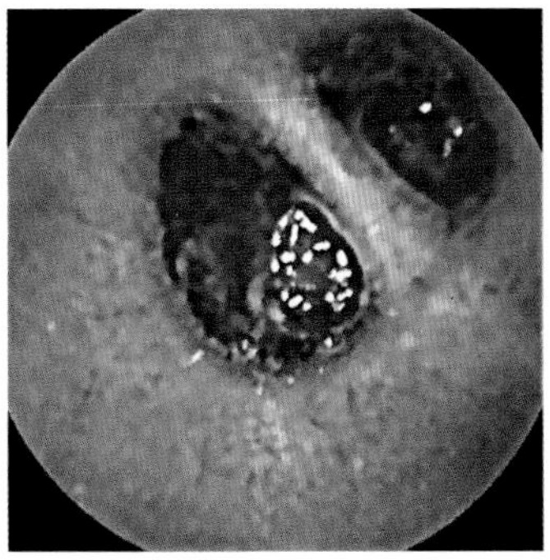

# Diverticula of Small Intestine

A *diverticulum* is a blind outpouching of a hollow viscus involving one or more layers of the bowel wall. Small intestinal diverticula are termed "false" or "true" depending on the layers of the diverticular wall. False or "incomplete" diverticula involve only two layers of the intestinal wall (mucosal and submucosal) and are found on the mesenteric border, where the vasa vasorum penetrate the bowel wall. True or "complete" diverticula involve all three layers and are found on the antimesenteric border. Additionally, false small bowel diverticula are believed to be acquired due to herniation at points of weakness, whereas true diverticula are congenital as in a Meckel diverticulum (see Plate 2.23). The term *small bowel diverticula* in this section refers to the false small bowel diverticula, which is the main type.

Small bowel diverticula usually occur in the duodenum (80%–90%) and become less frequent downstream. The true incidence is not known because the diagnosis is usually incidental, reported in over 5% of small bowel contrast studies and over 7% of endoscopic retrograde cholangiopancreatography procedures.

Diverticula of the small intestine may be single or multiple. Duodenal diverticula are commonly periampullary in location, occurring within 2 to 3 cm of the ampulla of Vater. Jejunal diverticula, although rare, are usually multiple and are located almost always along the line of mesenteric attachment, with sizes varying from a few millimeters up to several centimeters in diameter. The latter are frequently associated with disorders of intestinal motility, such as progressive systemic sclerosis, visceral neuropathies, and myopathies.

Diverticula of the small intestine are frequently asymptomatic and are found incidentally on imaging or endoscopy or at autopsy. Symptoms can range from vague abdominal pain and postprandial bloating and flatulence to acute complications including acute diverticulitis, intestinal obstruction, perforation, and hemorrhage. Acute diverticulitis with enteroliths, inspissated food particles, or infection leads to increased intraluminal pressure that causes erosion of the diverticular wall with inflammation and focal necrosis, which can result in perforation and peritonitis mimicking acute appendicitis. The perforation may occur in the free abdominal cavity, the mesentery, or another intestinal loop, resulting in generalized peritonitis, a walled-off abscess, or an intestinal fistula. Intestinal obstruction may occur by strangulation, compression by an inflammatory tumor, or, more rarely, intussusception. Bleeding from small bowel diverticula can be caused by recurrent injury of the exposed vasa recta, which is only separated from the bowel lumen by mucosa, although this complication is much more common in colonic diverticula. Alternatively, the bleeding can arise from ulceration associated with diverticulitis. A phenomenon unique to large periampullary duodenal diverticula is extrinsic compression of the common bile duct that can lead to cholestasis, jaundice, and even recurrent acute pancreatitis. In rare instances, aberrant pancreatic tissue and benign or malignant tumors can be present in an intestinal diverticulum.

The presence of multiple diverticula in the small intestine can lead to bacterial overgrowth, which can seriously interfere with absorption, causing steatorrhea, megaloblastic anemia, and other symptoms that characterize the malabsorption syndrome (see Plate 2.29). The diagnosis of small intestinal diverticula depends on endoscopic or radiologic visualization. In patients with asymptomatic diverticula, no treatment is required. Small intestinal bacterial overgrowth can be treated with oral antibiotics, but this is rarely curative unless the underlying risk factor (diverticulosis) is removed, and patients often require intermittent antibiotic therapy. Acute diverticulitis and diverticular bleeding are managed similar to that for colonic diverticular disease.

Opening to ileal diverticula

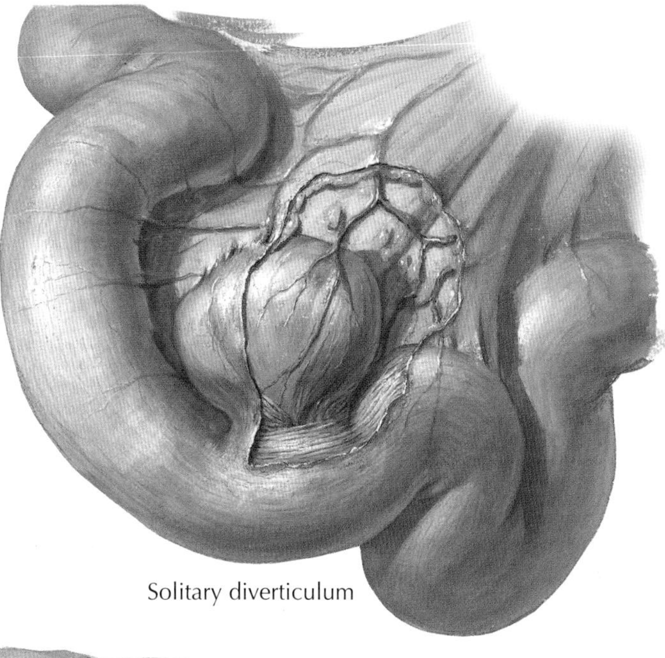

Solitary diverticulum

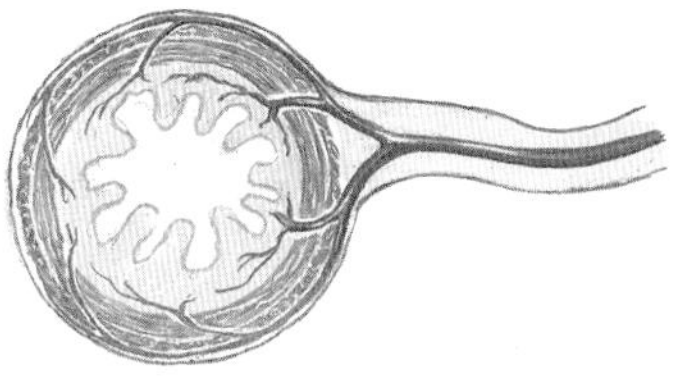

Arterial arrangement in bowel wall

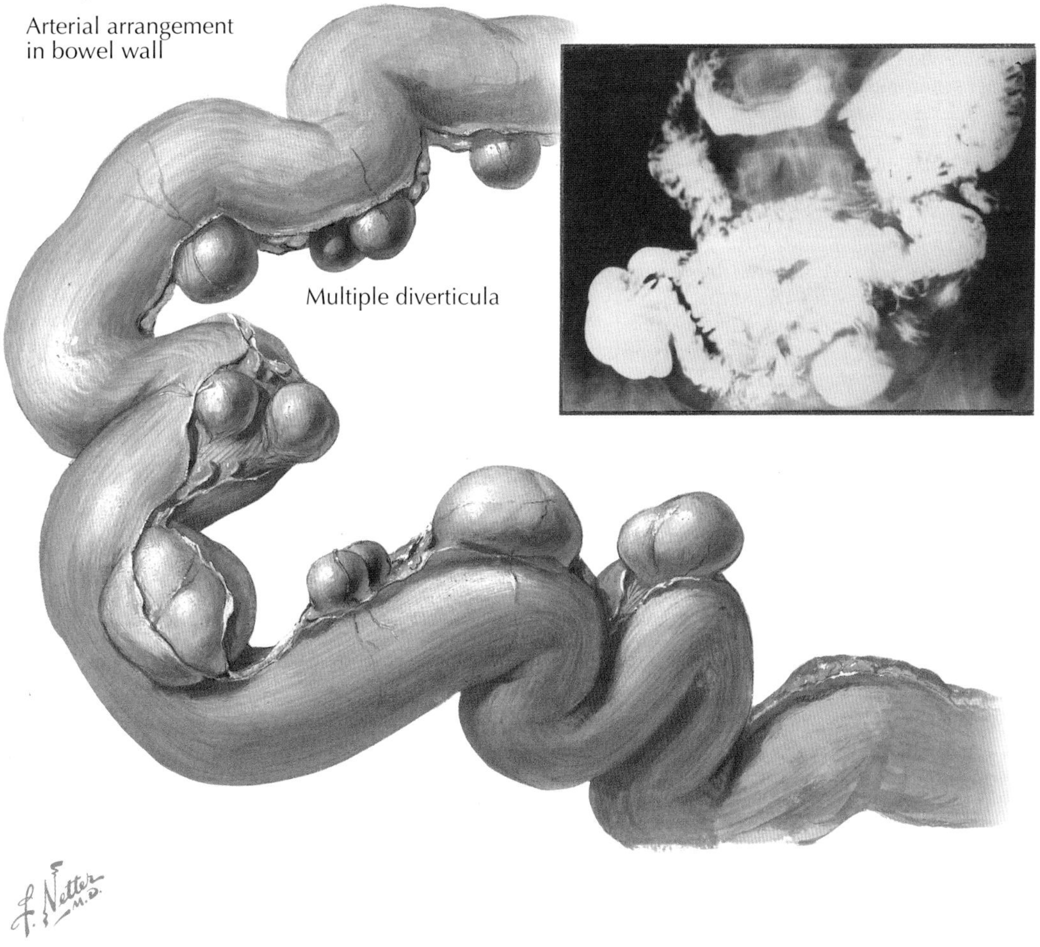

Multiple diverticula

## Celiac Disease

Celiac disease, also known as *gluten-sensitive enteropathy* or *nontropical sprue,* is a chronic immune-mediated enteropathy triggered by exposure to dietary gluten and related proteins in genetically predisposed individuals. The primary target of the disease is the small intestine; however, celiac disease can affect multiple systems.

The overall prevalence of celiac disease in the general population globally is estimated to be 1% based on serologic results and is increasingly recognized on almost every continent, with different rates observed with geographic and ethnic variations that parallel the distribution of human leukocyte antigen (HLA) genotypes. The prevalence appears to be slightly higher in females compared with males, and approximately two times higher in children than adults.

Celiac disease develops in genetically predisposed individuals as a result of the influence of environmental factors such as wheat consumption, age at gluten intake, GI infection, and antibiotic use. First-degree relatives of patients with celiac disease have a 10% to 20% risk of developing the disease. Individuals with certain autoimmune diseases, particularly those with type 1 diabetes and autoimmune thyroiditis, and with Down syndrome or Turner syndrome are also at an increased risk.

The HLA class II genes (HLA) DR3-DQ2 and DR4-DQ8, which are normally expressed on the surface of antigen cells in the gut, are the most important genetic susceptibility factors in celiac disease. HLA-DR3-DQ2 is found in 90% to 95% of patients with celiac disease, with HLA-DR4-DQ8 found in most of the remaining patients. These molecules are necessary variables predisposing a patient to the disease, which means that celiac disease is unlikely if neither molecule is present. The molecules are not, however, sufficient to cause celiac disease and occur in 30% to 40% of the general population of most countries.

Gluten is a storage protein of wheat. The alcohol-soluble fraction of gluten, gliadin, is toxic in celiac disease, along with similar proteins in barley (hordeins) and rye (secalins). These proteins are rich in glutamine and proline residues that even the healthy human intestine cannot fully digest. As a result, intact gliadin peptides are left in the lumen, but few cross the intestinal barrier. In individuals with celiac disease, these fragments come into contact with tissue transglutaminase, a ubiquitous intracellular enzyme that is released by inflammatory and endothelial cells and fibroblasts in response to mechanical irritation or inflammation. Upon contact, tissue transglutaminase cross-links with these glutamine-rich proteins and deamidates them. This process modifies glutamine residues into glutamic acid residues, which are ideally suited to interact with the HLA-DQ2 or HLA-DQ8 molecules. Once bound to HLA-DQ2 or HLA-DQ8, gliadin peptides are presented to the CD4+ T cells, triggering the inflammatory reaction. The result is an inflammatory state of the small intestine, causing a derangement in the architecture of the mucosa, with flattening of the villi, and infiltration of lymphocytes into the epithelium.

The stereotypic patient with celiac disease is a malnourished child with profound GI signs and symptoms; however, most patients are older and asymptomatic and the disease is discovered incidentally upon testing, whereas others present with atypical extraintestinal manifestations.

Classic celiac disease is characterized by chronic or intermittent diarrhea, often bulky and foul smelling, accompanied by abdominal pain, bloating, and flatulence.

A variety of extraintestinal manifestations have been described in atypical celiac disease and are often the presenting symptoms. Iron deficiency anemia, resistant to oral iron supplementation, is the most common extraintestinal sign and is considered the most frequent presentation among teenagers and adults. Nonerosive, polyarticular, or oligoarticular arthritis that promptly resolves with a gluten-free diet has been documented, and metabolic bone diseases, including osteopenia, osteoporosis, and, rarely, osteomalacia can present in the absence of GI symptoms. Neurologic symptoms such as headaches and psychiatric issues including depression and anxiety can also be associated with celiac disease.

*Dermatitis herpetiformis* is an uncommon cutaneous manifestation of celiac disease and presents as an intensely pruritic inflammatory papular and vesicular skin eruption involving the extensor surfaces of the elbows, forearms, knees, buttocks, back, and scalp. Direct immunofluorescence microscopy of a punch biopsy is the gold standard test for the diagnosis of dermatitis herpetiformis. Treatment consists of dietary gluten restriction and pharmacotherapy with dapsone. Long-term treatment lasting several years may be required to achieve complete remission.

The diagnosis of celiac disease requires a high index of suspicion and the identification of risk factors associated with the disease. Testing should be carried out for those with GI symptoms and those with unexplained iron deficiency anemia, folate deficiency, or vitamin $B_{12}$ deficiency. The presence of unexplained persistent elevation in serum aminotransferases, short stature, delayed puberty, recurrent fetal loss, reduced fertility, persistent aphthous

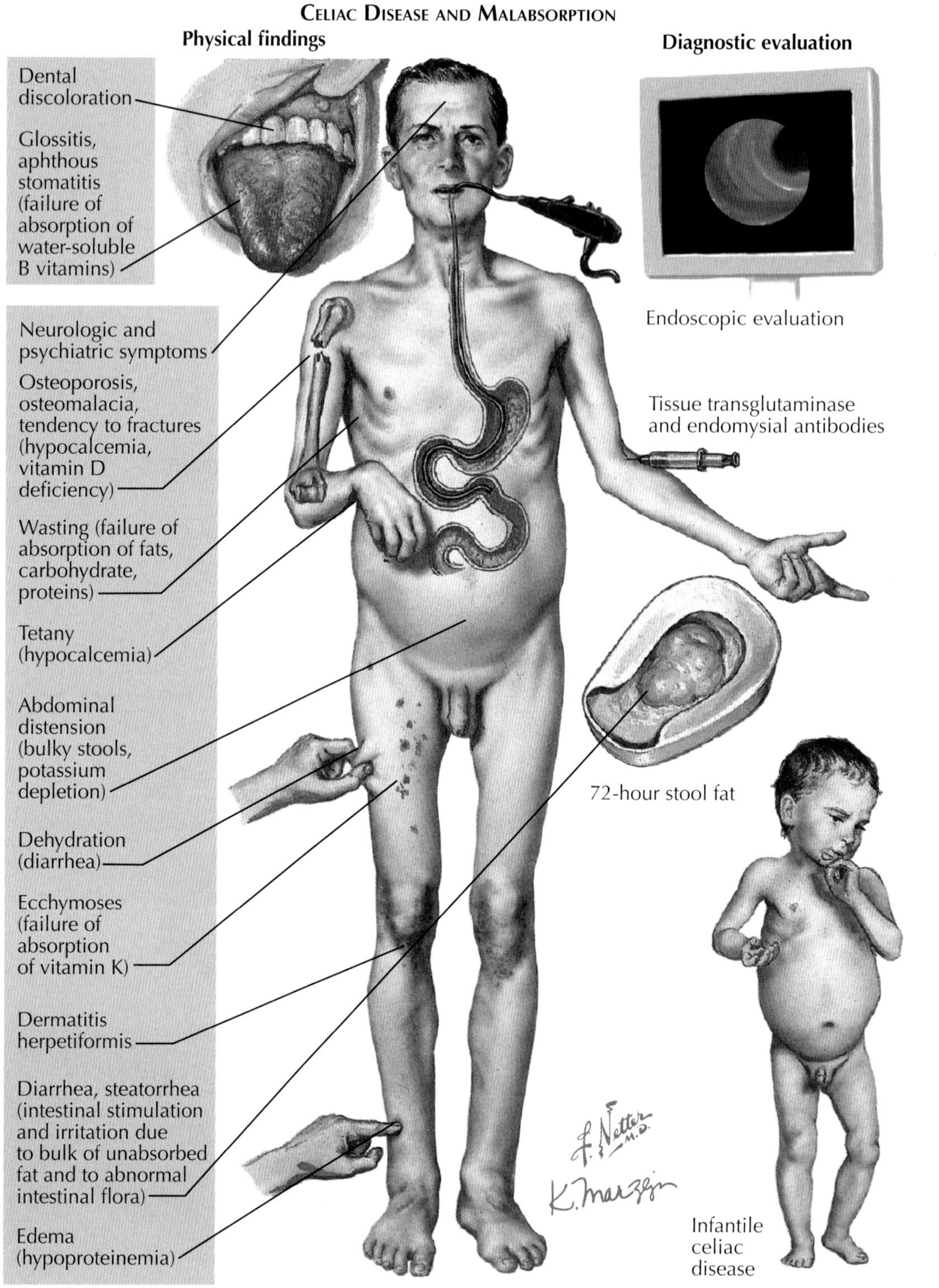

CELIAC DISEASE AND MALABSORPTION

Physical findings

Dental discoloration

Glossitis, aphthous stomatitis (failure of absorption of water-soluble B vitamins)

Neurologic and psychiatric symptoms

Osteoporosis, osteomalacia, tendency to fractures (hypocalcemia, vitamin D deficiency)

Wasting (failure of absorption of fats, carbohydrate, proteins)

Tetany (hypocalcemia)

Abdominal distension (bulky stools, potassium depletion)

Dehydration (diarrhea)

Ecchymoses (failure of absorption of vitamin K)

Dermatitis herpetiformis

Diarrhea, steatorrhea (intestinal stimulation and irritation due to bulk of unabsorbed fat and to abnormal intestinal flora)

Edema (hypoproteinemia)

Diagnostic evaluation

Endoscopic evaluation

Tissue transglutaminase and endomysial antibodies

72-hour stool fat

Infantile celiac disease

F. Netter M.D.

K. Marzen

## CELIAC DISEASE (Continued)

stomatitis, dental enamel hypoplasia, idiopathic peripheral neuropathy, nonhereditary cerebellar ataxia, or recurrent migraine headaches also merits testing for celiac disease. Testing should be considered for first-degree relatives of individuals with celiac disease and for individuals with disorders known to coexist with celiac disease.

Serum antitissue transglutaminase immunoglobulin A (IgA), the best initial test to screen for celiac disease in an individual consuming a gluten-containing diet, has high levels of sensitivity (98%) and specificity (96%). A total IgA level must be assessed concurrently because IgA deficiency is more common in celiac disease (2%–5%) compared with the rate in the general population (<0.5%), potentially leading to a false-negative test. In individuals with IgA deficiency, IgG-based assays should be substituted. Anti–endomysium IgA testing has a specificity of close to 100% and a sensitivity exceeding 90%, but this test has high interobserver variability and has higher costs. Antibodies to deamidated gliadin peptides (DGP-IgA and DGP-IgG) can also be used as screening tools and are especially useful in very young children, especially those younger than 2 years. Negative results on testing for HLA-DQ2 or HLA-DQ8 can also help exclude the diagnosis in this setting.

The diagnosis of celiac disease is confirmed by histologic changes in the small intestinal mucosa obtained by biopsy during an upper endoscopy in a patient with positive serologic studies, with the only exception being a biopsy-proven dermatitis herpetiformis where positive celiac serology is sufficient to make a final diagnosis. The classic finding of celiac disease on endoscopy includes atrophic duodenal mucosa with loss of the folds with or without scalloping or a nodular appearance. Such findings, however, are not universally present and the mucosa can appear normal. Histologic findings range from mild alteration characterized only by increased intraepithelial lymphocytes to crypt hyperplasia and complete villous atrophy and are reported using the Marsh-Oberhuber and Corazza classifications.

In certain scenarios, patients may have discordant serology and small bowel biopsy results due to falsely positive antitissue transglutaminase IgG or falsely negative small bowel histology due to the patchy nature of small bowel involvement. In these cases, genetic testing for HLA-DR3-DQ2 and HLA-DR4-DQ8 can sometimes be helpful to exclude celiac disease in those individuals who are negative for both HLA subtypes.

The treatment of celiac disease remains strict adherence to a gluten-free diet, which typically results in a complete return to health. Compliance with a gluten-free diet, however, is difficult at all ages but particularly for teenagers and younger adults. Dietary counseling with a skilled dietitian is one of the most important aspects of management and should be recommended to all patients with celiac disease. Patients should be monitored for deficiencies of vitamins, particularly A, D, E, and $B_{12}$; iron; and folic acid. Copper and zinc should be supplemented. Deficiency of magnesium and selenium may also occur, and signs or symptoms of a deficiency should be sought. Constipation can occur as a consequence of a gluten-free diet because the diet is low in roughage, and patients can benefit from regular use of psyllium seed husks.

The most common reason for persistent symptoms and/or abnormal serology and/or histology while a patient is on a gluten-free diet is poor compliance with the diet or inadvertent gluten ingestion. Alternative or concurrent disorders such as bacterial overgrowth, pancreatic insufficiency, and microscopic colitis should be considered and

### ENDOSCOPIC AND HISTOLOGIC FINDINGS

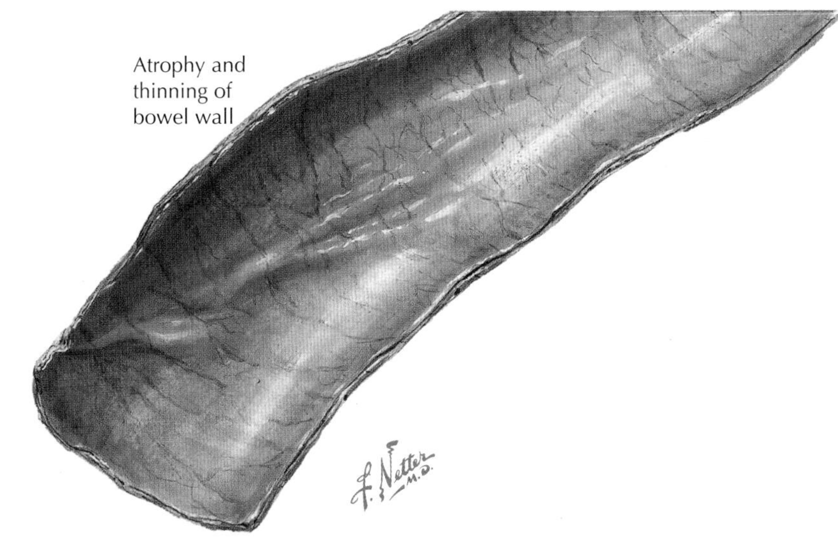


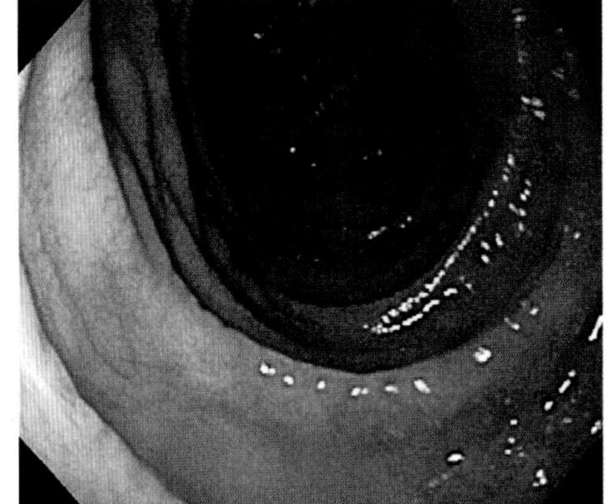
Endoscopic image of atrophic mucosa

Capsule endoscopic image of scalloping *(Courtesy Julio C. Bai.)*

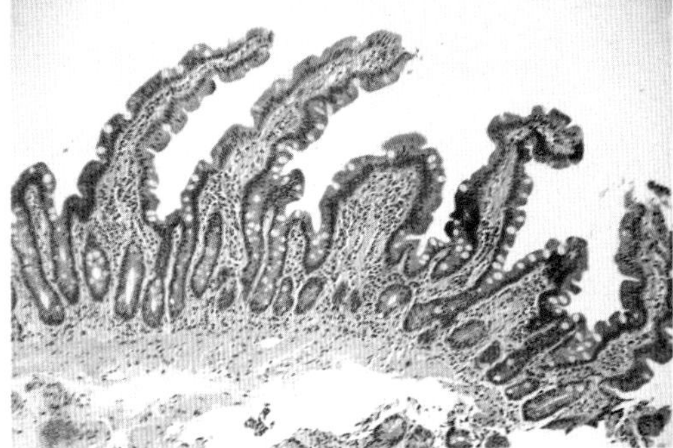
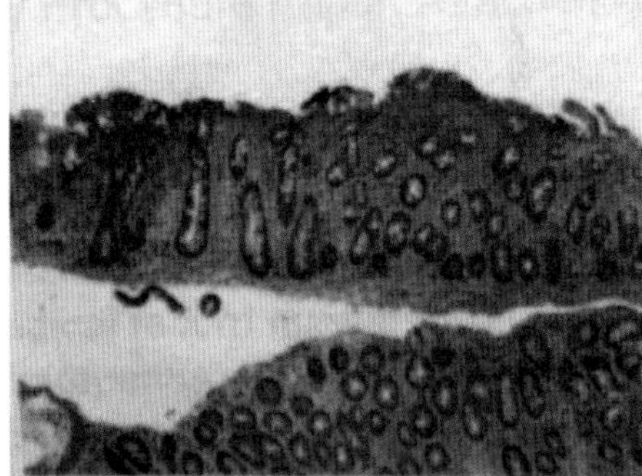
Normal *(left)* and abnormal *(right)* intestinal villi *(Left image from Wilcox CM, Munoz-Navas M, Sung JJ. Atlas of Clinical Gastrointestinal Endoscopy. Elsevier; 2012.)*

excluded appropriately. *Refractory sprue* is the persistence of symptoms and villous atrophy despite a strict gluten-free diet for at least 2 years. The cause is unknown, but the course can be severe, with progressive malabsorption and even death. Aggressive nutritional support is required, including parenteral nutrition if needed and pharmacotherapy focused on immunosuppression.

In patients unresponsive to immunosuppression, ulcerative jejunitis and lymphoma should be considered. Patients with ulcerative jejunitis have multiple chronic, benign-appearing ulcers, most frequently in the jejunum, which can rarely form strictures. These can be identified on cross-sectional abdominal imaging or on upper endoscopy and capsule endoscopy. Ulcerative jejunitis has an unfavorable prognosis, with a 30% mortality rate.

Distinction between ulcerative jejunitis and lymphoma is challenging because both have very similar symptoms and findings on imaging. Enteropathy-associated T-cell lymphoma is a rare but aggressive neoplasm that arises in the GI tract as a sequela of untreated celiac disease. Most patients present with stage IV disease. Treatment consists of chemotherapy with or without autologous hematopoietic cell transplantation.

Various malignant diseases are associated with celiac disease, and the gluten-free diet is protective against the development of certain malignant diseases. These include esophageal, head, and neck squamous carcinoma, small intestinal adenocarcinoma, and non-Hodgkin lymphoma.

## TROPICAL SPRUE

Tropical sprue is a chronic diarrheal disease seen in certain tropical areas and characterized by small intestinal damage causing malabsorption and nutritional deficiencies, particularly of folate and vitamin $B_{12}$.

Tropical sprue occurs in distinct geographic areas located within a narrow 30-degree band north and south of the equator and is particularly prevalent in southern India, the Philippines, and several Caribbean islands (Haiti, the Dominican Republic, Puerto Rico, and Cuba) but rarely seen in Jamaica, Africa, the Middle East, or Southeast Asia. It affects both native populations as well as visitors who stay for more than a month.

It is widely believed that infectious agents are responsible for the development of tropical sprue, which may follow an acute infectious diarrheal illness. Multiple microorganisms, including *Klebsiella pneumoniae, Enterobacter cloacae,* and *Escherichia coli,* have been identified in jejunal aspirates, but there is little consistency among studies. Bacterial overgrowth has also been documented in patients with tropical sprue, which can contribute to significant small bowel structural damage, by elaboration of toxins and fermentation products.

Intestinal injury causes loss of brush-border disaccharidase enzymes, which leads to carbohydrate malabsorption. The loss of normal villous architecture impairs fat absorption and causes steatorrhea. Vitamin $B_{12}$ and folate malabsorption leads to megaloblastic anemia. This contrasts with small intestinal bacterial overgrowth, where vitamin $B_{12}$ deficiency and increased or normal folate levels are seen. This phenomenon is probably related to a difference in the bacterial species colonizing the small bowel in the two conditions. Facultative anaerobic toxigenic coliforms in tropical sprue produce fermentation products such as ethanol that diminish folate absorption, whereas anaerobic nontoxigenic flora in the small bowel overgrowth generate folic acid.

The diagnosis of tropical sprue should be entertained in any individual with chronic diarrhea who is either residing in or has recently returned from a prolonged visit to a tropical country. Steatorrhea is often present and is accompanied by cramping abdominal pain, gas, and fatigue. Malabsorption is evident, with progressive weight loss, megaloblastic anemia, and signs of a low-protein state.

Chronic diarrhea in a tropical environment has extensive etiologic possibilities, primarily of an infectious nature. Therefore exclusion of these causes of diarrhea is necessary before invasive endoscopic studies can be performed. Careful stool and serologic testing should be performed to exclude parasitic infections such as *Entamoeba histolytica, Giardia lamblia,* and *Cryptosporidium parvum,* and serologic tests should be carried out to rule out celiac disease. In individuals at risk for human immunodeficiency virus (HIV) and in patients who are immunocompromised, HIV infection and associated opportunistic infections should be ruled out.

Once these are excluded, one should proceed with an upper endoscopy with biopsy of the duodenum. Gross findings at endoscopy are nonspecific and include flattening of duodenal folds and "scalloping." The histologic features are nearly identical to those of celiac disease, with shortened, blunted villi and elongated crypts and increased inflammatory cells. However, in tropical sprue there appears to be less villous architectural alteration and more mononuclear cell and eosinophilic infiltrate in the lamina propria, whereas in celiac disease, blunting of the villi is more severe with complete or nearly complete absence of villi.

Prolonged course of a broad-spectrum antibiotic and folic acid supplementation are most often curative for this disease, although relapse or reinfection can occur in up to 20% of patients living in the tropics. Folic acid alone can improve appetite and lead to weight gain and hematologic remission, and therapy with tetracycline, given for up to 6 months along with folic acid, completely reverses the intestinal and hematologic abnormalities of tropical sprue. Coexistent $B_{12}$ deficiency should be treated with intramuscular injections of cyanocobalamin.

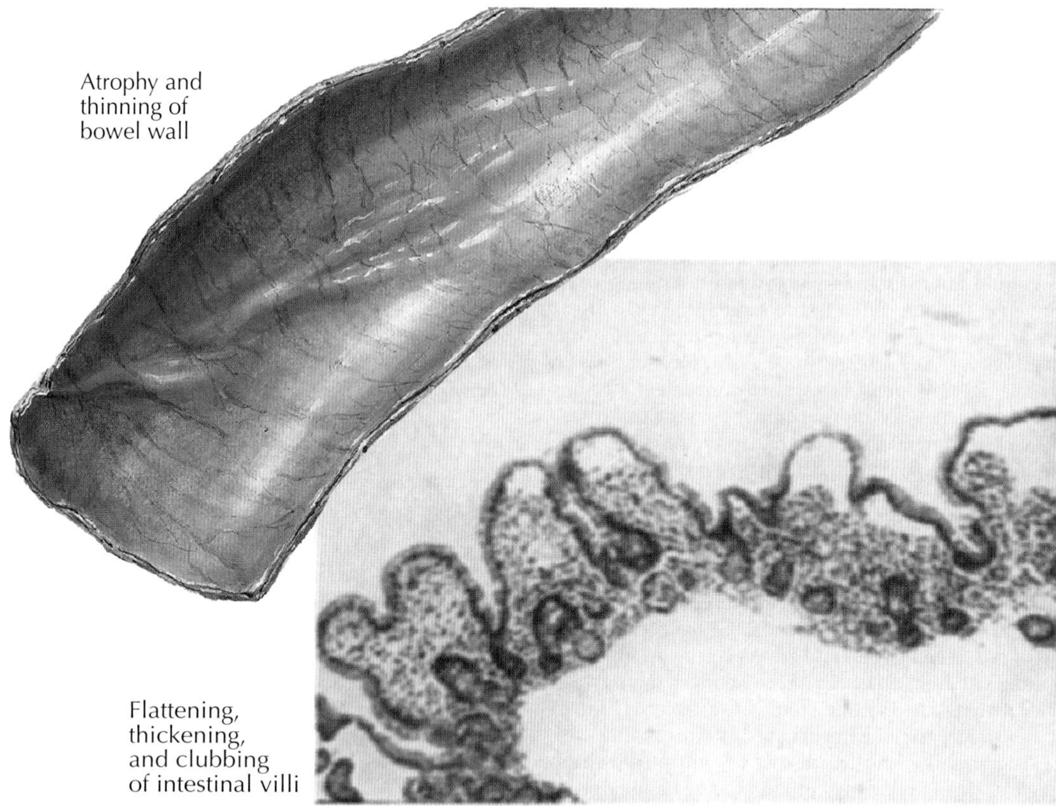


Geographic Distribution of Tropical Sprue

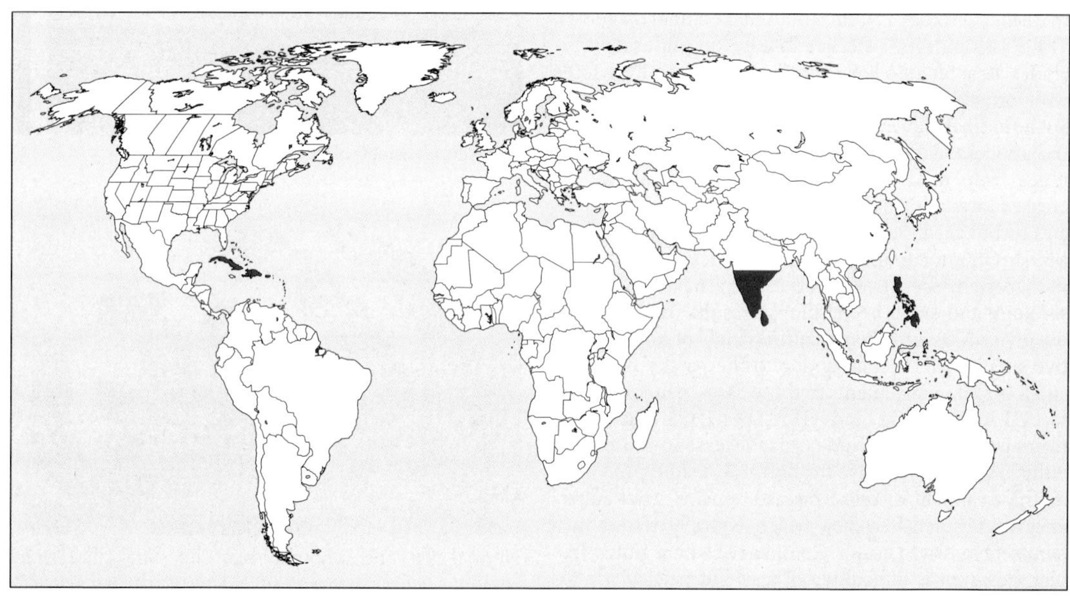

## Whipple Disease (Intestinal Lipodystrophy)

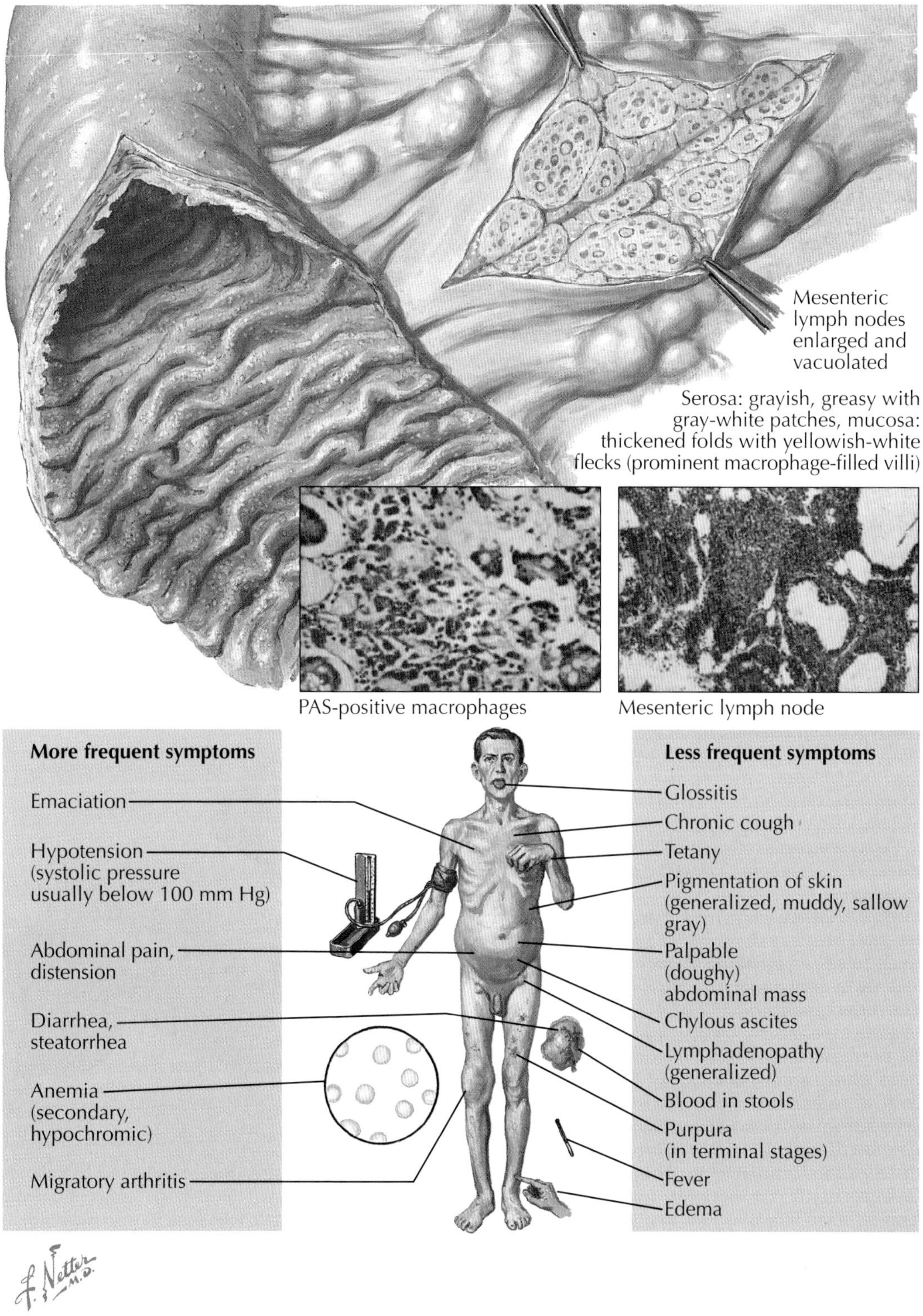

Whipple disease is a rare, chronic, multisystemic infectious disease caused by colonization with *Tropheryma whipplei,* a gram-positive bacillus. The disease was first described in 1907 by G.H. Whipple, who noted "large masses of neutral fats and fatty acids in the lymph spaces," but the infectious agent was not identified until 1991.

*T. whipplei* is ubiquitously found in the environment and is transmitted orally or feco-orally among individuals, where it can colonize healthy carriers or gradually lead to disease. Most cases have been reported from North America or Europe and suggest predilection to middle-aged White males of European ancestry with occupational exposure to soil or animal, suggesting an underlying genetic predisposition and/or immune defects that allow colonization with *T. whipplei* and development of the disease upon exposure to soil microbes.

The classic presentation is a 50-year-old White male who initially complains of intermittent migratory arthralgias and experiences chronic intermittent diarrhea with colicky abdominal pain and weight loss. Nonspecific symptoms such as fatigue, cough, and myalgia can occur. The bacterium can affect nearly all organs, including the eye, skin, lung, and even epididymis and testes. Lymphadenopathy, mainly mediastinal, is present in over 50% of cases, and neurologic symptoms are present in nearly one-quarter of patients. Cognitive changes such as dementia or memory impairment and psychiatric signs such as personality changes and depression are the most frequently observed signs. Whipple disease may rarely present as a chronic localized infection without intestinal and systemic involvement. This form can involve the endocardium, causing culture-negative endocarditis, or can infect the eye, causing corticosteroid-resistant uveitis. Additionally, *T. whipplei* has been implicated in acute infections such as pneumonia, gastroenteritis, and even bacteremia.

Because of the rarity of Whipple disease, the diagnosis requires a high index of suspicion. Routine laboratory findings include anemia with both iron and vitamin $B_{12}$ deficiency and hypoalbuminemia. Polymerase chain reaction (PCR) testing of saliva and stool lacks sensitivity, and in most cases, upper GI endoscopy with biopsies of the small intestine is necessary to make the diagnosis. Gross examination may reveal thickened small intestinal folds studded with yellowish-white flecks. The corresponding mesentery and retroperitoneal lymph nodes are often enlarged, appear yellow or gray in color, and have a soft, doughy consistency; on section, they show many vacuolated spaces (Swiss cheese, or honeycombed, appearance), which are filled with a yellowish-white creamy material.

The duodenal mucosa may appear atrophied during examination, although it appears normal in most cases. Histologically, the small intestinal mucosa shows a thickened lamina propria containing a large number of mononuclear macrophages with foamy cytoplasm and eosinophilic granularity. Demonstration of extensive periodic acid–Schiff–positive material in the lamina propria of duodenal biopsies confirms the diagnosis. However, periodic acid–Schiff staining can be positive in other circumstances, such as *Mycobacterium* infection, and biopsy specimens should also submitted for PCR testing. Immunohistochemical analysis using specific antibodies allows the direct visualization of bacteria in samples; it has a sensitivity and specificity superior to those of periodic acid–Schiff staining and can be used in cases where the diagnosis is still in question. In individuals without GI involvement, testing for *T. whipplei* should be carried out on specimens taken from relevant anastomotic sites, such as synovial fluid from patients with arthritis or lymph nodes from patients with lymphadenopathy. Additionally, lumbar puncture is recommended for all patients diagnosed with Whipple disease for PCR testing of cerebrospinal fluid (CSF) to evaluate CNS involvement, which dictates treatment.

The treatment of Whipple disease has evolved over the past 40 years. Before the use of antibiotics, the disease was uniformly fatal. With adequate treatment, however, most patients do well. Clinical improvement is often dramatic, occurring within 7 to 21 days. Current treatment regimens recommend use of a third-generation cephalosporin or penicillin followed by long-term maintenance with trimethoprim-sulfamethoxazole. The two major problems are CNS disease and relapsing infection. CNS disease is difficult to manage and requires longer use of an antibiotic that readily enters the blood-brain barrier. Relapse has been reported in up to 35% of cases and indicates incomplete eradication of the organism during the initial therapy. *Immune reconstitution inflammatory syndrome* is sometimes observed in the first few weeks of therapy and may be fatal. Therefore close monitoring during therapy, especially during the initial period, is essential and may require corticosteroid therapy.

## BACTERIAL OVERGROWTH

*Small intestinal bacterial overgrowth* refers to the excessive proliferation of native bacteria or the presence of colonic bacteria in the small bowel, leading to symptoms and interfering with absorption of nutrients. Although sterile at birth, the alimentary canal is populated by the maternal flora within a few hours after birth. The interaction among an infant's genes and microbiome and the nutrition the infant receives and environment surrounding the infant plays a role in the early establishment of the intestinal flora.

The proximal small bowel normally contains few bacteria, which provides a more challenging environment for microbial colonizers given the short transit times (3–5 hours) and the high bile concentrations. Farther down in the mid to distal jejunum, facultative anaerobes and oxygen-tolerant obligate anaerobes predominate with concentrations ranging from $10^3$ to $10^5$ CFU/mL, whereas the terminal ileum represents a transition zone between the aerobic flora of the proximal small bowel and the dense anaerobic population found in the colon, with concentrations reaching as high as $10^9$ CFU/mL. In individuals with resected or incompetent ileocecal valves, the microbiome composition can resemble that of the colon. The large intestine, which is characterized by slow flow rates and neutral to mildly acidic pH, harbors by far the largest and most diverse microbial community with concentrations exceeding $10^{12}$ CFU/mL. The organisms are predominantly anaerobes such as *Bacteroides, Lactobacillus, Clostridium,* and bifidobacteria, although multiple species coexist.

Enteric microbial composition is maintained by several defensive mechanisms that prevent excessive bacterial colonization of the small bowel. Gastric acid sterilizes ingested microorganisms, and proteolytic pancreatic and intestinal enzymes digest bacteria that escape into the small bowel. An intestinal mucous layer traps bacteria, and the sweeping action of small intestinal peristaltic movements, particularly the MMC prevents attachment to the mucosa and effectively sweeps residual debris from the proximal bowel to the colon. Gut immunity plays an important role through secretory IgA, which prevents bacterial proliferation. Last, an intact ileocecal valve prevents retrograde bacterial translocation. Therefore disorders that disrupt any or all these mechanisms permit the development of small intestinal bacterial overgrowth.

Anatomic abnormalities that lead to stasis, such as surgical blind loops, fistulas, and strictures related to CD; short bowel syndrome; and small intestinal diverticula, are common causes of small intestinal bacterial overgrowth. Small intestinal dysmotility, commonly seen in scleroderma, postradiation enteropathy, and small intestinal pseudoobstruction, can cause functional stasis that allows bacterial proliferation.

Certain endocrine disorders, such as diabetes mellitus (DM) and thyroid disease, can alter intestinal motility, and hypochlorhydria and immunodeficiency interfere with the host's ability to neutralize pathogens. Rarely, small intestinal bacterial overgrowth can occur in the absence of an underlying cause.

Once established, the bacterial overgrowth interferes with nutrient absorption and causes several digestive symptoms by elaboration of toxins, or direct mucosal injury. Deconjugation of bile accompanied by premature fermentation of carbohydrates contributes to bloating, flatulence, diarrhea, and steatorrhea. Nutrient deficiencies can occur owing to malabsorption of vitamin $B_{12}$ and fat-soluble vitamins. Notably, folic acid levels are normal or even increased due to anaerobic nontoxigenic flora, which can generate folic acid. In severe cases malabsorption can lead to weight loss, hypoalbuminemia, and peripheral edema and rarely, patients may present with xerophthalmia, perioral numbness, and neuropathy with paresthesias reflecting severe underlying deficiencies of vitamins A, D, and $B_{12}$, respectively.

The gold standard for the diagnosis of small intestinal bacterial overgrowth has traditionally been a jejunal aspirate culture demonstrating more than $10^3$ CFU/mL. This test, however, is cumbersome to perform and poorly reproducible. Carbohydrate breath tests rely on the principle that the premature fermentation of a test dose of carbohydrate in the presence of bacterial overgrowth leads to production of hydrogen and/or methane that is absorbed and exhaled in the breath. The sensitivity and specificity of breath tests compared with jejunal aspirate cultures are low, and testing protocols are not standardized; however, they are safe, inexpensive, and easy to perform and are currently widely used for the diagnosis of small intestinal bacterial overgrowth. Lactulose and glucose are the most common substrates used.

Treatment of bacterial overgrowth involves the use of antibiotics, but when an underlying disease is present, it should be corrected. Surgical resection of a blind loop and discontinuation of agents that reduce motility or suppress acid secretion are such measures that eliminate and prevent relapse of bacterial overgrowth. Several broad-spectrum antibiotics have been used, including tetracycline, metronidazole, amoxicillin/clavulanic acid, and cephalosporins. Recently the use of rifaximin, a nonabsorbable antibiotic that inhibits bacterial RNA synthesis, has been shown to be effective.

Recurrence is common after treatment, especially in patients with underlying disorders that have not been corrected. For recurrent symptoms, several antibiotic treatment strategies exist, including intermittent courses or the use of rotating antibiotics during the first week of every month or every other week. Dietary prescriptions include a dairy-free diet that is low in fiber and low in carbohydrates but high in fat. This type of diet reduces symptoms and ensures a good source of calories.

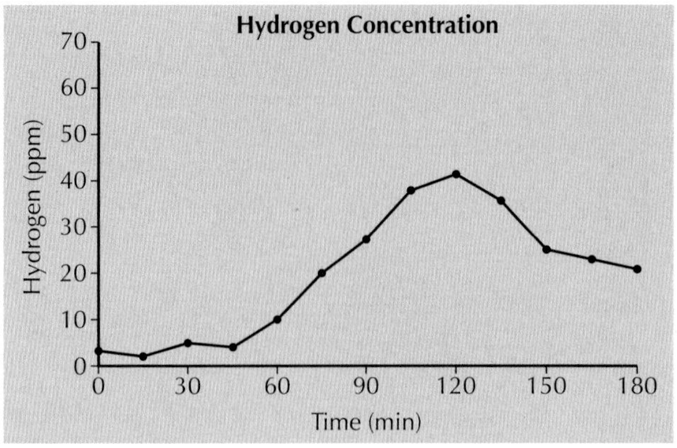

Hydrogen Concentration

Lactulose breath test

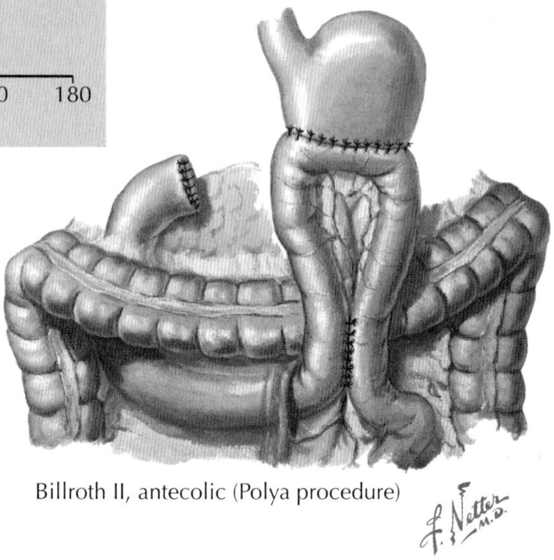

Billroth II, antecolic (Polya procedure)

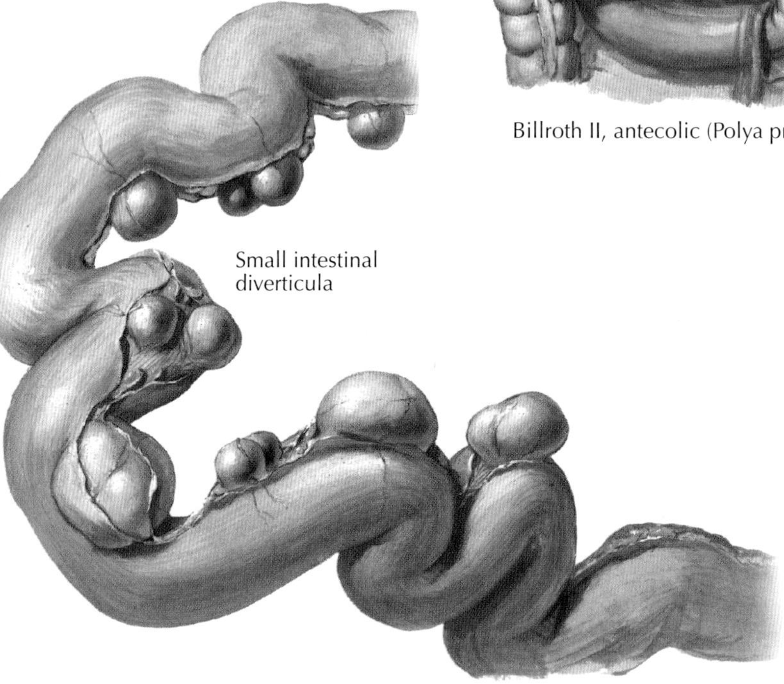

Small intestinal diverticula

# Carbohydrate Malabsorption, Including Lactose Malabsorption

Carbohydrate malabsorption is a frequent clinical condition caused by fermentation of unabsorbed carbohydrates by colonic flora, giving rise to digestive symptoms. Lactose is the most commonly malabsorbed sugar; however, other carbohydrates, including oligosaccharides, disaccharides, and monosaccharides such as fructose, can also cause symptoms related to malabsorption.

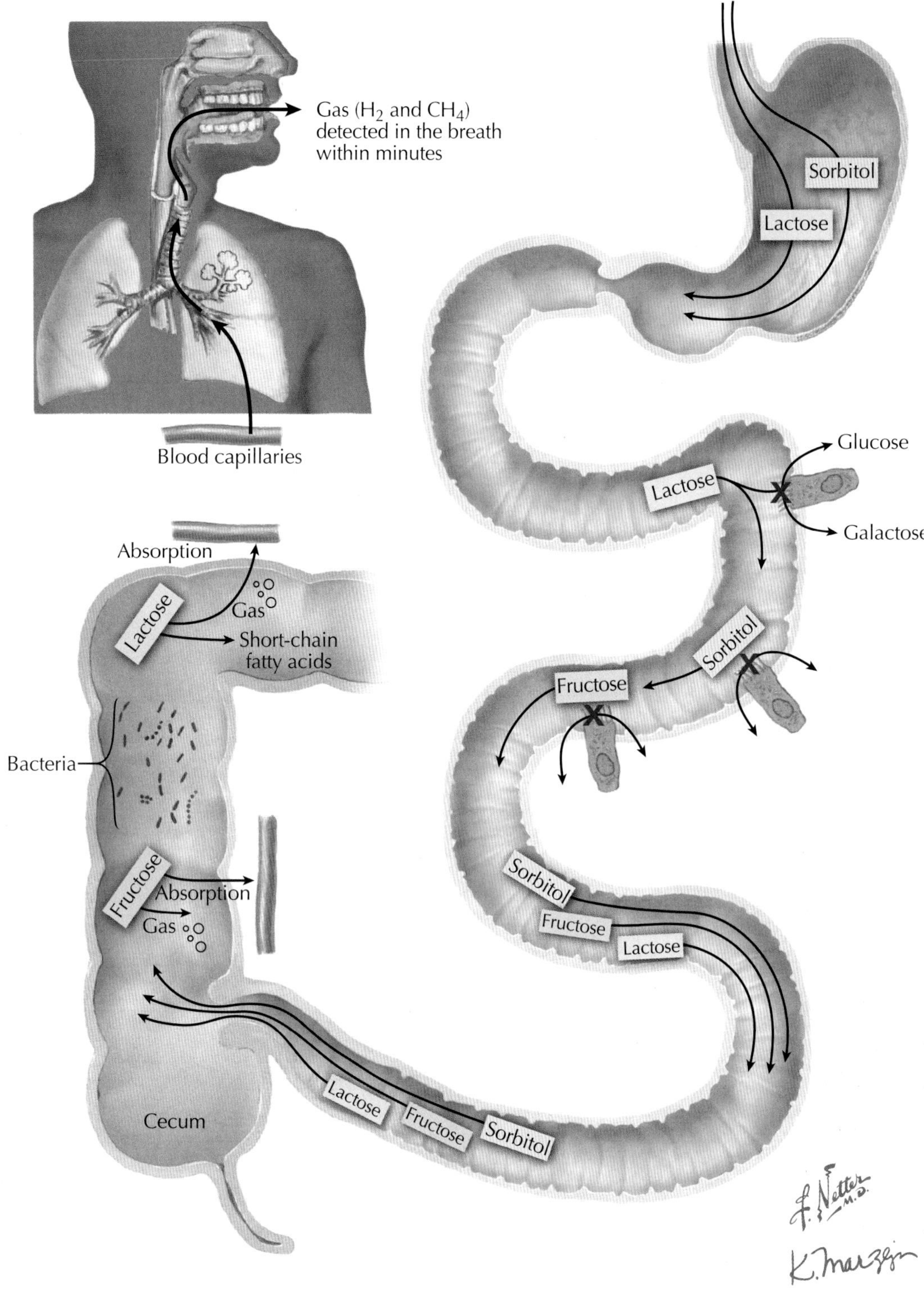


## LACTOSE MALABSORPTION

*Lactose intolerance* refers to the development of abdominal pain, flatulence, nausea, bloating, and diarrhea after ingestion of lactose, whereas *malabsorption* refers to the inefficient digestion of lactose, a disorder that may or may not cause symptoms. *Lactose* is the main source of sugar in milk and milk products for all mammals except the sea lion. It is hydrolyzed by *lactase,* an intestinal brush-border enzyme that cleaves lactose into glucose and galactose.

Intestinal lactase activity is maximal at birth but starts to decline after the age of 2 years, a process that might help weaning. Most people in the world (70%) have low lactase activity after childhood *(lactase nonpersistence).* The proportion is higher in Native Americans and some populations of Southeast Asia and Africa, where it reaches 95%. Low activity should be distinguished from *congenital lactase deficiency,* a rare autosomal recessive disease that affects infants from birth, and *acquired lactose intolerance,* which is a consequence of loss of intestinal brush-border enzyme activity associated with infectious enteritis or celiac disease. In approximately 30% of the population, the lactase activity level does not decline and continues at the maximal neonatal level well into adulthood *(lactase persistence).* This occurs mainly in people of Northern European descent and may indicate a natural selection in those populations who relied on mammalian milk in times of poor harvest.

Individuals with lactase nonpersistence can tolerate low doses of lactose. Studies indicate that symptoms are likely to be negligible if lactose intake is limited to 12.5 g, equivalent to 240 mL of milk per day. The average adult with a Western diet consumes approximately 15 g of lactose per day.

Lactose that is not absorbed by the small intestine rapidly reaches the colon and is fermented to short-chain fatty acids and hydrogen gas, which are responsible for the ensuing symptoms. Symptoms, however, are variable and may depend on the fat content of the food, the intestinal transit time, and the composition of the colonic flora. Furthermore, short-chain fatty acids can be used up as an energy source by colonocytes, and this is one mechanism whereby individuals who are lactose deficient adapt to ingestion of lactose.

The presence of lactose intolerance is usually suggested by the patient's history, and alleviation of symptoms with lactose elimination often confirms the diagnosis. The lactose breath test is widely used as a diagnostic tool that involves measurements of hydrogen in serial breath samples after ingestion of a measured amount of lactose and has largely replaced the lactose tolerance test where serum glucose level is serially assessed after ingestion of lactose. Lactase enzyme activity can also be assessed by obtaining jejunal biopsy via endoscopy and can distinguish between primary and secondary lactase deficiency.

The treatment of choice in symptomatic lactose malabsorption is avoidance of lactose in the diet. Initial strict elimination is recommended with gradual reintroduction to work up to a tolerated limit of lactose-containing foods. Preparations containing bacterial or yeast β-galactosidases are commercially available and can be added to foods containing lactose or ingested with meals to prevent symptoms. Products containing predigested milk or other dairy substances or nondairy milk products such as almond milk are possible alternatives. Live culture yogurt, which contains endogenous β-galactosidase, is well tolerated and can be a good source of calcium. Avoidance of dairy products has been associated with low calcium and vitamin D levels; therefore these levels should be monitored and properly supplemented.

## FRUCTOSE MALABSORPTION

A quarter of the general population is estimated to exhibit varying degrees of fructose malabsorption. This should not be confused with *hereditary fructose intolerance,* in which infants develop hypoglycemia owing to a deficiency of the enzyme fructose-1-phosphate aldolase. Fructose is naturally present in fruits such as apples but can also be produced from corn and is a major ingredient in high-fructose corn syrup. Fructose is not efficiently absorbed, and the capacity of the gut to absorb fructose can be easily overwhelmed when large quantities are ingested. Unabsorbed fructose can reach the colon, where fermentation by colonic bacteria leads to abdominal symptoms. Fructose malabsorption appears to be more common in patients with functional bowel disease and can be present in up to 80% of cases. Avoidance of fructose from the diet or even reduction of intake eliminates symptoms.

## PROTEIN-LOSING ENTEROPATHY

Protein-losing enteropathy (PLE) is a condition where excess protein is lost in the GI tract, leading to hypoalbuminemia and edema with or without anasarca. This condition can be caused by a diverse group of disorders that can be classified under three broad categories as primarily erosive or ulcerative mucosal disorders, such as IBD, or graft versus host disease; nonerosive mucosal disorders, such as celiac disease or Ménétrier disease; and disorders that obstruct lymphatics, such as primary intestinal lymphangiectasias or secondary lymphangiectasias caused by right-sided heart failure or lymphatic malignancies.

The clinical presentation of PLE depends on the underlying etiology and often includes nonspecific digestive symptoms such as flatulence, bloating, diarrhea, and steatorrhea. Peripheral edema is often present, and ascites, pleural effusion, or even anasarca can develop. Laboratory features reflect the loss of protein with low levels of albumin, gamma globulin, and deficiencies in minerals bound to albumin and other carrier proteins. Clotting factors are frequently reduced, but this rarely causes complications. Lymphopenia is a common feature, and deficiencies of fat-soluble vitamins may develop. The diagnosis of PLE is established by an increase in alpha-1 antitrypsin clearance, which requires a 24-hour stool specimen and a serum sample for simultaneous measurement of alpha-1 antitrypsin in plasma. The diagnostic evaluation often includes abdominal imaging and endoscopic evaluation and echocardiogram when underlying cardiac disorder is suspected. Management is focused on correcting the underlying disease with dietary therapy containing low fat, high protein, and high medium-chain triglycerides.

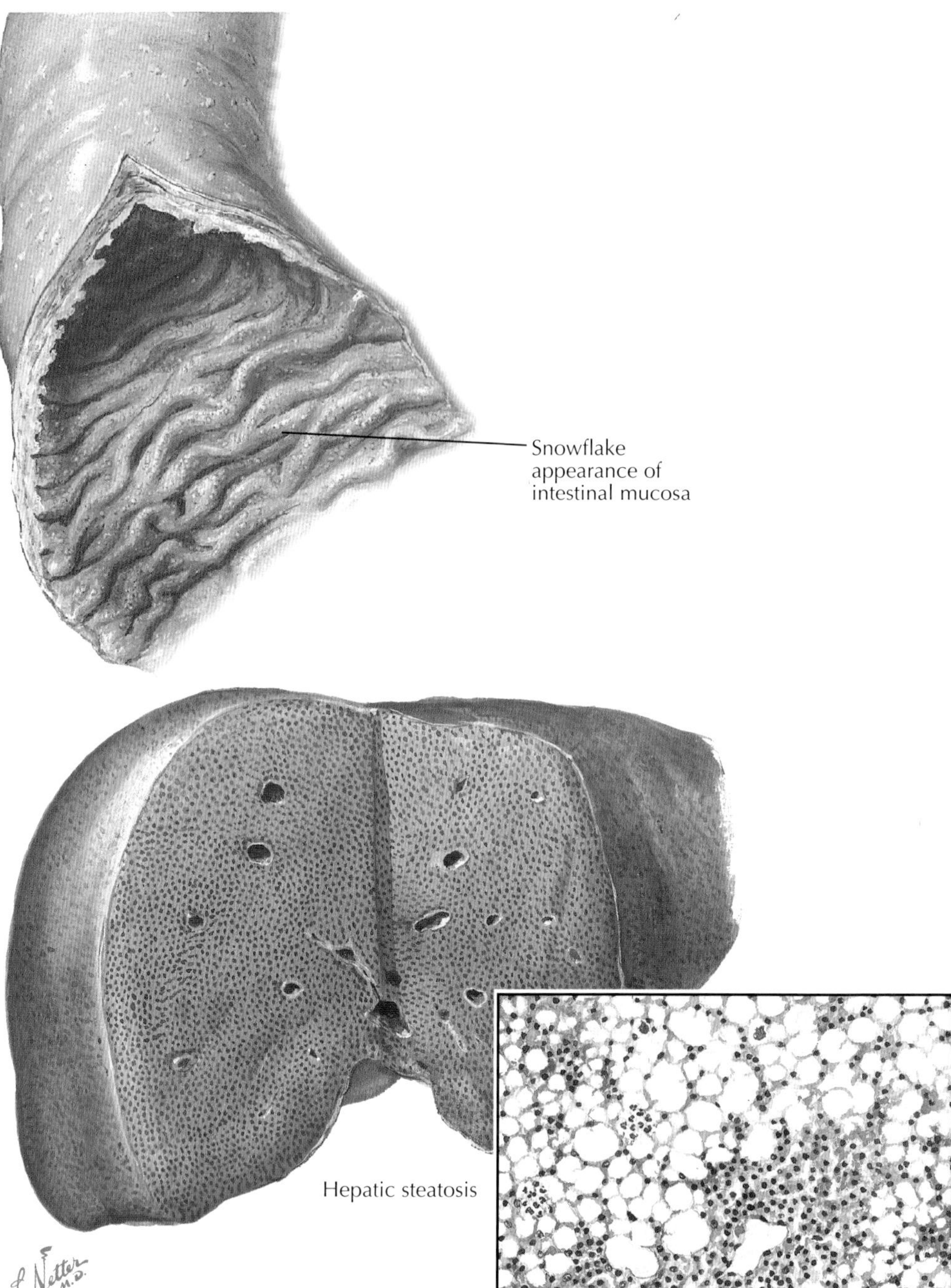


### INTESTINAL LYMPHANGIECTASIA

Intestinal lymphangiectasia is an unusual disorder characterized by dilated lymphatic channels in the mucosa, submucosa, or subserosa of the small intestine, leading to PLE. Waldman originally described an idiopathic form, *primary intestinal lymphangiectasia;* however, obstruction to the flow of lymph in certain cardiac diseases or hematologic malignant diseases and retroperitoneal lymph node enlargement due to chemotherapeutic, infectious, or toxic agents can secondarily lead to lymphangiectasias that present in the same manner as primary intestinal lymphangiectasia.

The worldwide prevalence of primary intestinal lymphangiectasia is not well known; it is more common in children but is also seen in adults. It appears to occur sporadically, but reports of familial clustering suggest an underlying genetic role. The clinical manifestations and laboratory evaluation mirror that of PLE.

CT enterography may show a characteristic *halo sign,* and MRI can also be suggestive; however, the diagnosis of intestinal lymphangiectasia is based on endoscopy findings that appear as white spots overlying the mucosa, described as a *snowflake appearance,* and is confirmed by histologic examination demonstrating markedly dilated lymphatic channels most apparent at the tips of the mucosal villi, with polyclonal plasma cells. Capsule endoscopy provides complete examination of the small intestine, but deep enteroscopy may be required to sample abnormalities detected past the duodenum.

The treatment of intestinal lymphangiectasia involves maintenance of nutrition and addressing an underlying disorder, if present. A diet rich in protein and low in fat is recommended to lessen lymphatic flow. Supplementation of medium-chain triglyceride (which is directly absorbed in the portal venous circulation, bypassing the intestinal lymphatics) provides extra energy and lessens lacteal congestion and lymph loss. In severe cases, total parenteral nutrition may be needed. Use of octreotide and tranexamic acid has been reported, and segmental small bowel resection for localized areas of lymphangiectasia may be beneficial.

### ABETALIPOPROTEIN DEFICIENCY

Abetalipoproteinemia is a rare, autosomal recessive disorder caused by a mutation in the transfer protein responsible for assembly of apolipoprotein B (apoB) and lipids in the liver and intestine. It is characterized by fat malabsorption, acanthocytosis, and hypocholesterolemia. Hypobetalipoproteinemia is another rare inherited disorder that results from improper packaging and secretions of apoB-containing lipoproteins.

Both disorders are characterized by defective secretion and transport of lipids that leads to intestinal fat malabsorption and fat-soluble vitamin deficiencies. If left untreated, they have profound consequences, including the development of retinitis pigmentosa, coagulopathy, posterior column neuropathy, and myopathy. Hepatic steatosis is also common. Clinical diagnosis is based on symptoms of chronic diarrhea and failure to thrive during infancy. Acanthocytosis on blood smear, and the virtual absence of apoB-containing lipoproteins in the case of abetalipoproteinemia, is diagnostic. Endoscopic examination performed while the patient is consuming a normal fat diet reveals a white, studded appearance of the intestinal mucosa. Histologic study of biopsied specimens shows distended enterocytes with a clarified cytoplasm that stains strongly positive with oil red O owing to the presence of intracellular neutral lipid.

The prognosis is good when the diagnosis is made early and the patient is maintained on the proper low-fat diet with adequate vitamin supplementation.

| Symptoms | |
|---|---|
| **Mucosal disease** | Abdominal pain<br>Nausea/vomiting<br>Diarrhea<br>Early satiety |
| **Muscular disease** | Intestinal obstruction<br>Pseudoachalasia<br>Gastric outlet obstruction<br>Bowel perforation |
| **Subserosal disease** | Ascites |

# Eosinophilic Gastrointestinal Diseases

Eosinophilic gastrointestinal diseases (EGIDs) are chronic, immune-mediated disorders characterized by pathologic eosinophilic infiltration of one or more layers of the esophagus, stomach, small intestine, or colon leading to clinical symptoms. Eosinophilic esophagitis is the most well-characterized EGID and has become increasingly prevalent; it is covered in another section. The other EGIDs, namely eosinophilic gastritis, eosinophilic gastroenteritis, and eosinophilic colitis, are rare and less understood.

EGID can occur at any age but appears to be more common between the third and fifth decades, and except for eosinophilic esophagitis, a male preponderance is not observed. The worldwide prevalence is not known, but hundreds of cases have been reported in the literature.

The pathophysiology of eosinophilic gastroenteritis is complex and not well understood, but several epidemiologic and clinical observations point to an allergic reaction triggered, perhaps by a food or an environmental allergen. More than half of patients have a history of asthma, eczema, or rhinitis, and peripheral eosinophilia and elevated IgE levels are seen in a significant proportion. Moreover, the role of an allergic component is further supported by the improvement seen with steroid therapy and with elemental diet.

Eosinophilic gastroenteritis commonly involves the stomach, followed by the small intestine, and is classified into different patterns based on the depth of involvement, including mucosal muscular, or serosal type.

The clinical presentation may vary, depending on the site of disease as well as the depth and extent of bowel wall involvement. The most common variety is mucosal disease, which presents with abdominal pain, nausea, vomiting, and diarrhea. Weight loss and anemia may be present with diffuse disease. Muscular infiltration presents with bowel wall thickening and impaired motility, whereas serosal disease, although rare, invariably causes ascites.

Peripheral eosinophilia is present in up to 80% of patients and is more commonly associated with muscular or serosal disease. Other laboratory features reflect fat and protein malabsorption that can develop and iron deficiency anemia with or without evidence of GI bleeding.

Imaging of the GI tract may allow detection of gastric and bowel thickening with mucosal disease or luminal narrowing with muscular involvement and ascites in serosal disease; however, these findings are nonspecific and only serve to exclude other diseases rather than confirm diagnosis of eosinophilic gastroenteritis.

The diagnosis is confirmed by the demonstration of an abnormal eosinophilic infiltrate in an endoscopically guided biopsy of the intestinal mucosa or in a laparoscopically guided full-thickness biopsy of muscular or serosal tissue. Eosinophilia is also encountered in the ascitic fluid and can be a clue to the diagnosis in cases of new-onset unexplained ascites.

**Biopsy appearance**

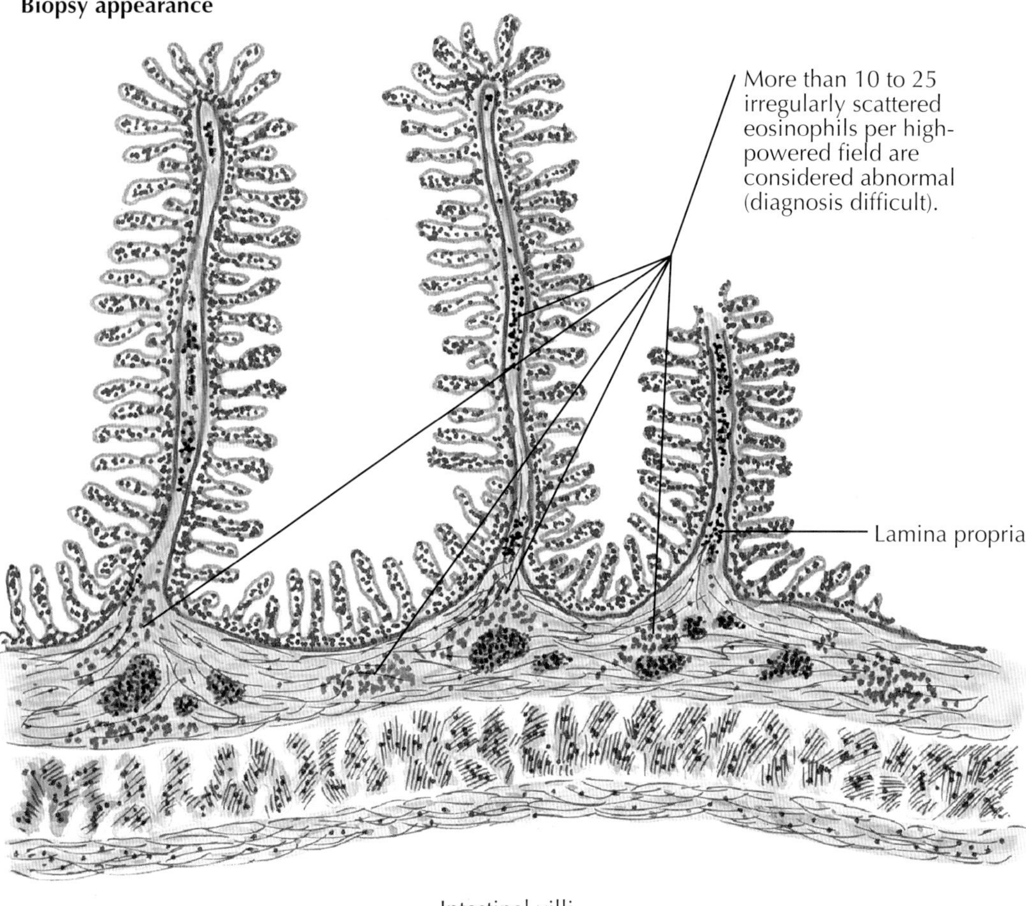
More than 10 to 25 irregularly scattered eosinophils per high-powered field are considered abnormal (diagnosis difficult).
Lamina propria
D. Mascaro

Intestinal villi

The diagnosis of primary eosinophilic gastroenteritis also requires a lack of involvement of other organs and an absence of other causes of intestinal eosinophilia, particularly drug-induced eosinophilia.

Treatment of eosinophilic gastroenteritis is limited and involves dietary and immunosuppressive therapy. A trial of a diet in which six foods are eliminated (soy, dairy, nuts, wheat, eggs, and shellfish) or an elemental diet for at least 6 weeks is recommended for the initial treatment, but patient compliance is an issue. In individuals who do not respond or who cannot tolerate dietary therapy, corticosteroid therapy is initiated. Improvement in symptoms usually occurs within a few weeks and then the dosage can be tapered; however, recurrence is common and some patients require long-term treatment. Other immunosuppressive therapies using azathioprine and monoclonal antibodies may play a role in refractory cases. Eosinophilic gastroenteritis has a chronic waxing and waning course, and most patients require close follow-up and long-term maintenance treatment of some kind.

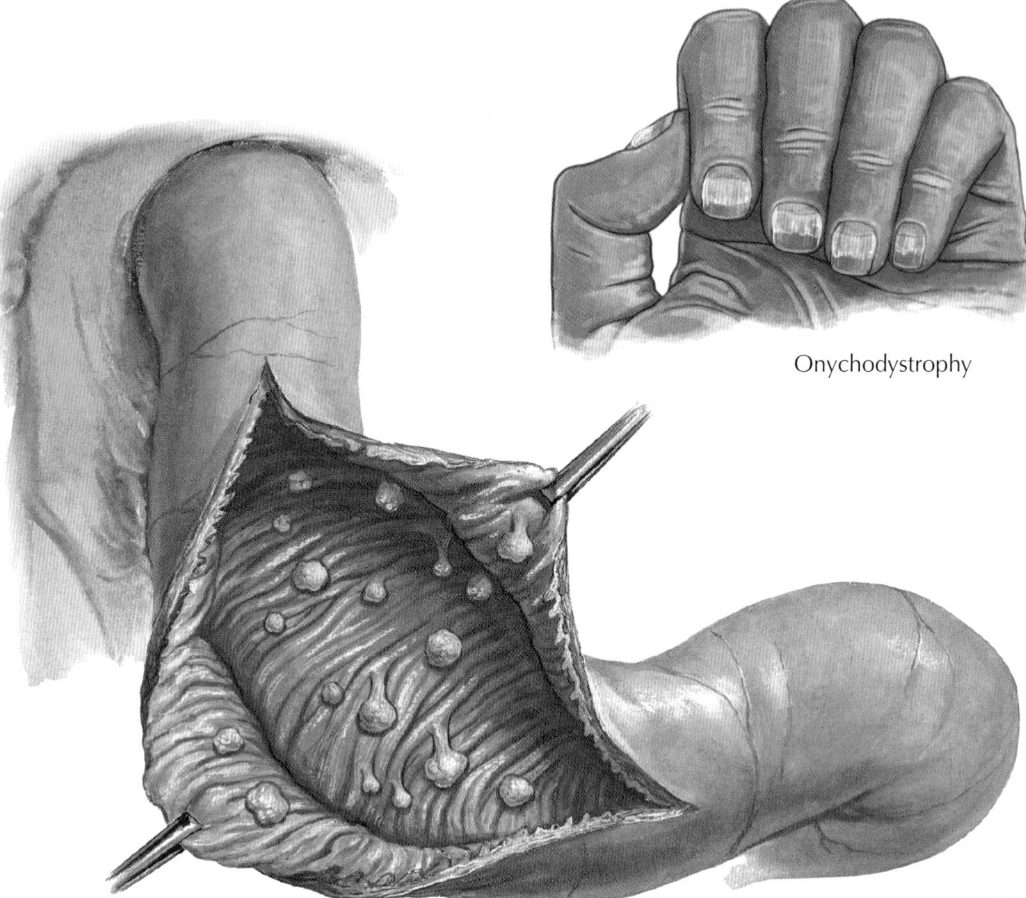


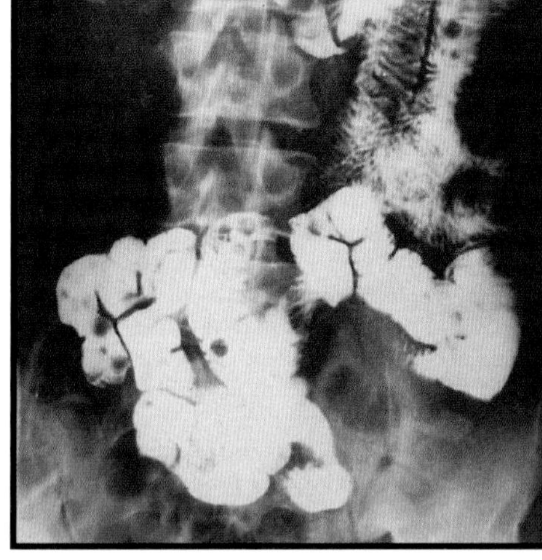

## Cronkhite-Canada Syndrome and Other Rare Diarrheal Disorders

### CRONKHITE-CANADA SYNDROME

Cronkhite-Canada syndrome is a rare, nonfamilial GI polyposis syndrome characterized by PLE and ectodermal abnormalities such as hyperpigmentation, hair loss, and dystrophic changes in the fingernails. It has been reported in all ethnic groups; however, more cases have been in individuals of European and Asian descent. The cause is not known, but the frequent association with other autoimmune diseases such as hypothyroidism, vitiligo, and systemic lupus erythematosus and the response to immunosuppressive therapy suggests an immune-mediated mechanism. The syndrome is characterized by development of innumerable polyps throughout the GI tract except in the esophagus. The polyps are hamartomas; however, there is an increased risk of colorectal cancer. Patients commonly present with diarrhea and weight loss accompanied by typical dermatologic manifestations that include hyperpigmentation and onychodystrophy. Management is largely supportive, with nutritional support accompanied by antisecretory and antiinflammatory treatment. Immunosuppressive therapy with glucocorticosteroids and azathioprine has also been reported to ameliorate symptoms, but the duration of treatment is not known and the prognosis remains poor with a 5-year mortality rate of over 50%.

### AUTOIMMUNE ENTEROPATHY

Autoimmune enteropathy is a rare malabsorptive disorder characterized by chronic diarrhea resulting from immune-mediated injury of the small intestinal mucosa. It presents more frequently in childhood but has been described in adults as well. The underlying cause is not well understood, but the disorder has frequent associations with immunoglobulin deficiencies and thymomas. The diagnosis is based on the presence of small intestinal villous blunting and circulating antienterocyte antibodies after excluding common malabsorptive disorders such as celiac disease. Immunosuppression with corticosteroids is the mainstay of treatment, and case reports suggest successful treatment with other immunosuppressive agents such as cyclosporine, azathioprine, and anti–tumor necrosis factor (anti-TNF) agents.

### DRUG-INDUCED DIARRHEA

Many medications have been implicated as a cause of chronic diarrhea with different pathophysiologic mechanisms. Certain medications can have a direct malabsorptive effect on the small bowel, as in alpha-glucosidase inhibitors (e.g., acarbose), or can alter the small bowel motility, such as selective serotonin reuptake inhibitors (e.g., sertraline). Others can lead to an enteropathy, as seen in angiotensin receptor blockers and purine antagonists (e.g., olmesartan, mycophenolate mofetil), or can promote dysbiosis (antibiotics). Diarrhea arising from small bowel disorders, from any cause, is often voluminous and watery. Weight loss may develop in severe or prolonged cases. Patients usually experience bloating and flatulence, but overt bleeding is rare. Physical examination and laboratory findings are nonspecific and reflect degree of fluid and electrolyte loss and malabsorption. Likewise, imaging is more useful to exclude the differential diagnoses such as CD. Endoscopy and small bowel histology may appear normal or reveal nonspecific findings consistent with enteropathy, often mimicking celiac disease. In the latter situation, celiac serologies and even a trial of a gluten-free diet may be necessary to distinguish between the two entities. Breath testing using a carbohydrate substrate (glucose or lactulose) can suggest small intestinal bacterial overgrowth. The diagnosis of drug-induced diarrhea is truly one of exclusion, and the history should focus on the onset and course of the diarrhea as well as medication use. Discontinuation of the offending agent is the first step in management and often leads to complete recovery. Supportive therapy to replace the fluid and electrolytes and repletion of micro- and macronutrient deficiency should also be instituted.

## Crohn's Disease

Crohn's disease (CD) is one disease in a larger group of inflammatory bowel disease (IBD) that includes ulcerative colitis and indeterminate colitis. It is a chronic, relapsing illness characterized by transmural inflammation within the digestive tract that may occur anywhere from mouth to anus, with the majority of cases involving the small bowel. It affects over 5 million individuals in the Western Hemisphere with rapidly rising incidence in newly industrialized countries in Africa, Asia, and South America.

Historically, a bimodal peak in age of onset between 15 and 40 years and 50 and 80 years has been observed in CD. Individuals of Jewish descent have a higher incidence compared with the non-Jewish population, and the incidence is lower in Black and Hispanic populations compared with White populations. There is a slight female predominance in patients who are diagnosed at an early age, which suggests a hormonal role in the pathogenesis.

Individuals with a first-degree relative with CD are up to 20 times more likely to develop the disease. Monozygotic twin studies indicate that genetics may contribute more to CD than to ulcerative colitis, with concordance rates of 50% versus 19%, respectively. Genome-wide association studies (GWAS) have been critical in identifying more than 160 susceptibility loci for inflammatory bowel disorders. Many signaling pathway defects in the innate immune system, autophagy pathway, and major histocompatibility complex have been identified as contributing to the pathogenesis. For instance, patients with CD who have a *NOD2 (CARD 15)* gene mutation exhibit a risk of ileal disease that is higher than those who lack the mutation. However, up to 20% of the general population carry this mutation and do not have underlying CD.

Indeed, there is considerable genetic variability between and within different CD phenotypes. The lack of 100% concordance in twin studies has increased inquiry into the contribution of diet and the environment to disease pathogenesis. Several studies demonstrate that Western diets high in processed foods, refined sugars, and fried foods and low in vegetables and fruits are associated with an increased risk for inflammatory bowel disorders. Whereas inflammatory bowel disorders in developing nations were rare in the past, major cities in such nations now demonstrate an increased or equal incidence of the disorders, possibly owing to expansion of Western diets into these regions. Likewise, consuming a pescovegetarian diet has been associated with a decreased trend toward flares and may thus confer antiinflammatory value.

Many of the aberrant signaling pathways elucidated through GWAS also demonstrate improper innate immune system interpretation of bacterial antigens within the intestinal lumen. Taken together, these studies suggest that individuals who are genetically predisposed may improperly interpret normal intestinal luminal antigens, made up of bacteria and/or dietary components, and instead immunologically react by increasing inflammatory cell activity within the intestine, leading to inflammatory bowel disorders.

Symptoms of CD are inherently variable, depending on the severity, location, and complications of the disease. Abdominal pain, diarrhea, lethargy, malaise, fatigue, and unintentional weight loss are common. The diarrhea is generally nonbloody, in contrast to the overtly bloody diarrhea of ulcerative colitis. In children, malabsorption from CD presents with growth failure, weight loss, or micronutrient deficiencies (vitamins A, $B_{12}$, D, and E, and zinc).

At initial diagnosis, most patients with CD will exhibit mucosal inflammatory disease. Approximately one-third of patients have focal ileal inflammation, up to 20% have colitis alone, and at least half have ileocolonic involvement. Nearly 75% to 80% of patients will, at some point, have small bowel involvement, whereas oral and duodenal lesions are present in a minority (5%–15%) of patients. One-third of patients exhibit perianal disease with or without fistulas, which may also occur further proximal in the large and small bowel, as detailed below.

Over time, uncontrolled transmural inflammation will result in fibrosis, leading to fibrostenotic (structuring) or fistulous disease. Natural history studies demonstrate that 20 years after the diagnosis of CD, more than half of patients develop a stricture more frequently

**Imaging and Regional Variations**

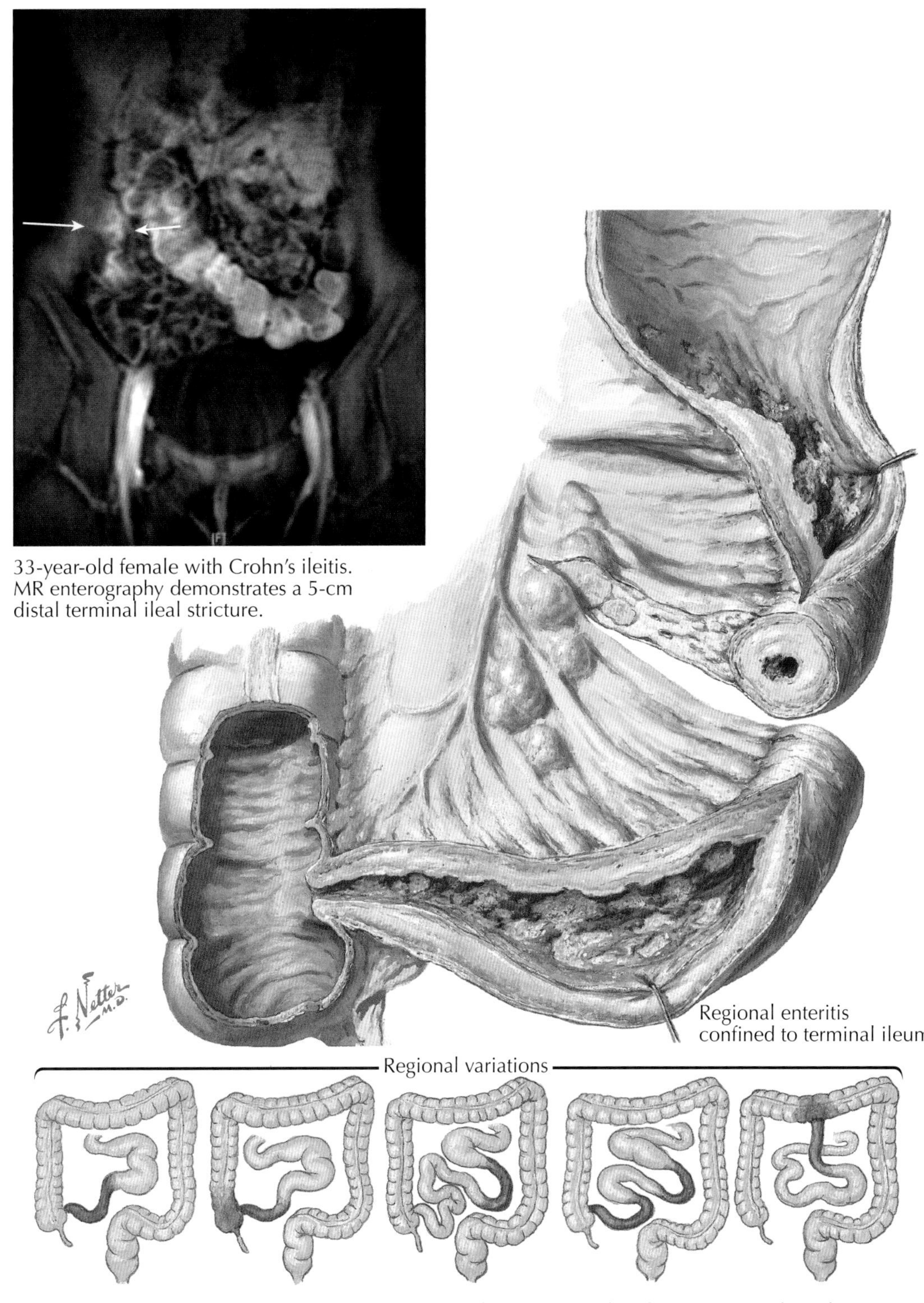


33-year-old female with Crohn's ileitis. MR enterography demonstrates a 5-cm distal terminal ileal stricture.

FISTULIZING (PENETRATING) CROHN'S DISEASE

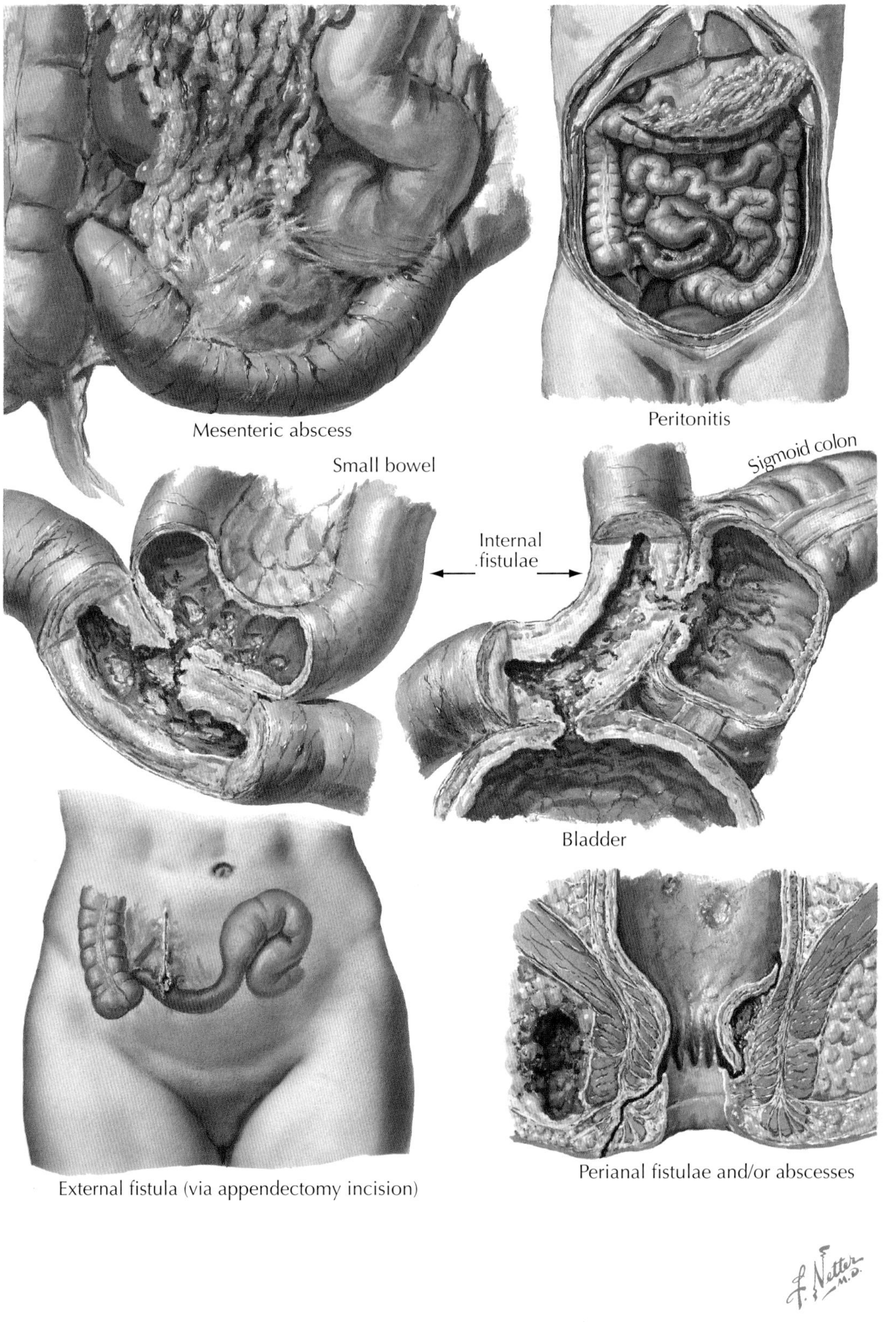

Mesenteric abscess

Peritonitis

Small bowel

Sigmoid colon

Internal fistulae

Bladder

External fistula (via appendectomy incision)

Perianal fistulae and/or abscesses

## CROHN'S DISEASE (Continued)

in the small bowel. Obstructive symptoms may ensue, or sometimes, the back pressure from stenosis may lead to the development of a secondary fistula proximal to the obstruction. Stenotic lesions may be fibrotic or inflammatory. The former may require serial endoscopic balloon dilation, whereas the latter may respond to antiinflammatory therapy. Failure to respond and/or clinical signs and symptoms of obstruction may warrant segmental bowel resection.

Approximately 20% to 50% of patients will develop predominant fistulizing (penetrating) disease. Over half of these will be perianal in location, with one-quarter characterized as enteroenteric and around 10% as rectovaginal. Notably, fistulas can extend from any loop of bowel to any other visceral, peritoneal, or cutaneous surface. This may result in simple or complex abscesses necessitating seton placement, surgery, or radiologically guided drainage. Regardless, the symptoms can be devastating and challenging to treat.

Inflammatory complications in IBD are not limited to the GI tract and are known as *extraintestinal manifestations* (EIMs). These can provide important insights, because they may precede the symptoms of a flare or herald uncontrolled disease activity.

The severity and occurrence of EIMs and their correlation with IBD activity vary. Certain conditions such as oral aphthous ulcerations, erythema nodosum, episcleritis, and pauciarticular arthritis occur directly associated with an ongoing intestinal flare, whereas other EIMs such as ankylosing spondylitis and uveitis are independent of intestinal activity.

Ophthalmic disease additionally involves keratopathy, and corneal ulcers that may require topical corticosteroids. Pulmonary involvement may be present in up to half of patients, who are often asymptomatic except for abnormal pulmonary function tests. However, interstitial lung disease, pulmonary fibrosis, and vasculitis can occur. Ileal disease promotes fat malabsorption, resulting in excess intestinal calcium reabsorption that ultimately precipitates with oxalate in the kidney, causing nephrolithiasis and pyelonephritis. Additional cutaneous lesions include pyoderma gangrenosum, Sweet syndrome, and rare primary cutaneous CD without intestinal involvement, whereas nutrient malabsorption can result in secondary cutaneous lesions, such as glossitis (with B complex deficiency) or acrodermatitis enteropathica (with zinc deficiency). Autoimmune (vitiligo) or atopic (psoriasis) lesions may also be associated with IBD. Other musculoskeletal manifestations include hypertrophic osteoarthritis with clubbing, sacroiliitis, or spondyloarthropathies. Elevated liver enzymes may herald primary sclerosing cholangitis, although this is more frequently observed in ulcerative colitis than CD.

Laboratory studies may demonstrate iron deficiency anemia from chronic occult blood loss, megaloblastic anemia from vitamin $B_{12}$ malabsorption with terminal ileitis, or anemia of chronic disease due to an inflammatory state. Serologic inflammatory markers such as the sedimentation rate and C-reactive protein levels are often elevated, although nonspecific. Elevated fecal calprotectin is more specific to intestinal inflammation; however, bacterial infections and use of proton pump inhibitors or nonsteroidal antiinflammatory drugs (NSAIDs) may falsely elevate this value. Notably, low vitamin D levels have been associated with severe disease and may have an immunologic role in disease pathogenesis.

Diagnostic imaging is a valuable tool to assess the small intestine, which is not easily accessible via endoscopy, and can identify bowel wall thickening, evidence of stricture, or bowel obstruction. Cross-sectional imaging is initially preferred, and CT scans afford excellent imaging; however, they expose patients to ionizing radiation that can increase the risk of secondary malignant disease, especially with multiple studies. For this reason, MRI is preferred when available; specifically, magnetic resonance enterography offers a highly sensitive assessment of small bowel inflammation, mucosal ulcers, luminal stricture, and fistulous disease.

Colonoscopy with intubation of the terminal ileum is the preferred study for evaluation of suspected ileocolonic CD and may demonstrate deep, cratered ulcers involving

## CROHN'S DISEASE (Continued)

the colon and ileum as *skip lesions*. Normal mucosa surrounded by inflamed and often denuded mucosa leads to a "cobblestoned" appearance, which is a classic finding in CD, and pseudopolyps signify long-standing inflammation as the natural disease activity waxes and wanes throughout life. An endoscopy and/or an enteroscopy should also be performed in individuals suspected to have proximal small bowel or gastric and esophageal involvement, and, with any endoscopic procedure, several biopsies should be obtained from abnormal and normal mucosa for histologic confirmation. Wireless video capsule endoscopy is a noninvasive test that allows visualization of the entire small bowel; however, it should be avoided in individuals with known or suspected stricture, which may lead to the capsule getting stuck and require additional endoscopic or surgical procedure to retrieve it.

The histopathology of affected mucosa demonstrates crypt abscesses and cryptitis with a focal, transmural inflammatory infiltrate of neutrophils, plasma cells, and lymphocytes within the mucosa and submucosa. Granulomas are neither necessary nor pathognomonic for diagnosis, and, when present, other entities such as tuberculosis (TB) should be excluded, especially in those with ileal disease.

The goal of therapy in luminally active CD is to control inflammation and modify the course of the disease. Systemic corticosteroids were employed in inducing mucosal remission in the past; however, the resulting steroid dependency often led to untold suffering via the consequences of chronic steroid use (e.g., infection, avascular necrosis, hirsutism, acne, adrenal insufficiency). Therefore noncorticosteroid antiinflammatory agents such as oral and rectal mesalamine were developed and were initially employed in CD and ulcerative colitis; these therapies have proven to be ineffective at inducing remission in CD, although they continue to be efficacious in ulcerative colitis. Immunomodulators such as methotrexate, azathioprine, and 6-mercaptopurine are used to maintain remission once it is achieved. Over the past two decades, enhanced understanding of the complex cascade in the inflammatory pathway has offered multiple immunologic and genetic targets and led the way to the biologic era, where several biologic antibodies have been developed to block or alter key signaling factors in the inflammatory pathway.

TNF inhibitors such as infliximab and adalimumab are well-established and effective treatment for the induction and maintenance of remission in patients with CD. The anti–alpha-4/beta-7 integrin vedolizumab and the anti–interleukin-23 agent ustekinumab are also well-studied biologic agents active against CD. More recently, small molecules, such as Janus kinase inhibitors and sphingosine-1-phosphate receptor modulators, and selective interleukin-23 antagonists have been approved for treatment of CD and offer additional modes of therapy. Another innovative and promising therapy is stem cell therapy, which may offer an effective avenue of treatment. Biologic agents alone or in combination with immunomodulators have demonstrated efficacy in inducing remission and promoting fistula closure in biologically naïve patients. Quinolone and metronidazole antibiotics are used in the setting of perianal fistulizing disease but are not intended for indefinite therapy.

Recalcitrant disease often responds to diversion via ileostomy or colostomy, resulting in mucosal healing. Surgical resection of diseased segments of intestine may improve the quality of life drastically but typically suggests the need for future surgical interventions due to recurrent disease. Hence early biologic immunosuppression is recommended to prevent insidious inflammation and consequences of recurrent disease in the form of stricture and/or fistula in the future. Tobacco use is discouraged because it increases CD flares, prevents wound healing, and can help promote the development of stricture.

Numerous quality measures have been established as goals in inflammatory bowel disorders. These include annual TB assessment, hepatitis B screening before anti-TNF induction, initiation of corticosteroid-sparing agents, prophylactic immunization (pneumococcal/influenza), bone density assessment and calcium and vitamin D supplementation, tobacco cessation education, venous thromboembolism prophylaxis, and ruling out *Clostridium difficile* infection during flares. Interdisciplinary coordination between adult and pediatric transitional providers, surgeons, social workers, dietitians, ostomy nurses, and mental health specialists optimizes the overall quality of care.

EXTRAINTESTINAL MANIFESTATIONS IN CROHN'S DISEASE

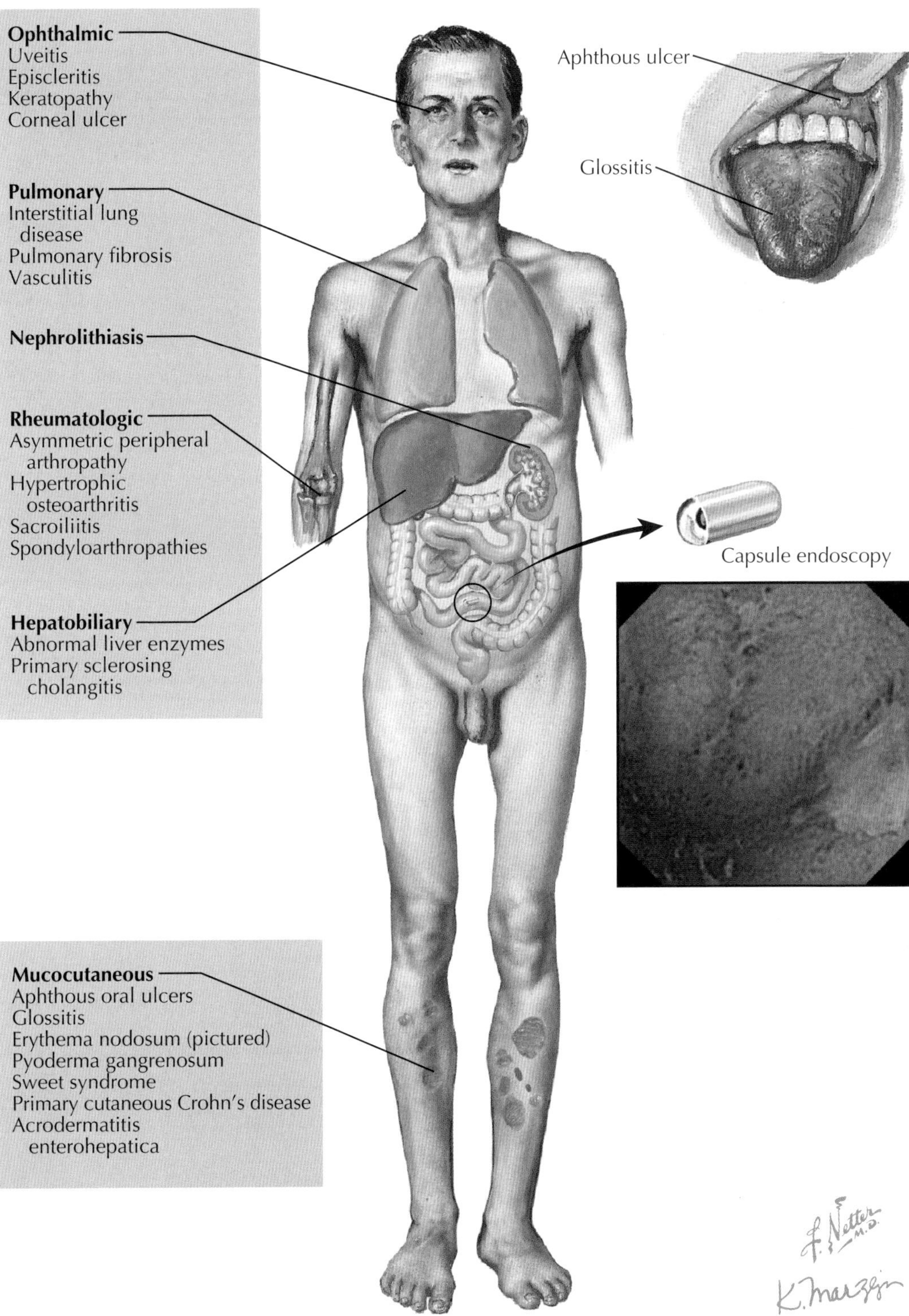

**Typhoid Fever: Transmission and Pathologic Lesions**

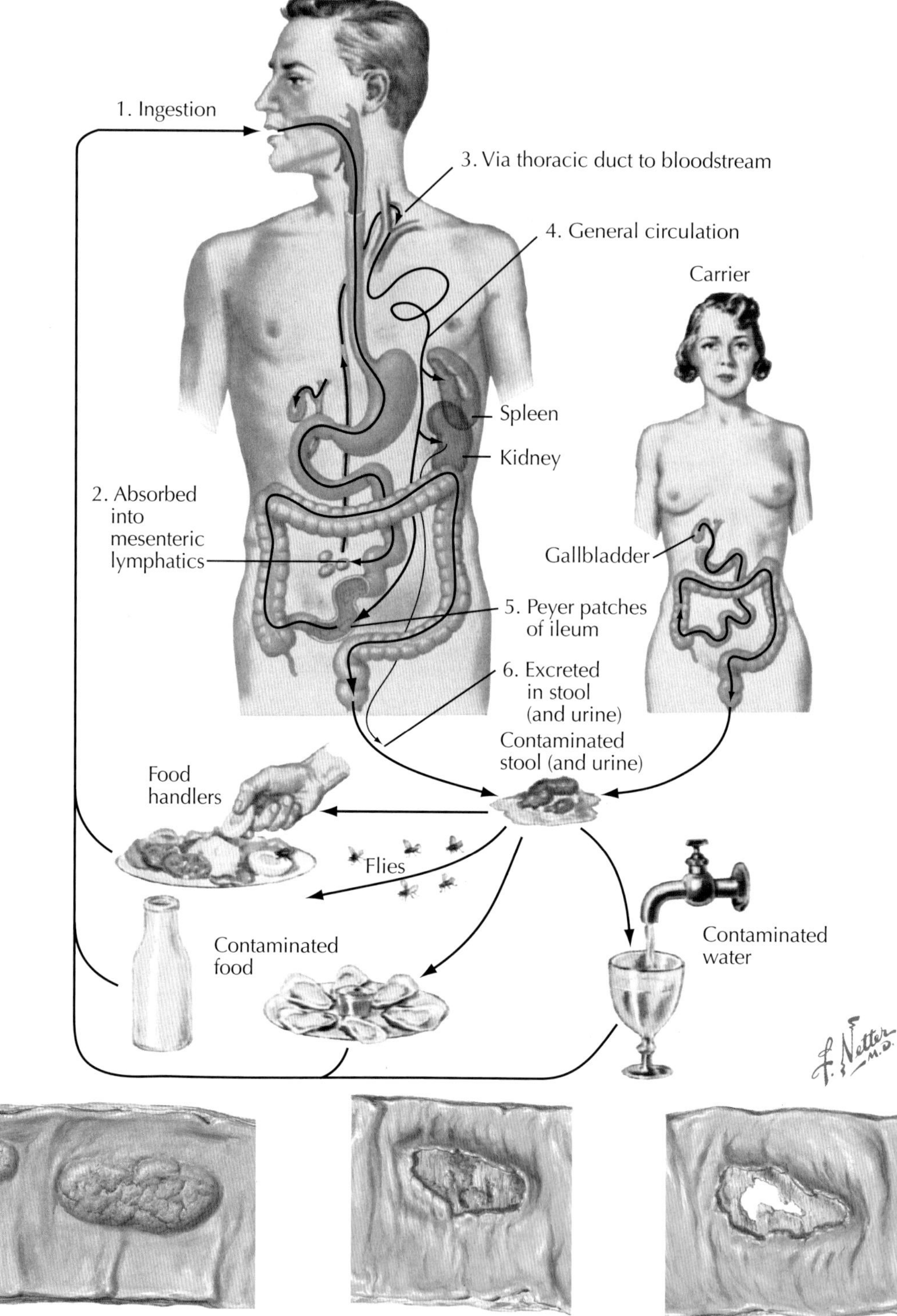


Early stage: Peyer patches of ileum swollen and inflamed

Advanced: slough cast off; ulcer base on muscularis

Perforation

## TYPHOID FEVER

In popular culture, the potential devastation of typhoid fever or enteric fever was well illustrated by the story of Mary Mallon, better known as Typhoid Mary, who was a personal chef to numerous affluent families in the greater New York City area in the early 20th century. She was an asymptomatic chronic carrier of the *Salmonella enterica serotype typhi* (previously *S. typhi*) and is believed to have caused approximately 50 deaths as she moved between families, initially unaware and later resisting to accept her role in their demise. She spent the bulk of her last 30 years of life in and out of quarantine.

Enteric fever, or typhoid fever, is a severe systemic illness characterized by fever and abdominal pain caused by *S. enterica serotype typhi.* Other *serotypes such as paratyphi A, B,* and *C* cause similar illnesses. The distinction is not relevant, however, because all are identically managed. Globally, an estimated 11 to 20 million cases and 200,000 related deaths are reported annually and are concentrated in densely populated impoverished areas with poor access to public sanitation in south central Asia; southeast Asia; southern, eastern, and western Africa; and some countries in Latin American and the Caribbean. *S. enterica serotype typhi* is uncommon in the United States, with only 200 to 300 cases reported annually. Most of these cases occur in travelers returning from endemic countries.

The organism is spread via the fecal-oral route, and optimal hygiene is paramount to preventing transmission. The organism is ingested in contaminated food or water and must survive the caustic gastric environment before invading the small bowel, where it is spread systemically via hematogenous and lymphatic routes. The higher the infectious load, the greater the symptoms.

A characteristic temporal pattern of illness then ensues. The incubation period may range from 5 to 21 days initially, manifesting with fever that can be prolonged up to 4 weeks due to bacteremia accompanied by relative bradycardia, and headache, chills, cough, myalgias, and arthralgias. During the second week of disease, submucosal tissue hypertrophy manifests as diffuse abdominal pain. Also, characteristic rose spots, described as salmon-colored macules, are distributed across the abdomen and upper torso. Dissemination during the third week manifests with hepatosplenomegaly. At this stage, progressive submucosal and lymphatic tissue hyperplasia may advance to tissue necrosis, presenting with intestinal bleeding and ileal perforation. The latter is more common in adults than children and can be potentially fatal if not promptly identified and treated. Although headache is a frequently reported symptom, nausea and vomiting, interestingly, are not. Also, individuals may experience either diarrhea or constipation with equal frequency, although this dichotomy is not clearly understood. In some cases, patients may develop delirium *(typhoid encephalopathy)*. Other extraintestinal manifestations of disease are infrequent but may include disease of the cardiovascular, respiratory, musculoskeletal, hepatobiliary, and central nervous systems and the genitourinary tract.

Even with treatment, symptoms may last for weeks to months, with 1% to 5% of individuals developing a chronic carrier state. This is defined as identification

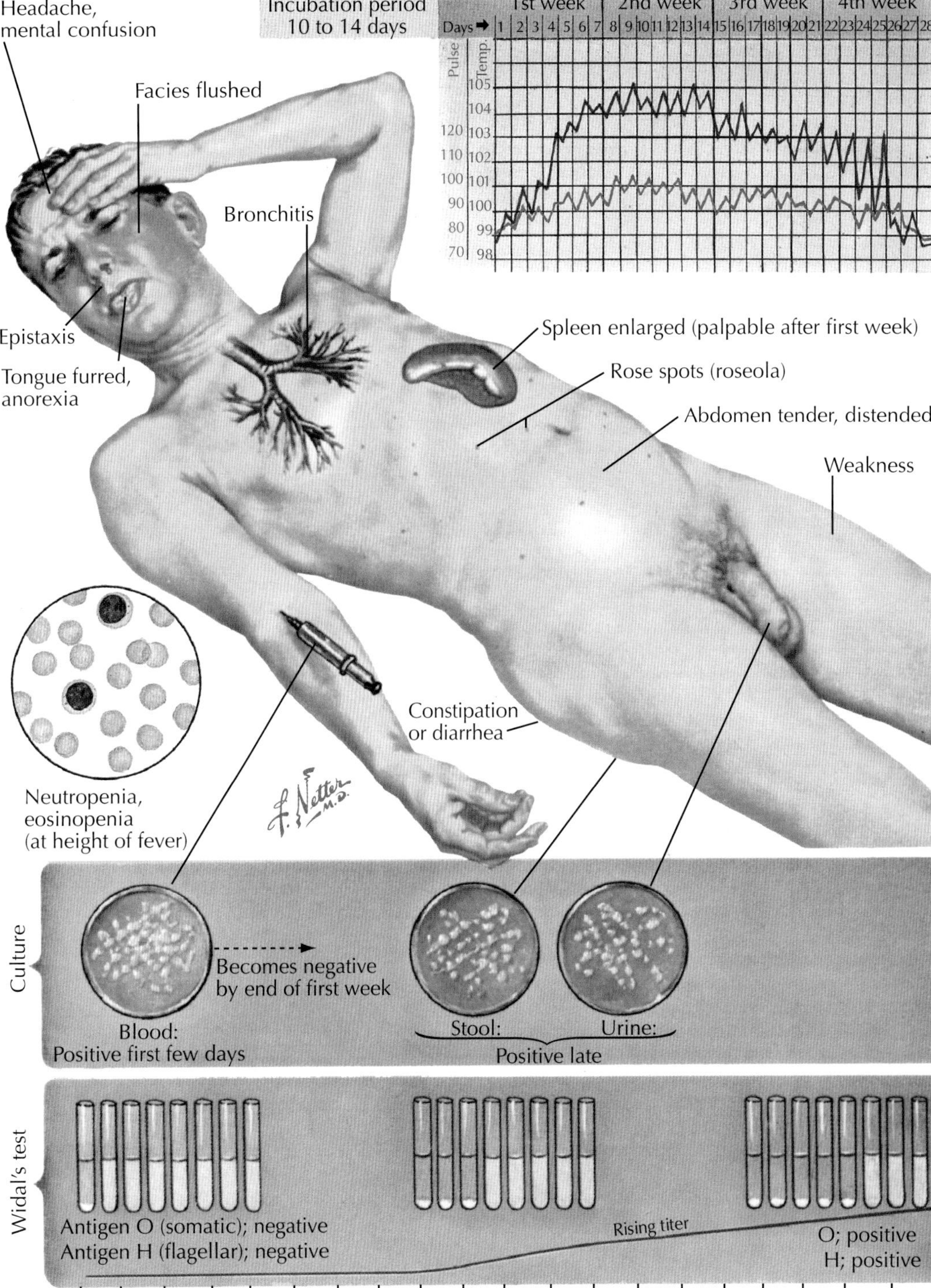


## Typhoid Fever (Continued)

of *S. enterica typhi* within urine or stool more than 12 months after established acute infection. Notably, the gallbladder is a known nidus for chronic colonization; this development may be an independent risk factor for gallbladder carcinoma. Hence individuals with recurrent infection may warrant cholecystectomy. Interestingly, *Schistosoma* bladder infection increases the risk of an *S. enterica typhi* chronic carrier state, suggesting a synergistic parasite-bacteria relationship. Mechanical defects in the genitourinary tree due to prostatic hyperplasia, urolithiasis, or stricture are also associated with a chronic carrier state. Notably, individuals with C282Y homozygous hemochromatosis are resistant to *Salmonella* infection but of course are very susceptible to infection with *Vibrio* species.

The diagnostic value of the Widal test, a serologic agglutination test commonly performed in endemic countries, suggests previous exposure rather than active infection, and more sensitive antigen and nucleic acid amplification tests have been developed. Definitive diagnosis of enteric fever requires isolation of *S. typhi* or *S. paratyphi* from the blood, bone marrow, stool, or rose spots and can also guide antibiotic selection. However, cultures may take several days to become positive. The most sensitive tissue source for diagnosis remains the bone marrow. Whereas blood cultures may return with negative results after several days of infection, bone marrow culture may be positive in up to 50% of cases. Hence the clinical history and physical examination are key to the initiation of lifesaving antibiotics.

Other diagnostic clues include the presence of leukopenia or anemia in adults; leukocytosis is more common in children during the first 10 days or may herald ileal perforation during the third week of disease. Elevated liver enzymes can often be high enough to suggest viral hepatitis, making the diagnosis challenging. CSF assays in those with mental status changes are often frustratingly normal.

In individuals who are thought to have contracted the organism in a nonendemic area, fluoroquinolones given for 7 to 10 days are a reasonable option. For individuals thought to have acquired infection from an endemic source, the culture isolates should be screened for nalidixic acid resistance, which has been associated with reduced fluoroquinolone susceptibility. In these individuals, azithromycin, beta-lactams, and chloramphenicol have demonstrated good clinical efficacy. Remarkably, relapse can occur even in healthy patients who are not immunocompromised 2 to 3 weeks after acute infection; therefore patients should be monitored closely even after they have demonstrated signs of improvement.

Two live vaccines exist, one oral and one parenteral, but neither provides protection against *S. paratyphi A* or *B*. Also, neither is completely effective at preventing *S. enterica serotype typhi* infection. Travelers to endemic regions are strongly encouraged to be vaccinated unless they are pregnant or immunocompromised. Handwashing and good hygiene and sanitation methods remain essential to preventing deadly outbreaks of infection.

# Infectious Enteritis

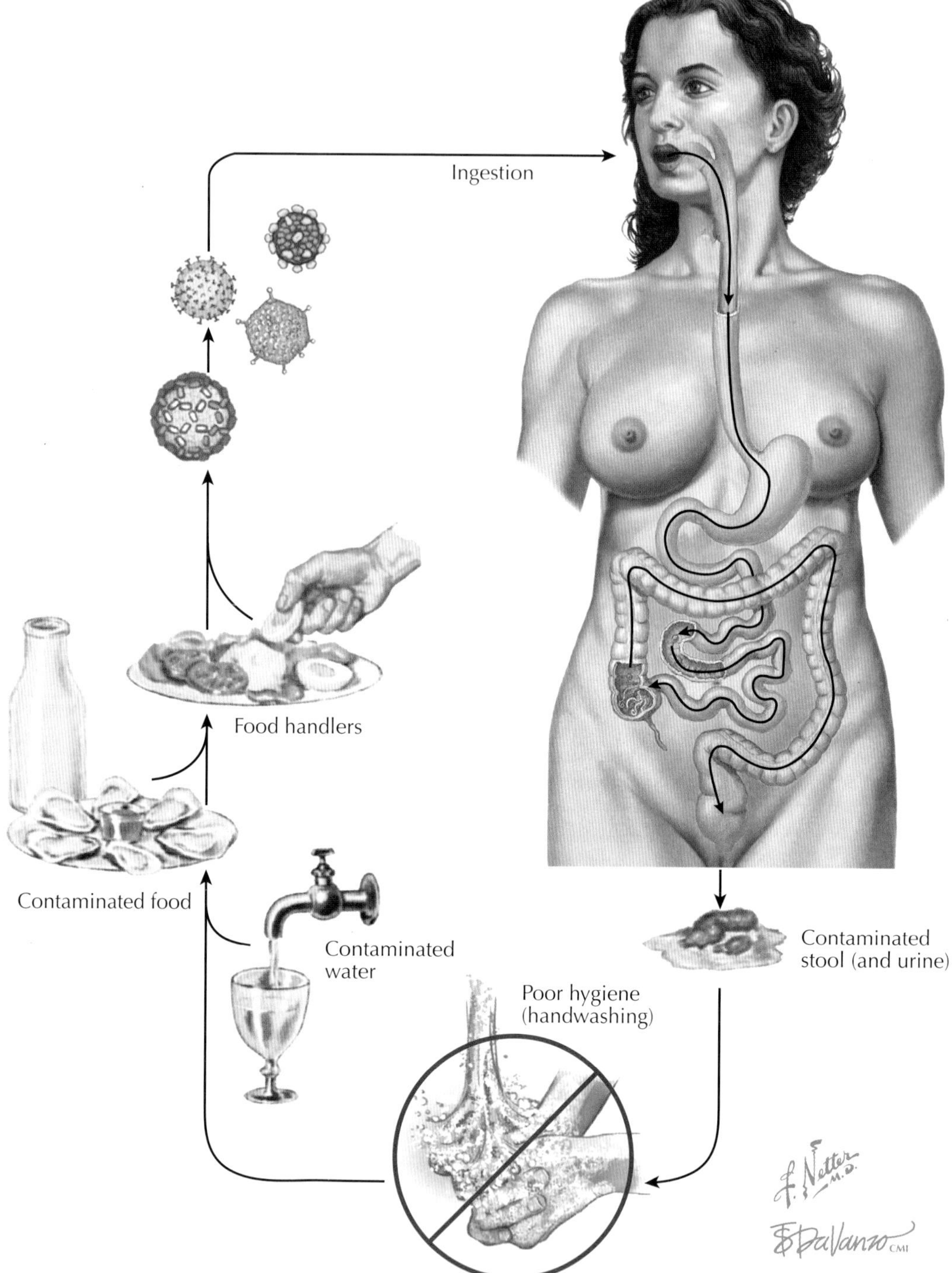


Infectious enteritis is a common worldwide illness caused by a wide variety of infectious agents including viruses, bacteria, and protozoa. The majority of infectious diarrheal diseases are acute in onset and duration (<2 weeks) and self-limiting. Globally, acute enteritis is the fifth leading cause of death across all ages. Viruses are responsible for 70% to 75% of acute diarrheal cases, bacteria cause approximately 15%, and protozoal organisms cause a lesser fraction of these cases.

In developing nations, overcrowding, poor sanitation, and a higher prevalence of HIV infections help propagate infectious causes and fuel worldwide mortality rates. In contrast, developed nations exhibit low mortality rates because medical resources are more readily available, although they still account for a significant amount of morbidity and healthcare expenditure.

## VIRAL GASTROENTERITIS

The leading cause of infectious gastroenteritis is norovirus followed by rotavirus, adenovirus, and astrovirus. Viral gastroenteritides classically exhibit short prodromes of fever, vomiting, and self-limited watery, nonbloody diarrhea. These viruses are generally spread via fecal-oral contamination. Notably, norovirus and enteric adenovirus can also be aerosolized.

Norovirus is notorious as a cause of epidemic diarrhea on cruise ships but is a factor in outbreaks in any facility in which people exist in close quarters, such as schools, hospitals, and prisons. Although the disease may occur throughout the year, a peak has been noted in the winter months. It demonstrates a short incubation period of 1 to 2 days, followed by acute onset of nausea, vomiting, and a high-volume, noninflammatory, nonbloody diarrhea. No enterotoxin unique to norovirus has been isolated, but marked jejunal villous blunting and impairment of brush-border enzymes have been observed that normalize approximately 2 to 3 weeks after the onset of symptoms. Symptoms can last anywhere from 2 to 4 days. Upon resolution of symptoms, marked reflux, dyspepsia, and, paradoxically, constipation have occurred.

Rotavirus has a minimum 2-day incubation period and specifically affects infants and toddlers, leading to severe dehydration with shedding known to last up to 2 weeks. Rotavirus can cause villous blunting with subsequent loss of brush-border enzymes (lactase, maltase, sucrase), resulting in severe osmotic diarrhea. This can stimulate an increase of intraluminal fluid secretion via the enteric nervous system and lead to electrolyte abnormalities. Transaminitis is an uncommon "red herring" feature, as also seen in celiac disease, caused by increased reabsorption via the damaged villi in the enterohepatic circulation. Diagnosis is generally a clinical decision, although assays based on PCR testing exist to identify the virus. Rare manifestations of rotavirus causing seizures and neonatal necrotizing enterocolitis have been reported. Infant rotavirus vaccination should be strictly maintained.

From over 60 subtypes of adenoviruses, the F subtype can lead to infantile gastroenteritis and rarely affects adults. The viruses may be transmitted via droplet aerosolization or fecal-oral contamination or may exist on fomites resistant to typical disinfectants. A minimum incubation period of 7 to 10 days is typical before the onset of diarrhea, which can last for 1 to 2 weeks. Antiviral agents are rarely required. In contrast to norovirus disease, vomiting is not a common feature in enteric adenovirus, which is the second most common agent, after rotaviruses, in causing acute diarrhea in children. They may be distinguished with a dedicated enzyme-linked immunosorbent assay kit.

Astroviruses generally affect children, although there have been cases in adults, in whom a much milder diarrheal presentation has been reported. The astrovirus incubates for 3 to 4 days, with diarrhea usually lasting up to 3 days. Again, PCR testing is more sensitive than immunoassays in identifying specific isolates. In acute viral gastroenteritis, the management should focus on supportive measures with aggressive IV fluid hydration and/or oral rehydration solutions (e.g., Pedialyte, coconut water, World Health Organization [WHO] oral rehydration solution). Symptomatically, antimotility agents (e.g., loperamide) and antiemetics may be used but no specific antiviral agents exist.

## BACTERIAL GASTROENTERITIS

Bacterial pathogens are abundant and should certainly be considered when the diarrhea is bloody or particularly severe with predominance of abdominal pain and volume depletion.

*Campylobacters* are gram-negative rods that are transmitted to humans in raw or undercooked food products or through direct contact with infected animals. *Campylobacter*

## INFECTIOUS ENTERITIS (Continued)

*jejuni* accounts for almost 90% of all cases of diarrheal disease. It is hyperendemic in many developing countries with the highest rates among children younger than 2 years, whereas all ages are affected in developed countries with a predilection to young children and young adults as well as those who are immunocompromised. The incubation period ranges from 1 to 7 days; often a prodrome of fever, headache, and myalgia is present 12 to 48 hours before the onset of diarrhea that varies from several loose stools to grossly bloody stools. Abdominal pain may be diffuse or localized to the right lower quadrant, simulating appendicitis. The bacteria may continue to be shed for up to 1 to 2 months after resolution of symptoms. Individuals who are immunocompromised may have local complications, including extension into cholecystitis, pericarditis, and peritonitis, or distant complications such as meningitis, endocarditis, and arthritis. Immune cross-reactivity can occur from bacteremia not only with *Campylobacter* but also *Salmonella* and *Shigella* and can lead to rare extraintestinal complications, including hemolytic-uremic syndrome, interstitial nephritis, and Guillain-Barré syndrome or its Miller Fisher variant.

Salmonellae are divided into organisms that cause typhoid fever (discussed separately) and those that do not (*nontyphoidal salmonellosis* [NTS]) and are responsible for a significant portion of gastroenteritis in both tropical and temperate climates. Five of the most common subtypes are *Salmonella typhimurium, S. enteritidis, S. Newport, S. Heidelberg,* and *S. javiana.* Infection is generally transmitted via contaminated food products of animal origin, such as egg yolks, poultry, dairy products, or undercooked ground meat; fresh produce contaminated with animal waste; and even contact with reptilian animals, such as turtles, lizards, and snakes. Centralization of food processing and widespread food distribution have contributed to *Salmonella* outbreaks that have led to mass recalls. Such outbreaks have been linked to packaged foods, ranging from peanut butter to infant formula, and to fresh produce such as tomatoes and peppers. Additionally, extensive use of antimicrobial agents in animal feed has led to antibiotic resistance to several conventional antibiotics against NTS and other enteric pathogens.

Infection with NTS results in gastroenteritis indistinguishable from other enteric pathogens. Nausea, vomiting, and watery diarrhea ensue within 2 days of exposure. Abdominal pain and fever are common, and the course is often self-limiting with symptoms usually resolving within 3 to 7 days. Rarely, diarrhea can be bloody, and patients can develop severe symptoms mimicking appendicitis or IBD. Bacteremia has been reported in less than 5% of cases, accompanied by osteomyelitis, myocarditis, endovascular infection (e.g., mycotic aneurysms), and hepatobiliary and respiratory infections. Antibiotics are not indicated unless infection is severe or complex and in fact may lead to a more symptomatic disease or prolong the carrier state. This is because *Salmonellae* have a unique ability to bypass the acidic environment of the stomach, and infection is naturally prevented by the normal enteric microbiome, which serves a protective role by competing for nutrition and villous binding sites and secreting locally toxic fatty acids and antibacterial peptides that can neutralize Salmonellae that reach the small bowel. Hence antibiotics may have a deleterious role by disrupting these protective microflorae.

### FOOD POISONING: INFECTION TYPE

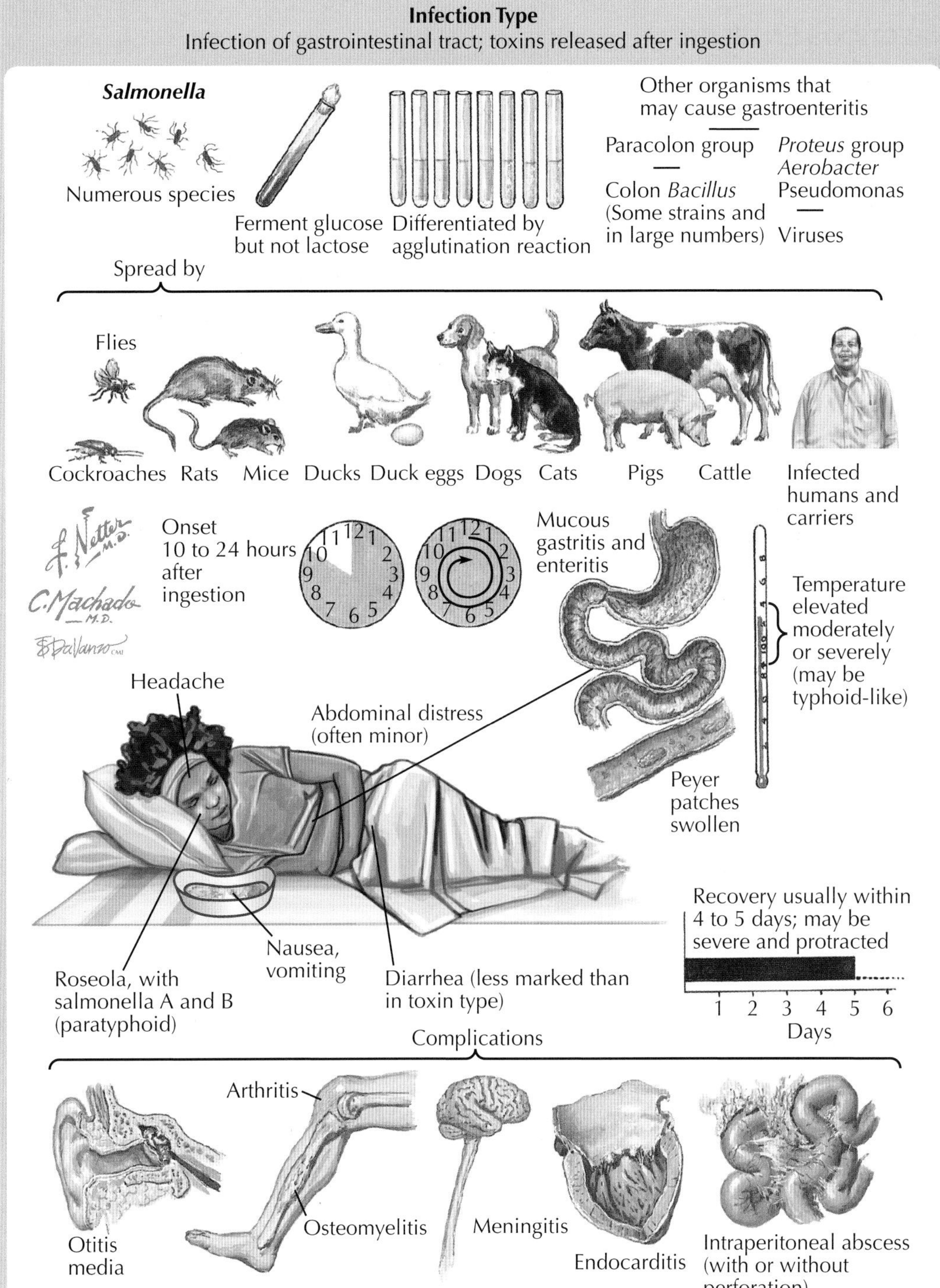


*Vibrio cholerae* and *Shigella* are common causes of diarrheal epidemics, although the latter primarily causes colitis. *V. cholerae* is the etiologic agent of cholera, a severe diarrheal disease that can result in profound fluid and electrolyte loss, hypovolemic shock, and death in a matter of hours. It is transmitted via contaminated bodies of water or feco-orally and rarely by consumption of fish and shellfish from contaminated aquatic reservoirs. It is endemic in some countries in Asia and Africa; however, epidemics and even pandemics can follow natural disasters or human conflict anywhere access to safe food, water, and basic sanitation is disrupted. *V. cholerae* is a toxin-mediated disease and possesses virulence factors allowing successful colonization of the small intestine. Once established in the small bowel, it secretes the potent cholera toxin, which leads to uninhibited adenylate cyclase stimulation and luminal chloride secretion, resulting in massive volume loss. The incubation period depends on the quantity of ingested inoculum and can range from 1 to 5 days. The subsequent voluminous diarrhea may take on the appearance of "rice water" with a malodorous, fishy odor and is often accompanied by vomiting, which can also be massive. Aggressive volume repletion is critical, without which severe dehydration, acidosis, and shock quickly ensue. *V. cholerae* responds well to fluoroquinolones, macrolides, and tetracycline antibiotics.

## INFECTIOUS ENTERITIS (Continued)

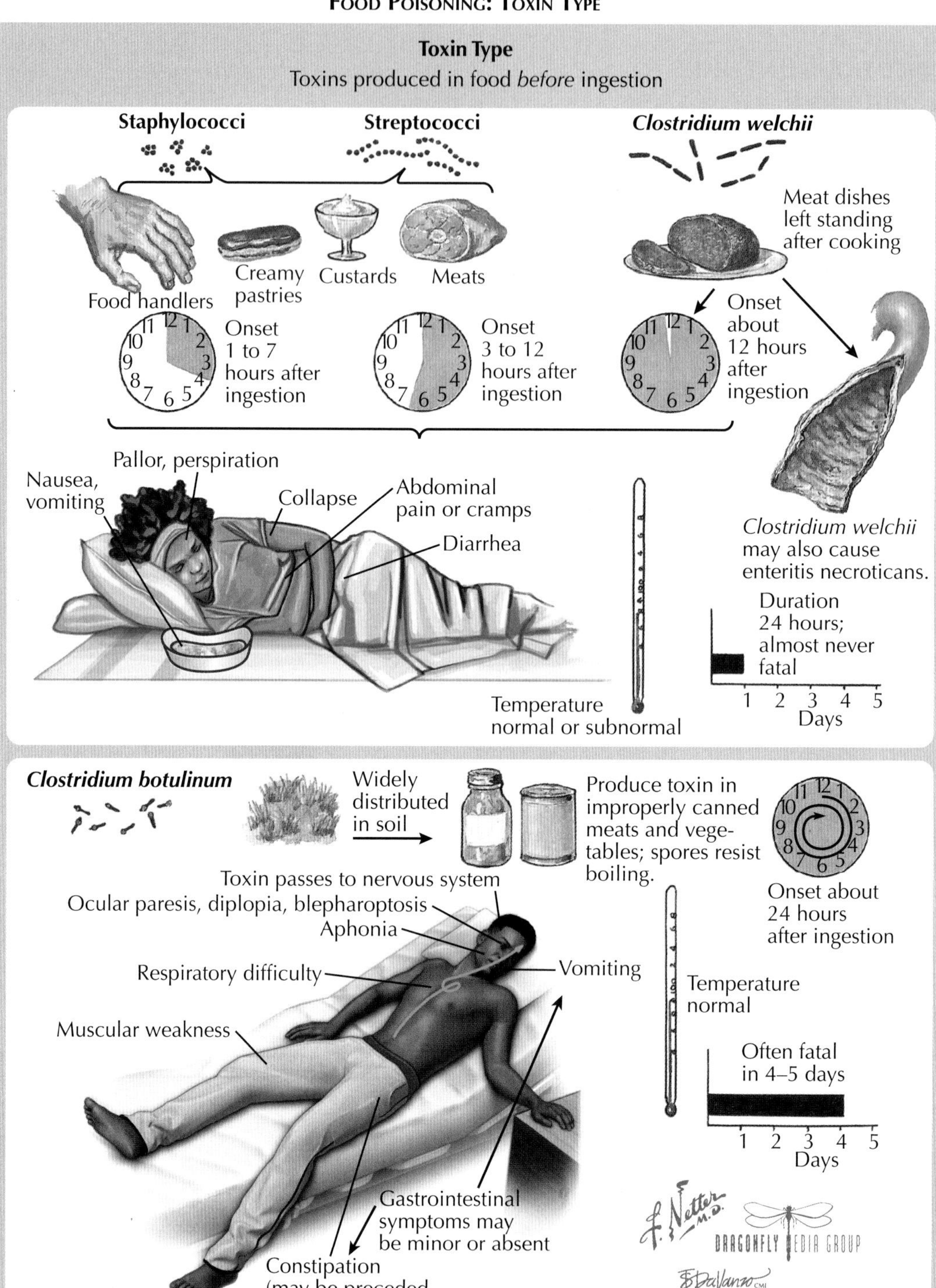


*Escherichia coli* is a gram-negative rod with >2000 strains, five of which are distinct intestinal subtypes responsible for diarrheal disease. *Enterotoxigenic E. coli* (ETEC) is a major cause of endemic diarrhea in least developed countries and the most predominant cause of traveler's diarrhea. After a brief incubation period, watery diarrhea develops and lasts 1 to 7 days. ETEC produces a heat-labile toxin (LT-1) and a heat-stable toxin (STa) and a net movement of fluid into the lumen via activation of adenylate cyclase (LT-1) and/or guanylate cyclase (STa) in the jejunum and ileum. *Enteropathogenic E. coli* (EPEC) primarily infects young children, including neonates, and breastfeeding seems to be protective. Rather than secreting toxins, this subtype directly adheres to the enterocyte, producing proteins that change signal transduction within the cell. This intracellular cascade changes intercellular and tight junction permeability, increasing electrolyte and water secretion into the lumen and producing watery diarrhea, often containing mucus but no blood. PCR assays can assess for ETEC toxin genes and the EPEC adherence factor gene. *Enteroaggregative E. coli* is a cause of diarrheal outbreaks in both developing and developed nations and contributes to traveler's diarrhea. It is exhibited to have a pattern of adherence in tissue culture adherence assays and elaborates a unique cytotoxin that causes mucosal tissue disruption and promotes mucosal spread. *Enterohemorrhagic E. coli* belongs to a group of pathogens that can cause hemorrhagic colitis and the hemolytic uremic syndrome, of which *O157:H7* is the most prominent serotype; *O104:H4* has been responsible for outbreaks. It is commonly transmitted via contaminated beef and fresh produce. The ability to produce Shiga toxin belies its pathogenicity. It may begin as nonbloody diarrhea but evolves into hemorrhagic enteritis and colitis. The ensuing inflammatory cascade can precipitate a microangiopathic hemolytic anemia and acute kidney injury known as *hemolytic-uremic syndrome.* This may not occur until 7 to 10 days after the bacteria have been naturally cleared by the immune system; this fact explains the ineffectiveness of antibiotics in ameliorating this condition. Antibiotics may even precipitate hemolytic-uremic syndrome and are generally avoided. *Enteroinvasive E. coli* is an uncommon cause of diarrhea in children and travelers, with self-limited symptoms lasting 7 to 10 days. It initially causes secretory small bowel diarrhea and may progress to an inflammatory colitis picture with abdominal pain, fever, and dysentery.

*Aeromonas* species are associated with diarrheal disease that ranges from watery, secretory choleretic-like diarrhea to bloody dysenteric-like diarrhea with mucus. *Aeromonas* can grow on routine microbiologic media cultures using specific identification protocols. Most cases are self-limited, and treatment is generally supportive with no need for antibiotics. When clinically indicated, fluoroquinolone and trimethoprim-sulfamethoxazole are generally effective. If the infection is acquired abroad, regional resistance patterns vary, and drug susceptibility testing becomes important.

Organisms such as *Staphylococcus aureus* and *Bacillus cereus* each possess a preformed toxin that causes gastroenteritis. *S. aureus* may contaminate dairy products, eggs, meat, and produce; when these foods are left at normal room temperature, bacteria may rapidly proliferate and synthesize the toxin. After ingestion, nausea, severe vomiting, and abdominal pain begin within 1 to 6 hours and resolve spontaneously over 24 hours. *B. cereus* also produces an enterotoxin commonly found in leftover or "take-out" rice that leads to symptoms and illness pattern similar to *S. aureus.*

### COMMON PROTOZOAL INFECTIONS

Protozoal causes of acute enteritis include *Cryptosporidium, Giardia, Cystoisospora, Microspora,* and *Cyclospora. Cryptosporidium* and *Giardia* are the most common protozoal enteric parasites. *Cryptosporidium hominis* is an *intracellular* protozoal parasite that causes a self-limited diarrhea in healthy hosts but can have a chronic and severe pattern in patients who are immunocompromised (especially those with AIDS) and may invade the hepatobiliary tree and cause symptoms of hepatitis, pancreatitis, cholecystitis, or cholangitis. Contaminated drinking water or recreational pool water commonly acts as a reservoir for transmission. Person-to-person transmission takes place feco-orally among household members or via anal-oral intercourse between partners. The life cycle involves liberation of sporozoites from excystation, which then infects small

## INFECTIOUS ENTERITIS (Continued)

intestinal epithelium and reproduces via asexual and sexual modes, after which new oocysts are passed in the feces. Symptoms begin after an incubation of 1 to 2 weeks with watery diarrhea, abdominal cramping, nausea, and fatigue that generally subside within 2 weeks. Because of the need for multiple samples, immunoassay has supplanted microscopy as the test of choice for its ease of use and convenience. Nitazoxanide is generally effective at clearing the infection except in patients with AIDS, in whom immune reconstitution with antiviral therapy is necessary to help clear the infection. *Giardia* infection is discussed separately.

*Cystoisospora belli* (formerly *Isospora belli*) is an opportunistic protozoan that exists as a sporulated oocyst in fecally contaminated food and water supplies. The microbes must exist outside the host to undergo successful sporulation after 1 to 2 days. Upon ingestion, the sporulated oocysts invade the small and large bowel epithelial cells to complete their life cycle and thereafter be released into the host lumen. Intestinal biopsies reveal an inflammatory infiltrate, blunted villi, and crypt hyperplasia. Stool microscopy will demonstrate thin-walled ellipsoidal oocysts. The course is typically self-limited in immunocompetent hosts, but the secretory diarrhea that results can cause significant dehydration, with prerenal kidney injury and electrolyte abnormalities. Treatment is reserved for individuals with severe dehydration, unrelenting disease, or immunocompromised state; a course of 7 to 10 days of trimethoprim-sulfamethoxazole is generally effective.

*Microsporidium* is a poorly understood intracellular spore-forming organism, with over 1300 species identified. *Enterocytozoon bieneusi* and *Encephalitozoon intestinalis* are the most common species causing infection in humans, particularly those with AIDS. Spores have been observed in respiratory, fecal, and urine specimens and may be inhaled or ingested. Intestinal symptoms include watery diarrhea, nausea, fever, and abdominal pain. Extraintestinal infection of the brain, eyes, and muscles has been reported in healthy patients, with severe presentations in AIDS. The diagnosis can be confirmed with detection of microspores in small bowel biopsy, stool, or body fluids. Most infections will respond to a short course of albendazole except *Enterocytozoon bieneusi,* which may require a macrolide or tetracycline.

*Cyclospora cayetanensis* is an obligate intracellular parasite that is passed in a noninfective state in the stool and is only known to be pathogenic in humans. *C. cayetanensis* awaits in hot, humid climates to undergo sporulation. Hence an increased incidence in tropical climates such as those of southeast Asia, India, and Latin America is observed. Once the organism has sporulated, its ingestion in contaminated water or foodstuffs leads to excystation within the intestinal tract and the release of sporozoites, which infiltrate the epithelial cells where they undergo replication. Acute watery diarrhea, fatigue, anorexia, and weight loss are common. Stool microscopy will identify the oocysts, which may be indistinguishable from *Cryptosporidium,* except for *Cyclospora, which* is almost double the size of *Cryptosporidium.* A short course of trimethoprim-sulfamethoxazole or nitazoxanide results in prompt diarrheal resolution.

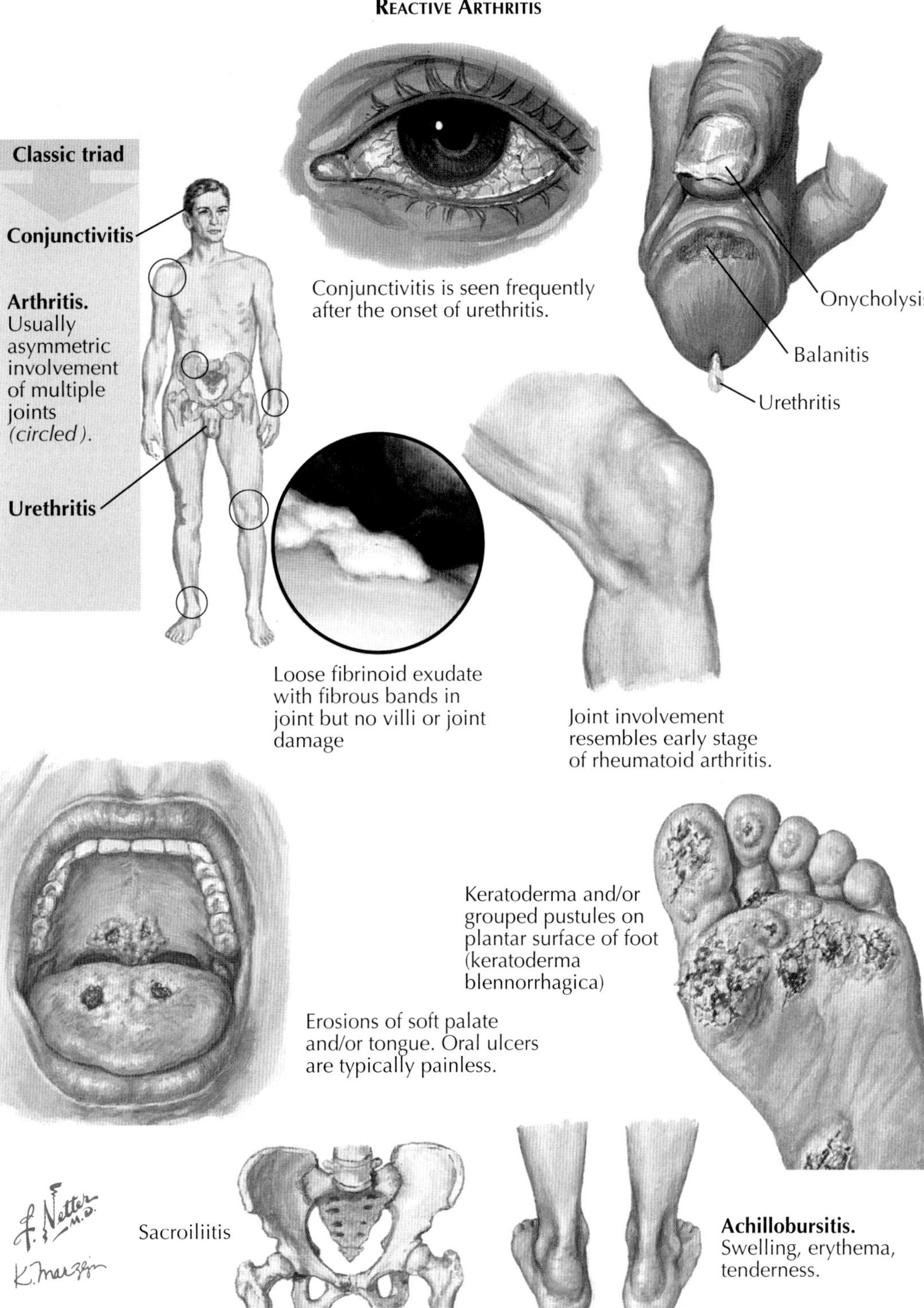


It is worthwhile to note that some bacterial (e.g., *Salmonella, Campylobacter*) and protozoal organisms *(Giardia, Cryptosporidium)* may lead to acute persistent (2–4 weeks) and even chronic diarrhea (>4 weeks) and should be considered in the differential diagnosis, especially in immunocompromised populations. The diarrhea in these cases may also result from a postinfectious irritable bowel syndrome, although this is often a diagnosis of exclusion.

Standard cultures will not detect all pathogens and only test for the most common bacterial causes of enteritis, such as *Campylobacter, Salmonella,* and *Shigella.* Instead, careful history taking and an understanding of the risk factors for these pathogens are required to direct assessment for the appropriate organisms by the microbiology department. PCR testing and immunoassay have made detection much easier. However, some organisms still require multiple stool microscopy specimens to ensure detection. Assessment of ova and parasites need not be ordered routinely but should be reserved for the clinical settings where the patient may be immunocompromised, immunosuppressed, or chronically ill.

Prevention is key in many of these illnesses. It begins with promoting adequate breastfeeding to ensure maternal-infant transfer of immunoglobulins. Availability of safe drinking water, modern sanitation, and frequent handwashing can reduce fecal-oral transfer of many of these illnesses.

## HIV/AIDS ENTEROPATHY

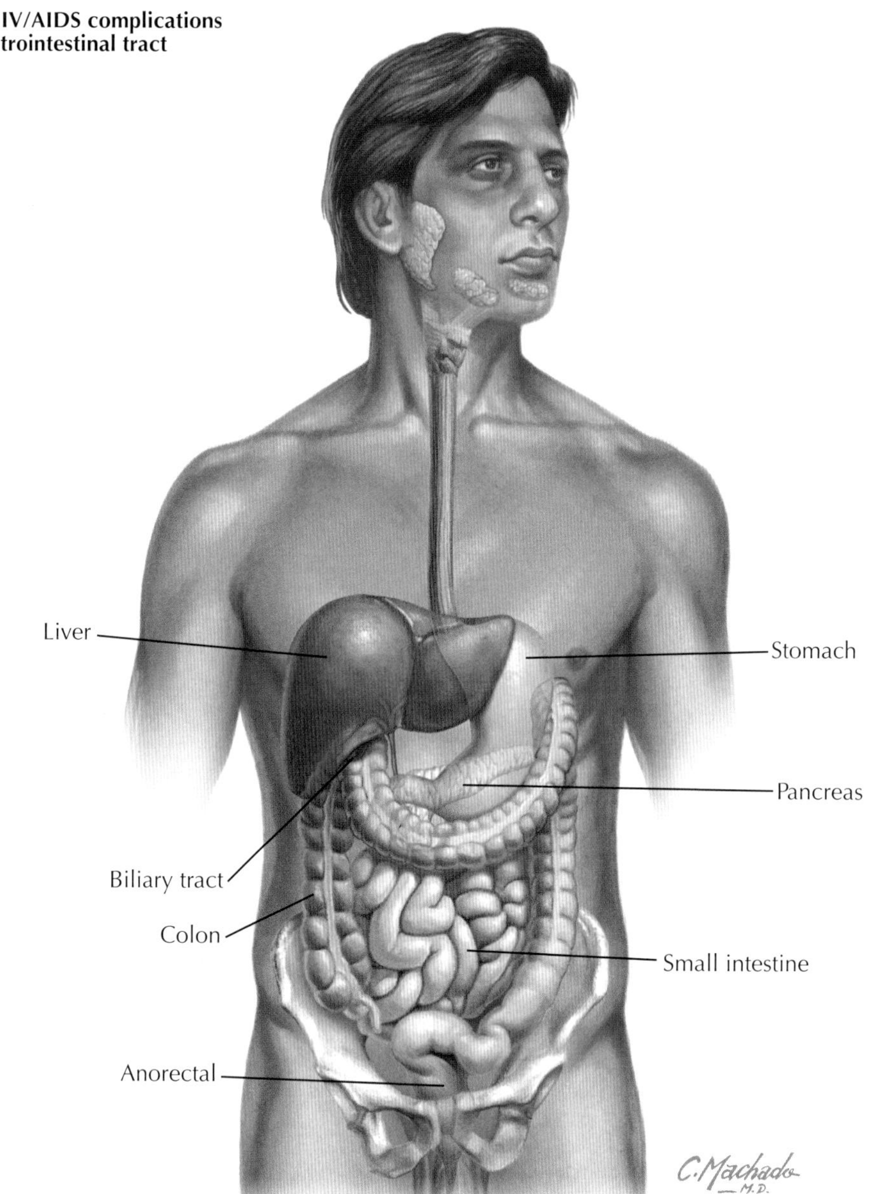


Diarrhea is reported in over half of patients who are infected with HIV, yet a distinct cause such as infection, malignancy, or medication is identified in only two-thirds of these cases. A portion of these idiopathic cases may be attributed to HIV enteropathy, which is characterized by chronic diarrhea lasting more than 4 weeks and accompanied by malabsorption and abdominal discomfort. As is characteristic of small bowel diarrhea, stools are typically voluminous and may occur postprandially. There may be marked electrolyte disturbances, severe dehydration, and unintentional weight loss.

The mechanism by which HIV exerts its effect remains unclear and may involve effects of the virus on the GI tract and the gut-associated lymphoid tissue (GALT). Mucosal biopsies demonstrate an increase in stem cells leading to crypt hyperplasia with encroachment of crypt cells into the villi, causing a decrease in the surface area–to-volume ratio. HIV may cause a transient decrease in the activity of several brush-border enzymes, including lactase activity, as well as diminished sodium/glucose cotransporter activity, causing carbohydrate malabsorption. Together these suggest an osmotically mediated mechanism at play. Additionally, a profound decrease in $CD4^+$ T lymphocytes is observed within the lamina propria and Peyer patches within GALT, which is responsible for the defense against intestinal pathogens and the development of tolerance to food antigens and normal commensal microbiota. In vitro studies have demonstrated a delay in epithelial cell differentiation, which may contribute to tight junction disorganization and a *leaky gut phenomenon,* which may promote microbial translocation across the intestinal wall. Also observed are elevated levels of plasma lipopolysaccharide, an endotoxin produced by bacteria in the serum of patients with HIV, creating a proinflammatory state that stimulates immune activation and perpetuates chronic inflammation.

HIV enteropathy is a diagnosis of exclusion; therefore initial stool assessment should include routine stool culture and testing for *C. difficile* infection. Stool analysis for ova and parasites should be performed on at least three stool samples separated by at least 24 hours, with additional assays for *giardiasis* and *cryptosporidiosis.* Anal receptive intercourse increases the risk for the latter as well as other sexually transmitted diseases such as *Chlamydia* and *Neisseria gonorrhoeae,* which can lead to proctitis characterized by urgency, tenesmus, and bloody diarrhea. In the presence of AIDS, additional specific tests should be considered, including *Microsporidium, Cystoisospora, Cyclospora, Mycobacterium avium complex,* and *Entamoeba histolytica.* Viruses such as adenovirus, echovirus, and cytomegalovirus are found with increasing frequency in patients with HIV. Candidal overgrowth is rare but has been reported in the literature, and other fungal infections should be ruled out (see table at right).

If laboratory or stool testing is nonrevealing, endoscopic evaluation is warranted. The mucosa often appears normal; therefore multiple biopsies should be obtained from the duodenum, ileum, and colon. If inflammation or focal lesions are observed, staining for acid-fast bacilli should be performed to exclude the great masquerader, *Mycobacterium tuberculosis.* Rarely, intestinal Kaposi sarcoma or lymphoma may be discovered. In the event of a negative work-up, careful attention should be focused on the individual patient's antiretroviral therapy regimen. Multiple protease inhibitors have demonstrated diarrhea as a potential adverse reaction that is reversible upon drug withdrawal.

**Differential Diagnoses of Diarrhea in HIV Enteropathy**

| Bacterial | Protozoal | Viral | Fungal | Intestinal neoplasm | Drug-induced diarrhea |
|---|---|---|---|---|---|
| *Campylobacter*<br>*Salmonella*<br>*Shigella*<br>*Clostridium difficile*<br>*Mycobacterium avium-intracellulare* (MAI)<br>*Mycobacterium tuberculosis* | *Entamoeba histolytica*<br>*Cyclospora*<br>*Cystoisospora belli*<br>*Cryptosporidium*<br>*Giardia lamblia*<br>*Leishmania donovani*<br>Microsporidium | Enteric adenovirus<br>Norwalk virus<br>Rotavirus<br>Cytomegalovirus (CMV) | *Candida albicans*<br>Coccidiomycosis<br>Histoplasmosis | Kaposi sarcoma<br>Lymphoma | Didanosine<br>Pentamidine |

The cornerstone of treatment in HIV enteropathy remains antiretroviral therapy to manage the underlying viral infection. Supportive measures to replace the volume and electrolytes are equally important, as is nutritional therapy. Lactose avoidance and fiber supplementation may lessen diarrheal losses and frequency; symptomatic control with antimotility agents such as loperamide, diphenoxylate with atropine, or codeine phosphate may also prove useful. Crofelemer, a novel chloride secretion antagonist, has demonstrated a decrease in noninfectious secretory diarrhea in patients with HIV. Limited data exist regarding the use of octreotide for this population.

Ultimately, HIV enteropathy diagnosis demands careful scrutiny of the patient's clinical history, individualized risk factors, laboratory studies, stool studies, and medications. Immune reconstitution will help ameliorate the condition.

## Posttransplant Lymphoproliferative Disorder

Solid-organ and allogeneic hematopoietic cell transplantation have revolutionized the ability to treat disease; however, the obligatory immunosuppression has several negative consequences, one of which is an increased frequency of early onset malignancies. *Posttransplant lymphoproliferative disorder* (PTLD) is one such entity, referring to a group of primarily B-cell–mediated lymphoid and/or plasmacytic cell proliferations that have the potential for malignant transformation. PTLD accounts for only a minority of cancers seen after hematopoietic cell transplantation but has emerged as the most common cause of malignancy after solid-organ transplantation. The risk is highest in the first year and then drops significantly, but it remains a significant cause of early graft failure and death.

Genetic, immunologic, morphologic, and clinical factors are used to identify three subtypes of PTLDs: (1) *plasmacytic hyperplasia and infectious mononucleosis-like PTLD,* (2) *polymorphic PTLD,* and (3) *monomorphic PTLD.* Epstein-Barr virus (EBV) has been implicated in most of these malignant diseases, a fact that highlights the risk of T-cell immunosuppression.

Mononucleosis caused by EBV is normally characterized by a polyclonal B-cell proliferation, which is held in check by T-cell suppressor cells. By downregulating antigenic expression, some B cells evade T-cell suppression and can lay dormant throughout life until a period of immunosuppression.

In patients who have undergone solid-organ transplant, recipient T cells are inhibited by calcineurin inhibitors, promoting dormant B-cell proliferation. In allogeneic hematopoietic cell transplant recipients, the T cells are inhibited by administration of antithymocyte globulin and other cytotoxic agents. Interestingly, most allogeneic hematopoietic cell transplant PTLDs are derived from donors positive for EBV, which had been dormant in the donor until the time of transplant, after which T-cell inhibition allows B-cell expansion.

*Plasmacytic hyperplasia and infectious mononucleosis-like PTLD* can occur early in the course after transplant with a viral prodrome of fever, fatigue, and weight loss, much like that of infectious mononucleosis. No atypical architectural distortions are demonstrated on histologic studies. Symptoms may resolve with time as immunosuppression is slowly reduced and the recipient recovers from the initial transplantation.

*Polymorphic PTLDs* do not meet all the criteria for malignant lymphoma but can demonstrate malignant transformation. They commonly present with complications of a focal mass effect, such as bowel obstruction, lymphadenopathy, or focal lesions.

*Monomorphic PTLD* generally presents as disseminated malignant lymphoma of which the majority are non-Hodgkin lymphomas of B-cell origin. Clinical presentations mirror those with indolent or aggressive disease.

In patients undergoing solid-organ transplant, PTLD arising from the donor is generally focused within the allograft tissue and presents a great risk for allograft dysfunction and/or loss. However, when the PTLD arises from host tissue cells, distant organs such as the skin, liver, or lung or the CNS are typically involved.

Up to 95% of the general population are positive for EBV, accounting for most cases of PTLD. However, EBV-negative PTLD has been documented in up to 30% of patients, which represents genetically and immunologically distinct tumors that are poorly understood.

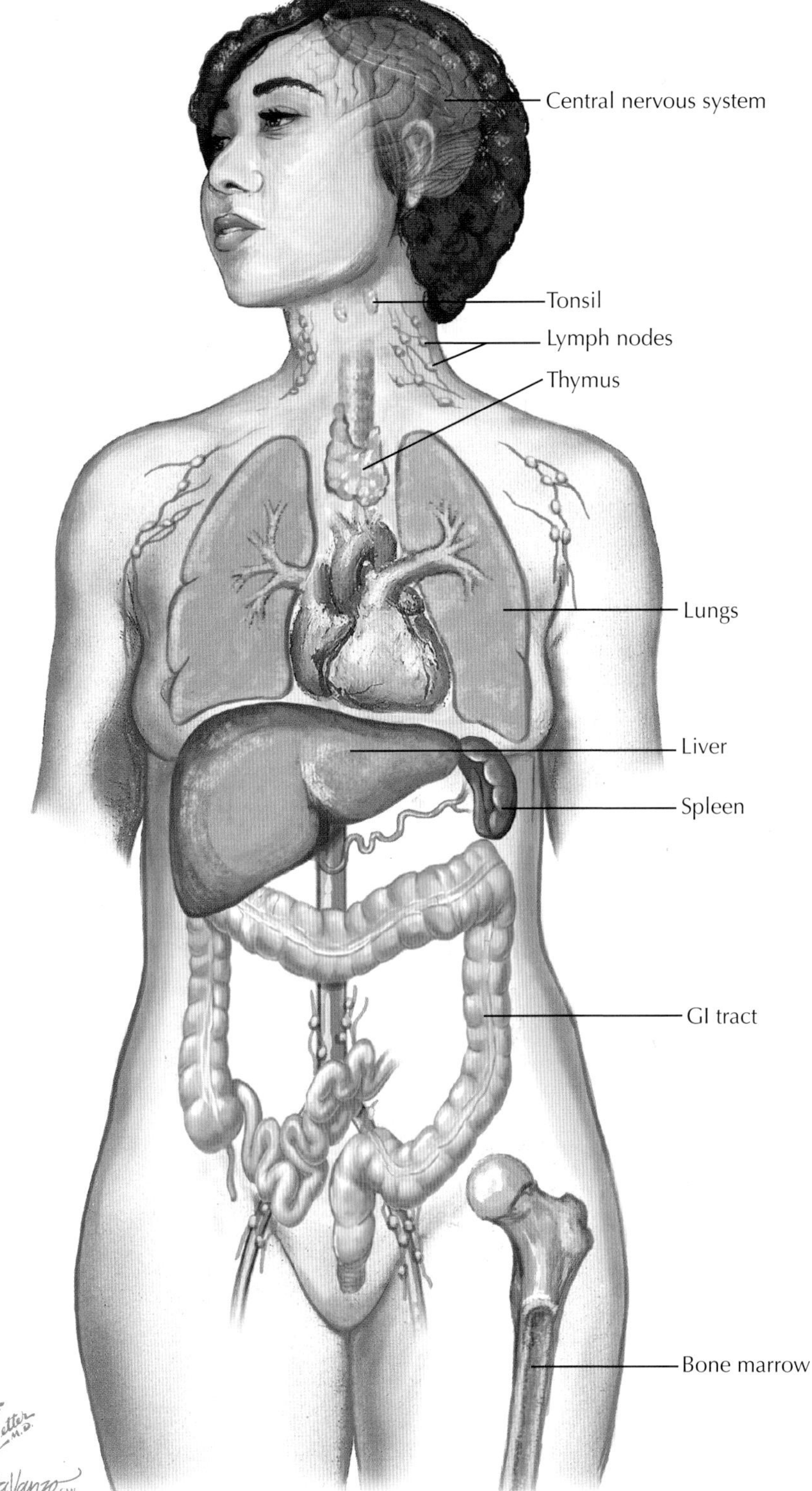


Accurate diagnosis of PTLD requires a high index of suspicion, and strict monitoring of the donor/recipient EBV status is important. Laboratory abnormalities, such as hypercalcemia, hyperuricemia, or elevated lactate dehydrogenase levels, and unexplained anemia, thrombocytopenia, or leukopenia may suggest PTLD. Elevated monoclonal serum and urinary protein levels and radiologic studies, including positron emission tomography scanning, MRI, or US studies, may favor PTLD and guide tissue biopsy, which is required to make an accurate diagnosis.

Treatment should initially be directed toward reduction of T-cell immunosuppression while minimizing the risk of allograft loss. Patients with polymorphic PTLD or monomorphic PTLD that express CD20 may respond to monoclonal antibody rituximab, whereas CD20-negative monomorphic PTLD is best treated with CHOP (cyclophosphamide, doxorubicin, vincristine, prednisone). A novel therapy, termed *adoptive immunotherapy,* is used in refractory cases where EBV-specific cytotoxic T lymphocytes are infused into the donor to treat PTLD. Antiviral therapies such as ganciclovir are typically used for cytomegalovirus prophylaxis and also demonstrate activity against EBV, with the unfortunate risk of bone marrow suppression. Focal lesions are successfully treated with chemotherapy and radiation therapy.

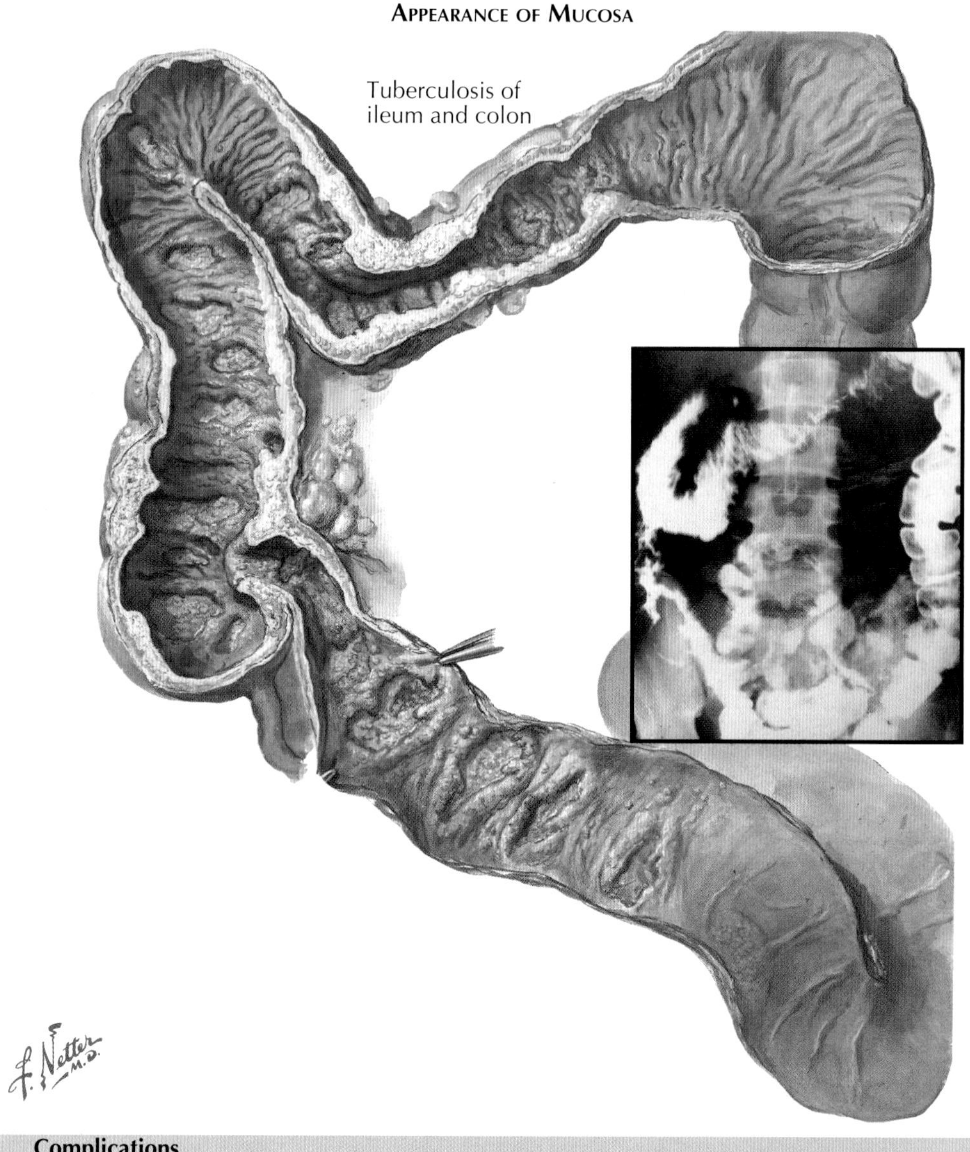


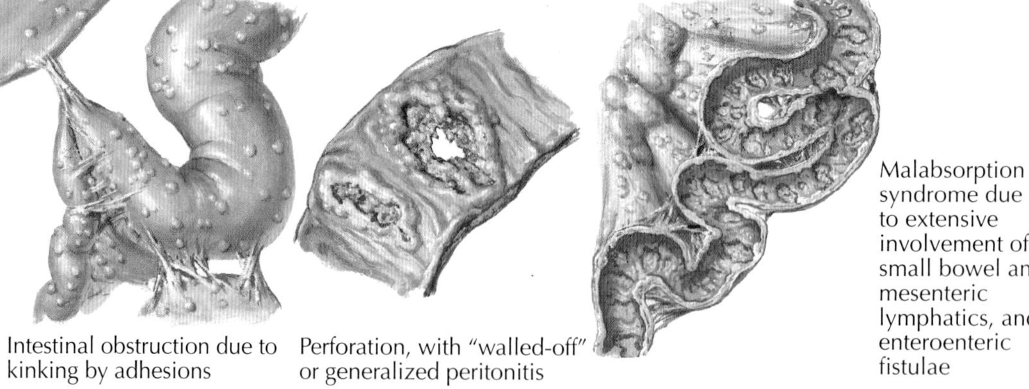

Complications
Intestinal obstruction due to kinking by adhesions
Perforation, with "walled-off" or generalized peritonitis
Malabsorption syndrome due to extensive involvement of small bowel and mesenteric lymphatics, and enteroenteric fistulae


## Abdominal and Intestinal Tuberculosis

Worldwide, tuberculosis (TB) has an annual incidence of 7 to 10 million, infecting almost 22% of the world population. According to the WHO, the incidence has gradually been declining since 2003. Abdominal TB can involve the peritoneum, stomach, intestinal tract including the perianal area, hepatobiliary tree, pancreas, and lymph nodes. TB peritonitis and intestinal TB are two of the more prevalent extrapulmonary manifestations and can mimic CD.

The principal cause of intestinal TB is *Mycobacterium tuberculosis* and may arise from reactivation of latent TB or as a primary infection from ingestion of tuberculous mycobacteria or via hematogenous spread during active pulmonary TB. Contiguous spread to direct adjacent organs is also observed.

M cells are found in the follicle-associated epithelium of intestinal Peyer patches of GALT, which provide a route of entry for pathogens into the mucosa, which then localize in the submucosal lymphoid tissue. The ensuing inflammatory reaction is often indolent, with severe consequences resulting in both acute and subacute symptoms. The ileocecal region is the most common site of involvement, with symptoms resulting from complications of ulcerative, hypertrophic/ulcerohypertrophic, or fibrous disease. Abdominal discomfort, altered bowel habits, anemia, and constitutional symptoms herald insidious disease. Fibrous or hypertrophic disease can present with obstruction from stricture, or the inflammatory reaction may lead to obstruction purely due to mass effect *(tuberculoma)*. Ulcerative disease may manifest with malabsorption and/or

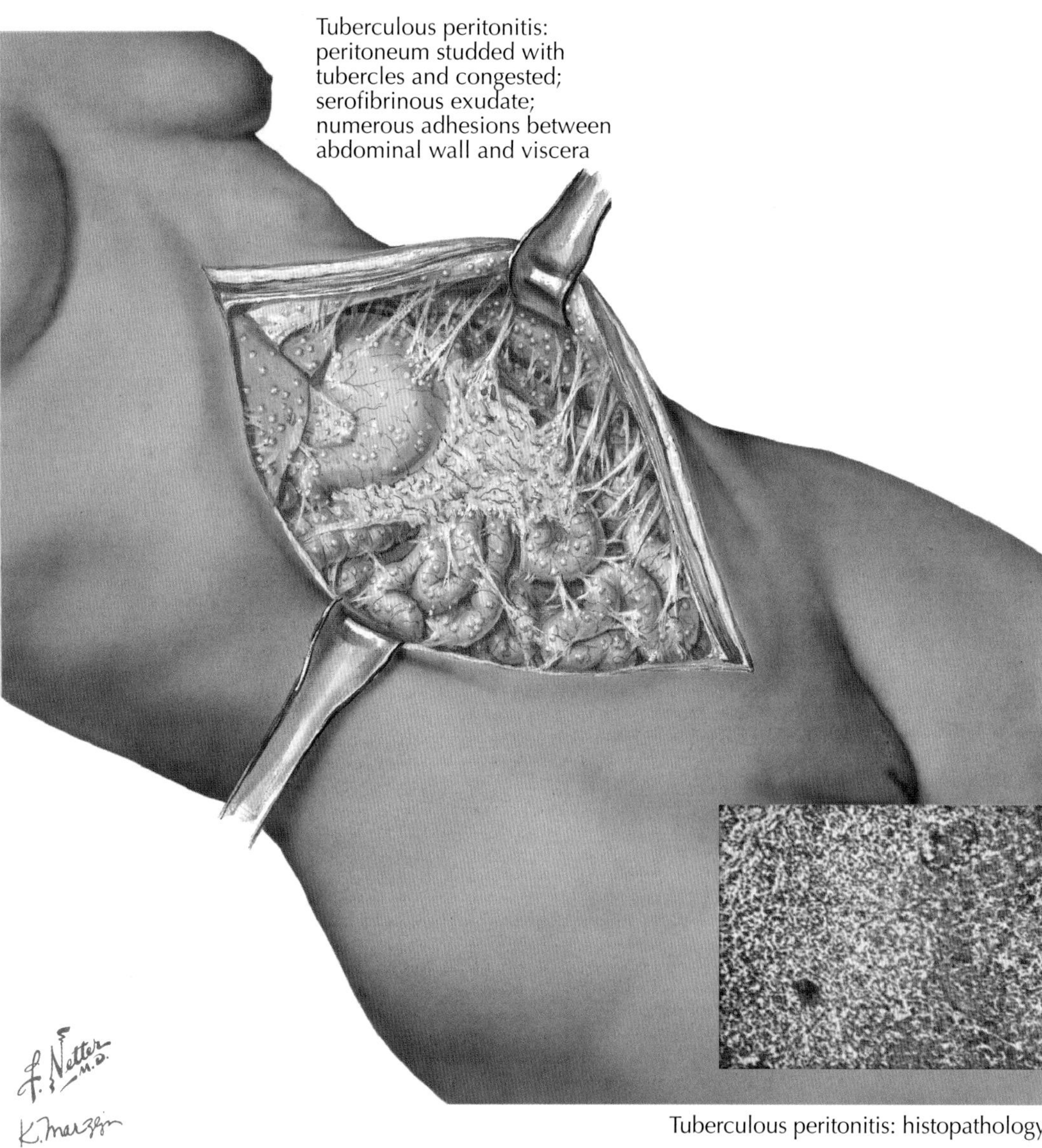

CHRONIC PERITONITIS
Tuberculous peritonitis: peritoneum studded with tubercles and congested; serofibrinous exudate; numerous adhesions between abdominal wall and viscera


Tuberculous peritonitis: histopathology

## ABDOMINAL AND INTESTINAL TUBERCULOSIS (Continued)

perforation. Peritoneal TB often manifests with ascites and/or fever of unknown origin.

Although uncommon, esophageal TB may present as an esophageal pseudotumor. Gastroduodenal TB can masquerade as peptic ulcer disease. Alternatively, it can simulate an adenocarcinoma with pyloric mass obstruction. Intestinal amebiasis and *Yersinia enterocolitica* have clinical manifestations similar to that of intestinal TB. The colon is involved in a minority of intestinal TB and can mimic colon cancer or ulcerative colitis. Rectal TB manifests with bleeding, whereas anal TB presents commonly with fistulous complications. CD and intestinal TB share similarities that often make it difficult to differentiate between the two; however, certain distinctions are present. The mucosal ulcers seen in TB can be superficial or deep, and circumferential as opposed to the deep, linear ulcers of CD. In developing nations, enteric disease is more likely to be caused by TB, whereas in developed nations, the small bowel findings are more likely to suggest CD, although TB should always be ruled out appropriately.

Initial diagnostic studies should include radiography with cross-sectional imaging. Imaging may reveal mesenteric or paraaortic lymphadenopathy, asymmetric bowel wall thickening ("white bowel sign" from lymphatic infiltration and "sliced bread sign" from bowel wall edema), ileal stricture, fistulas, masses, or ascites. Ultimately, tissue biopsy is necessary to confirm the diagnosis, and endoscopic evaluation allows tissue sampling where acid-fast staining, culture, and PCR testing can be used extensively. Tissue sample diagnosis may also be obtained via laparotomy or percutaneous biopsy of peritoneal nodes. Histologic analysis will classically reveal findings of caseating granuloma. When investigating a case of peritoneal TB, paracentesis or laparoscopic biopsy may be necessary, which will demonstrate multiple yellow-white tubercles on the peritoneal surface and/or visceral organs. Analysis of ascitic cell count demonstrates a lymphocytic predominance (lymphocytes $> 250$ cells/mm$^3$) with a serum ascites albumin gradient $< 1.1$ g/dL and high protein content consistent with an exudative process. Elevated adenosine deaminase in the ascitic fluid is evidence that supports tuberculous ascites. Measurement of peritoneal fluid interferon-gamma concentration is more specific to latent and/or active TB infection but is not available for routine testing. Early diagnosis, especially in nonendemic regions, is critical to prevent unnecessary surgical resection and intervention. Notably, patients with IBD taking immunosuppressive medications are at risk for acquiring TB and/or for its latent reactivation. These patients should be screened for TB annually, whereas those receiving immunosuppressant agents and patients found to have latent TB should be treated for 3 months before induction of immunosuppression.

Standard antituberculous treatment is extremely effective for abdominal TB. It involves using rifampicin, isoniazid, pyrazinamide, and ethambutol for 2 months, with rifampicin plus isoniazid daily or three times weekly for 4 to 7 months more.

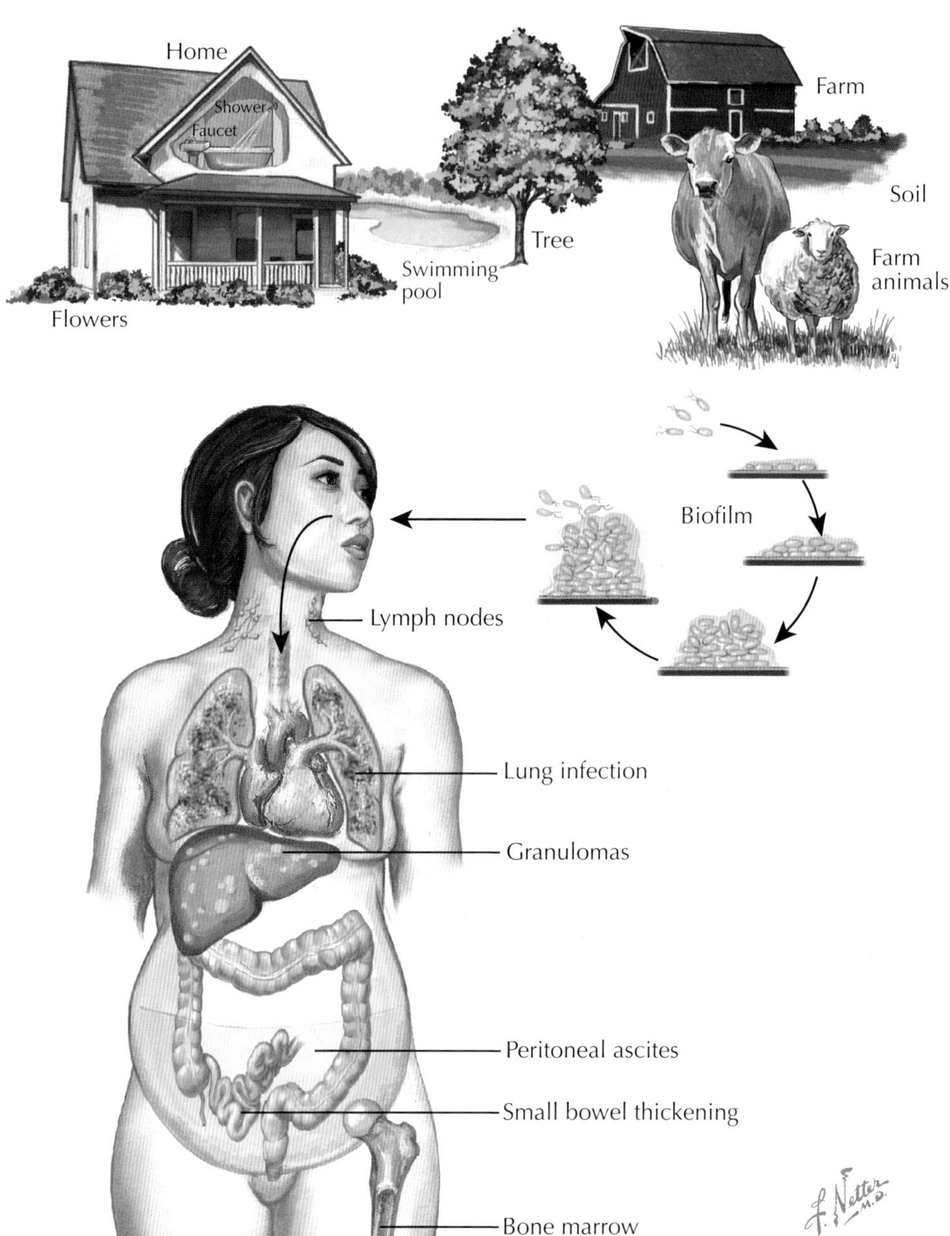


## *MYCOBACTERIA AVIUM-INTRACELLULARE* INFECTION

Nontuberculous mycobacteria (NTM) are free-living mycobacterial species other than those belonging to *Mycobacterial tuberculosis* complex and *Mycobacterial leprae* (causative agent of leprosy). NTM can cause four clinical syndromes: pulmonary disease, superficial lymphadenitis, skin and soft tissue infection, and disseminated disease. *Mycobacterium avium-intracellulare* complex (MAC) encompasses multiple species and is the most common NTM responsible for pulmonary and disseminated disease.

Potable water and soil are main reservoirs and provide surfaces for biofilms that harbor MAC and other NTM species. MAC has been isolated from residential drinking water, faucets, swimming pools, domesticated farm animals, produce, and even potting mix. These biofilms consist of complex communities of bacteria, viruses, fungi, protozoa, and other organisms, all held within a polysaccharide matrix, rendering routine disinfectants ineffective. When protozoa are present on a biofilm surface, MAC can parasitize them. After exposure, infection is slow to develop, and disease ensues if the host immune response fails to contain or eliminate the infecting microbes, such as in patients with primary immunodeficiency or autoantibodies to interferon-gamma, and lymphopenia due to hematologic malignant disease or HIV infection. Disseminated disease occurs via hematogenous and lymphatic spread in those with very low CD4 counts.

MAC is routinely aerosolized, promoting pulmonary infection in individuals with or without preexisting lung disease (e.g., CF, interstitial lung disease, emphysema). Children may demonstrate superficial lymphadenitis, particularly along the cervical chain. Soft tissue and cutaneous infections (e.g., in a wound) occur with direct inoculation. Individuals who are immunocompromised, such as those with hematologic malignancies, solid-organ transplant recipients, those taking immunosuppressive therapy (e.g., anti–TNF-α agents), and those with AIDS (particularly those with a CD4 count <50 cells/mL), are at increased risk of developing MAC infection and disseminated disease. Fortunately, MAC has not been demonstrated to be contagious.

Pulmonary disease presents with a dry or a productive cough, lethargy, dyspnea, chest discomfort, and, rarely, hemoptysis. The presence of fever, weight loss, and night sweats may suggest disseminated disease. Bone marrow infiltration may manifest with leukopenia or anemia. Lymphatic involvement presents as lymphadenopathy or hepatosplenomegaly, sometimes with transaminitis, whereas intestinal involvement can lead to diffuse, dull, intermittent abdominal discomfort without evidence of obstruction. Patients with AIDS who have a CD4 cell count <50 cells/mL may develop acute or chronic diarrhea.

The cornerstone of diagnosis rests on identification of the organisms on mycobacterial culture-specific media from sputum or other tissue specimens. In disseminated disease with GI involvement, imaging may reveal bowel wall thickening and endoscopic biopsy is indicated for histologic confirmation. Infrequently, MAC may present with a nonspecific peritonitis with or without high-protein ascites and, if inconclusive, laparoscopic biopsy can be helpful to obtain tissue sample. Both *M. tuberculosis* and MAC may manifest with hepatic lesions that contain caseating granulomas on histology. In this case, culture becomes critical for differentiation. MAC disease has been implicated in AIDS cholangiopathy, and the diagnosis is made by isolation of the organism in culture of the blood or lymph node.

In a select group of patients with pulmonary disease, prolonged anti-TB medication is indicated as the first-line therapy, whereas patients with cavitary disease and treatment failure should be evaluated for surgical resection. Disseminated disease requires multidrug regimens with typical antitubercular agents (rifabutin, ethambutol, isoniazid). Treatment continues until cultures are negative for at least 12 months, and lack of a therapeutic response at 6 months of therapy or a relapse after therapy should trigger repeat mycobacterial culture to assess sensitivity and susceptibility.

# SMALL BOWEL MANIFESTATIONS OF SYSTEMIC DISEASES

## CONNECTIVE TISSUE DISORDERS

*Scleroderma* frequently involves the small bowel, primarily causing dysmotility with reduced peristalsis leading to stasis and dilated bowel that often promotes development of small intestinal bacterial overgrowth. Scattered wide-mouthed diverticula throughout the small bowel is a common feature and in severe cases, small intestinal pseudoobstruction and malabsorption can be present.

*Ehlers-Danlos syndrome* is a term used for a group of inherited diseases affecting collagen synthesis that can involve the intestine in various ways. Bleeding from mucosal lesions can be a feature in the classic-like I subtype, whereas the vascular subtype can predispose to life-threatening intraabdominal bleeding from ruptured splanchnic artery aneurysms. Irritable bowel syndrome and delayed gastroparesis are often present in patients with the hypermobile subtype.

*Dermatomyositis* and *polymyositis* can affect the entire GI tract but commonly involve the proximal esophagus. *Systemic lupus enteritis with or without terminal ileitis* is not uncommon and can be confused with CD. Rarely, malabsorption and PIL with lymphangiectasia can be seen.

In *rheumatoid arthritis* (RA), the small intestine may rarely be involved with intestinal ischemia, bleeding, or infarction due to vasculitis of the mesenteric vessels. Patients with long-standing RA are at risk for secondary amyloidosis that can lead to chronic diarrhea. More commonly, chronic use of medications such as NSAIDs causes erosions and ulcers.

In *Behçet disease,* there is GI involvement in up to 50% of patients and ulcerative lesions throughout the GI tract, in particular the ileocecal region, which can imitate CD. Similarly, patients with reactive arthritides may have endoscopic or histologic evidence of ileocolonic inflammation that sometimes resembles CD.

## ENDOCRINOLOGIC DISORDERS

Diarrhea is reported in over 25% of patients with DM. Visceral autonomic neuropathy plays an important role in association with segmental small intestinal dilation often seen in long-standing DM, both of which promote small intestinal bacterial overgrowth and the resulting diarrhea. Furthermore, certain drugs used for DM, such as metformin, or the presence of concomitant subclinical pancreatic insufficiency, or celiac disease (commonly associated with type 1 DM) may exacerbate the diarrhea. *Hyperthyroidism,* which causes rapid intestinal transit, may lead to diarrhea or hyperdefecation, whereas intestinal motility is slowed in *hypothyroidism.* Likewise, *hypoparathyroidism* can lead to neuromuscular irritability that manifests with abdominal pain, intestinal tetany, and diarrhea, whereas hyperparathyroidism can lead to bowel hypomotility and constipation or peptic ulcer disease and pancreatitis.

### CONNECTIVE TISSUE DISORDER AND DERMATOLOGIC DISEASES

**Connective tissue disorders**

**Scleroderma**

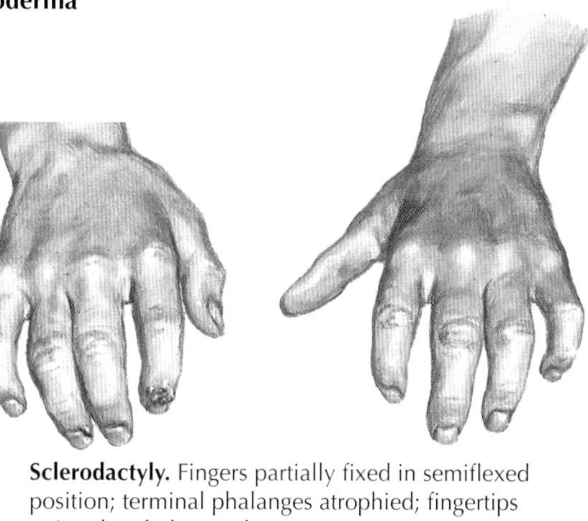

**Sclerodactyly.** Fingers partially fixed in semiflexed position; terminal phalanges atrophied; fingertips pointed and ulcerated.

**Characteristics.** Thickening, tightening, and rigidity of facial skin, with small, constricted mouth and narrow lips, in atrophic phase of scleroderma.

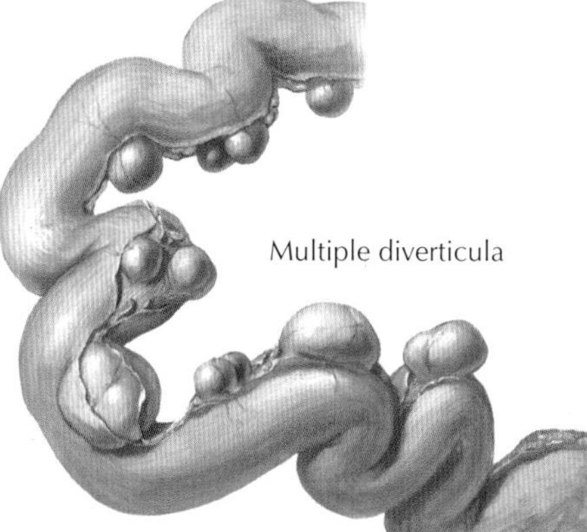

Multiple diverticula

**Dermatologic diseases**

**Blue rubber bleb nevus syndrome**

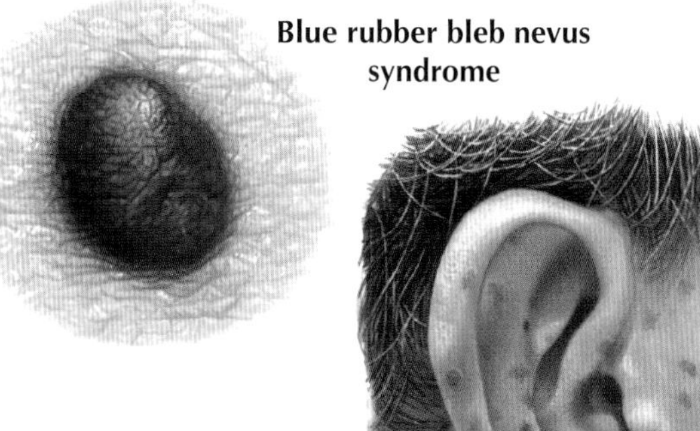

**Pellagra**

Erythematous hyperpigmented and scaly skin rash in the distribution of a broad collar (dermatomes C3 and C4) in sun-exposed areas; "Casal's shawl."

F. Netter M.D.
C. Machado M.D.

## DERMATOLOGIC DISEASES

*Blue rubber bleb nevus syndrome* is characterized by blue nevi on the skin and GI hemangiomas, can present with iron deficiency anemia or overt GI bleeding, and can also act as the lead point of intestinal intussusceptions. *Neurofibromatosis (von Recklinghausen disease)* is associated with polypoid neurofibromas that can be present throughout the GI tract and cause GI bleeding, obstruction, or both.

*Acrodermatitis enteropathica* is a rare autosomal recessive disorder that impairs sufficient intestinal zinc absorption but can also result from severe zinc deficiency secondary to CD. It typically presents at the time of weaning, with eczematous pink scaly plaques on the hands and feet and around the mouth and anus, in addition to paronychia and nail dystrophy. GI symptoms are often intermittent and consist of diarrhea and malabsorption. The small bowel shows patchy villous lesions of

## Small Bowel Manifestations of Systemic Diseases (Continued)

### Miscellaneous Disorders

**Endometriosis**

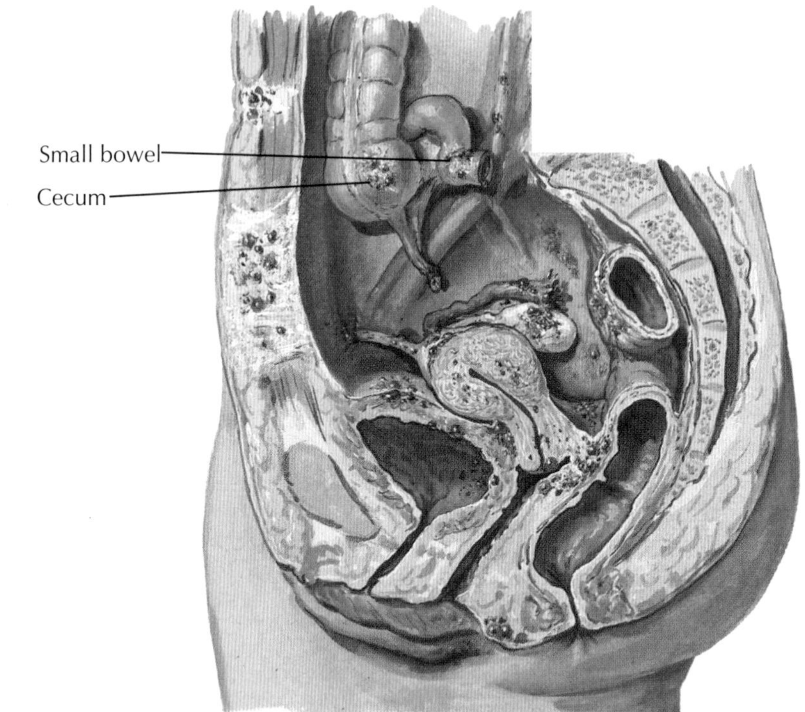


Possible sites of endometriosis

**Graft-versus-host disease**

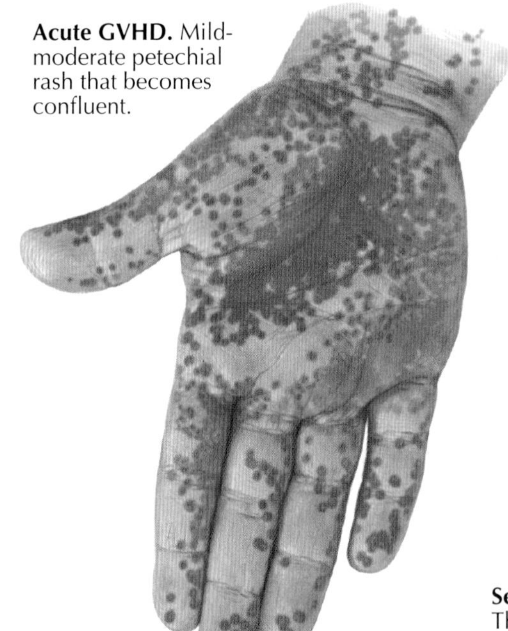

**Acute GVHD.** Mild-moderate petechial rash that becomes confluent.

**Severe acute GVHD.** The skin peels off in large sheets due to necrosis of the skin and subsequent blistering.

variable severity, with abnormal inclusions in Paneth cells. It can be reversed by giving zinc orally. *Pellagra* is a disease caused by niacin (vitamin $B_3$) deficiency manifested by the 4D's: dermatitis, diarrhea, dementia, and death. The dermatitis is a hyperpigmented rash that affects sun-exposed areas giving the characteristic "Casal necklace" appearance. Deficiency of niacin is seen in chronic alcoholism or as a complication of bariatric surgery, anorexia nervosa, or other malabsorptive disorders.

### CARDIOVASCULAR DISEASES

*Aortic stenosis* has long been associated with angiodysplasia *(Heyde syndrome)* resulting from an acquired deficiency of von Willebrand factor. *Congestive heart failure* can lead to congestion of the splanchnic venous bed, causing anorexia, nausea, bloating, and abdominal pain. Rarely, it can lead to mesenteric ischemia of the bowel and weight loss, diarrhea, malabsorption, and PIL.

### HEMATOLOGIC DISORDERS

Solitary *plasmacytomas* most frequently occur in the bone *(plasmacytoma of bone)* but can also be found outside bone in the GI tract. *Waldenström macroglobulinemia* can involve the GI tract where monoclonal IgM protein is deposited as extracellular amorphous material in the lamina propria, producing severe malabsorption with diarrhea and steatorrhea. Similarly, *heavy-chain disease* commonly leads to infiltration of the jejunal mucosa with plasmacytoid cells, resulting in abdominal pain, malabsorption with chronic diarrhea, steatorrhea, and loss of weight.

### MISCELLANEOUS DISORDERS

*Endometriosis* is characterized by the presence of endometrial glands, stroma, or both outside the uterine cavity. Intestinal endometriosis commonly takes the form of plaques of tissues on the serosal surface of the bowel lying in the pelvis, but the plaques can rarely infiltrate into the deeper layers of the bowel, causing intestinal obstruction and GI bleeding.

*Sarcoidosis* is a systemic disorder that is characterized by noncaseating granulomas. Involvement of the small bowel is extremely rare, and the presence of typical granulomatous ileocolitis even in a patient known to have sarcoidosis should prompt a search for CD.

*Graft-versus-host disease* (GVHD) can be acute or chronic and commonly involves the GI tract. Small bowel involvement causes diarrhea that can often be severe.

CF is associated with unique intestinal disorders that arise as a result of inspissated thick and viscous mucus secretions. MI occurs exclusively in newborns and is often the first manifestation of CF, whereas DIOS is the adult equivalent and can cause intestinal obstruction. Amyloidosis is caused by extracellular deposition of "amyloid" proteins, and GI involvement manifests as an occult or overt GI bleeding or with diarrhea and malabsorption as a PIL or GI dysmotility.

*Coronavirus infection 2019* (COVID-19) is a widespread respiratory infection caused by severe acute respiratory syndrome coronavirus 2 (SARS-CoV-2) and is responsible for almost 6.5 million deaths worldwide. Symptoms are primarily respiratory in nature with fever, cough, and upper respiratory symptoms that can progress to acute respiratory distress syndrome; GI manifestations with diarrhea, abdominal pain, nausea, and vomiting occur in up to 40% of patients.

**Obstruction and Adynamic Ileus of Small Intestine**

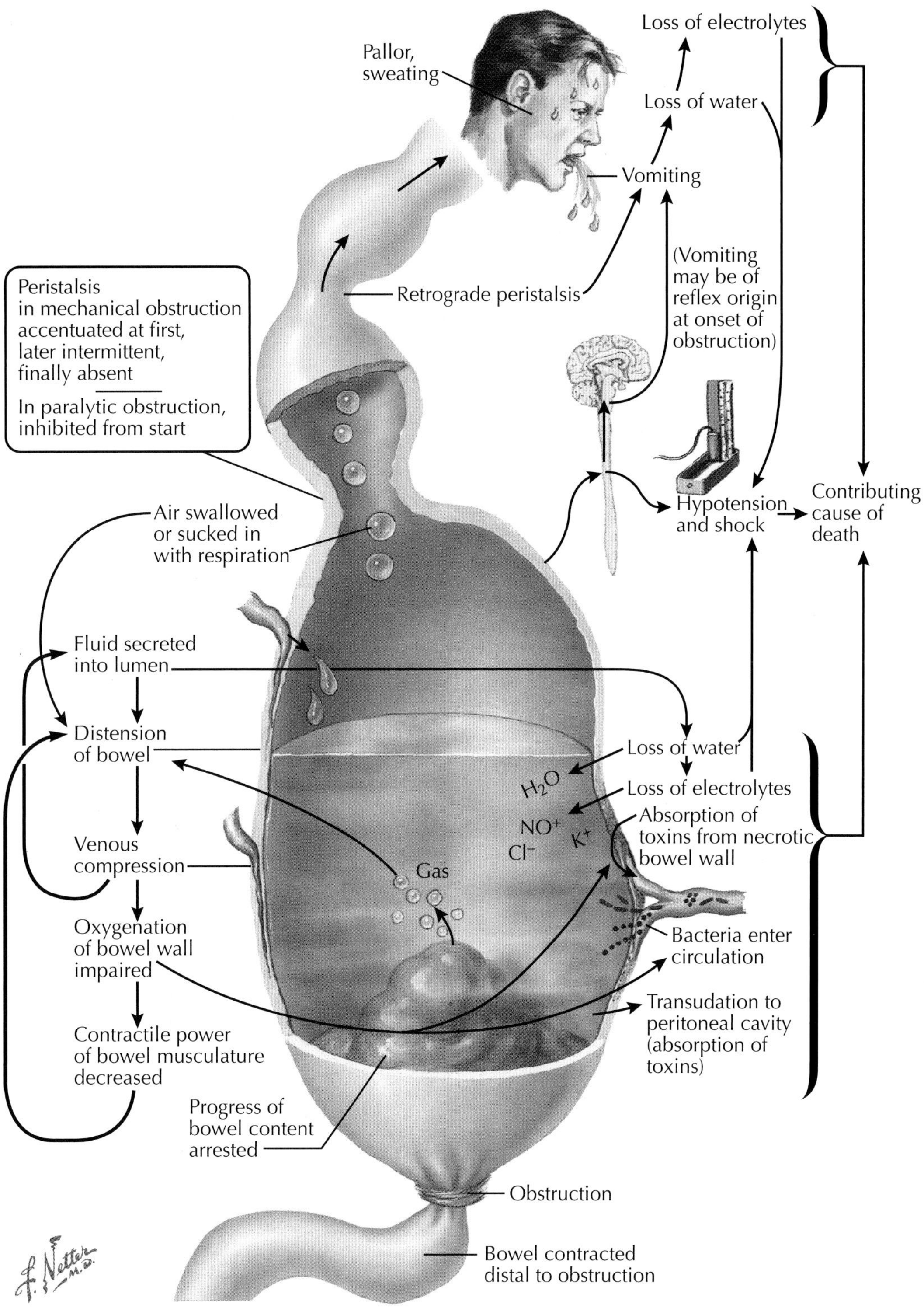

## INTESTINAL OBSTRUCTION

Small intestinal obstruction occurs when the normal propulsion of luminal contents is hindered by either mechanical obstruction or abnormal intestinal motility. The obstruction may be partial or complete and can occur at any level of the small bowel.

### MECHANICAL OBSTRUCTION

The majority of mechanical intestinal obstructions are caused by adhesive bands or incarceration of a loop of small bowel within an internal hernia formed by previous surgery. Intestinal obstruction can occur in the absence of previous surgery in cases of intussusception, abdominal wall hernia, volvulus, or congenital malrotation. Strictures related to tumors, CD, prior intestinal ischemia, or radiation are common luminal causes of obstruction, whereas peritoneal inflammation as seen in TB peritonitis and peritoneal carcinomatosis can lead to adhesive bands causing obstruction. Impaction by foreign bodies such as gallstones, enteroliths, or parasites can also cause mechanical obstruction. Irrespective of the cause, obstruction of the small intestine leads to distension of the segment proximal to the blockage while the distal bowel remains decompressed. Early in the course, intestinal contractility increases to propel luminal contents past the obstructed point. This explains the diarrhea seen early in partial or complete obstruction. Later in the course, the intestine becomes fatigued and dilates, with rapid accumulation of gas and fluid. The gas is mainly swallowed air in addition to gas produced from bacterial fermentation as gastric, intestinal, and biliary secretions are added to the luminal contents. With progression of the obstruction, the distended proximal intestine loses its absorptive function and sequesters electrolyte-rich fluid (sodium, chloride, potassium) with further influx of fluid and electrolytes. The emesis that invariably ensues leads to loss of electrolyte-rich fluid and metabolic alkalosis, aggravating the hypovolemia, which can progress to renal insufficiency and circulatory collapse. In cases with severe bowel distension, as in closed loop obstruction where a loop of bowel is occluded at two points by an internal hernia or in cases where there is torsion of bowel, the excessive stretching of the bowel wall can impair venous return and interfere with normal perfusion. Unless treated, this can progress to ischemia, necrosis, and frank perforation. Abdominal pain, vomiting, and distension are the hallmarks of acute intestinal obstruction. The onset of these symptoms varies depending on the cause of the obstruction, the location (proximal vs. distal), and the degree of obstruction (partial vs. complete). Proximal obstruction tends to cause early and severe vomiting, whereas more distal locations present with abdominal distension and failure to pass flatus or feces. The pain is typically located in the periumbilical area and is "colicky" in nature, with cramping episodes occurring at certain intervals. The progression to a more constant pain and focal localization may be an indication of complications with peritoneal irritation, ischemia, and gangrene. The physical examination should include assessment for dehydration and for clues to the cause of the obstruction. Abdominal inspection will assess the degree of distension and identify surgical scars or abdominal wall hernias. Examination of the groin is key in these cases because an incarcerated indirect inguinal

**Computed Tomography of Small Intestine Obstruction**

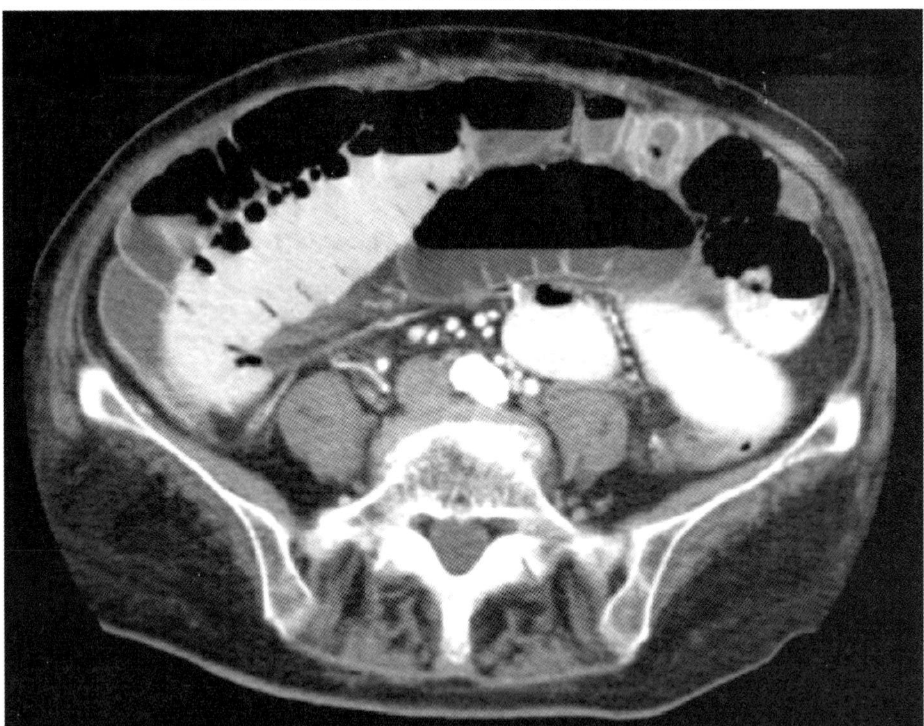

CT image of the abdomen of a patient with small bowel obstruction. Note the large dilated loops of small bowel with fluid levels.

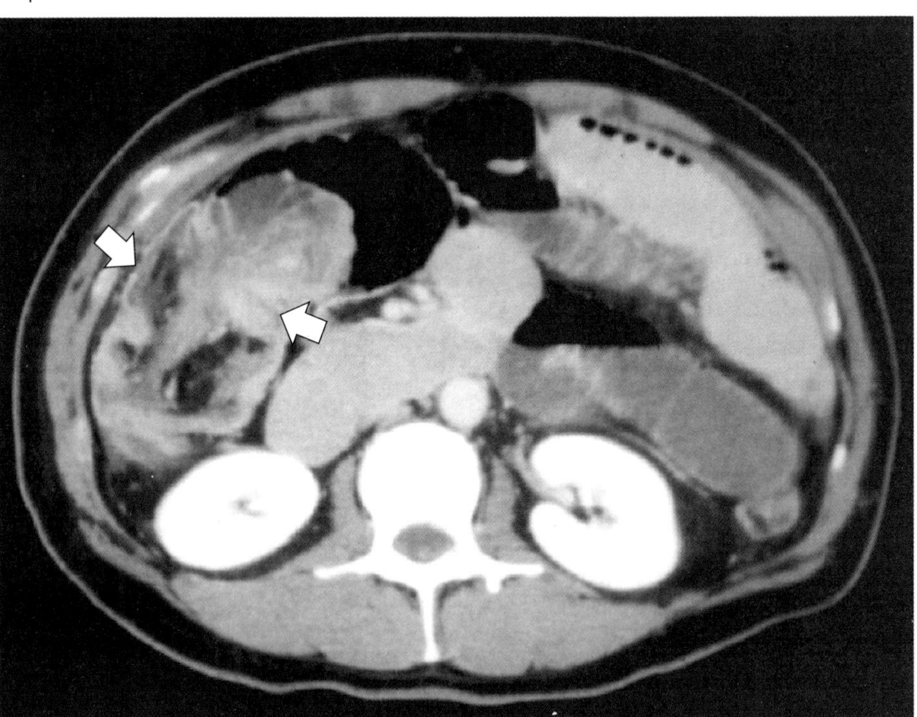

CT image of the abdomen demonstrating small bowel obstruction caused by intussusception *(arrows)*

## Intestinal Obstruction (Continued)

hernia can easily be missed without close attention. Abdominal auscultation may reveal a high-pitched "tinkling" sound typically found in acute obstruction, and as the bowel progressively distends, the sounds become muffled and eventually disappear. Bowel distension results in tympany upon percussion, but areas with fluid-filled bowel can be dull to percussion. In early obstruction, the abdomen may be soft with minimal tenderness; therefore the presence of significant tenderness and rigidity indicates the setting of peritonitis and compromised bowel.

Laboratory studies can assess the degree of fluid and electrolyte abnormalities, whereas leukocytosis and acidosis may indicate complications. There are no reliable laboratory markers for ischemia; however, an elevated serum lactate level can be suggestive of hypoperfusion. Plain abdominal radiography is the first-line imaging modality for suspected intestinal obstruction. The presence of air-fluid levels with fluid- and gas-filled loops of small intestine and a paucity of gas in the colon is pathognomonic for small bowel obstruction. Abdominal CT scanning can identify the specific site of obstruction and often determine the cause.

The initial management should be directed toward volume resuscitation and correction of metabolic derangements. Conservative management of the obstruction with nasogastric suction may be successful in patients with partial obstruction while they are closely monitored. Patients with signs of complicated bowel obstruction and evidence of ischemia, necrosis, or perforation require emergent surgical exploration.

### PARALYTIC ILEUS

*Paralytic* or *adynamic ileus* refers to the bowel distension and obstipation caused by nonmechanical factors that disrupt the normal coordinated propulsive motor activity of the GI tract. This is commonly seen after abdominal or nonabdominal surgery; however, a wide variety of conditions, including peritoneal or retroperitoneal inflammation caused by blood, chemicals, or intestinal juices, can lead to paralytic ileus. Infections, such as pneumonia and sepsis, and use of drugs such as opiates and anticholinergics are also frequent causes of ileus.

The clinical presentation of paralytic ileus is similar to that of mechanical obstruction, but certain distinctions exist. Abdominal distension is usually present without accompanying colicky abdominal pain. Nausea and vomiting may or may not be present, and patients may continue to pass flatus and even have diarrhea. Plain abdominal radiographs typically reveal distended small and large bowel with no transition point. The diagnosis can further be confirmed with orally enhanced CT scanning.

The management of ileus is mainly supportive, with IV hydration and bowel rest. Underlying conditions such as electrolyte imbalance and sepsis should be sought and treated. Offending drugs should be discontinued, and opiate use should be minimized. If vomiting persists, nasogastric decompression can offer relief. Pharmacologic agents that stimulate gut motility, such as the sympatholytic guanethidine or the parasympathomimetic neostigmine, have been used to treat ileus but have mostly been ineffective. Prokinetic therapy using erythromycin (motilin receptor agonist) and dexloxiglumide (cholesystokinin-1 stimulator) has been evaluated but does not appear to alter intestinal ileus.

# Vascular Malformation of Small Intestine and Other Causes of Small Intestinal Bleeding

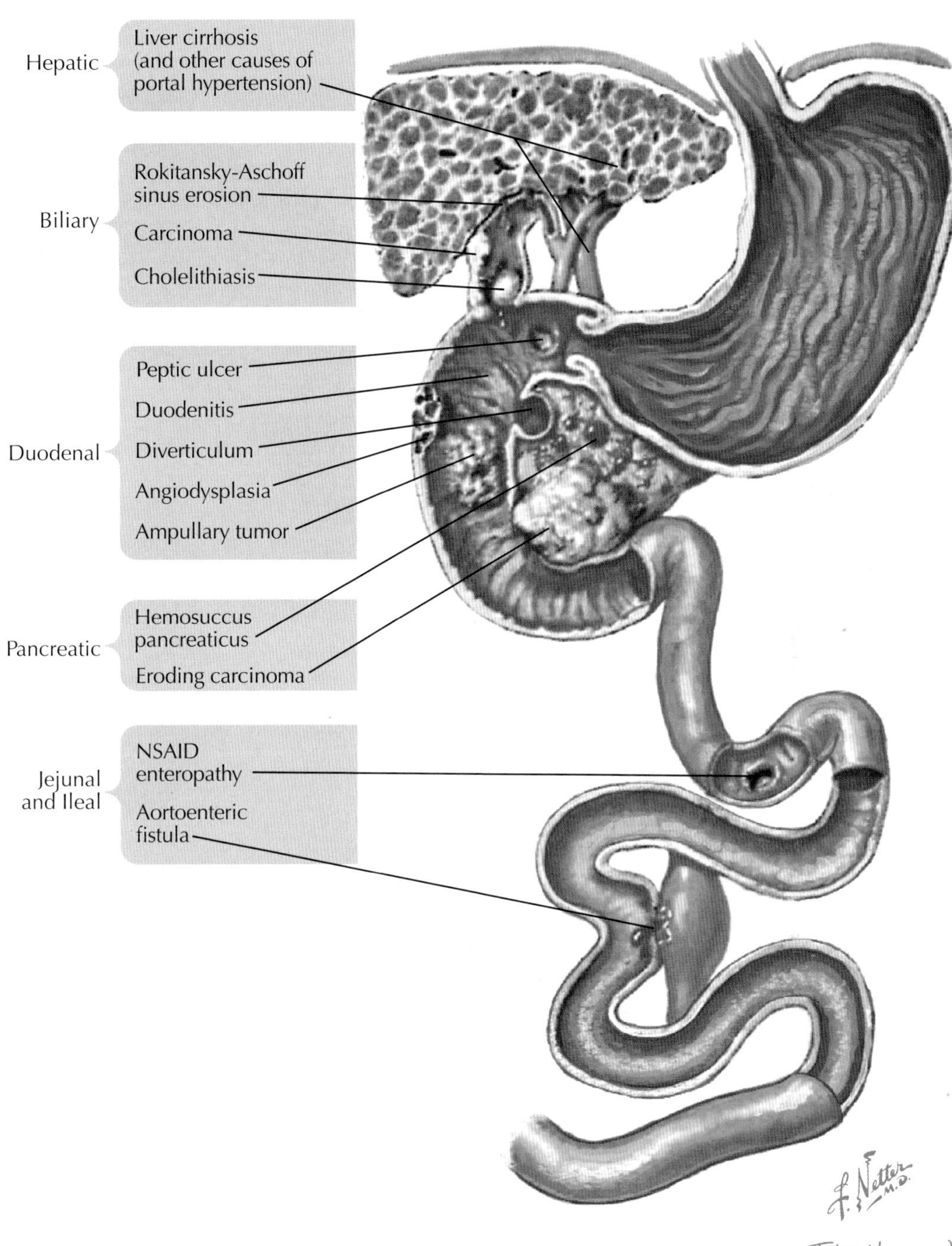


Approximately 5% of cases of GI bleeding originate in the small bowel, between the ampulla of Vater and the ileocecal valve. Small intestinal vascular malformations are responsible for the majority of small intestinal bleeding followed by enteropathy induced by NSAIDs, both of which are more often seen in elderly patients. Small intestinal tumors, CD, and nonspecific enteritis are more common in individuals younger than 40 years. Rarer causes include Meckel diverticulum, hemobilia, hemosuccus pancreaticus, and aortoenteric fistula.

## SMALL INTESTINAL VASCULAR MALFORMATIONS

*Vascular malformations of the small bowel* are rare and more commonly encountered in elderly persons and vary in size and distribution. Most vascular lesions present with obscure GI bleeding, but the severity of the symptoms and signs ranges from heme-positive stool to profound anemia requiring recurrent blood transfusion.

## ANGIODYSPLASIA (ANGIOECTASIA OR VASCULAR ECTASIA)

Angiodysplasias are pathologically dilated and tortuous, thin-walled vessels involving small capillaries, veins, and arteries and are visualized within the mucosal and submucosal layers of the gut. They are the most common cause of small bowel bleeding, accounting for 50% of cases. The jejunum is the most common location for angiodysplasias in the small intestine, followed by the ileum and duodenum. Approximately 40% to 60% of patients will have more than one lesion. Aortic stenosis has long been associated with angiodysplasia *(Heyde syndrome)*. The high stress in aortic stenosis was thought to cause shear-dependent cleavage of high-molecular-weight multimers of von Willebrand factor, leading to acquired deficiency of the factor; findings in recent large-scale studies have questioned this association, however. Chronic renal failure with or without hemodialysis is another condition associated with increased frequency of GI angiodysplasia. Other reported risk factors include hypertension, ischemic heart disease, arrhythmias, valvular heart disease, congestive heart failure, chronic respiratory conditions, previous venous thromboembolism, and use of anticoagulants.

Angiodysplasias commonly present with anemia with or without iron deficiency. The stool is frequently heme-positive, and it is rarely melenic. Capsule endoscopy has a high diagnostic yield and allows visualization of the entire small intestine. Small intestinal angiodysplastic lesions typically have a round, stellate, or spidery mucosal appearance with a distinct zone of pallor surrounding the margins. Biopsy is not recommended and carries a bleeding risk.

Device-assisted enteroscopy is the best choice for short-term and initial therapy. Single-balloon enteroscopy, double-balloon enteroscopy, or spiral enteroscopy can be used to identify and cauterize the lesions using argon plasma coagulation. For patients with diffuse lesions or those who are unfit to undergo invasive procedures, various pharmacologic agents have been studied. Hormonal therapy (estrogen and progesterone), thalidomide (a vascular endothelial growth factor inhibitor), and octreotide have been shown to be beneficial in several case series, but randomized trials are lacking.

## TELANGIECTASIA

Telangiectasias of the small bowel are essentially similar to angiodysplasias, but they can involve all the layers of the bowel, unlike angiodysplasias, which are limited to the mucosa and submucosa. Additionally, telangiectasias often occur as part of a systemic disorder and involve cutaneous and other mucous membrane surfaces.

GI telangiectasias are associated with hereditary hemorrhagic telangiectasia, scleroderma, CREST syndrome, and, possibly, Turner syndrome. *Hereditary hemorrhagic telangiectasia (Osler-Weber-Rendu syndrome)* is an autosomal dominant disorder with a prevalence of 1:5000 to 1:8000. Individuals with the disease can have vascular lesions, including GI telangiectasias and arteriovenous malformations of the liver,

## Vascular Malformation of Small Intestine and Other Causes of Small Intestinal Bleeding (Continued)

lung, and CNS. The most common clinical findings are epistaxis and iron deficiency anemia, but patients may be asymptomatic. Life-threatening bleeding can arise from visceral vascular lesions. The management is directed toward the organ involved and requires a multidisciplinary team approach. Endoscopic ablation is used to manage bleeding from GI lesions. Surgery or embolization may be useful for life-threatening hemorrhage from localized lesions. A vascular endothelial growth factor antagonist such as bevacizumab, sprayed topically or injected locally, has shown promise in reducing bleeding episodes.

### NSAID ENTEROPATHY

Intestinal injury related to the use of NSAIDs is common and is one of the most frequent causes of obscure GI bleeding. The distal small bowel is often involved, but lesions can be diffuse and range from erosions or ulcers to stricture or frank bowel perforation. Enteric-coated aspirin was originally designed to decrease adverse effects on the stomach, but its use may have shifted the damage to the distal small bowel. The pathogenesis of NSAID-induced enteropathy is distinct from that of NSAID-induced gastropathy. Local mucosal damage induced by NSAIDs appears to increase intestinal permeability and weaken the mucosal barrier, allowing bile acid, proteolytic enzymes, intestinal bacteria, or toxins to penetrate epithelial cells, resulting in mucosal injury.

Findings on capsule endoscopy or enteroscopy include reddened folds, a denuded area, red spots, or a sharply demarcated ulcer with or without bleeding. The pathognomonic finding of NSAID enteropathy, however, is a diaphragm-like stricture. These strictures are caused by scarring from recurrent ulcerative injury and appear as thin, concentric, diaphragm-like septa with pinhole-sized lumen. They are usually multiple and are found mostly in the mid small bowel, but they have also been described in the ileum and colon. They are histologically characterized by submucosal fibrosis and thickening of the muscularis mucosa, with normal overlying epithelium. These strictures can lead to entrapment of a capsule endoscopy, necessitating additional procedures for retrieval. Endoscopically accessible strictures or diaphragms may be amenable to through-the-scope balloon dilation, with retrieval of the retained capsule; otherwise, surgical intervention may be required. Cessation of NSAID use is the mainstay of management, with complete resolution of most lesions.

Angiodysplasias and Pigmentation

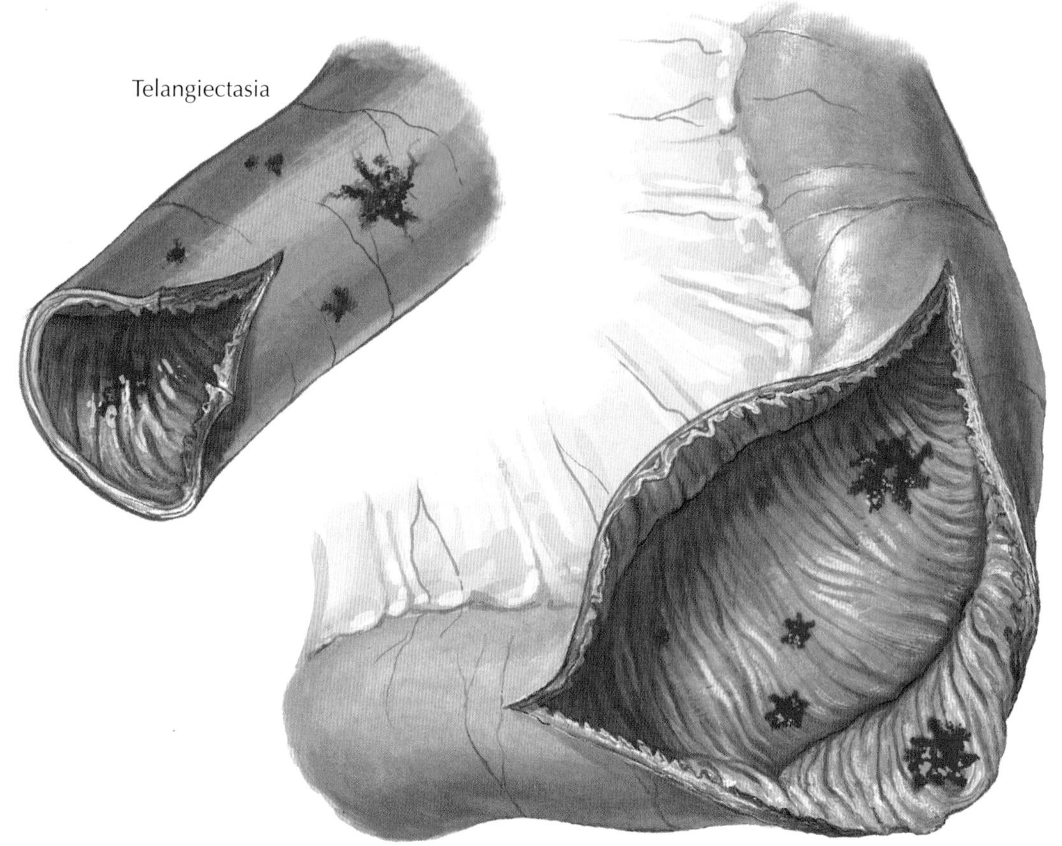


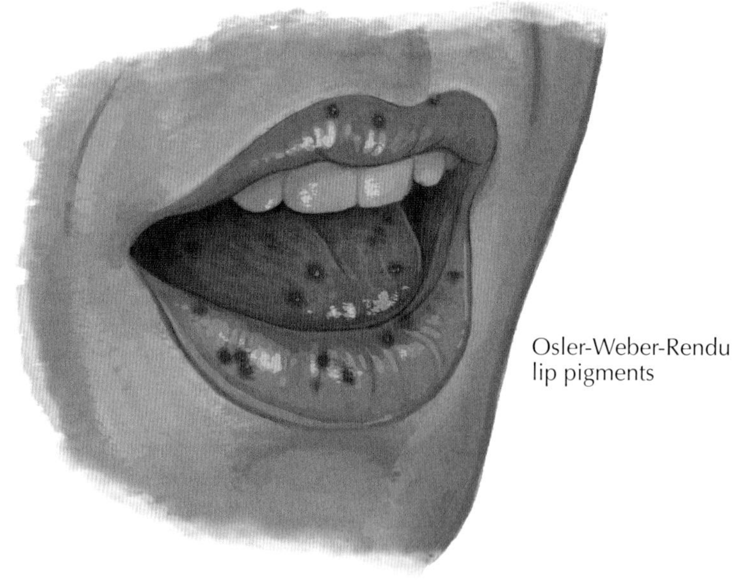


*Hemosuccus pancreaticus* refers to bleeding from a peripancreatic blood vessel into the pancreatic duct, most often in the setting of acute or chronic pancreatitis. Rarely this can be complication of therapeutic endoscopy of the pancreas. Selective arteriography of the celiac trunk and SMA is the most sensitive diagnostic tool. *Hemobilia,* or bleeding from the hepatobiliary system, usually presents as melena, hematemesis, biliary colic, or jaundice and should be suspected after recent instrumentation of the hepatic parenchymal or biliary tract or after blunt trauma to the abdomen. Side-viewing endoscopy can directly visualize the clot extrusion or blood oozing from the papilla of Vater.

*Aortoenteric fistula* is a rare life-threatening condition and is almost always seen secondary to reconstructive aortic aneurysmal surgery. It typically involves the third portion of the duodenum and presents with herald bleeding, followed by massive life-threatening hemorrhage. The best diagnostic modality is abdominal CT scanning.

# Indirect and Direct Inguinal Hernias

*Hernia* (a word derived from the Greek, meaning "sprouting forth") has been defined, from the time of A. Cornelius Celsus (2nd century CE), as a protrusion of an organ from its natural place in a cavity through an abnormal opening. Hernias are classified by the cause or the anatomic location of the defect. Approximately 75% of hernias occur in the groin region. Groin hernias are classified as *indirect inguinal, direct inguinal,* or *femoral hernias* based on the site of herniation in relation to the surrounding structures. An inguinal hernia that has direct and indirect components is referred to as a *pantaloon hernia.*

## INDIRECT INGUINAL HERNIAS

*Indirect inguinal hernia* is the most common type, irrespective of sex. It is characterized by the propulsion of the hernia sac through the internal inguinal ring toward the external inguinal ring and, at times, into the scrotum. The incidence of inguinal hernias has a bimodal distribution (<1 year and >60 years). Inguinal hernia is 3 to 4 times more common in males than in females, and this fact points to a causative relationship, namely, a developmental process connected with the descent of the testes in fetal life. As the testes descend from the intraabdominal space into the scrotum in the third trimester of pregnancy, they are preceded by the gubernaculum and a fold of peritoneum, known as the *funicular process* (see Plate 2.55) or processus vaginalis. This process is normally obliterated during the eighth month of intrauterine life, becoming a thin, solid strand of connective tissue (ligamentum vaginale). If the process is not obliterated, a peritoneal pouch or sac termed the *patent processus vaginalis* persists, which accounts for the high incidence of indirect inguinal hernias in preterm babies. Normally, the deep (internal) inguinal ring (see Plates 2.1 to 2.3) serves as a perfect closure against the egression of any structure within the abdominal cavity. If, however, the funicular process is not obliterated completely, the sac may enlarge or may be the object of pathologic changes resulting in damage to fascial and muscular elements and leading to incompetence of the ring. A patent processus vaginalis does not necessarily indicate an inguinal hernia. Numerous individuals of both sexes have been found with a patent funicular process without ever having had any signs of a hernia. Others "acquire" a complete hernia only late in life.

Epidemiologic studies have identified risk factors that play a role in the formation of a hernia in the presence or absence of a patent processus vaginalis. Inherent collagen weakness as in Ehlers-Danlos syndrome or acquired weakness due to chronic glucocorticoid use is associated with an increased incidence of hernia. A chronic increase in abdominal pressure and enhanced tension on the wall, as seen in pregnancy or with ascites or chronic obstructive pulmonary disease (COPD), can force abdominal contents through the inguinal canal. Alternatively, strenuous physical activity or a sudden increase in abdominal pressure caused by lifting heavy objects can exert increased pressure against the abdominal wall, producing a clinically detectable hernia.

To understand the cause, clinical manifestations, and, particularly, surgical repair of an indirect inguinal hernia, a detailed knowledge of the anatomy of this region is critical. The anatomy is illustrated and discussed in Plates 2.1 to 2.3. In *acquired inguinal hernia,* the ring becomes dilated over time, or is already wide enough as in a congenital hernia, and permits passage of the small or large intestine, omentum, or bladder. The size of the sac depends on its contents and always lies anterosuperior to the spermatic cord. The narrow proximal part of the sac is called the *neck* of the sac, whereas the distal part is known as the *fundus.* The coverings of the hernial sac are the same as those of the spermatic cord under normal conditions. The peritoneal innermost layer is covered by areolar tissue, the internal spermatic (infundibuliform) fascia derived from

Indirect Inguinal Hernia

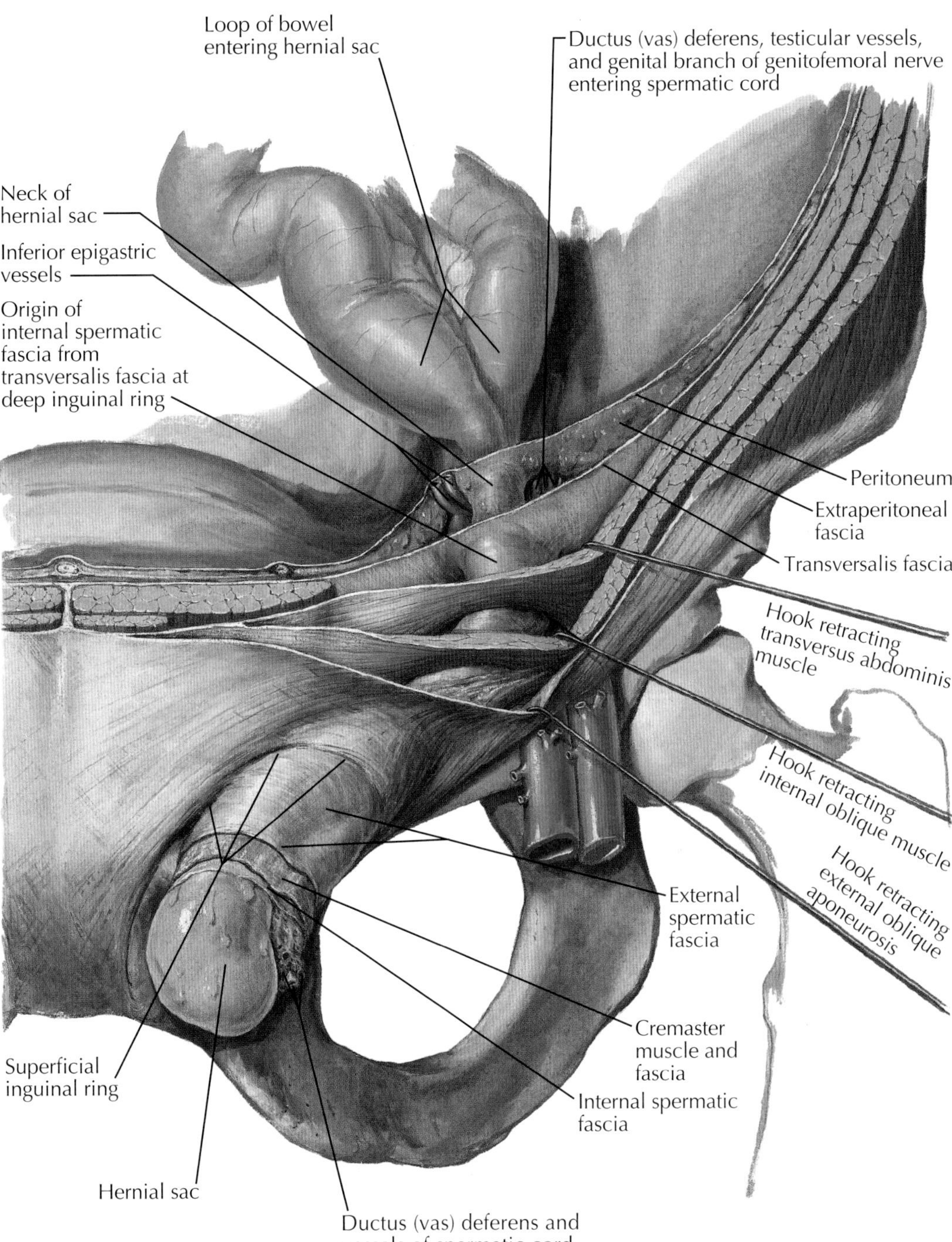

## INDIRECT AND DIRECT INGUINAL HERNIAS (Continued)

the transversalis muscle and the musculofascial cremasteric layer, essentially derived from the internal oblique muscle and aponeurosis. In moderate-sized to large indirect inguinal hernias, the obliqueness of the inguinal canal is mostly lost. With the widening of the deep (internal, abdominal) ring and the increased masses filling the canal, the two inguinal rings (deep and superficial) start to lie more and more perpendicularly above each other. Medial displacement of the inferior epigastric vessels is another consequence of this directional shift of the inguinal canal.

Indirect inguinal hernia has a wide range of clinical presentations. It may be incidentally detected during physical examination in an individual who is otherwise asymptomatic or it can cause a life-threatening mechanical bowel obstruction with incarceration and strangulation. At times patients, especially middle-aged or elderly, may describe pain or discomfort in the lower abdominal quadrants, or they note the appearance of a swelling after an accident or abdominal strain. The frequency and intensity of pain, however, vary greatly from individual to individual. In general, chronic moderate or even extensive protrusion of abdominal contents through an enlarged deep inguinal ring usually produces less discomfort than do those cases with a sudden onset, except for cases with incarceration. The diagnosis of an uncomplicated indirect inguinal hernia is made by inspection and palpation. A male patient should be examined in the supine as well as the erect position, first with the flat hand over the inguinal region and the fingertips resting over the superficial (subcutaneous) inguinal ring and exerting a slight pressure along the inguinal canal. Then, with the palmar surface of the hand resting over the patient's thigh, the fifth finger should be gently pushed forward through the superficial ring invaginating the scrotal skin. The protruding abdominal tissue can thus be felt while the patient is completely relaxed. A patent but empty sac cannot be detected; therefore the patient needs to be made to contract the abdominal musculature to increase the abdominal pressure or asked to cough. This will force a part of the abdominal contents to enter the canal where the palpating finger can feel it directly or at least feel a change or shift of the tissues within the canal "cough impulse." In infants, the examination is naturally not so simple, and a hernia, when reduced, is hardly recognizable. Thickening of the cord at the superficial ring is said to be a reliable sign of a hernia, provided it is unilateral so that the cord on both sides can be compared. Children with a left-sided congenital inguinal hernia often develop a right-sided hernia soon after. Oddly, this is not true of a right-sided hernia.

In females, the best diagnostic method consists of placing two fingers over the subcutaneous inguinal ring and palpating for an expansile impulse on coughing or with steadier increase of intraabdominal pressure as produced by voluntary contraction of the abdominal musculature.

### FUNICULAR PROCESS AND HERNIA IN INFANCY

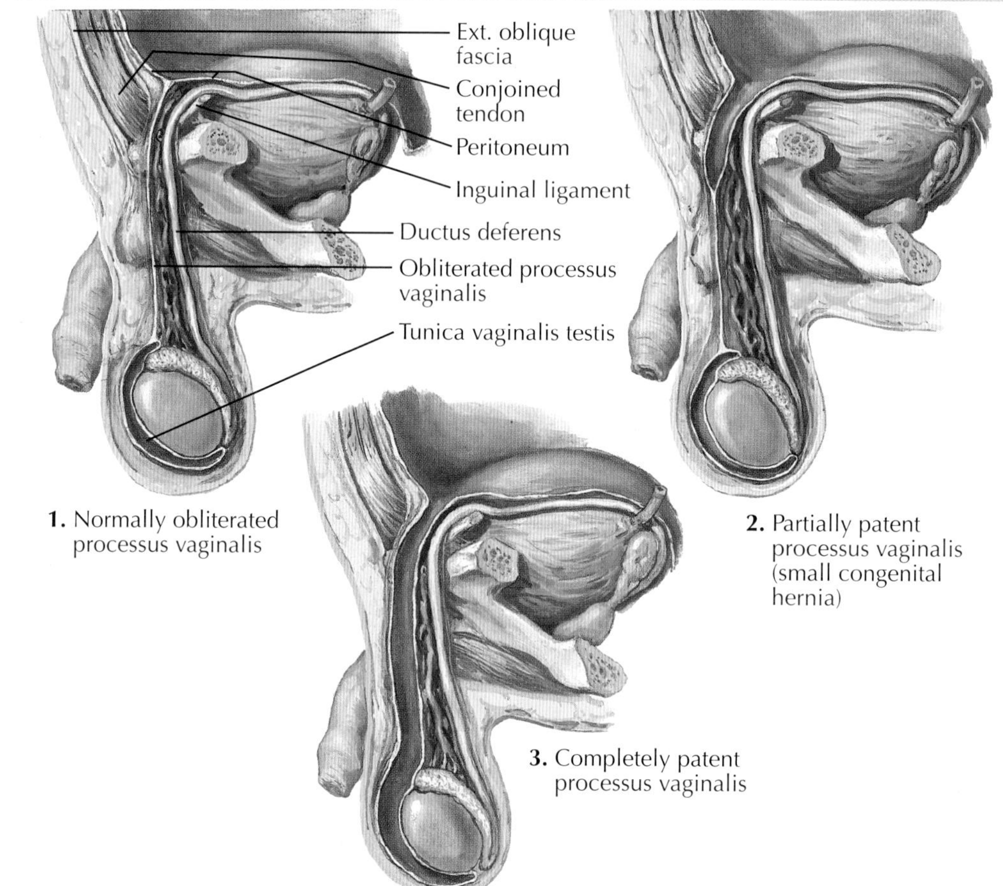


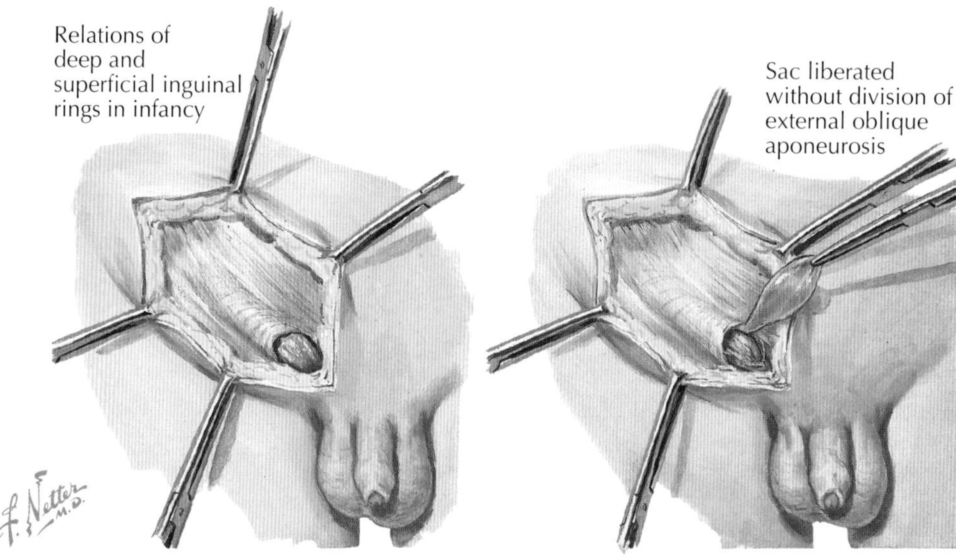


Distinction between indirect and direct inguinal hernias can be made by occluding the internal inguinal ring with a finger as the patient coughs. An indirect inguinal hernia should be blocked, but a direct hernia should freely bulge. Additionally, transmission of the cough impulse to the tip of the finger implies an indirect hernia, whereas an impulse palpated on the dorsum of the finger implies a direct hernia. Unfortunately, these physical findings help distinguish between direct and indirect hernias only 50% of the time. If the herniated organ has protruded as far as the scrotum, consideration must be given to the possibility of other scrotal swellings, such as a hydrocele, epididymitis, testicular torsion, varicocele, or even testicular tumors. In females, labial cysts, abscesses, or tumors should be considered.

Laboratory testing is generally not helpful in the diagnosis of inguinal hernias. Incarceration and bowel ischemia may be associated with nonspecific leukocytosis and elevated lactic acid. When the history strongly suggests a hernia, but none can be elicited on an exam

# INDIRECT AND DIRECT INGUINAL HERNIAS (Continued)

or in situations where body habitus makes physical examination limited, then a radiologic investigation may be warranted. Radiologic modalities include US, CT, and MRI. Under a skilled technician, US can detect an inguinal hernia with a sensitivity of 86% and a specificity of 77%. CT imaging is more beneficial in excluding other etiologies of groin mass or in cases of complicated hernias. MRI has the highest sensitivity (95%) and specificity (96%) in the detection of an inguinal hernia, but its use should be reserved for difficult cases due to limited access and its exorbitant cost.

## DIRECT INGUINAL HERNIAS

*Direct inguinal hernia* has an etiologic and pathologic background quite different from that of indirect inguinal hernia. It is rarely seen in children, and it more frequently presents at 40 to 50 years of age, with a strong preponderance in males. Although considered an acquired disease, it nevertheless must be traced back to a congenital condition characterized by a poorly developed musculofascial wall in the lowermost portion of the internal oblique muscle, where the fibers, instead of coursing obliquely, are arranged more transversely. Furthermore, partly as a result of the transverse course of the fibers, the conjoined tendon is attached to the sheath of the rectus muscle at a variable distance above the pubic crest. The predisposing factor of a direct hernia is thereby assumed to be deficient protection of the inguinal (Hesselbach) triangle, particularly at the lateral angle. The characteristic anatomic feature of a direct inguinal hernia is that it protrudes medial to the inferior epigastric vessels instead of lateral to them, as with the indirect hernia. In other words, the direct hernia does not pass through the deep ring but bulges through the posterior wall of the inguinal canal. The precipitating causes may be strenuous and/or prolonged exertion in the erect position that produces a marked increase in intraabdominal pressure, or progressive distension of the abdomen as in ascites, or a progressive atrophy of abdominal muscles owing to advanced age or a wasting disease.

The clinical manifestations of the direct inguinal hernia are even less noticeable than are those of the indirect type. It is often asymptomatic and incidentally discovered as a painless bulge in the inguinal area by the patient or a physician. The mass is reduced instantly when the patient lies down and can reappear upon arising or with straining. As it enlarges, the direct inguinal hernia remains in the area above the inguinal ligament, expanding medially, in contrast to the indirect variety, which, as a rule, enlarges downward into the scrotum in males or the labia majora in females.

The protrusion only rarely emerges from the subcutaneous ring and usually remains small and incomplete. The globular mass is found close to the lateral border of the os pubis, the spermatic cord resting superficially and laterally upon the protrusion. With the hernia reduced, the same maneuver outlined for the diagnosis of indirect hernia (see above) should be carried out. When the patient coughs, impulse detected by the index finger rather than the tip of the fifth finger suggests a direct inguinal hernia arising from the floor of the canal.

## TREATMENT OF INGUINAL HERNIAS

Surgical repair remains the definitive treatment of inguinal hernia and is among the most common procedures performed by surgeons. Nonoperative management, namely the use of a truss, can be used to manage the pain, pressure, and protrusion of abdominal contents in the patient who is symptomatic and is not able to undergo surgery. In newborns, the application of a simple yarn truss for a period of 2 to 6 months is sometimes sufficient to prevent the protrusion of the abdominal contents and to allow for the spontaneous closure of a funicular process not obliterated at birth, but this method is not used much today, and surgical repair is preferred at any age.

TENSION-FREE HERNIA AND McVAY REPAIRS

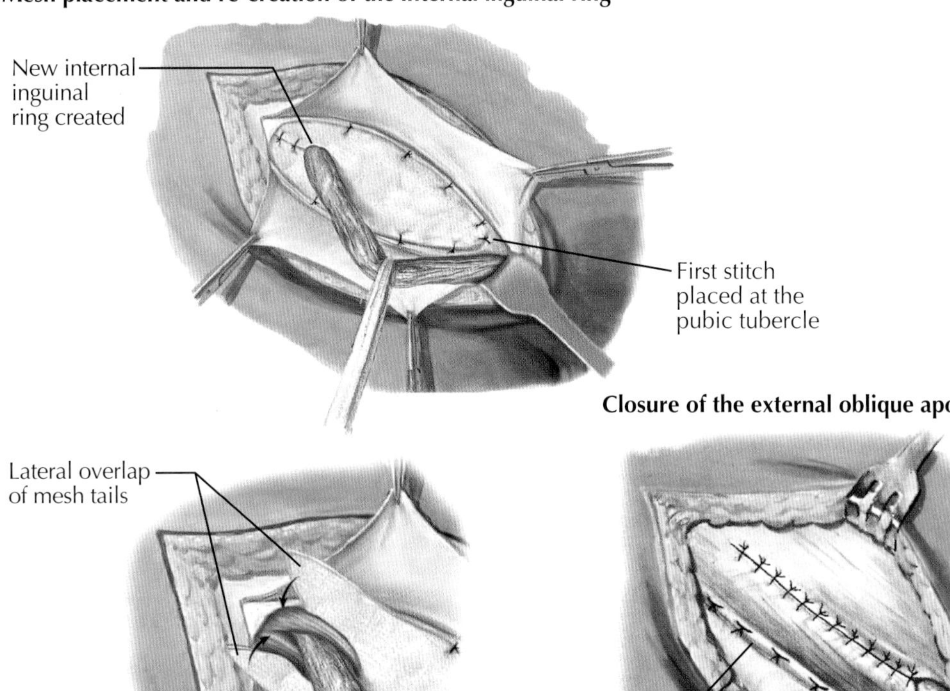


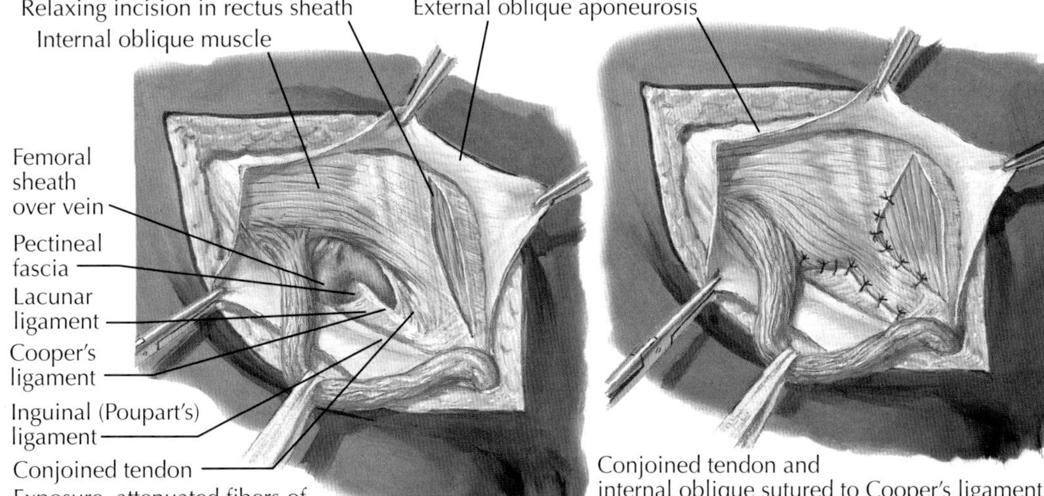


Exposure, attenuated fibers of posterior wall of inguinal canal (conjoined tendon and transversus abdominis trimmed away, Cooper's ligament cleaned)

Conjoined tendon and internal oblique sutured to Cooper's ligament, pectineal fascia, and anterior wall of femoral canal. Lateral margin of incision in rectus sheath sutured to rectus muscle and tendon.

TRANSABDOMINAL PREPERITONEAL AND TOTALLY EXTRAPERITONEAL APPROACHES TO INGUINAL HERNIA

**Transabdominal preperitoneal (TAPP) approach**

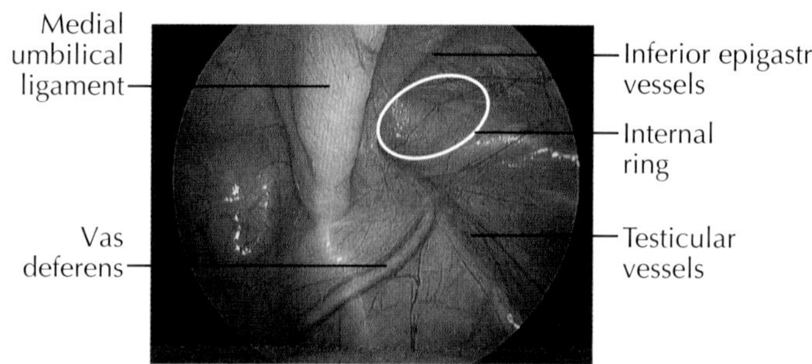


**A. Laparoscopic view of right groin**

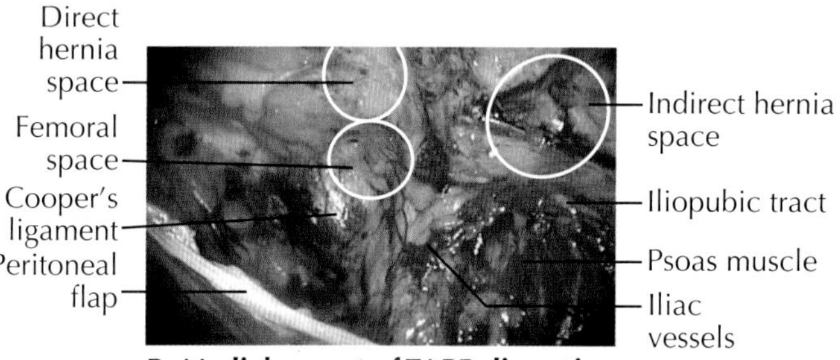


**B. Medial aspect of TAPP dissection**

**C. Mesh coverage prior to reperitonealizing**

**Totally extraperitoneal (TEP) approach**

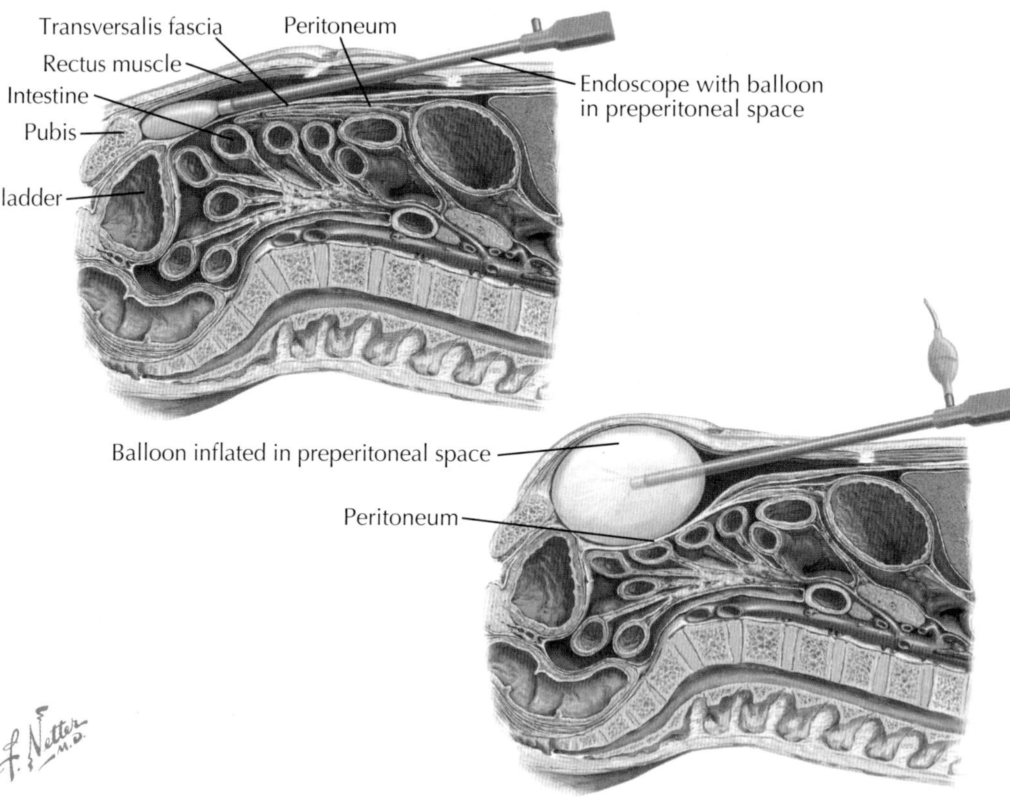


## INDIRECT AND DIRECT INGUINAL HERNIAS (Continued)

The surgical treatment of an inguinal hernia in infants is a relatively simple and low-risk procedure especially when the hernia is small and of recent onset. Ligation and excision of the sac is all that is required, because in infants the deep inguinal ring is almost adjacent to the superficial ring, and it is not necessary to divide the external oblique aponeurosis. Surgical intervention is urgently required in infants with an extroverted urinary bladder; an undescended testis, with or without torsion; or an ectopic testis. In girls, the presence of the ovary, fallopian tube, or uterus in the hernia sac must be ruled out before ligation.

Surgical repair of indirect inguinal hernias in adults can be performed using an open or minimally invasive technique (laparoscopic or robotic approach) with the latter preferred over the open approach because of faster recovery and reduced pain. Modern surgery of inguinal hernias began in the 1890s when Bassini (in Italy), Halsted (in the United States), and Ferguson (in Canada) simultaneously and independently developed operative techniques, the fundamental principles of which were identification and excision of the persistent sac, reparation of the defective deep ring, and strengthening of the posterior wall of the inguinal canal. Whether open, laparoscopic, or robotic, successful hernia repair depends on a tension-free closure that can be achieved either with a primary approximation or with the use of a mesh. Open repair is generally indicated for strangulated or large inguinal hernias or in cases where there is ascites or previous pelvic surgery. The open approach is also preferred for repair of unilateral inguinal hernias in males. If the open approach is planned, the use of tension-free mesh must be considered. The use of mesh generally reduces recurrence, but the risk of infection is increased if the hernia is complicated by incarceration or strangulation. The most common open mesh repair techniques used are the Lichtenstein repair and the "plug and patch" repair. When the mesh cannot be used, as in wound infection, primary approximation can be achieved using traditional open techniques such as the Bassini, Shouldice, and McVay repairs.

Laparoscopic hernia repair is increasingly popular, and under expert hands, recurrence rates are low. In the absence of the contraindications listed above, the laparoscopic approach is minimally invasive, with less postoperative pain and a fast recovery time. The two commonly performed laparoscopic inguinal hernia repair techniques are the transabdominal preperitoneal patch (TAPP) repair and the totally extraperitoneal (TEP) repair. The use of mesh to create a tension-free repair is recommended for all laparoscopic techniques. The choice of which laparoscopic technique to use mainly depends on the expertise of the surgeon. The TEP technique is generally recommended for male patients, whereas in females with indirect inguinal hernias or individuals who have undergone prior pelvic surgery, the TAPP approach offers an easier and safer method.

Robotic-assisted surgery has been well established as a technique that provides improved three-dimensional (3D) visualization and enhanced dexterity with articulating instrumentation. It has similar efficacy as conventional laparoscopic surgery under ideal circumstances, with placement of mesh an essential step. However, it is more costly, and relative contraindications include previous laparoscopic repair, ascites, peritoneal dialysis, and large inguinoscrotal hernias. Both TEP and TAPP repairs are feasible using a robotic approach (rTEP and rTAPP); however, the rTAPP is done with considerably more frequency than rTEP.

**ANATOMY OF FEMORAL HERNIA**

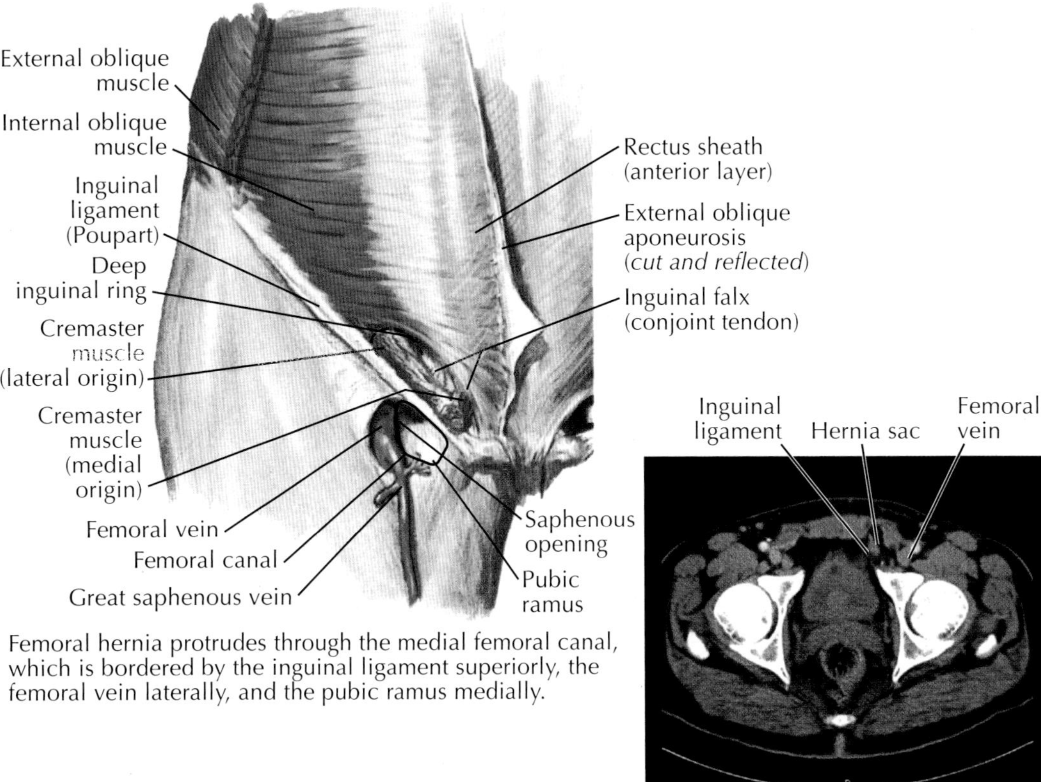


Femoral hernia protrudes through the medial femoral canal, which is bordered by the inguinal ligament superiorly, the femoral vein laterally, and the pubic ramus medially.

CT scan showing a femoral hernia. In this cut the femoral vein and inguinal ligament, which serve as boundaries for the femoral canal, can be seen.

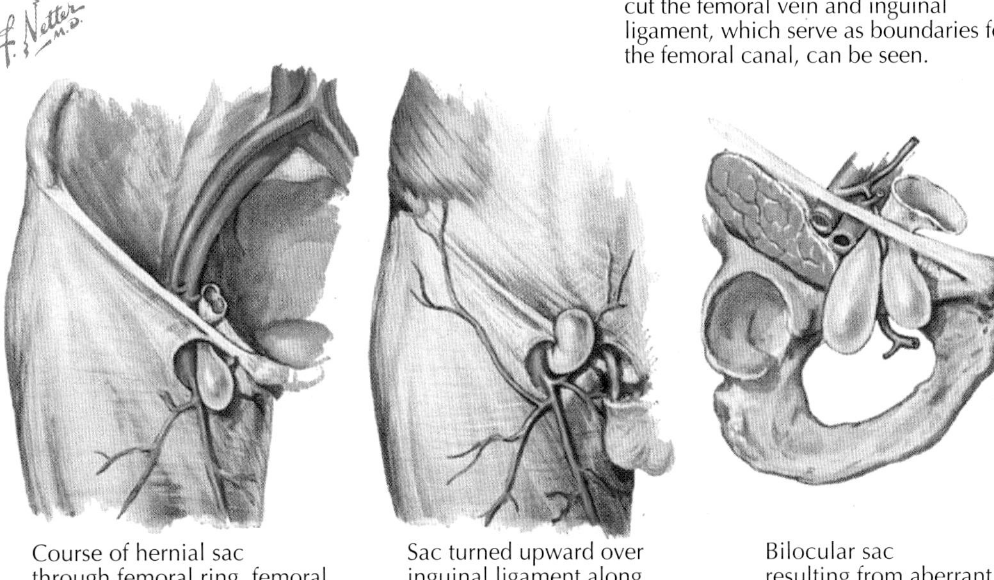

Course of hernial sac through femoral ring, femoral canal, and fossa ovalis

Sac turned upward over inguinal ligament along superficial epigastric vein

Bilocular sac resulting from aberrant obturator artery

Figures demonstrate different courses that the hernia sac can take after it protrudes through the femoral canal. If the sac is turned upward as in the second picture, this can mimic an inguinal hernia on physical examination.

## FEMORAL HERNIA

A protrusion of parts of the abdominal viscus or of peritoneal fatty tissue through the femoral ring is termed a *femoral hernia.* Its incidence is far lower than that of inguinal hernias and is very seldom seen in children. The right side is affected twice as frequently as the left, and females are four times more likely to develop a femoral hernia than males. Femoral hernias appear to be an acquired condition resulting from weakening or disruption of the fibromuscular tissue due to an underlying connective tissue disorder or after injury or from increased intraabdominal pressure. The higher incidence in parous females suggests muscular weakening related to pregnancy or childbirth; however, this finding is not always demonstrated in studies.

The protruding structures descend almost vertically behind and beneath the inguinal ligament and through the femoral ring. This ring presents the superior margin of the only potential space in most persons, known as the *femoral canal,* which is the most medial portion of the venous compartment of the femoral sheath. Anteriorly, the femoral sheath is flanked by a downward prolongation of the transversalis fascia over the femoral vessels, and posteriorly by the continuation of the pectineal fascia derived from the iliac fascia. Medially, these two fascial layers are adherent to each other, and as they descend, they blend with the adventitia of the vessels so that the sheath assumes a funnel-like configuration around the vessels. Just below the inguinal ligament, the femoral sheath (and its most medial portion, the femoral canal) lies under cover of the fascia lata, except in the region of the *fossa ovalis,* where the cover consists of the much weaker cribriform fascia. An advancing femoral hernia, after having entered the femoral ring, opens the femoral canal, *displacing and narrowing the femoral vein.* The hernial sac usually emerges through the fossa ovalis, pushing the cribriform fascia ahead of it. The *sac may then turn upward* and extend to the region in front of or above the inguinal ligament by following the *superficial epigastric vessels,* or it may turn medially toward or into the scrotum or labium majus, respectively. Laterally, the sac may pass over the femoral vessels or may descend downward along the saphenous vein. The neck, however, remains always below the inguinal ligament and lateral to the pubic tubercle, and the fundus of the sac lies usually in the medial part of the Scarpa triangle (trigonum femorale). A rather surprising number of varieties, some indeed very rare, have been described. The *sac may rest*

### Surgical Repair of Femoral Hernia

**Operation from above**

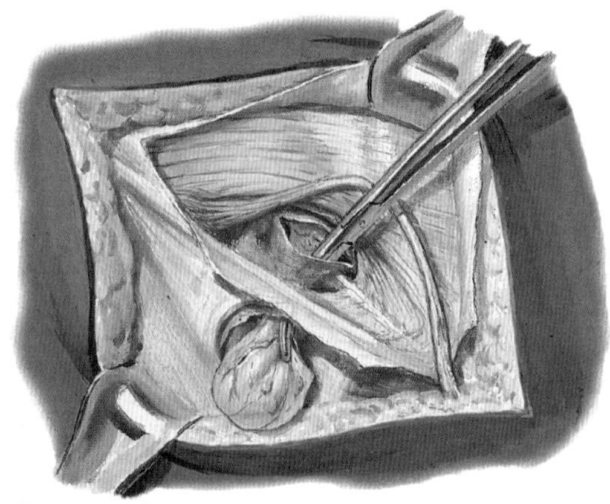

Liberation of sac: conversion of femoral to inguinal hernia through incision in transversalis fascia

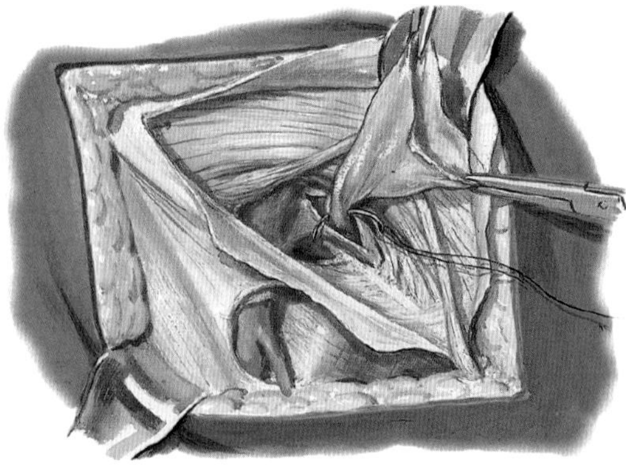

Sac drawn up, twisted, and transfixed preparatory to ligation and excision

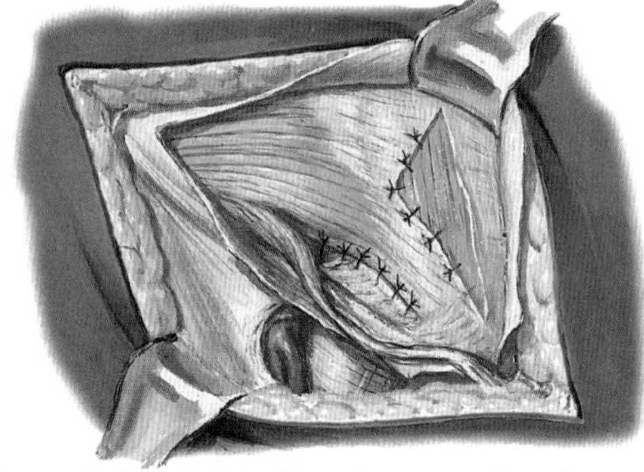

Internal oblique muscle and conjoined tendon sutured to Cooper's (pectineal) ligament and pectineal fascia

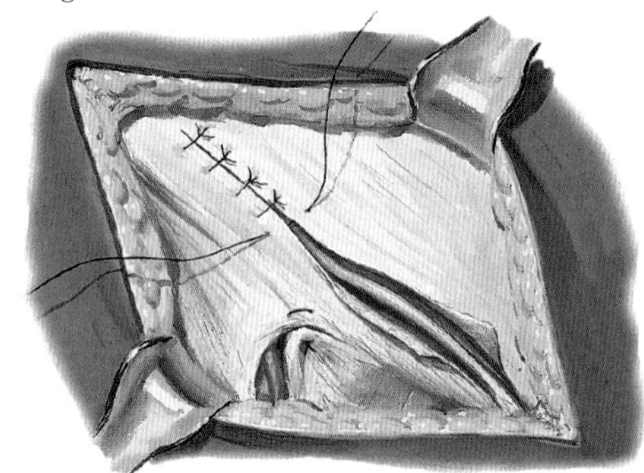

Closure of external oblique aponeurosis *over* round ligament or cord. Inguinal ligament sutured to pectineal fascia.

**Operation from below**

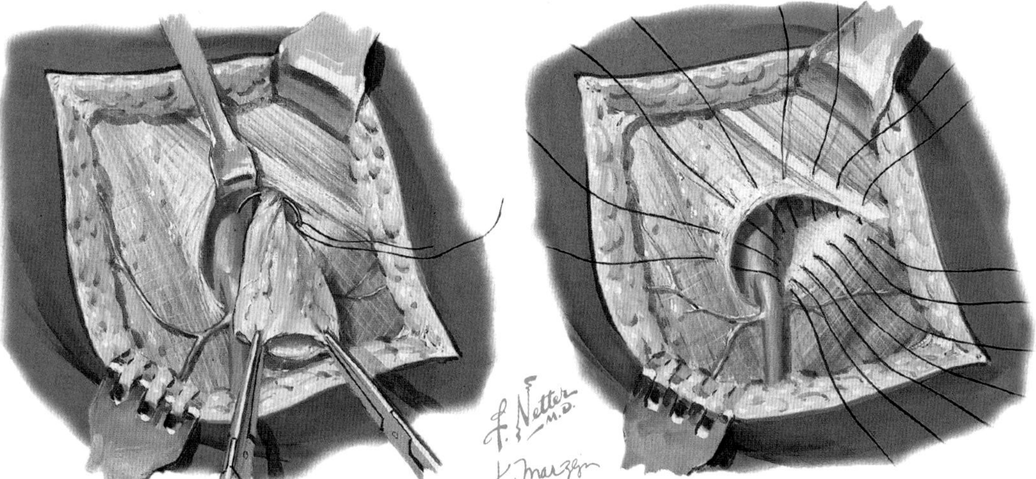

Sac freed, opened, emptied, twisted, and transfixed high up

Bassini's closure of femoral canal

## Femoral Hernia (Continued)

*on the femoral sheath* anterior to the femoral vessels *(prevascular hernia)* or may descend behind the vessels *(retrovascular hernia).* The sac may become divided at the femoral ring, one part following the normal route, and another being directed toward the obturator foramen. A *femoral hernia* may also become *bilocular* by virtue of an aberrant obturator artery. It also has been observed that a direct inguinal hernia may shift to the femoral region instead of descending into the scrotum *(cruroscrotal hernia),* thus simulating a femoral hernia.

Femoral hernias can be easily overlooked if small, but when part of the intestine is contained in the sac, pain is likely to be severe. Complications occur with great frequency, with 40% of cases presenting as emergencies with strangulation or incarceration. The diagnosis can usually be made upon finding a soft bulge at the femoral fossa inferior to the inguinal ligament and medial to the femoral artery. This finding may not be evident if the hernial sac has turned upward over the inguinal ligament along the superficial epigastric vein. In diagnosing a femoral hernia, reducible or not, one must exclude also inguinal adenitis, lipoma, varicosities of the saphenous vein, psoas abscess, obturator hernia, hydrocele of the femoral sac, hydatid cysts, dermoid cysts, and other processes that can present as a localized soft or fluctuant swelling. Commonly, hernia contents include the omentum and small bowel but rarely, the appendix (usually inflamed), a Meckel diverticulum, or a portion of the bladder (type of sliding hernia), ureter, or broad ligament have been observed to herniate.

Surgical repair is recommended for all patients with a femoral hernia. Early elective surgical repair is recommended to avoid urgent surgery for a strangulated femoral hernia necessitating bowel resection. Posterior repair using laparoscopic (either TAPP or TEP) approach is favored rather than an open anterior repair of femoral hernias for both technical and patient outcomes. The use of mesh reduces recurrence, and various mesh repair techniques can be used except for Lichtenstein repair, which does not cover the femoral ring. Laparoscopic repair (using TAPP or TEP) of femoral hernias is also possible. However, an open approach is still preferred to treat complicated femoral hernias, especially when bowel resection is expected. Open repair under local or regional anesthesia may also be favored in patients who cannot tolerate general anesthesia because the latter is often required for laparoscopic groin hernia repair.

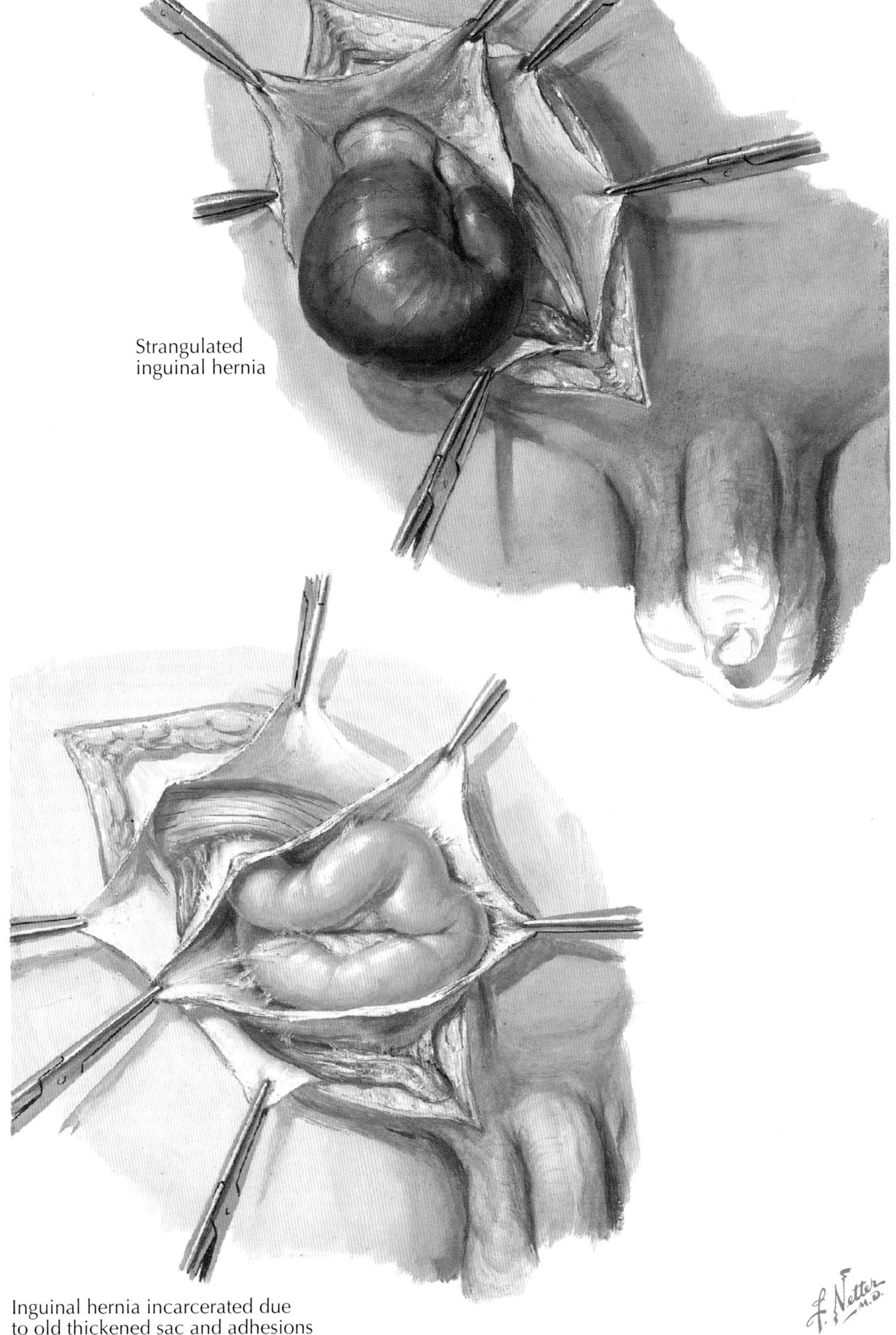


Inguinal hernia incarcerated due to old thickened sac and adhesions

## Complications of Inguinal and Femoral Hernias

### Hernial Incarceration and Strangulation

If the sac and the contents of a hernia cannot be replaced within the peritoneal cavity, the hernia is termed an *irreducible* or *incarcerated hernia.* Left untreated, edema develops, leading to obstruction of venous blood flow and then arterial blood flow, with subsequent ischemia and necrosis of the hernial contents *(strangulation).* A sharp pain over the very tender hernial area is usually present, and the pain may also be referred to the umbilicus. Vomiting of gastric contents begins early, but its character soon changes to bilious and finally to feculent vomiting. Systemic signs of acute circulatory collapse ensue, with bowel necrosis and frank perforation; however, generalized peritonitis may not occur, because the necrotic tissue is trapped within the hernial sac. In such cases, surgical intervention is urgently required. For incarcerated and strangulated groin hernias, the operating table may be placed in the reverse Trendelenburg position during induction of anesthesia to decrease the likelihood that the hernia will reduce spontaneously. The first operative step upon opening the hernial sac is inspection of the herniated intestinal loop to determine the viability. If the incarcerated loop is deemed to be viable (return of red color, restoration of elasticity, firmness, and shiny appearance), it is permitted to return into the peritoneal cavity. If deemed nonviable (black, green, or yellowish patches; loss of peritoneal luster; flabby consistency), then it must be resected. The decision to perform primary anastomosis or to exteriorize the loop through an ostomy depends on the health of the rest of the intestine and the patient's condition. Likewise, the use of mesh when repairing an acutely strangulated or incarcerated hernia depends on the wound classification. A synthetic mesh should be used for class 1 (clean) and class 2 (clean contaminated) hernias, whereas it should be avoided in class 3 (contaminated) and 4 (dirty infected) hernias.

### Recurrent Hernia

The incidence of recurrent hernia appears to have declined over the past several decades, likely due to the more frequent use of mesh in primary hernia repair, and currently ranges from 0.5% to 15%. This wide range is dependent on patient factors, such as age, obesity, and duration of the hernia and technical issues, such as the surgeon's experience, type of anesthesia, clinical circumstances (elective or emergency) type of repair, use of mesh, and type of suture material. Recurrence can be early (within 5 years of the repair) or late (>5 years after the repair). Earlier recurrence suggests technical problems, whereas late recurrence is associated with patient-related issues. Repair of a recurrent hernia can be approached through an open or a laparoscopic method. Most surgeons incorporate mesh to create a tension-free repair, even for recurrent hernias. Additionally, an anatomic approach that avoids previously dissected tissues is recommended. Failed anterior repairs should be approached using a posterior approach, and vice versa. If mesh was used for the primary repair, attempts should not be made to remove the mesh used previously, unless there is evidence of infection, or the mesh used previously was believed to be causing pain.

## Special Forms of Hernia

*Sliding hernia (en glissade)* is a special type of inguinal hernia in which an extraperitoneal viscus such as the cecum (on the right) and sigmoid (on the left) and occasionally the ovaries and fallopian tubes form the posterior wall of the hernia sac. This appears to result from partial detachment of the parietal peritoneum from the underlying structure, permitting the parietal peritoneum to "slide" on top of the viscus and its visceral serosa through the hernial opening. The herniated viscus is thus only partially enclosed in the sac because the posterior margin of the sac is reflected onto the viscus itself to form the visceral peritoneum. It should be noted, however, that the majority of herniations involving the colon are not of the sliding variety. In most instances, the large bowel in a hernial sac is entirely covered with peritoneum and is, therefore, freely movable, and readily reducible unless adhesions are present. The procedures recommended to repair this type of sliding hernia differ from those for an indirect or direct hernia. The peritoneal protrusion, including the contiguous bowel, is drawn into the wound. The sac is then opened, and the herniated intestine is freely mobilized by dividing its peritoneal attachment to the peritoneal wall of the sac, carefully avoiding injury to subjacent vessels. After the visceral organ has been replaced into the peritoneal cavity, the neck of the sac is obliterated by approximating it to the transversalis fascia below. The remainder of the operation corresponds to the traditional open McVay technique.

The bladder may herniate through the internal deep inguinal ring as an indirect inguinal hernia, or it may pass medial to the deep inferior epigastric vessels as a direct hernia. The protruding part of the bladder may be enclosed in a peritoneal fold *(intraperitoneal)* or the peritoneal fold may only partly accompany the protruding organ, lying above it *(paraperitoneal)*. A portion of the bladder not covered by peritoneum may herniate, usually by the direct pathway *(extraperitoneal hernia)*. Finally, a peritoneal hernial sac may form, entering the inguinal canal through the deep ring, whereas the bladder, usually an extraperitoneal part, protrudes medial to the inferior epigastric vessels *(pantaloon* or *saddlebag hernia)* where the vessel forms the "crotch" of the pantaloon. The bladder may enter the hernial sac by becoming adherent to the lateral aspect of the medial wall of the sac, so that the bladder forms one of the sac's covers, particularly in massive hernias. The history presented by patients with bladder protrusion is usually that of a long-standing, large, irreducible hernia, which diminishes or disappears after urination. Besides the bladder, the sac often contains intestine and/or omentum. Operation of a bladder hernia involves special techniques, beginning with a rather wide suprapubic incision. If the hernia is of moderate size, it has been customary merely to plicate the redundant part, but, in view of the frequent recurrences in this variety of hernia, it seems advisable to excise the diverticular protrusion and to close the aperture. The remainder of the operation is then the same as with any other direct hernia. The preoperative insertion of a catheter into the bladder is important if any suspicion exists that the bladder participates in the contents of the hernial sac.

A rare type of hernia called *reduction en masse (displaced hernia)* occurs when the contents of the hernial sac return to the peritoneal cavity while within the sac, the neck of which is so small and unable to dilate that the intestinal loop cannot retreat. Other complications arise when the sac's contents become inflamed, as may happen especially with the appendix vermiformis, a Meckel diverticulum, or when only a part of the intestinal wall (*partial enterocele,* sometimes called *Littré hernia*) gets caught in the sac. Another rare variety of hernia, termed the *hernia-in-W,* or *Maydl hernia,* develops when the sac contains two intestinal loops but the connecting portion between them is left in the peritoneal cavity and subsequently gets squeezed, strangulated (retrograde strangulation), and finally becomes gangrenous as a result of a narrow neck.

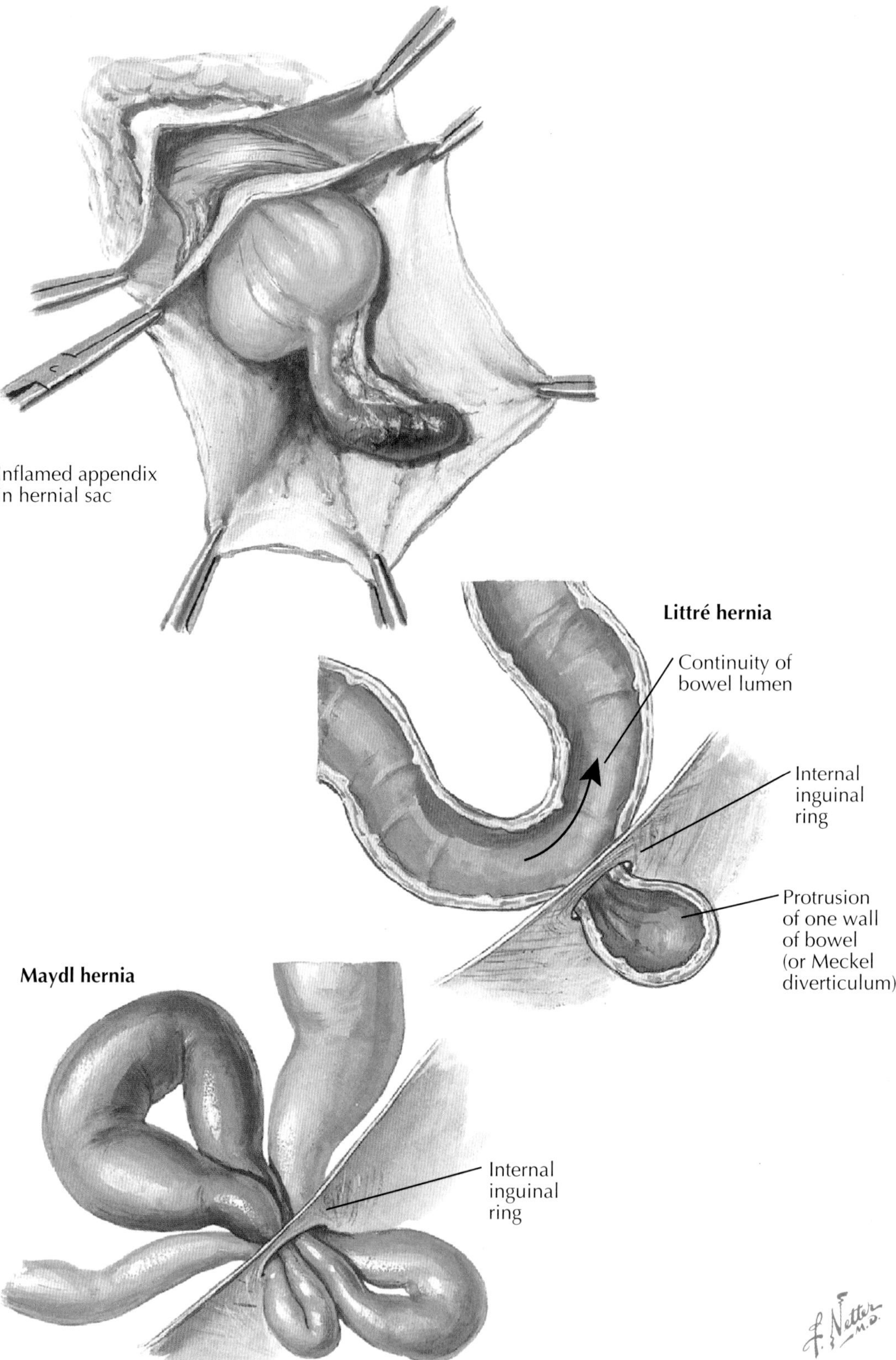

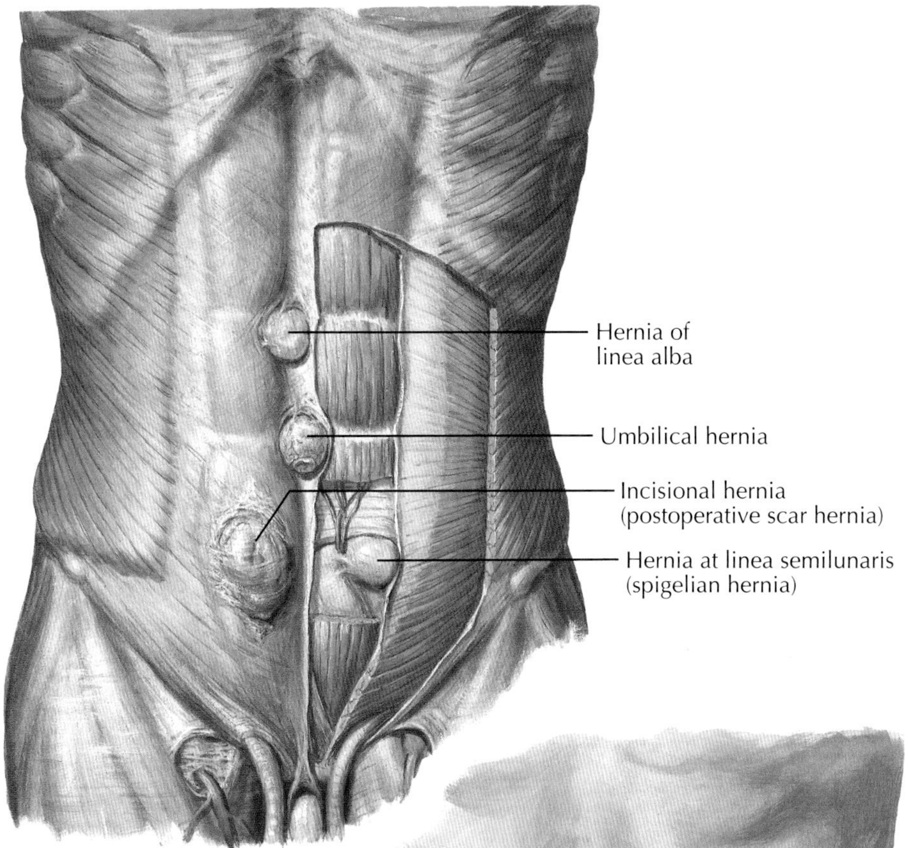

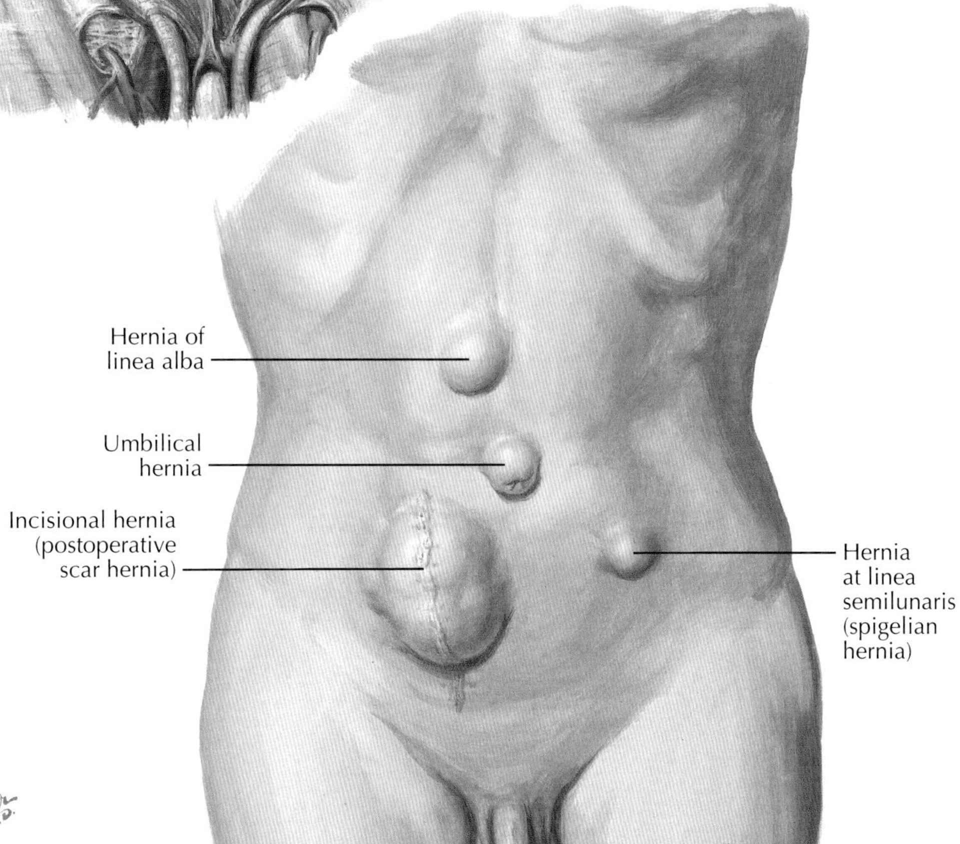

## VENTRAL HERNIA

*Ventral hernias* represent defects in the parietal abdominal wall fascia and muscle through which intraabdominal or preperitoneal contents can protrude. They include hernias that arise at the linea alba (*umbilical hernia* and *epigastric hernia*) and at the semilunar line *(spigelian hernia)*. Ventral hernias may be congenital or acquired from poor healing of an anterior abdominal wall incision *(incisional hernia)*.

*Epigastric hernias* are primary hernias of the linea alba that occur above the umbilicus just to the left or right of the midline. These types of hernias are uncommon and appear more often in males than in females. They develop as a result of a weakness in the fascial wall where the ventral cutaneous blood vessels emerge and rarely have a peritoneal sac or contain a viscus organ. Hernias located to the right of the midline usually contain fat of the falciform ligament, whereas those located on the left contain properitoneal fat. Most epigastric hernias are symptom-free and are discovered only upon routine physical examination. Occasionally, they may cause colicky pain or a "dragging" sensation in the epigastrium, with nausea, dyspepsia, and even vomiting. In children, epigastric hernias tend to close spontaneously with age.

*Umbilical hernias* occur at the umbilical ring and may present at birth or later in life. Umbilical hernias occur in 10% of newborns and are more common in premature infants. The hernia is often first noticed when intraabdominal pressure increases when the infant is crying, causing a protrusion. These hernias are usually small and disappear spontaneously by the fifth year. If closure does not occur, elective surgical repair is usually advised. In adults, these hernias may also be small; however, they may enlarge and cause a variety of symptoms, particularly when a peritoneal sac contains omentum and/or viscera or in cases of uncontrolled ascites. Furthermore, large hernias may become irreducible and incarcerated. Small and asymptomatic umbilical hernias in adults can be followed clinically, but larger ones require operation by primary sutured repair or placement of prosthetic mesh using open or laparoscopic methods.

A *spigelian hernia* appears at the point where the linea semilunaris and the linea semicircularis join and where the inferior epigastric vessels pierce the posterior wall of the rectus sheath, a transverse 6-cm-wide zone, referred to as the "Spigelian hernia belt." They generally appear in midlife, with an equal incidence in males and females. This type of hernia is assumed to be acquired and develops slowly. Spigelian hernias always have a peritoneal sac, with an overlying lipoma, and seldom grow more than 2 to 3 cm in diameter. The presentation and the management are similar to those of an umbilical hernia.

*Incisional hernias* develop at the site of a previous abdominal procedure, including laparoscopic port sites. The incidence ranges from 10% to over 20% in patients who develop wound infections. Obesity, smoking, malnutrition, chronic use of glucocorticoids, postoperational strain, and poor surgical technique are all factors that interfere with adequate wound healing and predispose to the development of incisional hernias. The management of incisional hernias can be expectant or surgical depending on the size, presence of symptoms, and comorbidities of the patient.

*Diastasis of the rectus abdominis muscles* cannot be considered a true hernia. It is caused by a separation of the two rectus muscles with widening of the linea alba more than 2 cm. It can be seen in newborns shortly after birth as a bulge and can sometimes extend from the xyphoid process to the umbilicus. It also occurs in adults, mostly in multiparous middle-aged females. In infants, the diastasis disappears with development and growth. In adults, this condition is usually asymptomatic with only cosmetic consequences. If symptomatic, then surgical repair with plication of the rectus sheath with or without abdominoplasty can be performed.

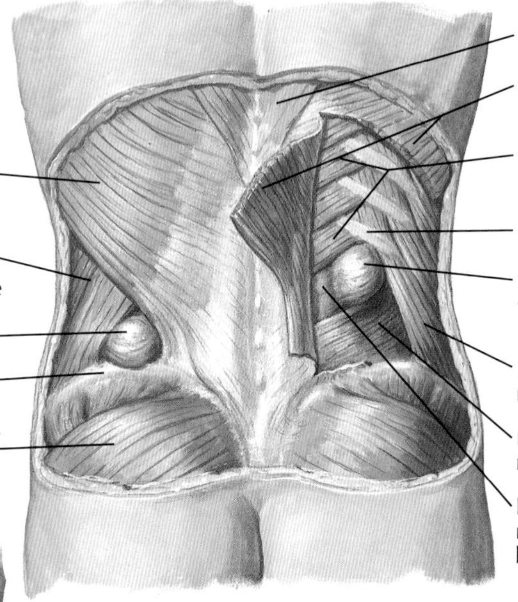

## LUMBAR AND PARASTOMAL HERNIAS

*Lumbar hernias* can develop in one of two naturally occurring defects in the lumbar region. One of these defects is the *inferior lumbar space,* or *Petit's triangle,* located above the iliac crest and bordered laterally by the posterior margin of the external oblique muscle and medially by the latissimus dorsi muscles. The other defect, the *superior lumbar space,* also known as the *Grynfeltt* or *Grynfeltt-Lesshaft triangle,* is an inverted triangle formed by the 12th rib and the serratus posterior inferior muscle superiorly, the erector spinae muscle medially, and the internal oblique muscle inferolaterally. *Lumbar hernias* as a rule contain a sac that consists of peritoneum, extraperitoneal tissue, or fat and omentum. Rarely, they may contain large or small intestine or the kidney, the latter, of course, without any peritoneal investment. Lumbar hernias can be congenital or spontaneous, but most are related to a prior abdominal trauma or urologic surgery. The most common clinical presentation is a posterolateral bulge that enlarges upon coughing. Occasionally, the patient may complain of pain in the loin or vague back pain. The hernia is usually easily reducible, and strangulation is rare. Surgical repairs, using a mesh, can be performed laparoscopically or via an open approach.

*Parastomal hernia* is a type of an incisional hernia that is formed at or adjacent to a stoma and is reported to be the most frequent complication occurring after the construction of an ileostomy or a colostomy. The incidence of parastomal hernias depend upon the type of ostomy and the definition used to identify the hernia; thus the reported incidence varies from zero to 50%. It typically occurs within a few years after creation of the ostomy but may also develop up to two to three decades after surgery. Patient factors such as ascites, obesity, and diabetes as well as technical factors have been implicated as risks for parastomal hernia formation. Most patients have typical symptoms and signs of peristomal bulging upon coughing, with pain or discomfort around the stoma. It is often difficult to maintain a seal between the stoma and the ostomy cover, with leakage of the effluent resulting in significant peristomal dermatitis, especially in patients with ileostomies and urostomies. Abdominal imaging with CT can confirm the diagnosis and characterize the hernia further.

Most patients with mild symptoms can be managed conservatively with the use of stomal support or abdominal belt and skin protective sealants. When available, a wound ostomy care nurse is an invaluable resource to help manage peristomal dermatitis and improve quality of life. Surgical management is indicated when there is obstruction, incarceration, or strangulation of the hernia. Surgery should also be considered for patients with recurrent pain, disfiguring hernias, and failure to manage leakage around the stoma with conservative measures.

Various surgical techniques have been described in the literature over the past few decades. The main techniques have included suture repair of the fascial defect, translocation of the stoma, and mesh repair. Several different approaches also have been described that include laparotomy, lateral approach, and laparoscopic methods, each with varying rates of success. Regardless of repair technique, emergent repair appears to be an independent risk factor for parastomal hernias.



**Anatomic relations of lumbar hernias**

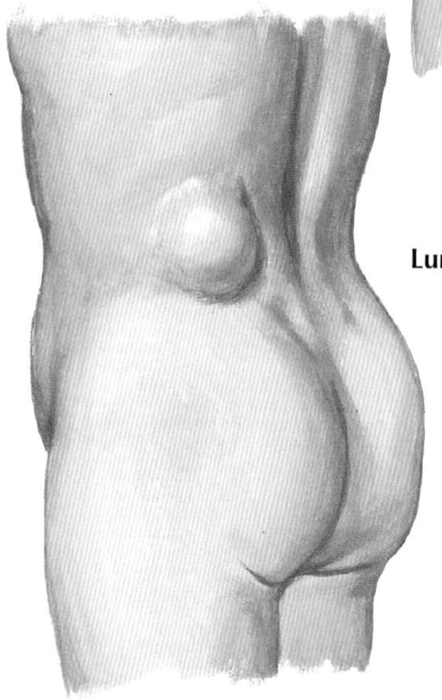

**Lumbar hernia**

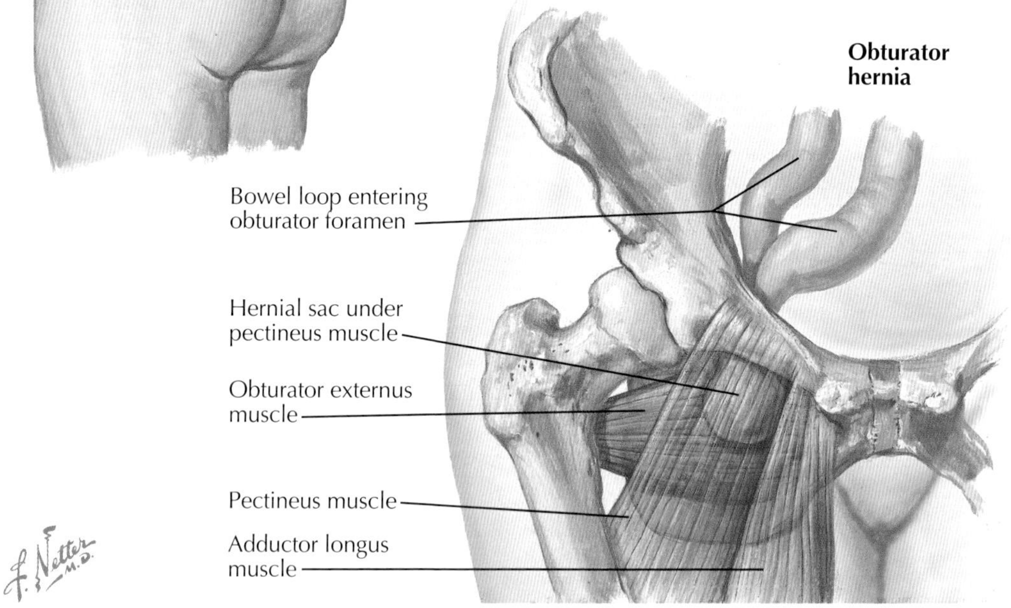

**Obturator hernia**

# Pelvic Hernias

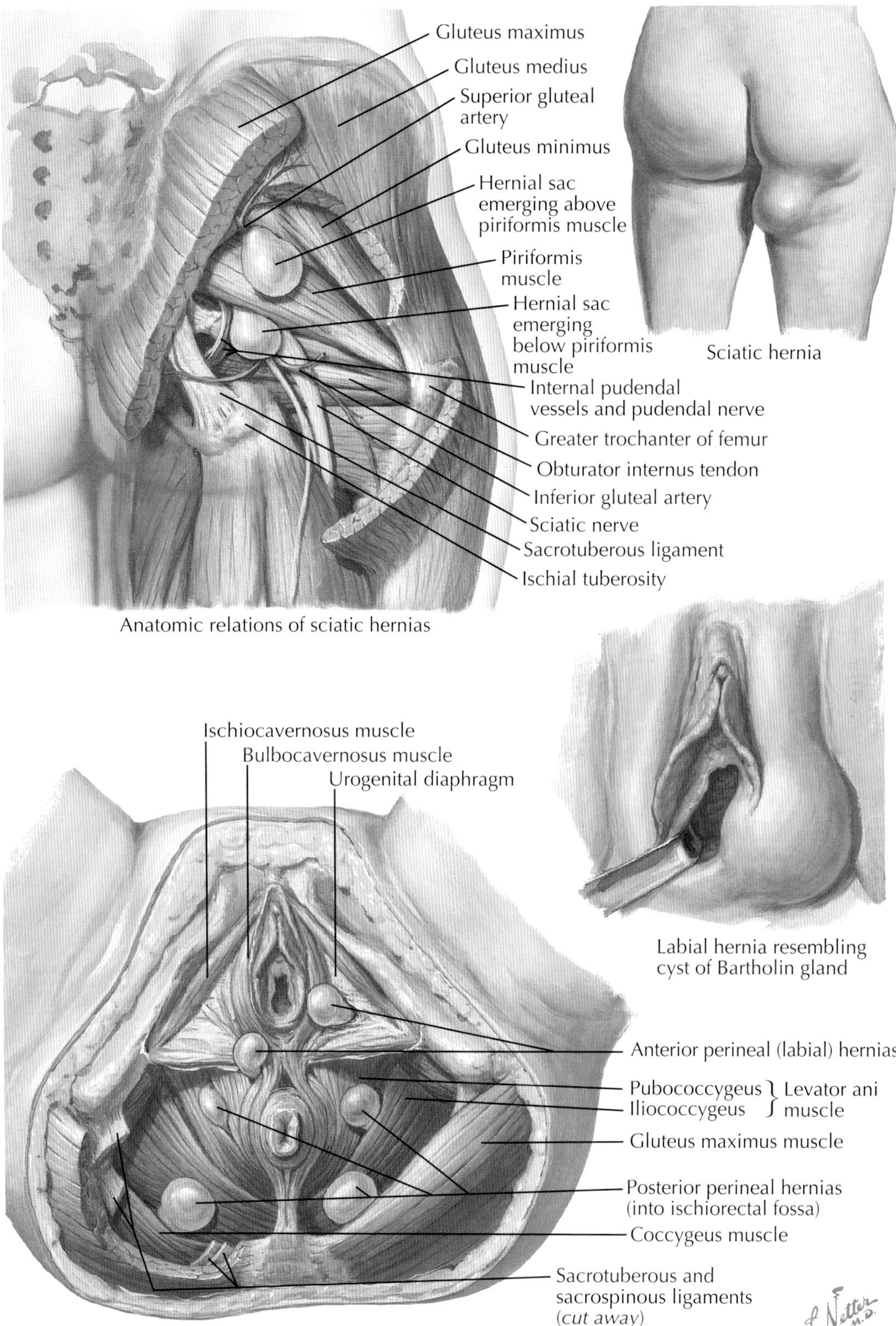


Anatomic relations of sciatic hernias

Anatomic relations of perineal hernias

*Obturator hernia* is a rare type of abdominal wall hernia that develops through the obturator foramen alongside the obturator vessels and nerve. It is caused by weakening of the obturator membrane, resulting in enlargement of the canal. It is often seen in the right side but can be bilateral and appears to be more common in females. The *obturator hernia* usually consists of a peritoneal sac and may contain small or large intestine, appendix, omentum, bladder, ovary, fallopian tube, or uterus. The sac may pass completely through the foramen and come to lie upon the obturator externus covered by the pectineus muscle. In some instances, it may pass between the fasciculi of the obturator externus muscle or even insert itself between the layers of the obturator membrane. Given the depth at which it lies, the diagnosis of an obturator hernia can be extremely difficult. A slight bulge may be noticeable as a tender, tense mass in the upper obturator region (i.e., the upper, inner part of the femoral [Scarpa] triangle) when the patient is in the dorsal position with the thigh flexed, adducted, and rotated outward so as to relax the pectineus, adductor longus, and obturator internus muscles. The *Howship-Romberg sign* is pathognomonic of an obturator hernia (when present) and is characterized by pain that extends from the inguinal crease to the anteromedial aspect of the thigh radiating to the knee. The neck of the sac may be palpated during rectal or vaginal examination when the hernia is sufficiently large. GI symptoms (nausea, vomiting, colicky pain, constipation) rarely appear before complications arise. The differential diagnosis must take into consideration inguinal adenitis; psoas abscess; obturator neuritis; diseases of the hip joint; internal, perineal, and femoral hernias; and other causes of intestinal obstruction. The treatment of obturator hernias is surgical repair using an abdominal, inguinal, or obturator approach. If strangulation is suspected, however, an abdominal approach is preferred.

*Sciatic hernias* pass through the greater sciatic foramen above *(suprapiriform hernia)* or below *(infrapiriform hernia)* the pyriformis muscle, or through the lesser sciatic foramen *(spinotuberous hernia)*. Diagnosis of a sciatic hernia or obturator hernia is difficult unless the hernia is large and bulges into the thigh. Patients occasionally complain of pain that radiates along the path of the great sciatic nerve. Lipoma, gluteal aneurysm, or abscess must be considered in the differential diagnosis. Strangulation of the hernial contents occurs frequently and may be the cause of intestinal obstruction. The surgical repair of a sciatic hernia is performed using a transabdominal or a transgluteal route, or a combined approach.

*Perineal hernias* are hernias that protrude through the floor of the pelvis and are usually seen in older multiparous females and/or after surgery. The *anterior variety* of perineal hernia, also known as a *pudendal* or *labial hernia,* which exclusively occurs in females, may pass through or behind the urogenital diaphragm and present as a bulge in the labia where it resembles a Bartholin gland cyst. The *posterior perineal hernias* may escape between the subdivisions of the levator ani muscle, or between the levator ani and coccygeus muscles, and ultimately present as a bulge over the gluteal region thus resembling a sciatic hernia (see above). Perineal hernias usually have a peritoneal sac containing omentum, a loop of the large or small gut, or other viscera. The mass may be palpated during a bimanual vaginal examination and confirmed via pelvic imaging. These hernias must be differentiated from vulvar masses and perirectal or anorectal abscesses or masses. The perineal hernias are usually reducible but may occasionally become strangulated. Surgical repair can be achieved via an abdominal, a perineal, or a combined abdominoperineal approach.

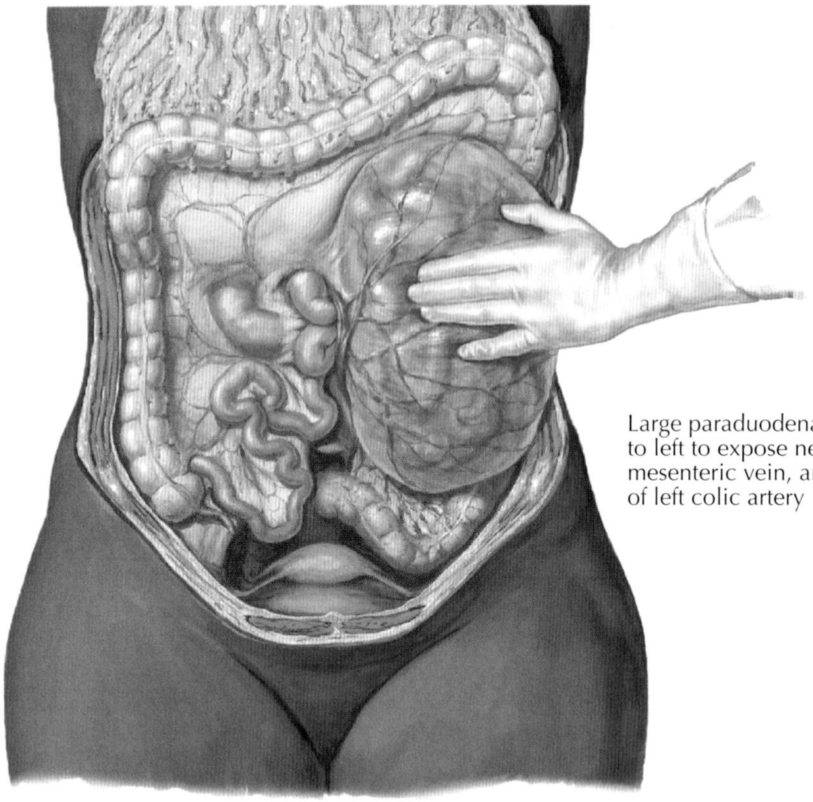

Large paraduodenal hernia sac drawn to left to expose neck, inferior mesenteric vein, and ascending branch of left colic artery

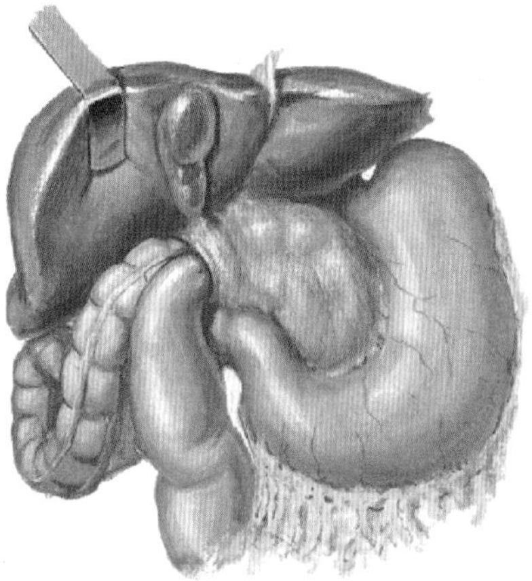

Hernia through epiploic foramen (Winslow) into lesser peritoneal sac (omental bursa)

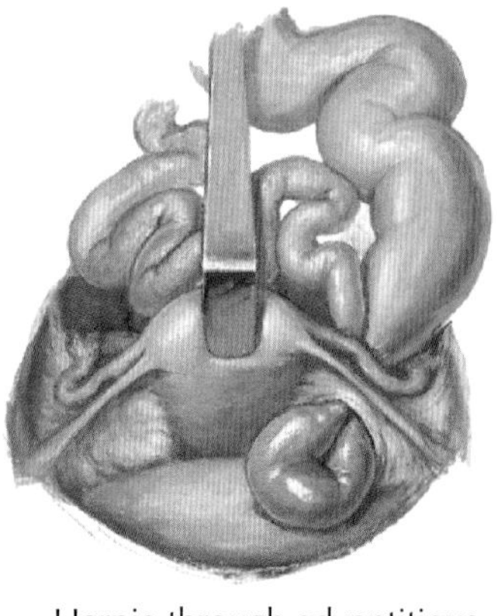

Hernia through adventitious opening in broad ligament

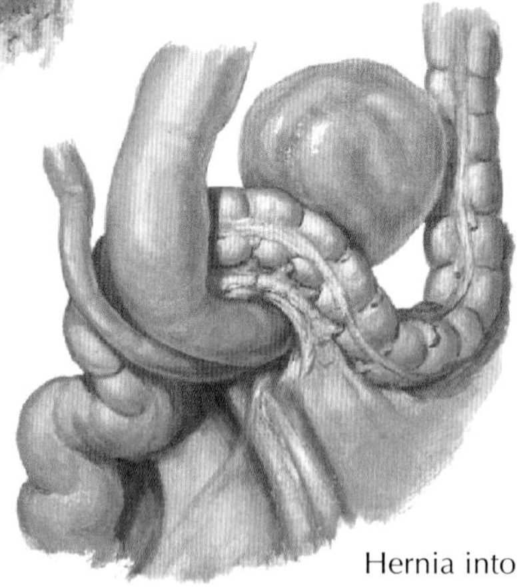

Hernia into intersigmoid fossa

## Internal Hernia

Internal hernia is a protrusion of a viscus through a normal or abnormal peritoneal or mesenteric aperture confined within the peritoneal cavity. These defects may be congenital, or they can be a result of iatrogenically created defects in the mesentery. Peterson's space is one such defect that is created during a roux-en-Y gastric bypass procedure. Internal hernias can be classified according to the anatomic distribution into paraduodenal, pericecal, intersigmoid, or transmesenteric hernias. The most common type is the paraduodenal hernia, which occurs on the left side in 75% of patients. Paraduodenal hernias are believed to occur because of congenital herniation of small bowel into the fossa of Landzert, located to the left of the fourth portion of the duodenum. The herniated bowel can extend into the descending mesocolon and distal transverse mesocolon. Twenty-five percent of paraduodenal hernias are right sided, involving the mesentericoparietal fossa of Waldeyer, located in the jejunal mesentery inferior to the third duodenum.

Internal hernias may remain asymptomatic, with incidental diagnosis made during an unrelated abdominal surgery or during autopsy. The clinical symptoms could be nonspecific with nausea and postprandial bloating and distension, or it can present acutely with life-threatening volvulus and intestinal obstruction. The presence of an internal hernia may be suspected when signs of intestinal obstruction set in and when a mass in the corresponding region can be palpated. Plain abdominal radiographs reveal signs of intestinal obstruction. Small bowel follow-through can be a useful aid for diagnosis. The typical finding on a small bowel follow-through is crowding of bowel loops in an abnormal location in the abdomen or pelvis, often appearing as though they are contained in a sac or confining border, and usually with varying degrees of small bowel obstruction. CT reveals a cluster of small-bowel loops mainly at the level of the ligament of Treitz or behind the pancreas.

Prompt surgical repair is indicated soon after diagnosis, and exploratory laparotomy is mandatory. It is useful to note that practically every case of internal hernia contains a major blood vessel coursing across the anterior margin of the hernial neck; therefore the steps of operation include adequate incision of the sac at the level beyond the neck, decompression followed by reduction of the hernia content, and repair of the defect. Removal of the sac remains controversial, and the decision to remove the sac should be made on a case-by-case basis.

## ABDOMINAL WOUNDS OF SMALL INTESTINE

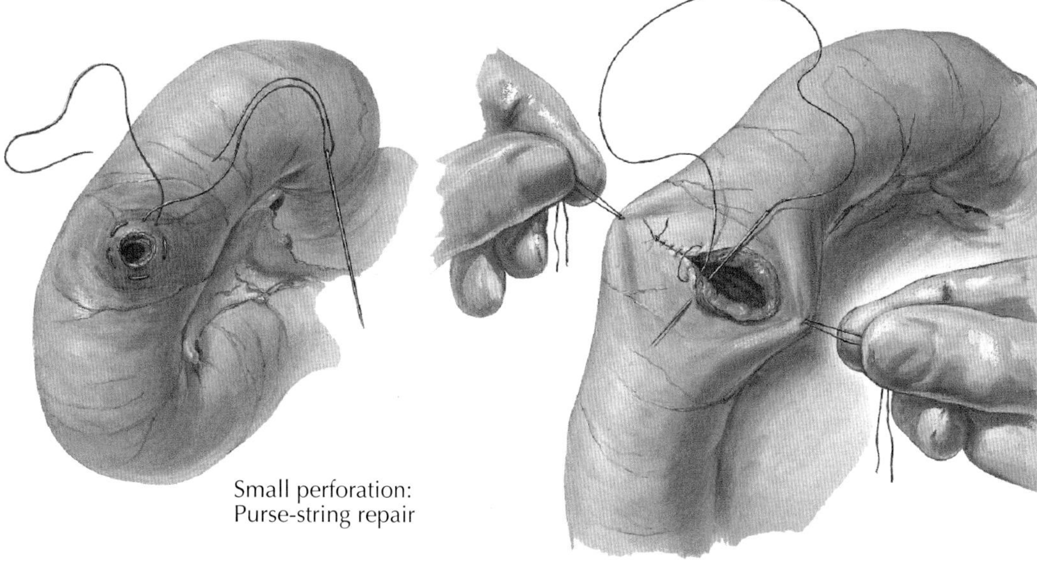

Small perforation: Purse-string repair

Small laceration: Transverse suture

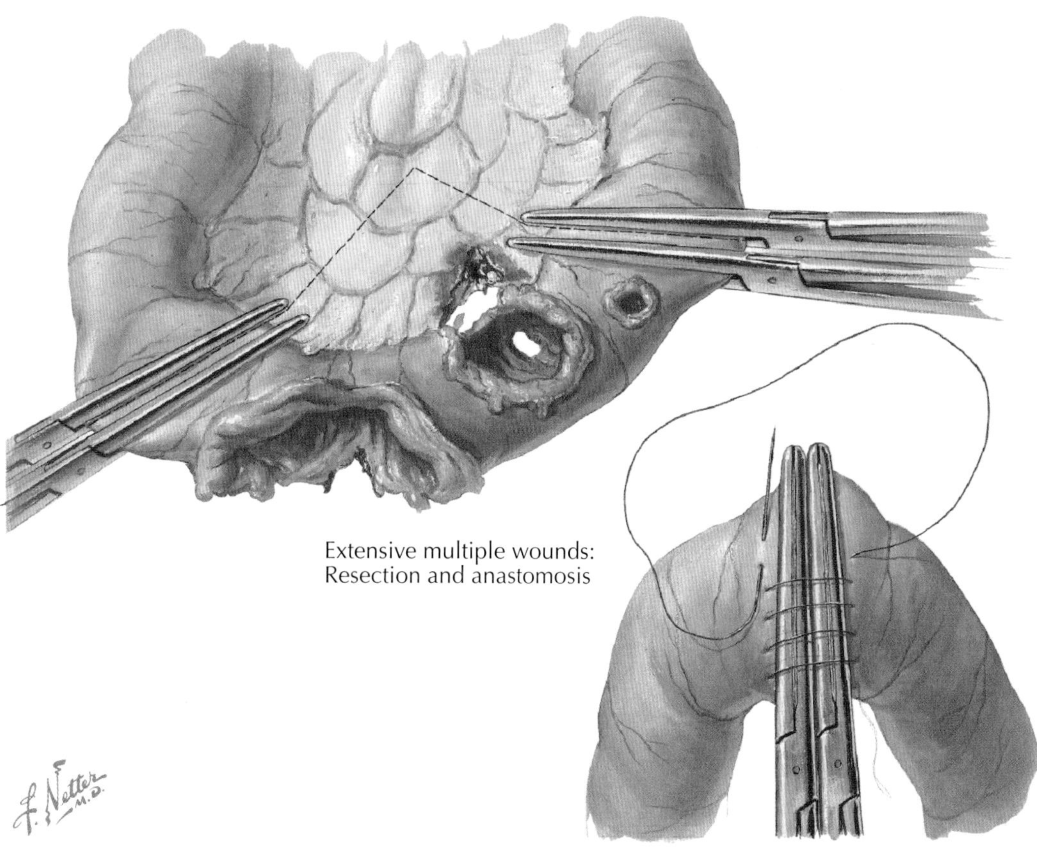

Extensive multiple wounds: Resection and anastomosis

Intestinal injuries can result from blunt or penetrating trauma. The small intestine is the most commonly injured organ in penetrating abdominal trauma with the ileum accounting for 70% of cases, followed by the jejunum then duodenum. Penetrating trauma can be broadly categorized under two groups: high-velocity injuries (projectiles) and low-velocity injuries (stabbings).

High-velocity injuries such as a gunshot wound can lead to multiple injuries, even with a single entry. Among abdominal war injuries, those of the small intestine are perhaps the most important, because of their relative frequency and high mortality rates. Although injuries of the duodenum are the least common, they are associated with the highest mortality rates. Bullets may cause contusion of the outer intestinal coat but usually produce small punctate wounds, one on each side of the bowel, with everted mucosa giving the appearance of small rosettes. In other cases, especially when the path of the bullet has approximated the long axis of the bowel, the perforations are more extensive, varying from simple slits to large gaping wounds that almost completely divide the bowel. Fragments of shells and bombs usually produce greater tissue damage, with more variable and irregular wounds. Bayonet and knife wounds, which are almost nonexistent in modern warfare, vary from small slits to actual division of the bowel. The clinical manifestation depends on the location and extent of the injury. Abdominal pain and evidence of peritoneal irritation, with localized or diffuse tenderness and rigidity, are common. Hemorrhage occurs in all perforating wounds of the small intestine, but the amount depends on the degree of damage to the vessels of the mesentery. The causes of death are peritonitis, hemorrhage, and shock.

In blunt abdominal trauma, the small intestine is the third most common injury after liver and spleen.

*Injuries of the small intestine* demand surgical repair as early as possible. Careful inspection of the entire length of the small intestine is essential, beginning at either the ileocecal junction or at the duodenojejunal junction, whichever is more convenient. Evisceration of large portions of the bowel should be avoided, and the inspection should be made by withdrawing and replacing lengths of about 15 to 20 cm at a time. All abnormalities should be thoroughly evaluated and tagged (e.g., with a bowel clamp), but definitive repair should not be undertaken until the entire length of bowel has been examined. This not only prevents further trauma but permits the surgeon to examine a sufficient length of the intestine adjacent to the perforations and thus to determine whether the perforations should be repaired individually or the segment resected. The inspection and repair should be so thorough that reexamination is unnecessary. Practically all small perforations can be repaired by hand-sewn and stapled techniques. In small, lacerated wounds, closure should be made transverse to the long axis of the bowel to prevent narrowing of the lumen. Resection should be avoided as much as possible, and even when the perforations are closely situated, individual closure is preferable if this permits adequate repair. On the other hand, if the *perforations* are *large* and are *located near each other,* if the bowel is practically divided, or if the segment is destroyed, resection should be done. Resection is also necessary in cases in which a segment of bowel is devitalized because of interference with its blood supply as a result of detachment of its mesentery or division or thrombosis of the mesenteric vessels. When resection is necessary, primary anastomosis can be performed using a one-layer or two-layer hand-sewn or stapled technique.

The use of antibiotics to control infection and supportive measures with IV fluids and blood products is essential to successful therapy. Physiologic rest of the bowel for the first few days postoperatively should be established by avoiding oral feedings and by instituting GI intubation and suction.

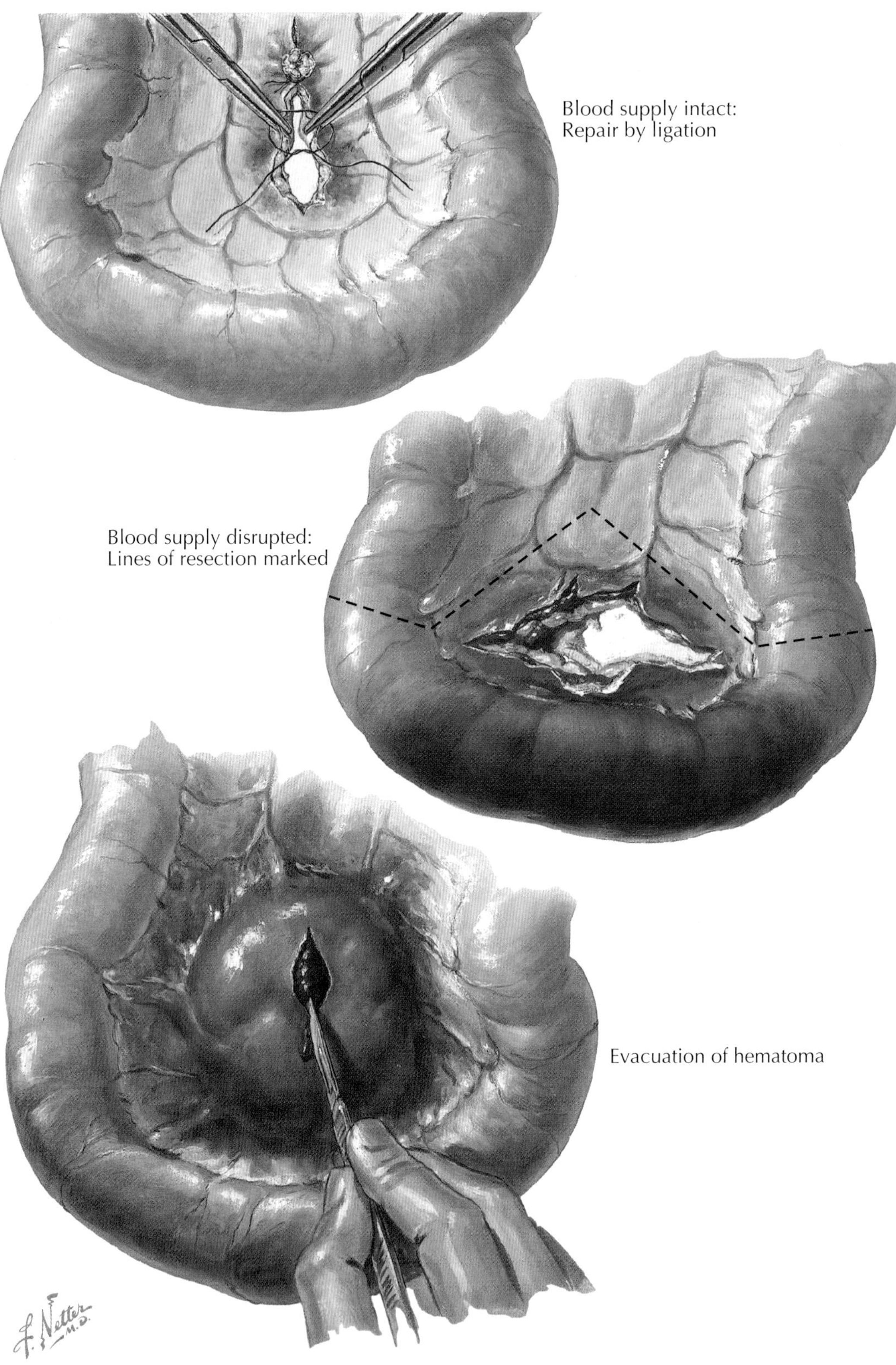


## Abdominal Wounds of Mesentery

*Wounds of the mesentery,* variable in type and extent, sometimes occur as independent lesions but are usually complications of intestinal wounds. They range from simple *hematomas* or *perforations* to irregular, jagged tears or *lacerations.* Their significance lies in the degree of damage to the vessels supplying the bowel. Damage to these vessels may result in hemorrhage between the leaves of the mesentery or into the retroperitoneal space with the formation of a hematoma, or into the peritoneal cavity. The mesentery may be torn in a relatively avascular area, with little hemorrhage, or it may be detached from the intestine, with consequent devitalization of the affected segment of bowel.

In dealing with wounds of the mesentery, the essential factors are arrest of hemorrhage and viability of the bowel. In cases in which the wound in the mesentery has not interfered with the blood supply of the intestine, hemorrhage is best controlled by individual ligation of the vessels at the torn edges. In such cases, closure of the wound by suturing is inadvisable and is best accomplished by grasping the edges with forceps and ligating the tissue at the tips of the approximated forceps. In the presence of a hematoma in which bleeding has apparently stopped and in which evidence of impairment of the blood supply of the nearby intestines can be excluded, nothing need be done. If, however, even a suspicion of continued bleeding remains or if the hematoma is enlarging, a careful search for the bleeding vessel must be undertaken.

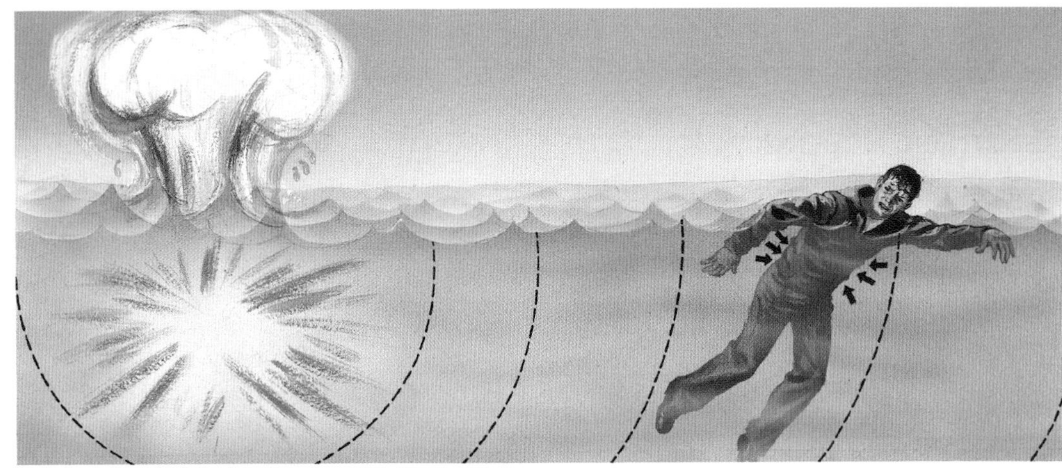

## Abdominal Wounds From Blast Injuries

*Blast-related injury* has traditionally resulted from one of four mechanisms. *Primary blast injuries* are caused when the impulse created by a detonated high-order explosive such as dynamite propagates from the detonation center through the victim, causing damage to predominantly air-filled organs. The small intestine is the most common visceral organ injured by such injuries causing immediate bowel perforation, hemorrhage (ranging from small petechiae to large hematomas) and mesenteric shear injuries. The injuries are far more pronounced in a closed space due to reverberation off surrounding surfaces. Immersion blast injuries is a type of primary blast injury that occurs in underwater explosions. The pressure waves created with the blast travel through water and strike a person floating nearby, injuring the intraabdominal organs and to some extent the intrathoracic organs. *Secondary blast injuries* are caused by flying debris and fragments leading to penetrating and/or blunt injuries. These, by far, can produce the most lethal injuries and are more common than primary blast injuries. *Tertiary blast injuries* occur when a victim is violently thrown by the blast of wind or is injured when a structure collapses. *Quaternary injuries* include explosion-induced injuries not classified under the previous three categories, such as burns and inhalational injury.

The type and extent of injuries depend on various factors such as the size of the charge, distance of the individual from the explosion, amount of gas in the hollow viscera, and, perhaps, position and degree of submersion. Blast abdominal injury should be suspected in anyone exposed to an explosion with abdominal pain, nausea, vomiting, hematemesis, rectal pain, tenesmus, testicular pain, unexplained hypovolemia, or any findings suggestive of an acute abdomen. Clinical findings may be absent until the onset of complications.

Victims of immersion blasts describe a temporary, paralyzing numbness of the abdomen and legs after the initial impact, followed by an urge to urinate or defecate. Symptoms usually abate by the time of rescue before a wave of severe, sharp, and stabbing, or colicky abdominal pain develops. These symptoms subside relatively rapidly in the absence of perforation, and escalation of symptoms with severe nausea, hematemesis, bloody diarrhea, diffuse abdominal tenderness, and rigidity point toward perforation and peritoneal irritation. Symptoms subside relatively rapidly in the absence of perforation. No laboratory tests can reliably demonstrate the presence of intestinal primary blast injury. Likewise, abdominal imaging may not reliably predict intestinal injury. On gross examination of the bowel, multiple intramural hematomas and petechiae can be evident involving the submucosal and subperitoneal layers of the small intestine, especially the lower ileum and the cecum. The size and shape of the injuries vary widely. The larger lesions can lead to gangrene of the bowel. Bleeding also occurs in the loose areolar retroperitoneal tissue and in fact, the hematomas are at risk of perforating up to 2 weeks after injury. Bowel perforations or tears are less frequent and are more likely to involve the small intestine, circular or linear, with everted edges, giving a blown-out appearance. Generalized or localized peritonitis often appears later.

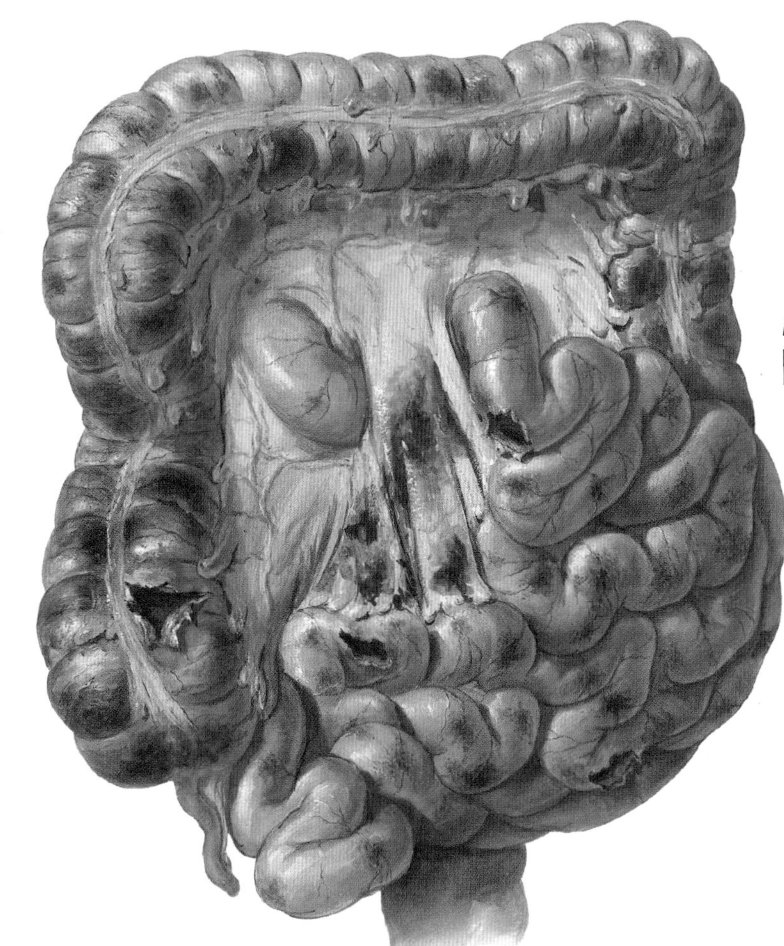


The prognosis depends on the extent of visceral injury and the time to intervention as well as the presence of associated injuries. Early deaths are due to shock, whereas late deaths are caused by infection and peritonitis.

In cases where perforation can be reliably ruled out, the treatment is conservative and like that of other nonpenetrating abdominal injuries. Resuscitative measures must be instituted early, but plasma and blood transfusions should be administered cautiously in cases of lung injury. For the same reason, anesthesia is challenging.

When perforation is obvious or could not be definitively ruled out, or if the patient becomes hemodynamically unstable, then abdominal exploration should be performed as early as possible. Surgical procedures for abdominal blast injuries are similar to those for abdominal injury from any other cause. Isolated small bowel lesions can be repaired unless they are multiple or are associated with significant mesenteric devitalization or mural hemorrhage. In addition to the customary pre- and postoperative measures, continuous gastroduodenal suction and antibiotic therapy are important.

# Mesenteric Ischemia

*Mesenteric ischemia* is an uncommon vascular disease that results from insufficient splanchnic blood flow that is unable to meet the metabolic demands of the small intestine. The mesenteric circulation is complex, with extensive collateralization between the primary mesenteric vessels: the celiac artery, SMA, and inferior mesenteric artery and their venous counterparts. Numerous classification systems exist based on the speed of onset (*acute* or *chronic*), the patency of the vessels (*occlusive* or *nonocclusive*), whether the affected vessel is *arterial* or *venous*.

*Acute intestinal ischemia* refers to the sudden onset of small intestinal hypoperfusion that often leads to catastrophic bowel infarction, sepsis, and death. It is commonly caused by acute arterial thromboembolism (70%) and can also be caused by acute venous thrombosis or be nonocclusive due to splanchnic hypoperfusion from focal vasospasm or widespread mesenteric vasoconstriction, as in dehydration or shock. *Chronic mesenteric ischemia,* on the other hand, develops over time in the background of atherosclerosis, which allows for development of collaterals and symptoms to occur when two or more primary vessels (usually celiac artery and SMA) are occluded. The classic presentation of chronic mesenteric ischemic is pain that starts soon after eating (30 minutes to 2 hours); it is located in the epigastric or periumbilical region and is termed "intestinal angina." This occurs due to the inability of the mesenteric vasculature to meet the increasing metabolic demands of a postprandial state. Patients learn to alleviate symptoms by eating smaller meals and gradually develop "sitophobia," which is an aversion to or fear of food accompanied by weight loss. A third of these patients may present with recurrent peptic ulcers, chronic diarrhea, or GI bleeding and even with an acute presentation if a thromboembolic event occludes the already narrowed segment of the vessel.

*Mesenteric arterial ischemia* is often an acute process and commonly involves an embolic (50%) or thrombotic (15%–25%) occlusion of the SMA. Emboli originate from the left atrium or ventricle or the aorta and get lodged at the narrow takeoff of the SMA. In patients with cardiac septal defects (patent foramen ovale, atrial septal defect, ventral septal defect) or an extracardiac shunt such as pulmonary arteriovenous malformation, a paradoxic emboli can originate in the systemic venous circulation and enter the systemic arterial circulation through these defects. Additionally, septic emboli, arising from septic cardiac valves, can lead to mycotic aneurysm. Thrombosis develops either from a vascular injury or hypercoagulable state or is superimposed on a preexisting atherosclerotic plaque.

*Mesenteric venous thrombosis* almost always involves the superior mesenteric venous circulation with distal ileal ischemia. The presentation can be acute, insidious, or asymptomatic identified by imaging or with complications of portal hypertension. The risk factors for developing mesenteric venous thrombosis correlate with the triad described by Virchow, namely, local intraabdominal infection causing endothelial damage (IBD, acute pancreatitis, acute diverticulitis), hypercoagulable states (myeloproliferative disorders, inherited thrombophilia, malignancy), and stasis (portal hypertension, abdominal mass).

Thrombosis of Mesenteric Artery

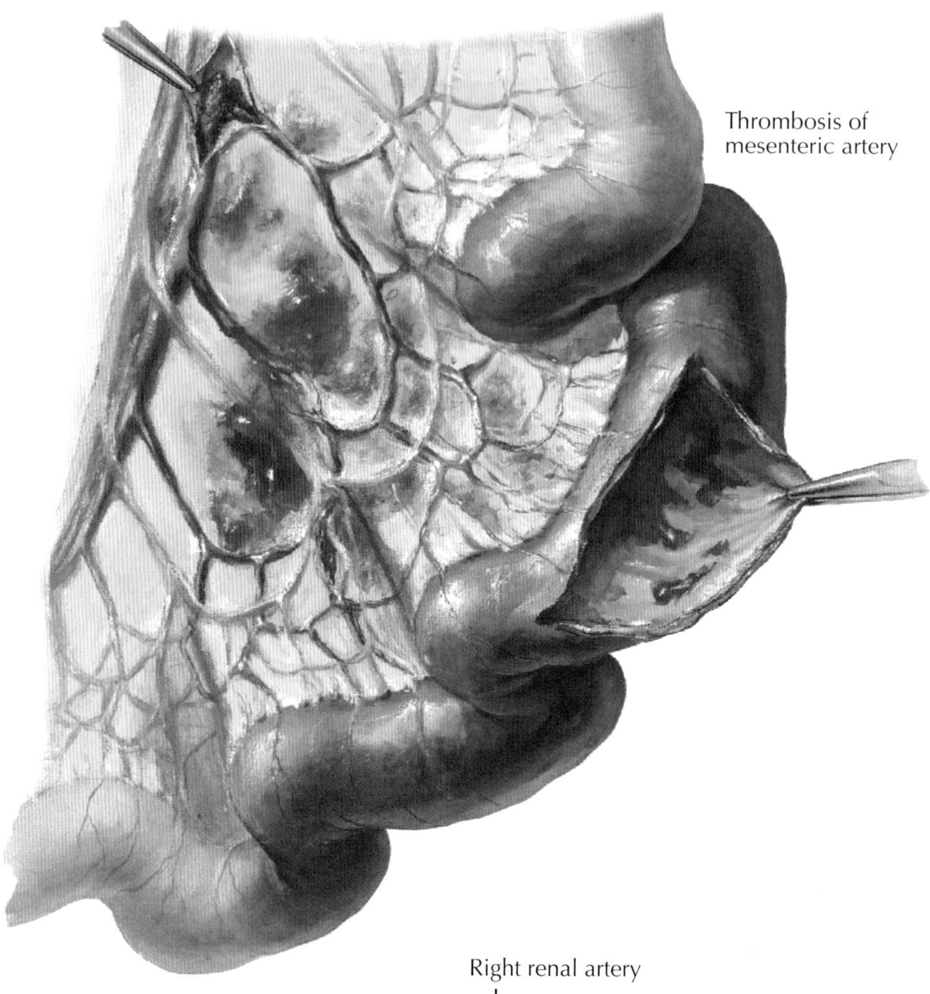


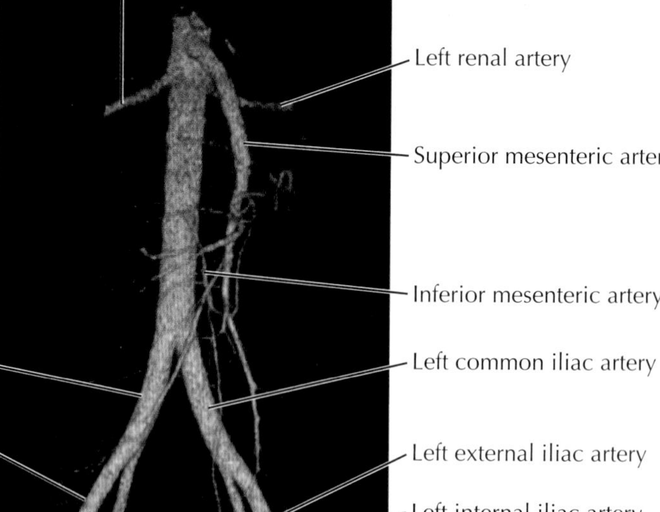


**Anterior view of 3D images reconstructed from axial CT angiogram studies of the superior and inferior mesenteric arteries.** Different colors can be assigned to the computer reconstruction of the different branches. *(From Cochard LR, Goodhartz LA, Harmath CB, et al. Netter's Introduction to Imaging. Elsevier; 2012.)*

*Occlusive ischemia* is caused by thromboembolic disease as outlined above, whereas *nonocclusive mesenteric ischemia* results from circulatory failure and vasoconstriction in the splanchnic circulation present in critically ill patients with severe shock. Other risk factors include congestive heart failure and any comorbidity that leads to profound hypoperfusion.

In acute mesenteric ischemia of any cause, the intestine is able to compensate for a reduction of approximately 75% in mesenteric blood flow for up to 12 hours without significant injury. Initially, vasodilation occurs and with prolonged period of ischemia, vasoconstriction sets in, which may persist even after intestinal blood returns. Early injury leads to bowel edema followed by mucosal and submucosal stress that can allow translocation of bacteria from the lumen. This in turn can activate a systemic inflammatory pathway that worsens the vasospasm, leading to ulceration and subsequent full-thickness necrosis of the bowel wall with eventual perforation.

# MESENTERIC ISCHEMIA (Continued)

The incidence of acute mesenteric ischemia is on the rise, in part due to an aging population with increased arteriosclerotic disease and in part due to prolonged survival of critically ill patients. The incidence of mesenteric venous thrombosis, on the other hand, has declined but still remains a major cause of acute intestinal ischemia in young individuals without cardiovascular risk factors.

*Acute occlusive mesenteric ischemia* typically presents with sudden onset of severe periumbilical pain that is out of proportion to findings on the physical examination, accompanied by nausea, vomiting, and diarrhea. Examination may show the abdomen to be normal or mildly distended early in the course, but as the bowel ischemia progresses, signs of peritonitis develop, with abdominal distension, tenderness, and hemodynamic changes indicating impending shock. Laboratory findings are nonspecific and may include marked leukocytosis, hemoconcentration, metabolic acidosis with an elevated lactate level, and an elevated amylase and D-dimer. These or any other serologic markers, however, should not be used to exclude or diagnose mesenteric ischemia. Plain radiographs are useful for excluding other causes, such as bowel obstruction and bowel perforation, rather than diagnosing mesenteric ischemia and can be normal in more than 25% of patients with ischemia. More specific signs, when present, indicate more advanced stages of ischemia and include thumbprinting resulting from edema and hemorrhage as well as pneumatosis and portal vein gas.

Duplex US can identify stenosis in the celiac artery or SMA; however, it is rarely useful for an acute ischemia because distended bowel loops easily interfere with the test, it is highly operator dependent, and it may not be available in an emergent setting. Abdominal CT is the best initial screening modality in patients with an acute abdomen. In those suspected to have acute mesenteric ischemia, a CT angiogram should be performed with no oral contrast and has a high sensitivity (85%–98%) and high specificity (90%–100%). Abdominal magnetic resonance angiogram is comparable to CT angiogram and can be helpful in individuals with serious allergies to iodinated contrast. Despite these advances, arteriography may still be necessary in patients with a high index of suspicion and negative imaging. Diagnostic laparoscopy should be limited to patients with obvious peritonitis or bowel perforation and those hemodynamically unstable to undergo imaging.

In contrast to acute occlusion, patients with *mesenteric venous thrombosis* may present with variable degrees of abdominal pain that depends on the location and timing of thrombus formation. Most have at least one obvious risk factor or a prior history of thrombosis; however, an antecedent event may not always be apparent. A subset of patients with chronic mesenteric venous thrombosis may be entirely asymptomatic until they develop complications of portal hypertension, such as variceal bleeding or ascites. A high index of suspicion based on the history and physical findings is necessary to make an early diagnosis. A magnetic resonance venography or CT venogram can be used to demonstrate thrombus within the mesenteric veins.

Patients with peritonitis or signs of bowel infarction should undergo surgical exploration without delay. In patients without an indication for urgent surgery, various options exist. In general, the goal of therapy is directed toward early revascularization and restoration of perfusion. In mesenteric arterial occlusive disease, this can be achieved via surgical thromboembolectomy or localized thrombolytic therapy. Anticoagulation should be initially instituted in patients with acute mesenteric venous thrombosis, although a subset go on to require venous thrombolysis. For patients with chronic mesenteric venous thrombosis, the decision to anticoagulate should be individualized, depending on the risk of bleeding. The management of patients with nonocclusive mesenteric ischemia is purely supportive with treatment of underlying causes and intraarterial infusion of vasodilators in selected cases. The prognosis in acute mesenteric venous thrombosis is more favorable than in arterial occlusion, but mortality rates in both can be as high as 75% once bowel infarction develops. Early diagnosis is the single most important factor in the prognosis of intestinal ischemia.

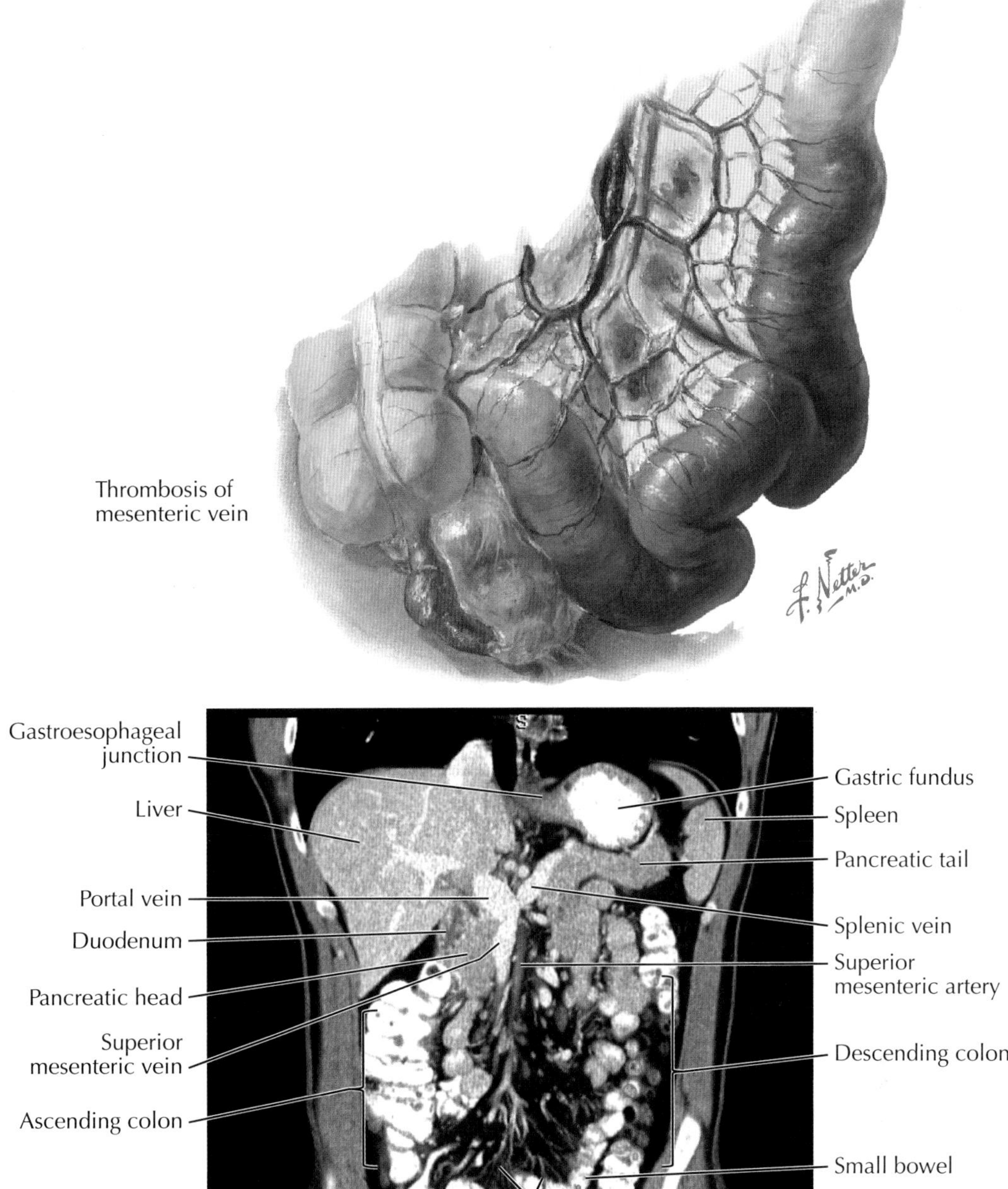


**Coronal CT reconstruction demonstrating the superior mesenteric artery and vein and vasa recta.** The inferior mesenteric artery is posterior and not seen on this image. *(From Cochard LR, Goodhartz LA, Harmath CB, et al. Netter's Introduction to Imaging. Elsevier; 2012.)*

## Superior Mesenteric Artery Syndrome

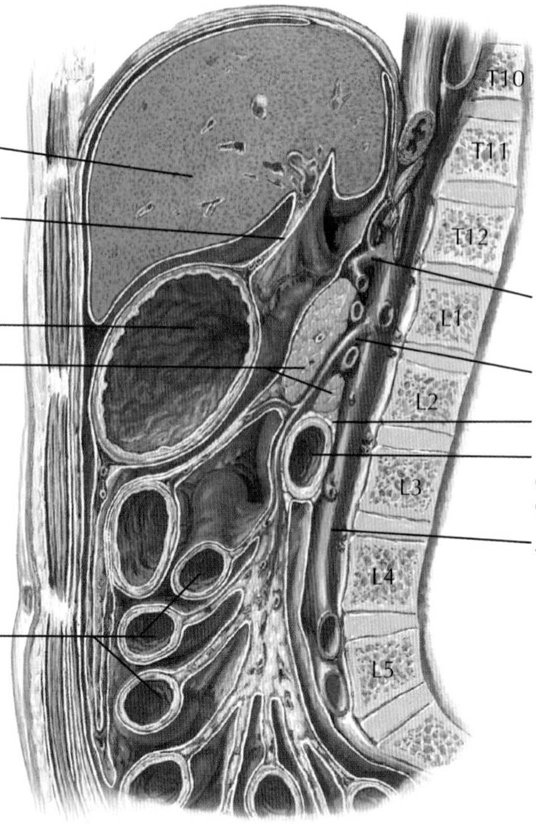

SMA syndrome, also known as *Wilkie syndrome, arteriomesenteric duodenal compression, chronic duodenal ileus,* or *cast syndrome,* is a rare form of proximal small bowel obstruction caused by extrinsic compression of the third portion of the duodenum between the SMA, anteriorly, and the abdominal aorta, posteriorly.

Normally, the SMA forms an angle of approximately 45 degrees (range, 38–65 degrees) as it comes off the aorta. This angulation produces an aortomesenteric distance spanning 10 to 28 mm without impingement on the duodenal lumen as the third portion traverses laterally toward the ligament of Treitz. Reduction in this angle to less than 25 degrees will decrease the aortomesenteric distance to less than 10 mm and lead to compression of the duodenum.

SMA syndrome was previously demonstrated in patients who underwent body casting (Risser cast) after orthopedic spinal surgery, hence the name *cast syndrome.* It has now been established that it can develop after any severe weight loss, such as in AIDS, cancer, or a psychological disorder that leads to the loss of the duodenal fat pad. Notably, SMA syndrome has been reported in patients without preceding weight loss, as demonstrated in young adults after corrective surgery for scoliosis, which can displace the SMA with lengthening of the spine, or in patients with a congenitally short ligament of Treitz.

This unusual entity can occur at any age but is often seen in younger individuals, with a slight female to male preponderance. Classically, patients present with nausea, vomiting with inability to tolerate an oral diet, and intermittent abdominal pain after a significant weight loss or corrective scoliosis surgery. Depending on the cause, the symptoms may be acute, with obvious proximal small bowel obstruction, or insidious, with only postprandial epigastric pain and early satiety. The findings on physical examination, likewise, can range from nonspecific distension to obvious signs of bowel obstruction.

The diagnosis of superior mesenteric syndrome can be challenging and requires a high index of suspicion. The evaluation often starts with exclusion of other common disorders that cause similar symptoms. A plain abdominal film may reveal gastric distension and dilated proximal small bowel loops but also can be normal. An upper GI series with oral contrast can suggest the diagnosis with evidence of proximal dilation and abrupt cutoff at the third portion of the duodenum, corresponding to the course of the SMA. However, conventional CT of the abdomen with oral and IV contrast has emerged as the modality of choice given its high diagnostic yield. In cases where the diagnosis remains unclear on imaging, arteriography may be necessary.

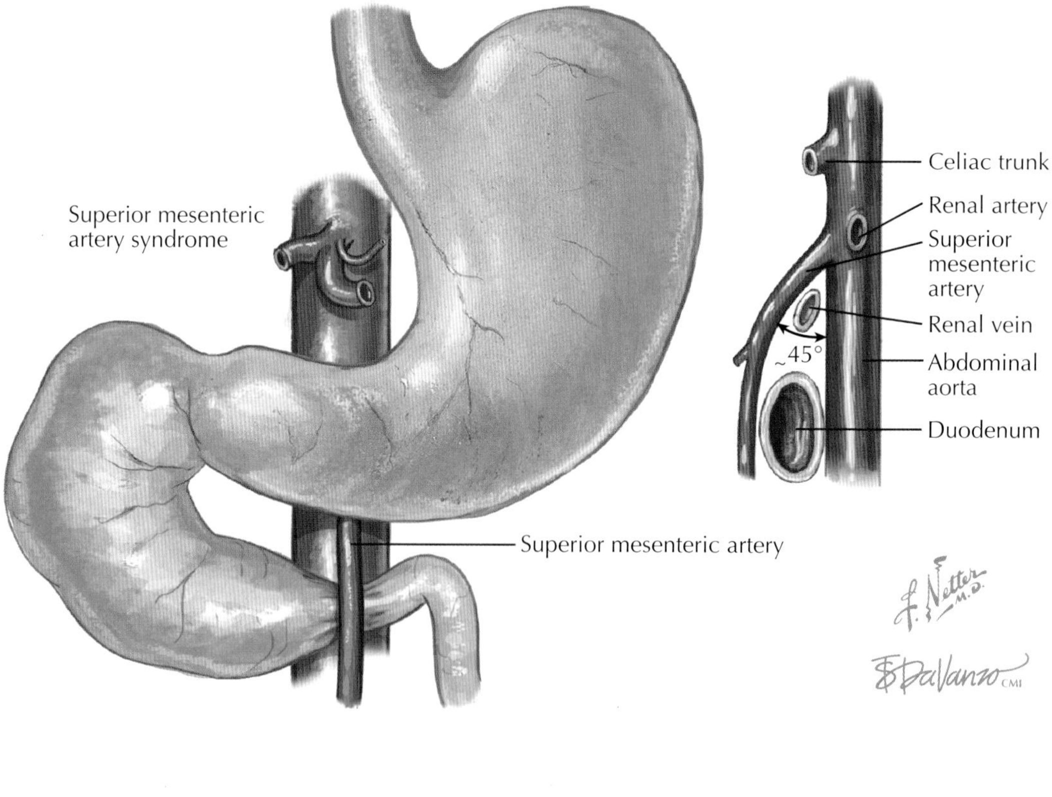

The initial management is supportive, with fluid resuscitation and correction of electrolyte abnormalities. Decompression of the stomach and proximal duodenum using a nasoenteric tube is often required and provides relief to the patient. Nutritional therapy is recommended as a first step to reverse the weight loss and recover the duodenal fat pad to increase the aortomesenteric angle. Enteral nutrition is preferred, which can be achieved by passage of a nasoenteric tube distal to the obstruction into the jejunum. If enteral feeding is unsuccessful, total parenteral nutrition may be necessary.

In patients who do not respond to nonoperative therapy, several surgical options exist. Strong's procedure involves mobilization of the duodenum outside the aortomesenteric angle by dividing the ligament of Treitz. This allows maintenance of the integrity of the bowel, but there is a 25% failure rate resulting from tethering of the inferior pancreaticoduodenal artery. Gastrojejunostomy is a feasible alternative because it alleviates the gastric obstruction; it does not, however, relieve the proximal duodenal obstruction and can perpetuate the symptoms. Open duodenojejunostomy provides the best results but is associated with significant rates of morbidity. Laparoscopic duodenojejunostomy, when feasible, offers fewer risks with reduced hospital stay and shorter recovery.

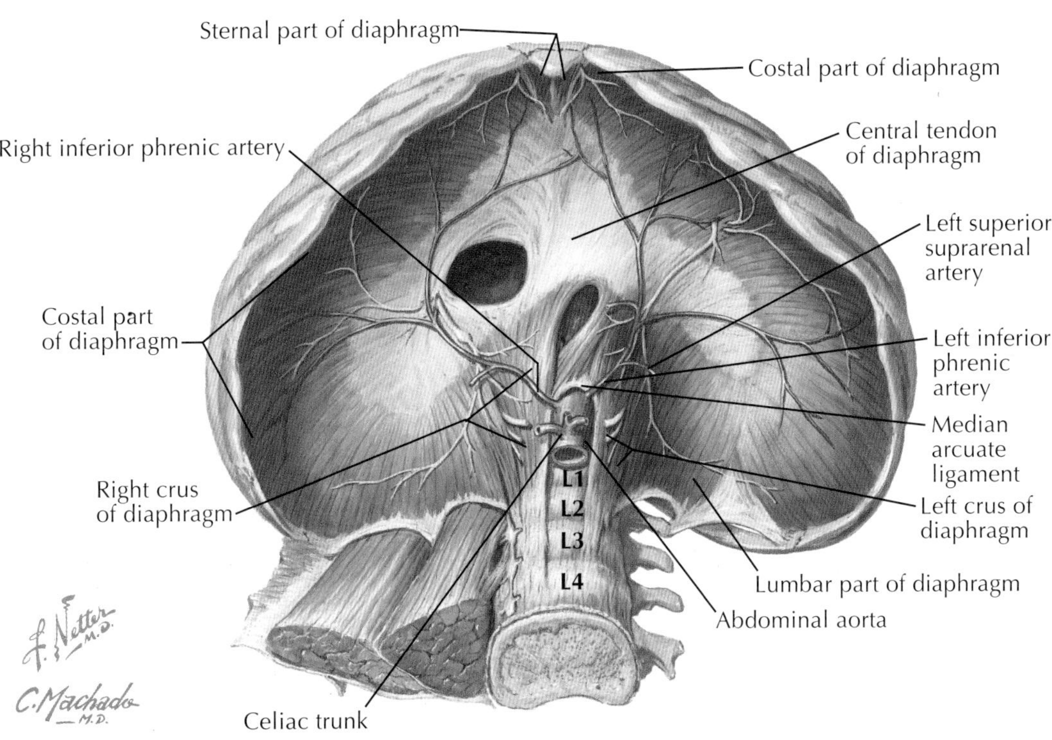


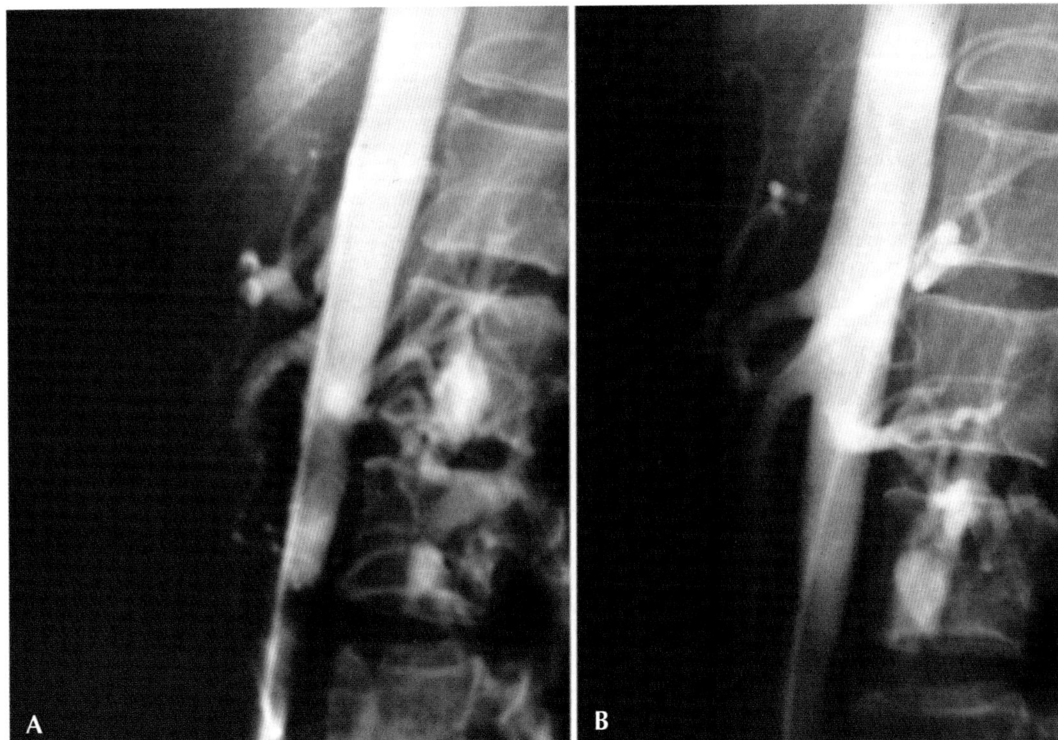


**A,** Preoperative appearance of celiac artery compression. **B,** Postoperative appearance of normal celiac artery after transection of the median arcuate ligament. *(From Escobar GA, Stanley JC. Current Therapy in Vascular and Endovascular Surgery. Elsevier; 2013:733–736.)*

## Celiac Artery Compression Syndrome (Median Arcuate Ligament Syndrome)

*Celiac artery compression syndrome,* or *median arcuate ligament syndrome,* also called *Dunbar syndrome,* is a rare disorder caused by compression of the celiac artery by the median arcuate ligament of the diaphragm. The median arcuate ligament is a fibrous band that borders the crura of the diaphragm anteriorly and arches across the aorta just above the origin of the celiac trunk. The celiac plexus (or ganglion) lies between the celiac trunk and the median arcuate ligament and supplies the preganglionic splanchnic nerves, somatic branches from the phrenic and vagus nerves, parasympathetic preganglionic nerves, and sympathetic postganglionic fibers.

The cause of the syndrome is not well understood. Under normal circumstances, occlusion of the celiac artery alone does not lead to mesenteric ischemia, which, due to the extensive collateralization of the mesenteric circulation, requires occlusion of two or more primary mesenteric vessels. In individuals with this disorder, however, compression of the celiac trunk by the fibrous median arcuate ligament leads to chronic abdominal pain and weight loss. Neuropathic pain caused by impingement of the celiac plexus is also suspected to contribute to the clinical presentation. Celiac artery compression syndrome is usually seen in middle-aged females, but cases have been reported in the pediatric age group. The classic triad (epigastric pain, weight loss, and abdominal bruit) is present in only a minority of patients. The epigastric pain is usually postprandial and is present in more than 80% of individuals with this syndrome. Delayed gastric emptying may be present, but physical examination is usually normal. The diagnosis is usually delayed by several months to years and requires a high index of suspicion. The gold standard for diagnosis is selective arteriography with inspiratory and expiratory maneuvers; however, noninvasive imaging techniques such as duplex US, CT scanning, or MRI may suggest the findings. Physiologic testing using gastric tonometry or ganglion nerve block has the benefit of predicting patients who might benefit from surgery and can be used when the diagnosis is unclear.

In patients who are symptomatic with confirmed diagnosis, surgical decompression is indicated with or without celiac artery revascularization. The surgery can be performed using open or laparoscopic (standard or robot-assisted) approaches. Outcomes after surgery are variable and are favorable in appropriately selected patients. Early complications include bleeding, pancreatitis, and splenic injuries. Recurrence rates of up to 10% can be seen over the long term.

## Cancer of the Peritoneum (Peritoneal Carcinomatosis)

Primary malignant tumors of the peritoneum (mesotheliomas or endotheliomas) are extremely rare. Extraovarian primary peritoneal carcinoma can resemble serous ovarian carcinoma and occurs almost exclusively in females aged 50 to 60 years. It is associated with a germline mutation in the *BRCA1* gene; therefore patients with familial breast cancer should be surveyed for serous peritoneal malignancy.

In contrast, secondary malignant tumors of the peritoneum are relatively frequent. Epithelial malignant tumors arising from abdominal organs, particularly the ovaries, stomach, and large intestine, are the most common cancers metastasizing to the peritoneum. Rarely, malignant neoplasms arising in the retroperitoneal connective, nervous, or muscular tissue, as well as distant sarcomas and teratomas, may spread to the peritoneum. Lymphomas and infections such as TB can also involve the peritoneum, mimicking peritoneal carcinomatosis. Disseminated peritoneal leiomyomatosis is associated with a high estrogenic state in postmenopausal females. Leiomyosarcoma is a secondary tumor occurring in Li-Fraumeni syndrome.

The spread of tumor cells into the peritoneum can occur by direct extension, by hematogenous spread, through the lymphatics, or via transcoelomic spread. The latter occurs when exfoliated tumor cells detach from the primary tumor and are transported throughout the peritoneal space by peritoneal fluid disseminating within the abdominal cavity, referred to as the "seed and soil" theory. The peritoneal stromal tissue provides a rich source of growth factors and chemokines, a favorable environment for tumor proliferation, which also leads to increased vascular permeability and blockage of lymphatic channels. These changes, in addition to fluids produced by certain tumor cells in the peritoneal cavity, lead to accumulation of excessive fluid in the peritoneum *(malignant ascites).* Proliferation of tumor cells can be observed as nodules scatter over the omentum, mesentery, and visceral and parietal peritoneum and are termed *metastatic implants.* Ovarian papillary serous cystadenomas most frequently exhibit this characteristic, followed by gastric carcinoma. Additionally, metastatic peritoneal implants from an appendicular adenocarcinoma or an ovarian pseudomucinous cystadenocarcinoma may lead to *pseudomyxoma peritonei,* which is characterized by accumulation of a large quantity of gelatinous material in the peritoneal cavity.

Symptoms of peritoneal carcinomatosis appear late in the stage and are initially nonspecific with vague abdominal pain, bloating, nausea, irregular bowel movements, or abdominal distension. Physical examination of the abdomen may reveal the presence of ascites with or without palpable masses. Diagnostic paracentesis should be performed in any patient with new-onset ascites, and ascitic fluid analysis reveals an "exudative" ascites with a low serum-ascites albumin gradient (<1.1 g/dL). The appearance can be clear or bloody, but chylous effusion may also be encountered. The white blood cell count in the fluid is often elevated with predominantly lymphocytes. Rarely, neutrophils may predominate as a result of a high burden of dying tumor cells, and the glucose may be low compared with the serum value. Cytologic analysis of the ascites fluid may reveal malignant cells, but the sensitivity is variable. The yield can be improved with repeated specimens and strict processing protocol. Abdominal imaging using US, CT scanning, or MRI can detect the ascites and peritoneal thickening or deposits, which can be a clue to the diagnosis. The best diagnostic procedure is *laparoscopy* (see Plate 2.76), which permits visualization and sampling of the peritoneal deposits.

Most frequent sites of primary tumor

1. Ovary
2. Stomach
3. Intestine

Less frequently other abdominal organs; rarely lung, breast, or other organs

Adenocarcinoma of appendix (malignant mucocele) and pseudomucinous carcinoma of ovary may give rise to pseudomyxoma peritonei.

Ascitic fluid cytology in peritoneal carcinomatosis: tumor cells, mesothelial cells, and lymphocytes (Leishman stain)

F. Netter M.D.

K. Marzen

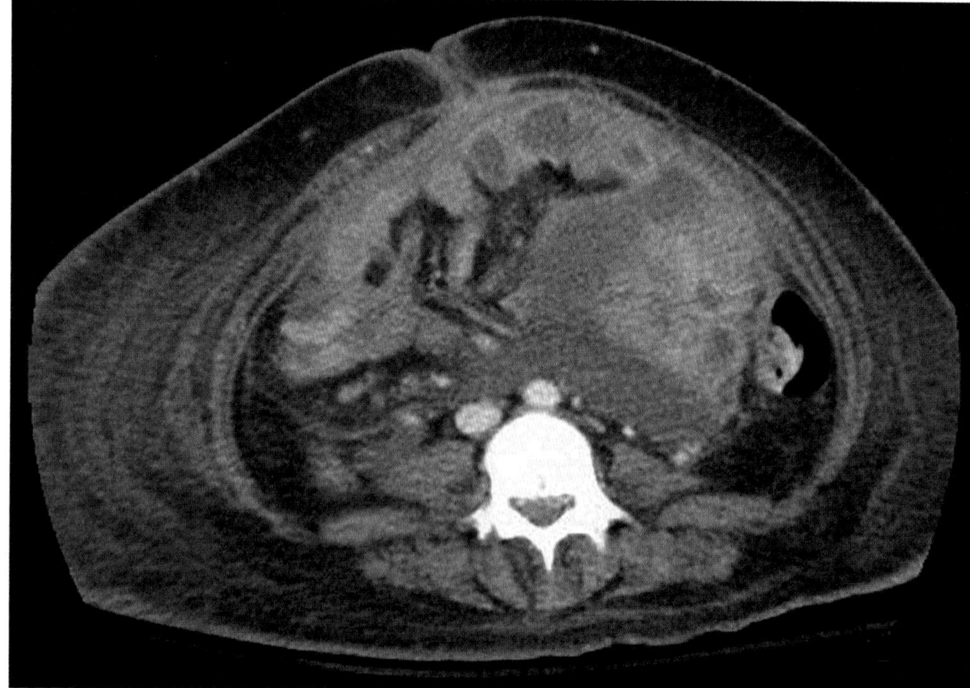

Peritoneal enhancement with peritoneal carcinomatosis from a gastric metastasis

The management of peritoneal carcinomatosis depends on the primary cause and the extent of the disease process. Supportive measures include removal of ascitic fluid and maintenance of nutrition. Bowel obstruction can be managed conservatively with bowel rest and nasogastric decompression, but surgical decompression may also be required. A combination of neoadjuvant intraperitoneal and systemic chemotherapy with cytoreductive surgery can be employed and has been shown to improve survival rates. The advent of hyperthermic intraperitoneal chemotherapy (instillation of heated chemotherapy directly into the peritoneum) has revolutionized the management of peritoneal carcinomatosis. This is performed in combination with cytoreductive surgery and allows the use of high doses of chemotherapy locally to the tumor while minimizing side effects and appears to prevent peritoneal recurrences.

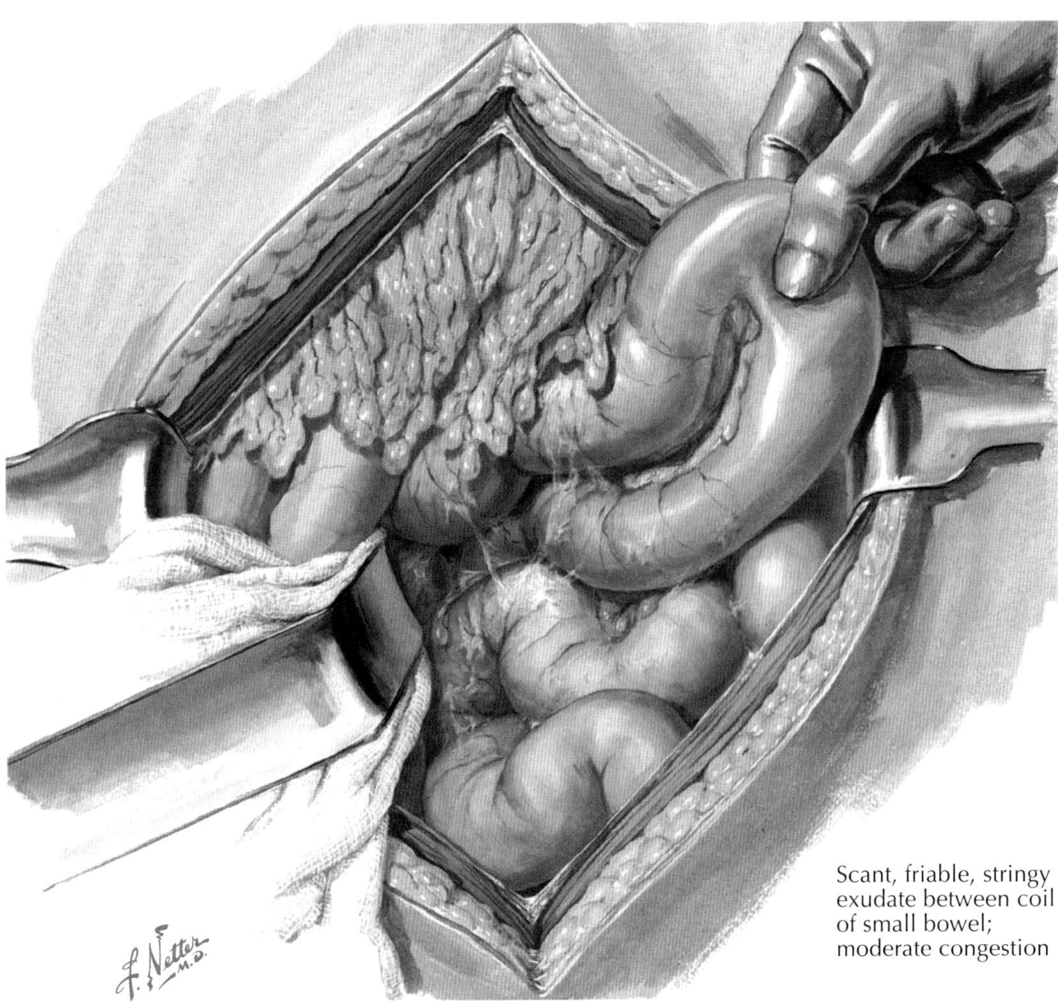

Scant, friable, stringy exudate between coil of small bowel; moderate congestion


# Familial Mediterranean Fever and Other Rare Etiologies of Abdominal Pain

## FAMILIAL MEDITERRANEAN FEVER

Familial Mediterranean fever (FMF) is a rare, inherited autoinflammatory disease characterized by recurrent attacks of fever and acute abdominal pain with polyserositis. The FMF gene, named the *MEFV* gene, was cloned in 1997 and encodes the protein pyrin, which is expressed predominantly in the cytoplasm in cells of neutrophils. Pyrin is thought to attenuate the activation of neutrophils in response to minor inflammatory perturbations that occur from time to time. Mutations of the *MEFV* gene allow a subclinical event (e.g., emotional stress) to rapidly evolve into a cascade of neutrophil recruitment and activation, resulting in a full-blown attack of FMF. It is assumed to be an autosomal recessive disease; however, up to 30% of individuals with FMF carry only one *MEFV* mutation, while 10% to 20% have no evidence of *MEFV* gene mutation. These facts and the varying expression of the disease suggest the presence of other genetic or environmental factors that could influence the expression of illness. As the name implies, FMF is common among people with eastern Mediterranean ancestry, particularly those of Sephardic Jewish, Middle Eastern, north Jewish, Turkish, and Arab descent. The carrier rate among these ethnic groups ranges from 1:4 to 1:8 with an observed disease rate of approximately 1:500. However, the disease has been reported in other parts of the world, including Japan, and among Ashkenazi Jews in Europe and the United States, and the diagnosis should be considered in any ethnic group if other clinical characteristics are present.

The first onset is usually during childhood and only rarely after the age of 40 years. Males are more frequently affected. In the beginning, the attacks may occur only once or twice a year, but the intervals soon shorten to every 1 to 2 weeks, sometimes with striking regularity, but more often irregularly. A typical crisis is characterized by severe abdominal pain that is initially localized but later becomes generalized with physical findings suggestive of peritonitis. Fever is a constant feature and may be mild and brief. The pleura and the joints may also commonly be involved, with dermatologic involvement present in a minority of patients, mimicking cellulitis of the leg or foot. The course usually lasts 1 to 4 days, and patients are symptom free in between intervals.

Neutrophilic leukocytosis with elevated inflammatory markers completes a clinical picture indistinguishable from that of acute surgical abdomen. Not surprisingly, exploratory laparotomy is often performed for these symptoms. Abdominal imaging is helpful to exclude other causes of an acute abdomen but is not used for the diagnosis of FMF. The pathologic findings in the peritoneum are those of an acute, nonspecific peritoneal inflammation, with *hyperemia* or even *edema* of the serosa and a small amount of serous or serofibrinous *exudate.* Cultures of the exudate are always sterile. A group of major and minor criteria have been developed to aid in the diagnosis FMF and confirmed by genetic testing, when present, and a positive response to colchicine therapy. The differential diagnosis of FMF includes hereditary angioedema, acute intermittent porphyria (AIP), acute recurrent pancreatitis, systemic lupus erythematosus, and abdominal migraine. In females, acute pelvic pathologies need to be considered. The attacks usually cease altogether during pregnancy. Rarely, they may occur only in the menstrual period, mimicking endometriosis.

The disease may be active for over 70 years, although occasionally, prolonged remissions occur and attacks may subside altogether in later life. However, secondary amyloidosis with eventual renal failure is a feared complication. Colchicine is the mainstay of treatment for FMF and can be used as a continuous, preventive therapy. It suppresses neutrophil recruitment and activation by binding to tubulin and other intracellular proteins and also by inhibiting neutrophil and endothelial cell adhesion molecules. An impending attack can be aborted by taking an extra dose of colchicine at the onset of the earliest prodromal symptoms. In the small subset of patients who do not respond to colchicine or do not tolerate the GI side effect, interleukin-1 inhibitor is a second-line therapy. Other agents such as interferon-alpha, infliximab, etanercept, and thalidomide have been shown to be effective, but control trials are lacking.

## Acute Intermittent Porphyria

AIP is a rare inherited condition that is characterized by recurrent attacks of abdominal pain associated with a variety of neuropsychiatric syndromes. It has an autosomal dominant inheritance with low penetrance. AIP is caused by mutations in the *porphobilinogen deaminase* (*PBGD*) gene that result in a catalytic deficiency of PBGD, the third enzyme in the heme biosynthesis cascade. All races are affected, but the condition is more commonly seen in individuals of northern European descent. There is no differences between the sexes and usually presents after the third or fourth decade. Acute attacks are usually triggered by medications (e.g., sulfa drugs, barbiturates), the use of contraceptive hormones, or reduced caloric intake and stress. The clinical presentation is highly variable but is characterized by recurrent attacks of abdominal pain that can be severe, steady, and poorly localized, often preceded by peripheral neuropathy. Involvement of the autonomic nervous system and CNS is common and can manifest as tachycardia, hypertension, or sweating, as well as seizures. Constipation, nausea, and vomiting, with signs of ileus, are common, but diarrhea can also be present. Dark reddish urine is an early symptom that results from the accumulation of porphyrins and/or porphyrin precursors in the urine. Most patients have complete resolution of their symptoms between attacks, but after multiple attacks, the abdominal pain, anxiety, and depression may become chronic.

The diagnosis of acute intermittent porphyria is challenging and requires a high index of suspicion. Elevated urinary levels of the porphyrin precursor porphobilinogen can be detected during an acute attack and should be the initial test. Other tests include urinary alanine aminotransferase, porphobilinogen, and porphyrins (including those in plasma and stool). The diagnosis of AIP is confirmed by a finding of decreased erythrocyte porphobilinogen deaminase activity and/or a mutation in the gene encoding it. The management focuses on prevention by avoiding known triggers and supportive treatment during an acute attack. Hospitalization is usually required during an acute attack, with administration of IV hemin with or without carbohydrate loading. Opioid analgesics, antiemetics, and anxiolytic therapies are often necessary to treat symptoms. Patients with AIP are at increased risk of long-term complications, including systemic hypertension, chronic renal failure, and hepatocellular carcinoma, and require long-term follow-up.

**Acute intermittent porphyria**

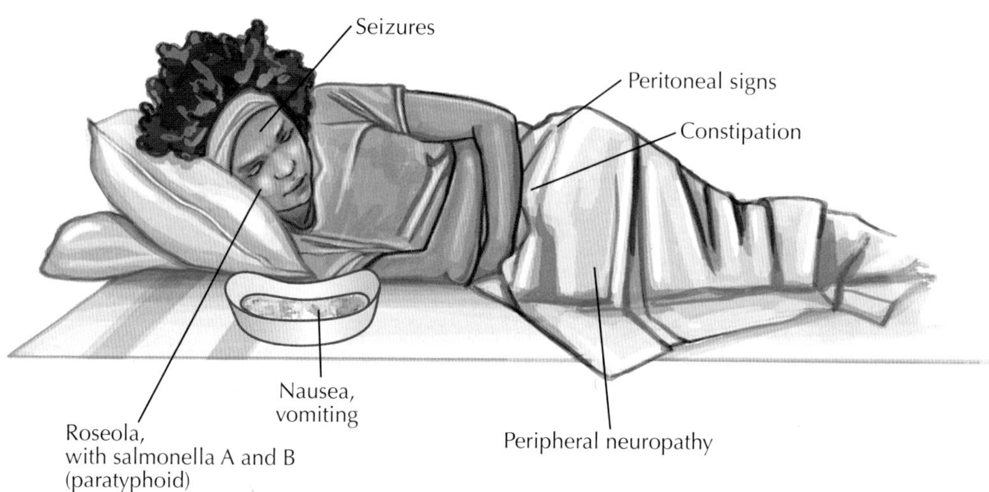


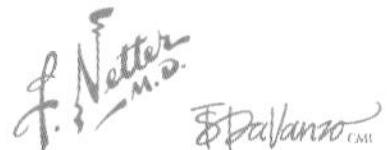

### HEREDITARY ANGIOEDEMA

Hereditary angioedema is a rare autosomal dominant disorder characterized by episodic attacks of angioedema and unexplained abdominal pain without urticaria or pruritus. It is caused by deficiency or dysfunction of the C1 inhibitor. Symptoms begin in childhood, and there are no appreciable racial or sex differences. An attack can involve any part of the skin or the upper airway. GI involvement is common and presents as recurrent colicky abdominal pain, distension, vomiting, and/or diarrhea caused by bowel wall edema. Reports have described isolated bowel wall angioedema triggered by angiotensin enzyme inhibitor therapy that resolves with its discontinuation. The diagnosis of hereditary angioedema is made by demonstration of specific abnormalities in complement proteins. The management involves prevention of acute attacks and supportive treatment of patients who are symptomatic. Specific therapies include human plasma derived or recombinant C1 inhibitor concentrate, a bradykinin, or kallikrein receptor antagonist.

**Hereditary angioedema**

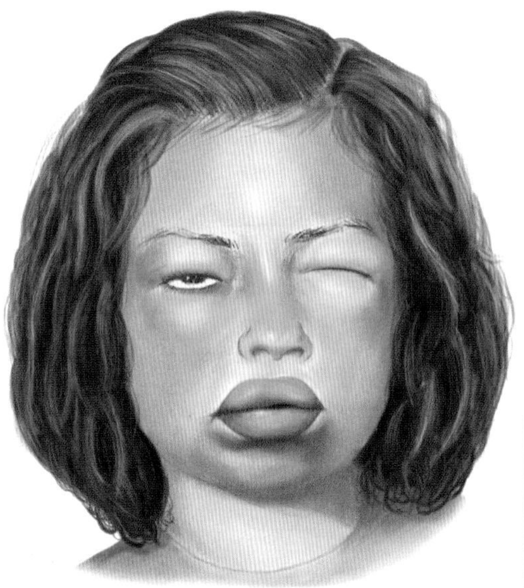

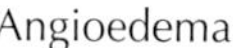

Angioedema

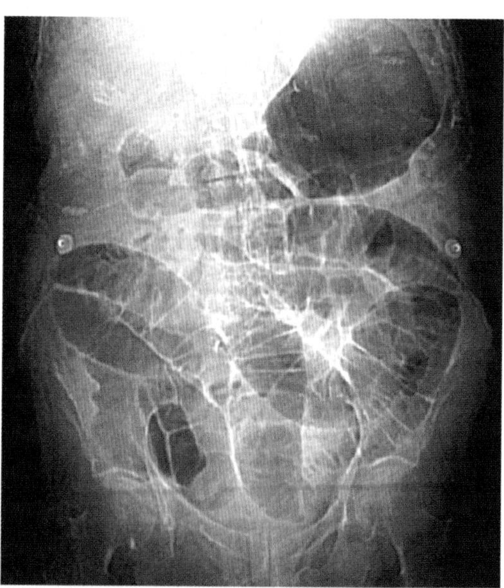

Dilated small intestinal loops

### MESENTERIC PANNICULITIS

*Mesenteric panniculitis* (also known as *mesenteric manifestation of Weber-Christian disease, isolated lipodystrophy,* and *mesenteric lipogranuloma*), is a benign chronic inflammatory disease that affects the adipose tissue of the mesentery of the small intestine. The specific cause of the disease is as yet unclear, but mesenteric panniculitis has been reported in a variety of conditions including pancreatitis, vasculitis, granulomatous disease, and malignant disease.

The most common clinical presentations include abdominal pain, vomiting, diarrhea, constipation, and a palpable abdominal mass or an intestinal obstruction. Contrast-enhanced abdominal CT can reveal a *fat ring sign* that reflects the preservation of fat around the mesenteric vessels or a *tumoral pseudocapsule,* which is highly suggestive, and histologic confirmation is diagnostic.

Mesenteric panniculitis can resolve spontaneously, and medical therapy (glucocorticoids, tamoxifen, azathioprine, thalidomide) can used for patients who are symptomatic. Surgical resection is reserved for those with obstructive or ischemic complications.

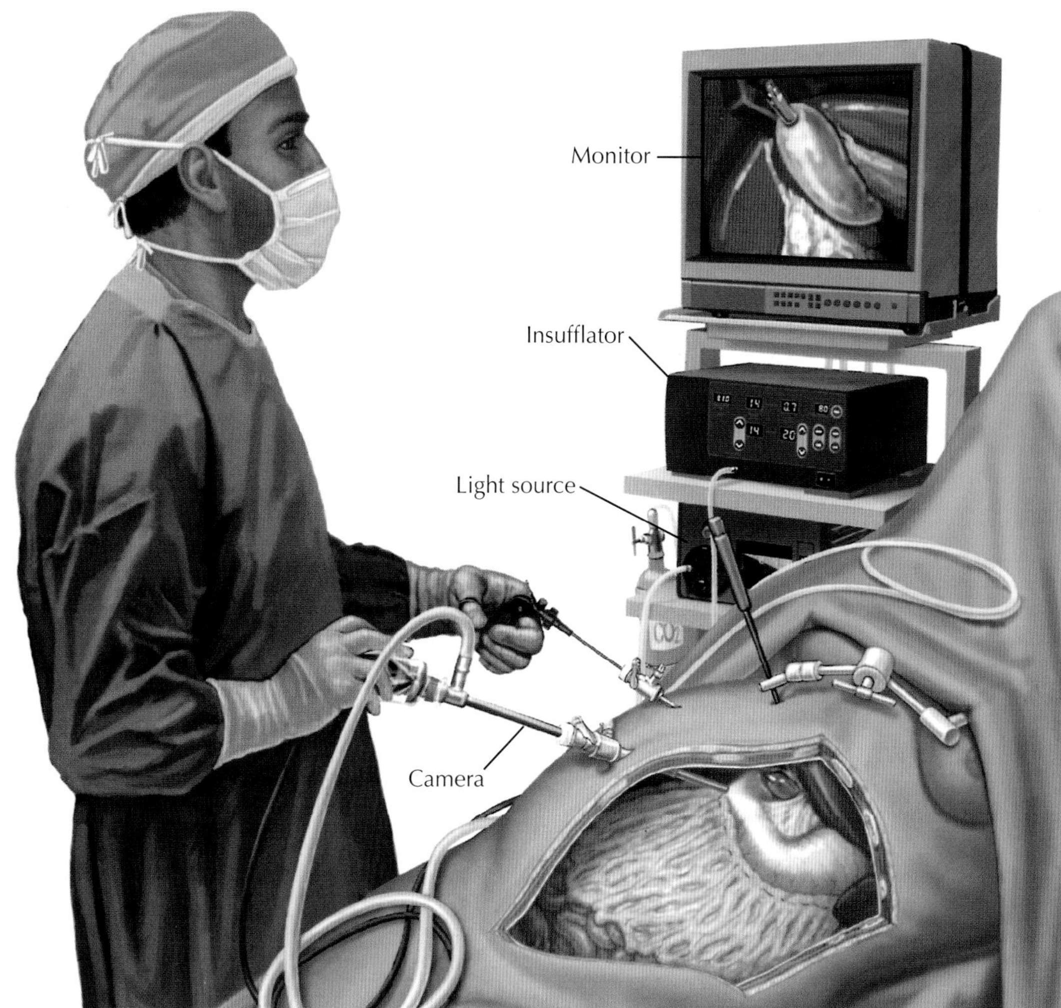


## LAPAROSCOPY

Laparoscopy is a minimally invasive surgical technique where a fiberoptic endoscope (laparoscope) is introduced through artificially made ports in the abdominal wall, allowing direct inspection of the peritoneal cavity and its contents. Laparoscopic techniques have transformed the field of surgery and have gradually replaced many conventional surgical procedures. Variations to the standard laparoscopic approach includes hand-assisted and robot-assisted laparoscopy. The latter is an innovative technique that offers enhanced 3D imaging and improved surgical exposure with increased instrument dexterity. Robot-assisted laparoscopy has been gradually gaining importance over conventional laparoscopy due to the shorter hospital stay and quicker recovery. Additionally, it offers better ergonomics to the surgical team who do not have to stand by the patient's side for the entire procedure. Limitations of this robotic technique include high cost, lack of tactile feedback, risk of mechanical failure, and prolonged operating time.

Diagnostic laparoscopy has a broad clinical applicability with the ability to visualize the surfaces of the peritoneum, the liver, the omentum, or the small bowel, as well as the pelvic organs. Intraabdominal adhesions, peritoneal carcinomatosis or TB, ascites, or hemorrhage can readily be recognized and sampled via a laparoscope. It is a useful tool in cases of malignancies, providing valuable information that directly impacts care.

Before the procedure, patients should undergo standard preoperative evaluation and testing as with any open surgery. The examination is conducted in an operating room under all aseptic precautions with the patient is positioned supine and secured to the operating table. After induction of general anesthesia, the initial step is establishing access using one of two methods. In the first, closed technique, a specialized spring-loaded (Veress) needle is placed into the abdominal cavity without damaging the underlying organs. The umbilicus usually is selected as the preferred point of access because, in this location, the abdominal wall is quite thin, even in patients with obesity. The other method is the open (Hasson) technique. With this technique, the surgeon makes a small incision just below the umbilicus. Under direct vision, the abdominal fascia is located, and a small incision is made through the fascia and underlying peritoneum. A finger is placed into the abdomen to make sure that there is no adherent bowel before insufflation. This technique is preferable for the abdomen of patients who have undergone previous operations in which small bowel may be adherent to the undersurface of the abdominal wound.

Next, a pneumoperitoneum is created by insufflation of carbon dioxide into the peritoneal cavity through a needle or cannula. An alternative to pneumoperitoneum is an abdominal lift device that can be placed through a trocar at the umbilicus. The usual site for initial insufflation is the umbilicus, with the primary trocar/laparoscope port placed at the same site. The locations of additional ports are chosen to triangulate the camera and instruments around a focal point within the abdomen, thereby maintaining optimal access for manipulation of the instruments. The number and size of additional trocars will depend on the need for biopsies and other interventions. Certain areas, such as prior operative scars, the upper right quadrant (because of the round ligament), and the midline of the rectus abdominis muscle (because of the course of the epigastric vessels), should be avoided. Alternative access techniques for laparoscopic surgery include single-incision surgery, single-port access, and natural orifice transluminal endoscopic surgery. In single-incision surgery, a single incision, usually at the umbilicus, is used to perform the procedure, as opposed to multiple incisions through multiple ports. Natural orifice transluminal endoscopic surgery involves an endoscopic/laparoscopic approach. A multichannel endoscope is used to gain access to the peritoneal cavity through the stomach, bladder, vagina, or rectum. The result is a truly "scarless" operation, with minimal pain.

Complications related to laparoscopic procedures appear to be few and are mainly related to abdominal access. Vascular injury most commonly occurs during access; laceration of the inferior epigastric artery has been reported. Other complications include injury to the bowel or bladder and injury to the nerves of the abdominal wall. Port site metastasis is a rare but serious complication, and port site hernia is a late complication seen in 3% to 5% of patients 5 years after the laparoscopic procedure.

Absolute contraindications to laparoscopic procedures include hemodynamic instability and inability to tolerate a laparotomy. Relative contraindications include the presence of COPD, generalized peritonitis, or bowel obstruction or a history of prior extensive surgeries; in these cases a frank discussion with the patient and family is needed to outline the relative merits and risks of laparoscopy.

# GIARDIASIS

Giardiasis is caused by an anaerobic, flagellated protozoal parasite (*Giardia intestinalis, Giardia lamblia,* or *Giardia duodenalis*). The CDC reported 15,000 confirmed cases of giardiasis in 2019, but estimates a much higher annual incidence of 1 million cases per year. Outside a host, *Giardia* exists as a remarkably resilient cyst that may survive for weeks to months; it is resistant to many disinfectants, including chlorinated agents. Beavers and deer serve as common wildlife reservoirs that contaminate streams, ponds, and soil with their excrement containing *Giardia.* A patient only needs to ingest as few as 10 to 25 cysts to produce illness, although a person who is infected may shed up to 10 billion cysts daily. After undergoing excystation, each cyst releases two trophozoites, which asexually replicate and multiply. *Giardia* possesses a ventral sucking disc allowing it to attach to the small intestinal mucosa without invading it but still can incite a severe inflammatory reaction. As the trophozoites approach the large intestine, they undergo encystation and are passed out once more in the host's feces.

Giardiasis is much more common in developing nations due to poor sanitation and limited access to safe, drinking water. In developed nations, campers, hikers, children in childcare, and even unconventional marathon runners in so-called "mud runs" are common victims of the disease. Poor handwashing techniques are notorious for spreading the infective cysts. Notably, anal-oral sexual activity has also been recognized as a mode of transmission.

The incubation period can range from 1 to 3 weeks and can have varying presentations. The infection can clear without any symptoms in half of exposed patients. In 35% to 45% of patients, acute symptoms develop. Profound diarrhea, steatorrhea, nausea, excessive belching, flatus, and abdominal cramping are predominant symptoms and can lead to weight loss. The rest can develop chronic symptoms that wax and wane for months. Additionally, an estimated 15% to 30% of individuals with acute infection will go on to experience chronic giardiasis. Long-term intestinal complications include the potentiation of functional GI disease, postinfectious irritable bowel syndrome, and lactose intolerance. Extraintestinal manifestations after giardiasis have been reported, including reactive arthritis, ocular disease, and hives. Pediatric chronic giardiasis can result in delay of both physical growth and mental development and in severe cases, the malabsorption leads to vitamin deficiencies (vitamin A, vitamin $B_{12}$, and folate). Cases of luminal invasion into the pancreaticobiliary tree and granulomatous hepatitis have been reported but are exceedingly rare.

Diagnosis of giardiasis historically relied on stool microscopy of a minimum of three samples from different bowel movements because the excretion of cysts can be highly variable and unpredictable. Hematoxylin and eosin stains uncommonly demonstrate the classic pear-shaped appearance on close examination. However, the advent of fecal immunoassays and nucleic acid amplification assays have since supplanted these insensitive microscopy tests. Endoscopy, often performed as part of the evaluation for abdominal pain and diarrhea, may appear completely normal or may reveal nonspecific erythema, nodularity, or granularity. The histology, likewise, may demonstrate nonspecific villous blunting and intraepithelial lymphocytes mimicking celiac disease or may appear normal. An increase in eosinophilic infiltration and lamina propria expansion have also been observed. Endoscopic duodenal aspirate can demonstrate *Giardia* trophozoites but has a low yield (20%).

Individuals with recurrent, relapsing giardiasis despite aggressive treatments need to be evaluated for underlying primary or acquired immunodeficiency (IgA deficiency, common variable immunodeficiency, HIV). A potential source of reinfection should also be sought.

An individual who is infected can shed infectious cysts for up to 6 months, so preventive measures are necessary to avoid further contamination. All individuals are encouraged to practice good handwashing hygiene. Campers and hikers should be encouraged to use iodine-based water disinfection because giardiasis is resistant to chlorine-based regimens. Individuals, especially children, with diarrhea should be placed on contact precautions.

Treatment with nitroimidazoles (tinidazole, metronidazole) and nitazoxanide is effective and should resolve symptoms and clear shedding of cysts within 1 to 2 weeks after treatment. Relapsing or refractory giardiasis may improve with longer duration of therapy or switching of agents; rarely, combination therapy is required, particularly in those who are immunodeficient.

Excystation to form trophozoites in upper small intestine

Trophozoites multiply by binary fission

Trophozoites attach to villous surface of small bowel mucosa, causing abdominal distress, cramps, and eructations.

Cysts and trophozoites pass in steatorrheic, foul stools (usually seen on microscopic stool examination).

Trophozoites disintegrate. Cysts survive and infect water.

Animals, particularly beavers, may also act as intermediate hosts.

Cysts ingested in contaminated, untreated stream water; in inadequately treated tap water; or via infected food handlers.

F. Netter M.D.

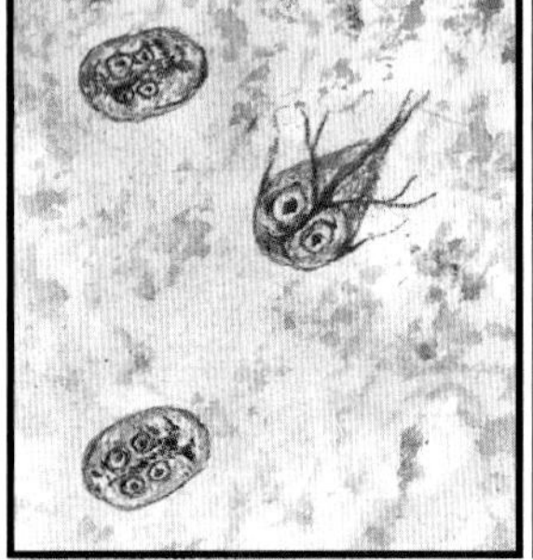

Cysts and trophozoite in stool

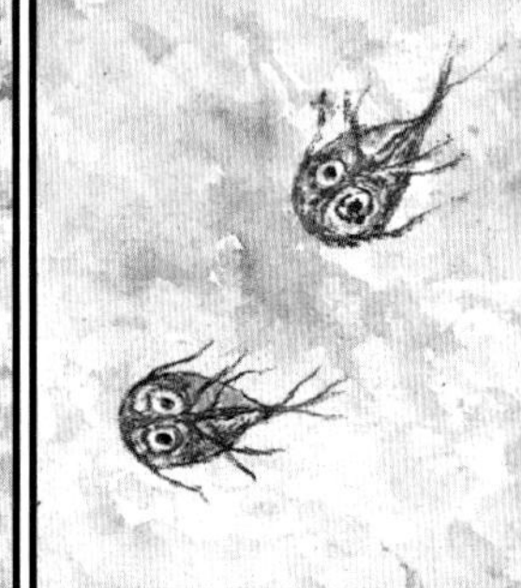

*Giardia* trophozoites in duodenal mucus

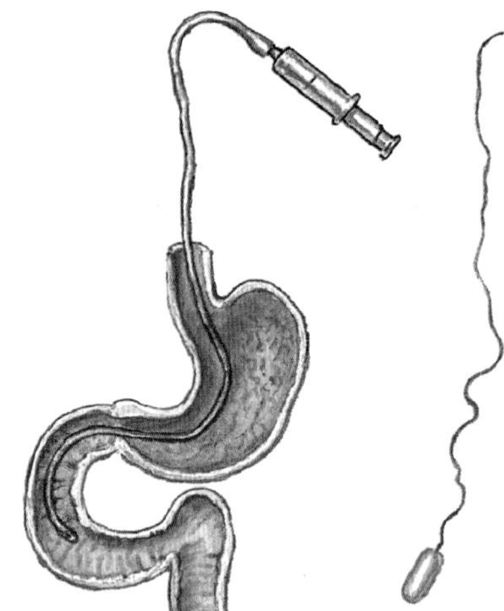

When infection is suspected but stool examination results are negative, duodenal or jejunal fluid (obtained by aspiration or gelatin capsule with string) should be examined.

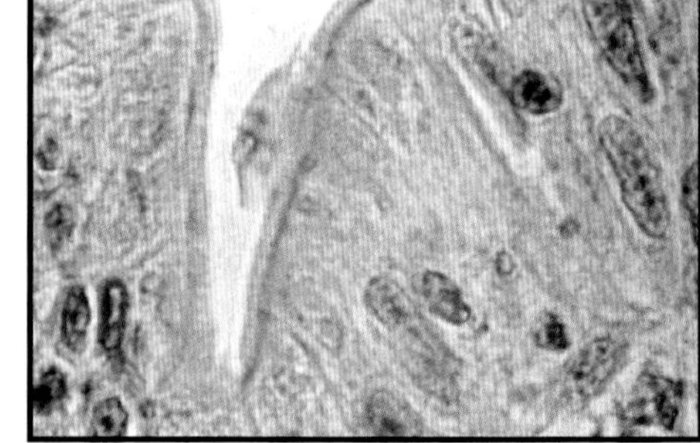

Jejunal biopsy specimen (obtained by suction or endoscopically) shows trophozoite on villous surface of mucosa.

## Benign Tumors of Small Intestine

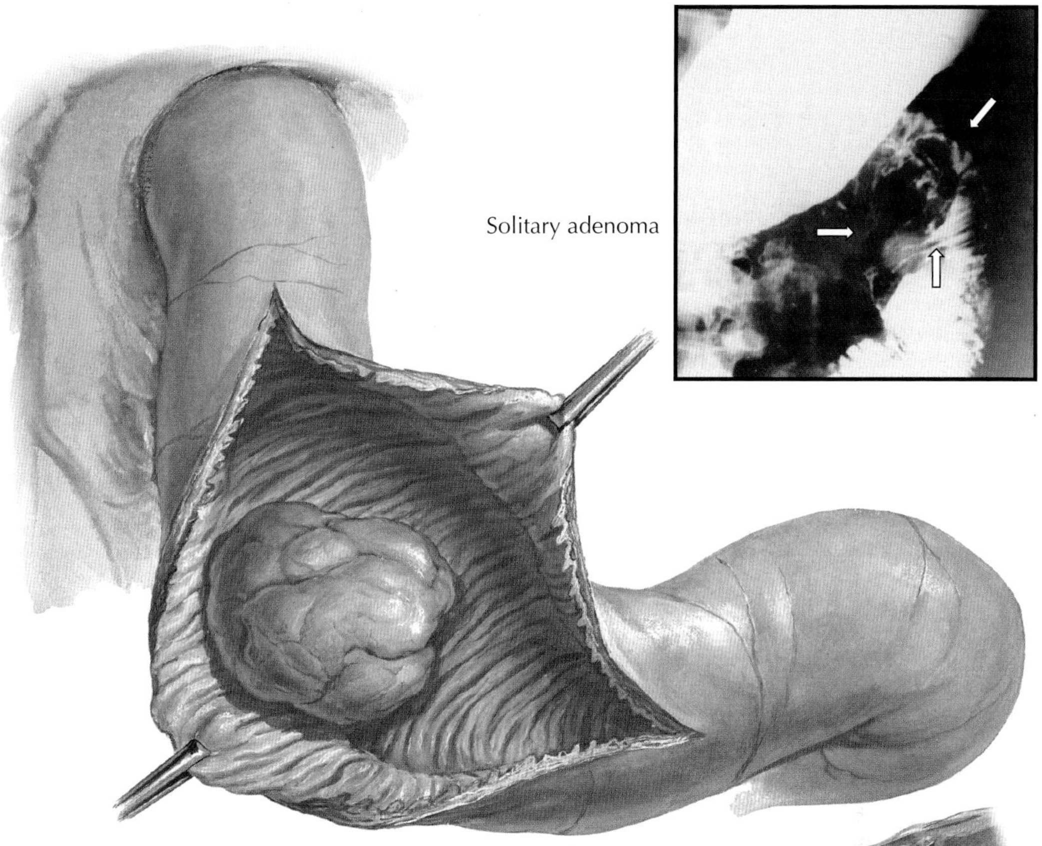

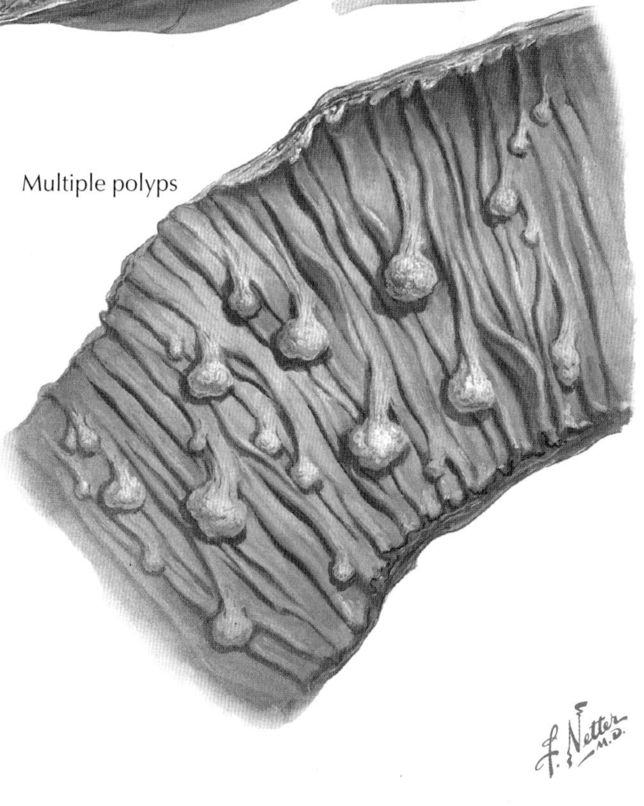

Benign tumors of the small intestine are a rare group of lesions that can affect any part of the small bowel from the duodenum to the ileum. Although the small intestine contains 75% of the length and 90% of the absorptive area of the GI tract, tumors of this area represent only a small percentage of all the primary GI tumors. Benign tumors account for around 35% of all tumors found in the small intestine. In a series of 22,810 autopsies, the incidence of these tumors was 0.16%. The incidence does not vary by race, ethnicity, or sex. These tumors have been documented in all age groups, but the mean age of presentation is typically between the fifth and sixth decades. For some types of benign adenomas, including neurofibromas and hemangiomas, there is a recognized familial occurrence.

Benign tumors of the small bowel may be single or multiple and may arise from any of its histologic elements. Neurogenic tumors appear in multiples, whereas adenomas, lipomas, and leiomyomas tend to appear as a single lesion. Benign tumors are commonly classified by location as intraluminal, extraluminal, and intramural types. Tumors may vary in size from a few millimeters to a few centimeters, and they can appear sessile, pedunculated, plaque-like, or annular. Adenomas, leiomyomas, and lipomas are the most common types of benign small intestine tumors. Other benign small bowel tumors include neurogenic tumors, myomas, hemangiomas, fibromas, lymphangiomas, myxomas, and osteomas. Neurogenic tumors in the small intestine may be part of a systemic syndrome, such as neurofibromatosis (von Recklinghausen disease). The incidence of benign small bowel tumors increases from the duodenum to the ileum. Adenomas are more common in the ileum, whereas stromal tumors or leiomyomas are more commonly found in the jejunum. Eighty percent to 90% of hemangiomas and neurofibromas are found between the jejunum and ileum.

*Adenomas* are the most common benign tumors of the small intestine, frequently located in the ileum. A majority of small intestine adenomas appear as single, sessile polyps and can range from few millimeters to a few centimeters, although larger tumors are rarely seen. Histologically, adenomas can be divided into three categories: tubular, villous, and tubulovillous tumors. Generally, adenomas are asymptomatic; however, they can rarely present with bleeding and abdominal pain with luminal obstruction. Similar to colon adenomas, they are subject to malignant degeneration. Overall, tubular adenomas have a low malignancy potential, whereas villous adenomas may undergo malignant degeneration in 40% to 50% of cases. Up to 90% of patients with familial adenomatous polyposis and Gardner syndrome have duodenal adenomas. The development of duodenal cancer from an adenoma in the setting of familial adenomatous polyposis is 5% to 10%.

*Lipomas* are the second most common benign tumor of the small intestine. They are commonly found in the ileum and arise from the submucosa. They tend to grow into the lumen and endoscopically appear as sessile or pedunculated polyps with normal or thin, atrophic-appearing mucosa. During endoscopy, lipomas can demonstrate a *pillow sign,* which refers to a soft indentation formed by a closed biopsy forceps pressed against the lipoma. On endoscopic US, lipomas will appear as hyperechoic, homogeneous lesions arising from the submucosa. Large lipomas can appear as a low-attenuating mass on CT. Lipomas are generally asymptomatic and do not have malignant potential; therefore no intervention is recommended unless they cause symptoms, which is rare (a lead point in intussusception, bowel obstruction, or obscure GI bleeding).

*Leiomyomas* arise from the smooth muscle wall of the muscularis mucosa or muscularis propria. They commonly appear as a single, firm, gray or white, well-defined mass. These tumors can grow into the lumen (intraluminal) or outside the bowel wall (extraluminal) undergoing necrosis. The histology of a leiomyoma is characterized by bundles of spindle-shaped smooth

Solitary adenoma

Multiple polyps

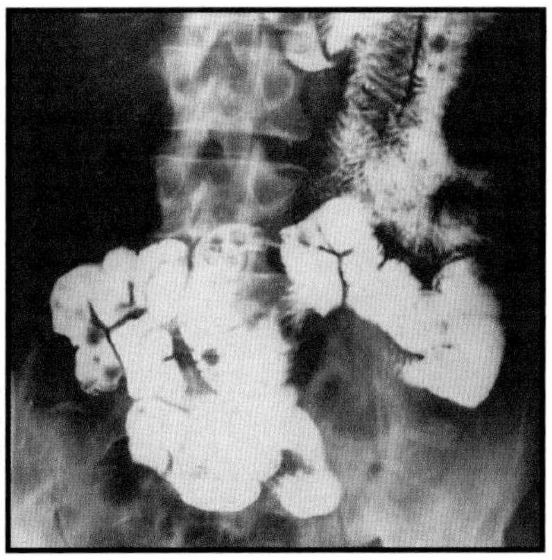

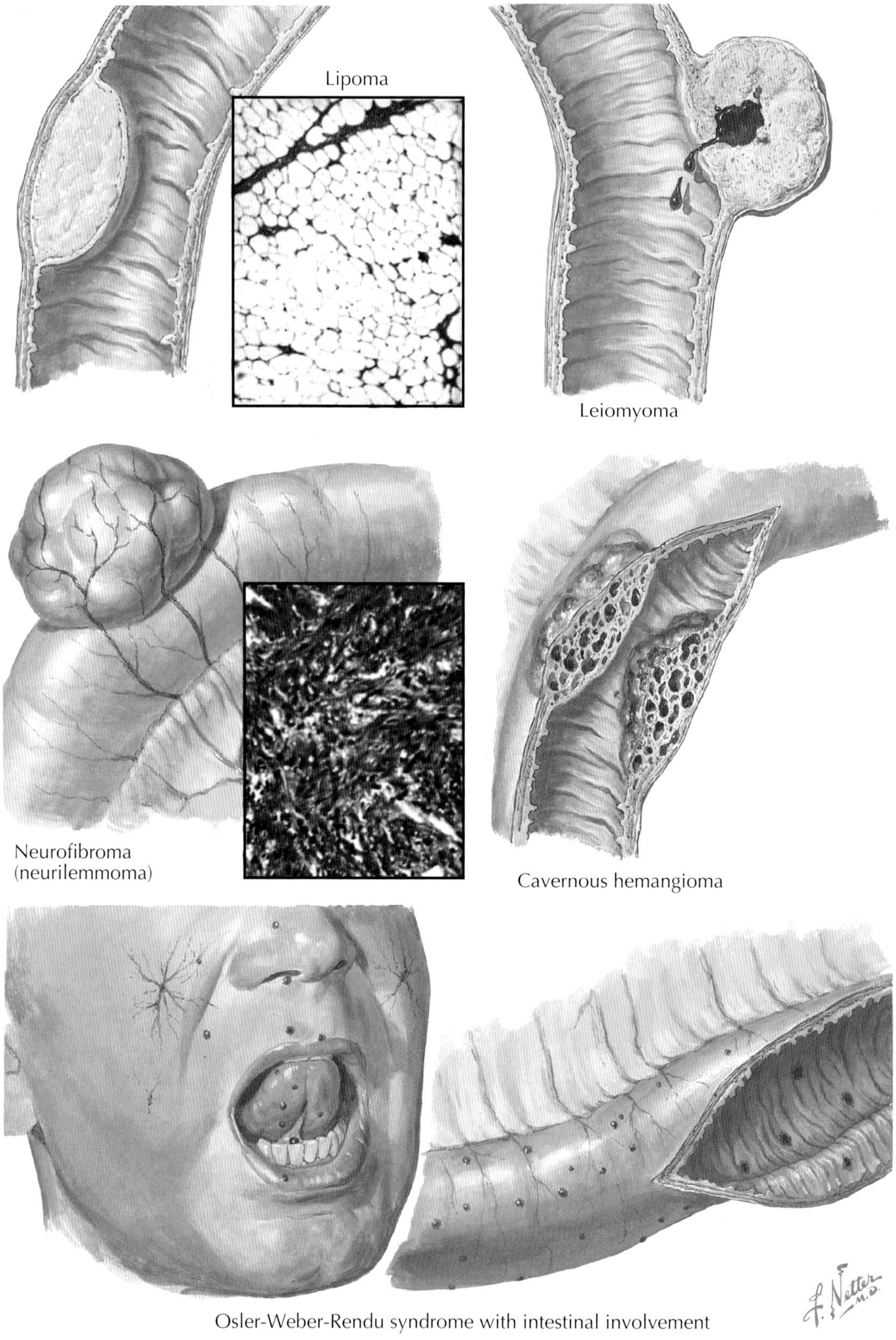

## Benign Tumors of Small Intestine (Continued)

muscle cells with rare or absent mitoses. A finding of more than two mitoses per high-power field (HPF) is indicative of a *leiomyosarcoma,* a malignant lesion.

Benign vascular tumors of the small intestine include tumors of blood vessels *(angiomas)* and congenital vascular malformations *(hamartomas).* It is difficult to differentiate between these two types of tumors. Small intestinal angiomas may present as single or multiple lesions and can be classified into capillary, compact, and cavernous types. *Cavernous hemangiomas* have large, blood-filled communicating spaces lined by endothelium and have little stroma. *Osler-Weber-Rendu disease,* also known as *hereditary hemorrhagic telangiectasia,* is an autosomal dominant disease of angiomas of the skin, mucous membranes, and viscera. The vascular lesions typically present as spider telangiectasias or nodular angiomas. Spider telangiectasias will partially fade with the application of pressure, whereas nodular angiomas will not. *Peutz-Jeghers syndrome* is another autosomal dominant disorder that is characterized by GI adenomas or hamartomas and mucocutaneous pigmentation.

Neurogenic tumors arise from neural tissue and occur anywhere along the small intestine and may appear as single or multiple lesions. The most common neurogenic tumor is a *neurofibroma.* Similar to most benign tumors of the small intestine, neurogenic tumors can grow in the extraluminal, intraluminal, or intramural space. Intraluminal tumors may be sessile or pedunculated, and the overlying mucosa may thin out and ulcerate, leading to GI bleeding. Neurogenic tumors in the small intestine may be part of *neurofibromatosis type I,* also known as *von Recklinghausen disease.* Histologic descriptions of such tumors typically display fasciculated spindle cells with palisading nuclei and thin-walled vascular spaces. Notably, neurogenic tumors can mimic other connective tissue tumors; specific immunohistochemical stains, such as S100, may aid in the diagnosis of a neurogenic tumor.

*Hyperplastic* and *hamartomatous polyps* are benign lesions that can also be found in the small intestine. Hamartomatous polyps can arise de novo or be associated with a polyposis syndrome such as *Peutz-Jeghers syndrome.*

In general, benign tumors of the small intestine are asymptomatic or cause vague symptoms that lead to a significant delay in the diagnosis. Intraluminal tumors tend to present earlier than extraluminal tumors due to luminal obstruction, ulceration, and bleeding. The bleeding arises from a necrotic erosion into a vessel and may be acute and massive or occult and chronic. Tumors that grow out of the serosal layer can result in intestinal obstruction or bleeding from an ulcerated tumor or malignant degeneration. In a subset of patients, extraluminal tumors grow to large dimensions and rupture into the peritoneal cavity, presenting with an acute abdomen. Rarely, intramural or extraluminal tumors can fistulize, leading to various clinical scenarios.

The diagnosis of benign tumors depends on the specific clinical scenario. Large tumors may be identified on contrast radiograph. In patients suspected to have a small bowel tumor, a wireless capsule endoscopy may be the best initial test to identify these lesions; however, lesions in the duodenum and proximal jejunum are easily missed due to the rapid transit through these areas, and CT enterography is more sensitive than capsule endoscopy for detecting small bowel tumors. Once identified, biopsy and/or removal should be attempted for tumors accessible via endoscopy (push enteroscopy or device-assisted enteroscopy).

Lipoma

Leiomyoma

Neurofibroma (neurilemmoma)

Cavernous hemangioma

Osler-Weber-Rendu syndrome with intestinal involvement

The management of benign small bowel neoplasms depends on the tumor size, location, malignant potential, and presence of symptoms. Resection can be accomplished via endoscopy (as in polypectomy of a tubular adenoma) or surgically (villous adenoma with high-grade dysplasia or small bowel leiomyoma). Overall, the prognosis for patients with benign tumors of the small bowel is excellent.

## CARCINOID

Carcinoid tumors are a type of well-differentiated neuroendocrine tumor that arise from enterochromaffin cells and represent nearly 40% of all malignant tumors of the small intestine. In recent years, the frequency of small bowel carcinoids has increased, which may in part be due to enhanced endoscopic and radiographic detection. The peak incidence is in the sixth decade, but the range of incidence is 20 to 80 years of age. Carcinoids are classified by their embryologic origin into foregut (bronchus, stomach, duodenum, and pancreas), midgut (jejunum, ileum, and proximal colon), and hindgut (distal colon, rectum, and genitourinary tract) types. This section will focus on carcinoid tumors involving the small intestine.

The most common location for a carcinoid tumor in the small intestine is the ileum, particularly within 60 cm of the ileocecal valve. Grossly, these tumors appear as firm intramucosal or submucosal nodules. Due to their indolent growth and lack of symptoms, most carcinoid tumors are found incidentally during surgery in the appendix or incidentally during a workup for another disease. In other cases, the carcinoid can cause mild abdominal pain, bleeding, or intussusception.

When these tumors secrete serotonin and other bioactive products, *carcinoid syndrome* can result. This syndrome is seen in approximately 10% of patients with carcinoid tumors. More than 90% of patients with carcinoid syndrome will have metastatic disease, which most commonly involves the liver. Typical symptoms of carcinoid syndrome include cramps with associated diarrhea, flushing, and bronchospasm or even cyanosis. An intense purplish rash that primarily involves the upper body and arms characterizes the flushing associated with carcinoid. Drinking alcohol or red wine, eating blue cheese or chocolate (high in amines), and exercise can precipitate flushing. If repeated attacks occur, permanent skin discoloration or telangiectasias may develop.

*Carcinoid crisis* is a life-threatening form of carcinoid syndrome that results from an overwhelming release of bioactive substances, usually in response to the administration of an anesthetic. Carcinoid crisis may present as intense flushing, diarrhea, tachycardia, hypertension or hypotension, bronchospasm, and altered mental status. Carcinoid crisis can also be precipitated by tumor manipulation during surgery or biopsy. Octreotide should be given before surgery to reduce the incidence of carcinoid crisis in patients with a history of carcinoid syndrome.

Carcinoid tumors of the small intestine are often asymptomatic. When symptoms develop, checking a 24-hour urine collection for 5-hydroxyindoleacetic acid may aid in the diagnosis. Further radiographic studies, such as CT scanning of the abdomen, contrast-enhanced MRI, and somatostatin receptor scintigraphy, allow for tumor localization and metastases if present. Regardless of tumor size, carcinoid tumors have the potential to metastasize. This is a unique feature of small bowel carcinoids. In the appendix and colon, for example, lesions greater than 2 cm in size have an increased risk of metastasis. The initial treatment of carcinoid tumors of the small intestine, regardless of size, is en bloc resection with adjacent mesenteric and lymph node dissection. Given that 40% of these patients will have a second GI tract malignant tumor, the entire GI tract should be examined before surgery. Unfortunately, chemotherapy has a limited role in metastatic disease. Somatostatin receptors are found in more than 80% of carcinoid tumors. Therefore when carcinoid syndrome develops, treatment with somatostatin analogs can effectively relieve symptoms. These medications do not reduce the tumor burden. Parachlorophenylalanine and methyldopa are inhibitors of serotonin synthesis and can also be used for symptomatic relief in carcinoid syndrome. Surgery plays a limited role in the treatment of carcinoid syndrome. The 5-year survival rate for carcinoid tumors of the small intestine ranges from 52% to 100% depending on the stage of the disease, size of the tumor, and organ affected. Even in the setting of distant metastasis, the 10-year survival rate has been cited at 40% to 60%. The overall prognosis for carcinoid tumor varies. Once carcinoids evolve into carcinoid syndrome, the prognosis is guarded.

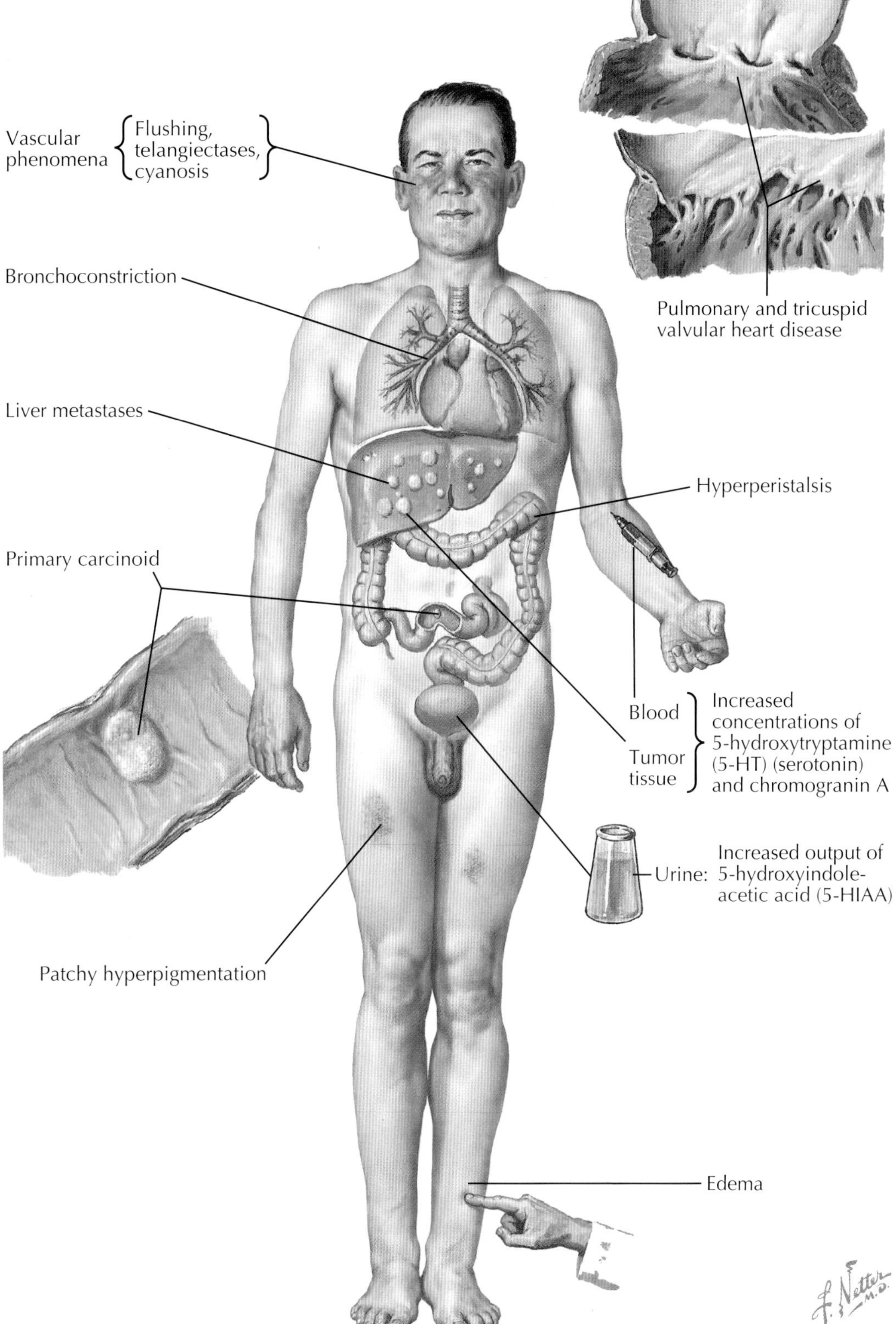

# PEUTZ-JEGHERS SYNDROME

Peutz-Jeghers syndrome

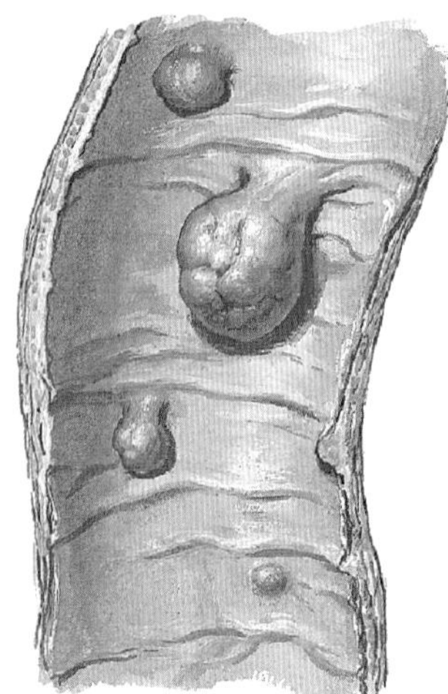

Polyposis of small intestine

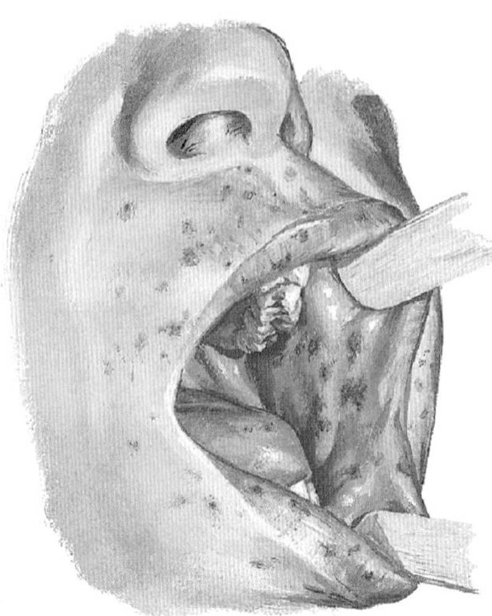

Mucocutaneous pigmentation

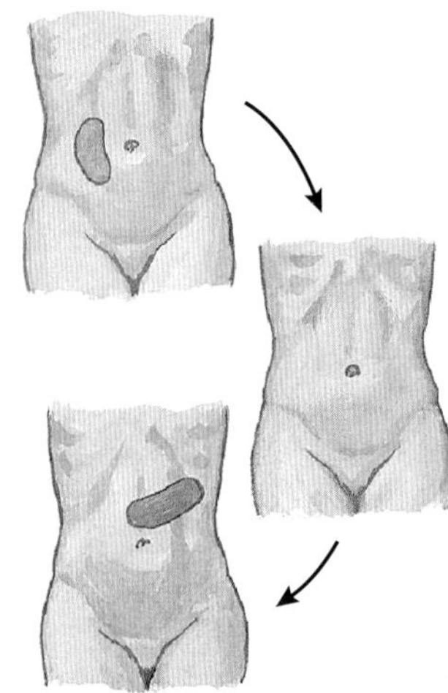

Intermittent, migrating mass (due to self-reducing intussusception)

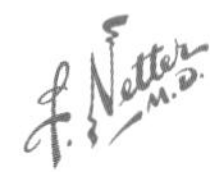

Complications of benign tumors

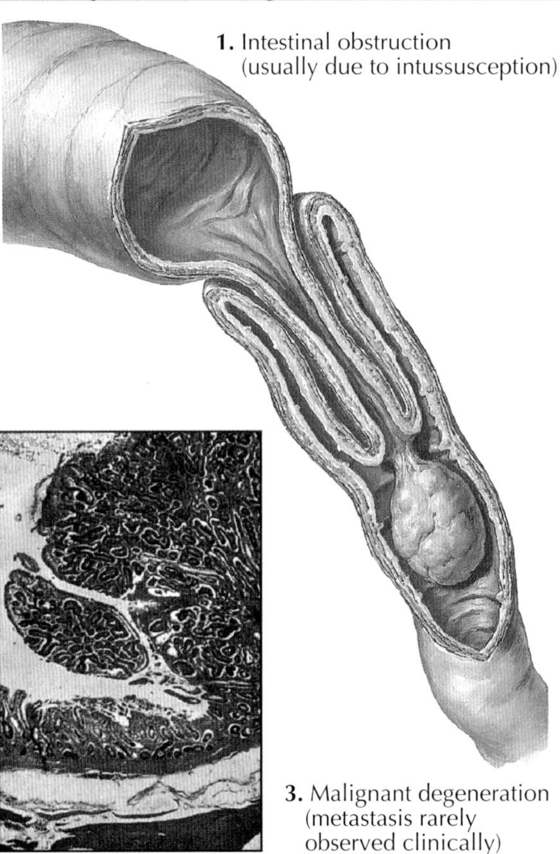


2. Hemorrhage (most often in leiomyoma)

First stage: interstitial hemorrhages

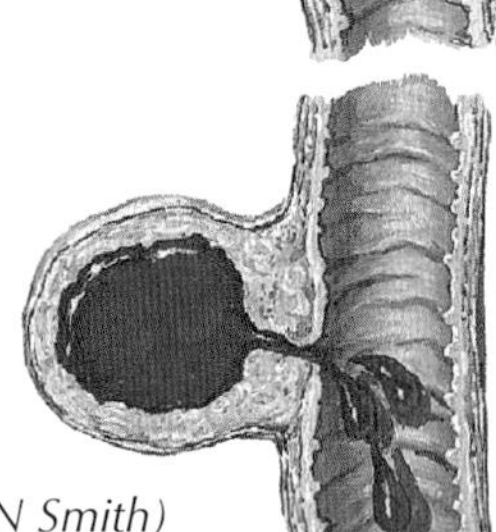

Second stage: confluence of necrotic, hemorrhagic areas

Third stage: evacuation into intestine, bleeding persists owing to firm, "noncollapsing" cavity walls. *(Modified after ON Smith)*

Peutz-Jeghers syndrome is an autosomal dominant syndrome consisting of mucocutaneous pigmentation and multiple GI hamartomatous polyps. Patients are at an increased risk for both GI and non-GI malignant disease. Germline mutations of the *STK11/LKB1* gene, located on chromosome 19p, are commonly implicated. Not all families with the syndrome are linked to this gene locus, suggesting that another mutation may be involved. An estimated 10% to 20% of patients have no family history of Peutz-Jeghers syndrome. Males and females are equally affected. The prevalence is not well reported and has been cited at 1:8000 to 1:200,000 births.

The two characteristic findings of Peutz-Jeghers syndrome are pigmented mucocutaneous macules and multiple hamartomatous polyps. *Pigmented mucocutaneous macules* are deposits of melanin that are seen in more than 95% of patients with the syndrome. The macules typically appear as flat, bluish-gray to brown spots less than 5 mm in size. These macules are present around the mouth, nose, lips, buccal mucosa, hands, feet, and perianal and genital regions. They are most commonly seen on the lips and perioral region. During the first 1 to 2 years of life, the macules typically increase in size and number until puberty, at which point they begin to fade. The one exception are macules of the buccal mucosa, which do not fade after puberty. It is prudent to distinguish these macules from freckles. Freckles are absent at birth, never appear on the buccal mucosa, and are scant around the nostrils and mouth. The presence of pigmented mucocutaneous macules is very sensitive for Peutz-Jeghers syndrome. It is important to remember, however, that these lesions can also be associated with other syndromes.

*Hamartomatous polyps* may occur in infancy and can be located throughout the GI tract, with a predilection for the small intestine. Patients are generally asymptomatic, but symptoms can range from abdominal pain to intussusception and bleeding. On endoscopy, hamartomatous polyps do not have gross identifiable features that allow for diagnosis. They may be sessile, pedunculated, or lobular; there may be a single polyp or multiple polyps. On histologic studies, these polyps appear as smooth muscle proliferations in the lamina propria, with arborization and normal overlying epithelium. Histologic studies are necessary for the diagnosis of a hamartomatous polyp.

Peutz-Jeghers syndrome is associated with an increased risk of both GI and non-GI malignant diseases. The average age of cancer diagnosis in these patients is 42 years, and the lifetime risk for developing cancer is between 37% and 93%. The most common GI malignant tumors associated with Peutz-Jeghers syndrome are colon and pancreatic cancers, whereas breast cancer is the most common site for non-GI malignant disease. The risk for developing breast cancer in Peutz-Jeghers syndrome is significant and parallels the risk with *BRCA1* and *BRCA2* germline mutations. Females with the syndrome are at an increased risk for cervical tumors, ovarian cysts, and ovarian sex cord tumors. Males with the syndrome are at an increased risk for Sertoli cell testicular cancers. In both males and females, these tumors occur at a younger age.

The diagnosis of Peutz-Jeghers syndrome can be made clinically if any one of the following criteria is met: (1) two or more histologically confirmed Peutz-Jeghers polyps, (2) any number of Peutz-Jeghers polyps in an individual who has a family history of the syndrome in a close relative, (3) characteristic pigmented mucocutaneous macules in a patient who has a family history of the syndrome in a close relative, or (4) any number of Peutz-Jeghers polyps in an individual who also has characteristic mucocutaneous pigmentation. Patients who meet the clinical criteria for the syndrome should undergo further testing for a mutation in the *STK11* gene. In a patient who meets the clinical criteria for the syndrome but lacks a mutation in the *STK11* gene, the diagnosis cannot be excluded, given that other genetic mutations likely exist.

The management of patients with Peutz-Jeghers syndrome is centered upon screening and surveillance protocols for both GI and non-GI malignant diseases.

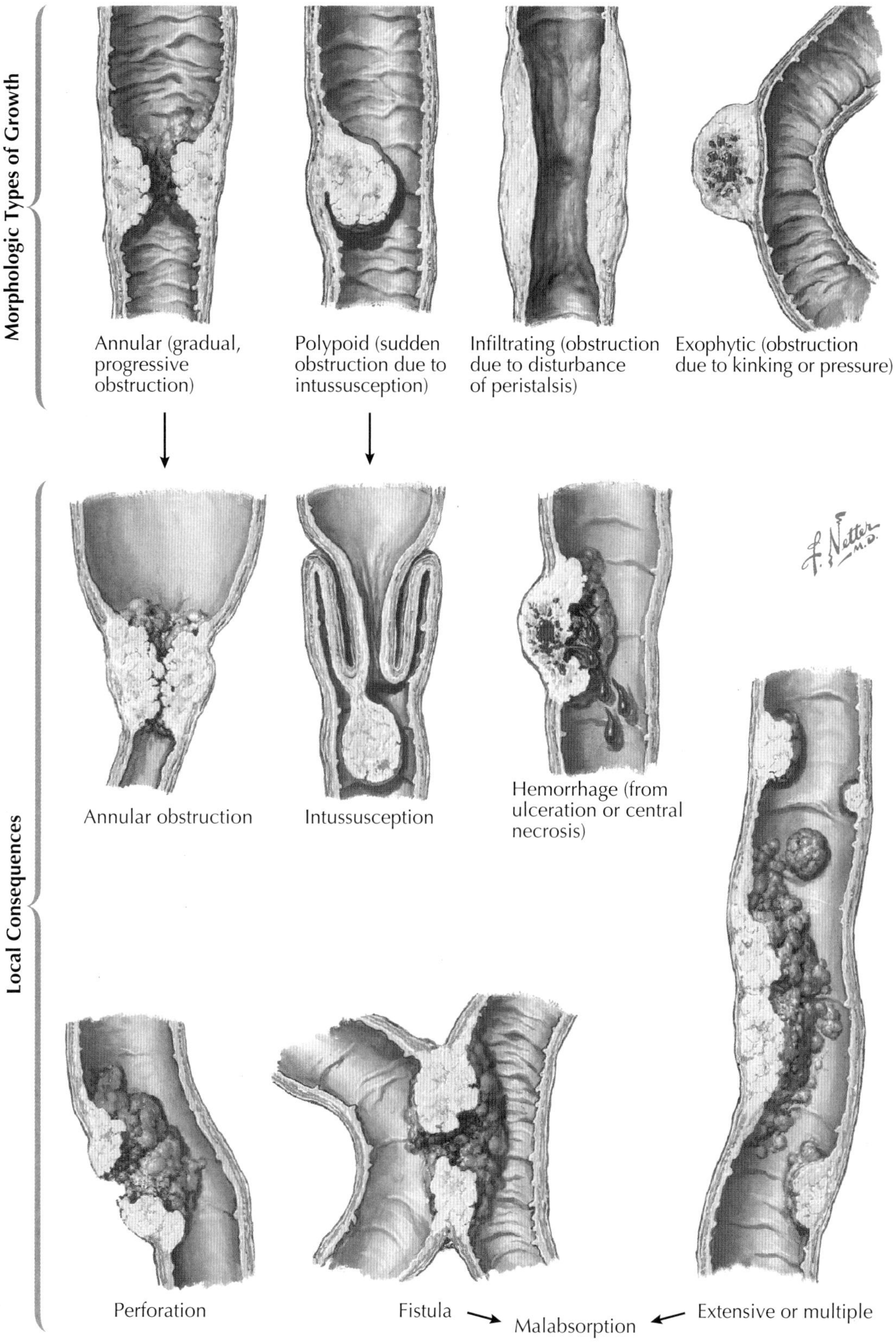

## Malignant Tumors of Small Intestine

Although malignant small bowel tumors account for only 0.5% of all cancers in the United States, they account for 65% of all tumors in the small intestine. Of all the neoplasms in the GI tract, around 5% originate in the small intestine. Even though malignant tumors of the small intestine are rare, a number of risk factors have been well described. Hereditary cancer syndromes such as familial adenomatous polyposis, Peutz-Jeghers syndrome, and hereditary nonpolyposis colorectal cancer (Lynch syndrome) are associated with an increased risk of adenocarcinoma. Chronic inflammation from diseases such as CD and celiac disease can lead to an increased risk of adenocarcinoma and lymphoma. Increased consumption of meals rich in refined carbohydrates, sugar, salt-cured or smoked foods, and red meats confers an increased risk for adenocarcinoma of the small intestine.

The four most common types of small bowel malignant diseases are adenocarcinoma, carcinoid, lymphomas, and sarcomas/gastrointestinal stromal tumors (GISTs). These lesions account for 95% of malignant small intestine tumors. Adenocarcinomas are commonly found in the duodenum, whereas carcinoid tumors and lymphomas are frequently found in the jejunum and ileum. Sarcomas, including GISTs, are equally distributed throughout the three segments of the small intestine. Carcinoids have surpassed adenocarcinomas as the most common malignant tumor of the small intestine. Carcinoid tumors of the small intestine are discussed in Plate 2.80.

Malignant small intestine tumors are more frequently found in males than females (1.5:1) and African Americans than Whites. The mean age of diagnosis is 65 years old. Adenocarcinomas and carcinoids tend to present slightly later than lymphomas and sarcomas.

Like benign tumors of the small intestine, malignant tumors can present in two forms, either as a tumor infiltrating the bowel wall or as a polypoid mass growing into the lumen. They can be differentiated based on histologic findings. Adenocarcinomas arise from glandular mucosa, carcinoid tumors from enterochromaffin cells, lymphomas from clonal proliferation of lymphocytes, and GISTs from the interstitial cells of Cajal.

*Nonampullary adenocarcinomas* account for about 40% of malignant small bowel tumors. They are most commonly found in the duodenum, except when they are associated with CD, in which case they are predominately found in the ileum. Presenting symptoms are vague, and the most common complaint is abdominal pain. Due to the vague nature of symptoms, diagnosis is frequently delayed and the majority of patients are diagnosed with advanced-stage disease. This lack of initial symptoms can be attributed to the distensibility of the small bowel lumen and the predominately liquid contents that inhabit it.

*Lymphomas* of the small intestine can be a primary tumor or be part of a systemic process. They make up about 15% to 20% of all malignant tumors of the small intestine, of which *non-Hodgkin lymphomas* are the most common. Lymphomas generally occur in adults and peak in the seventh decade of life. They are slightly more common in males than females. Lymphomas typically manifest as an infiltrating, constricting growth with or without ulcerations. The most commonly affected region is the ileum, which is the part of the small intestine with

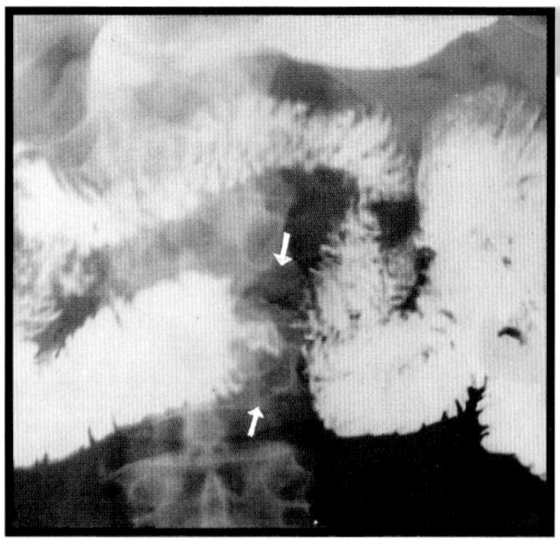

Contrast radiograph. Constriction of jejunum (*arrows*) due to carcinoma

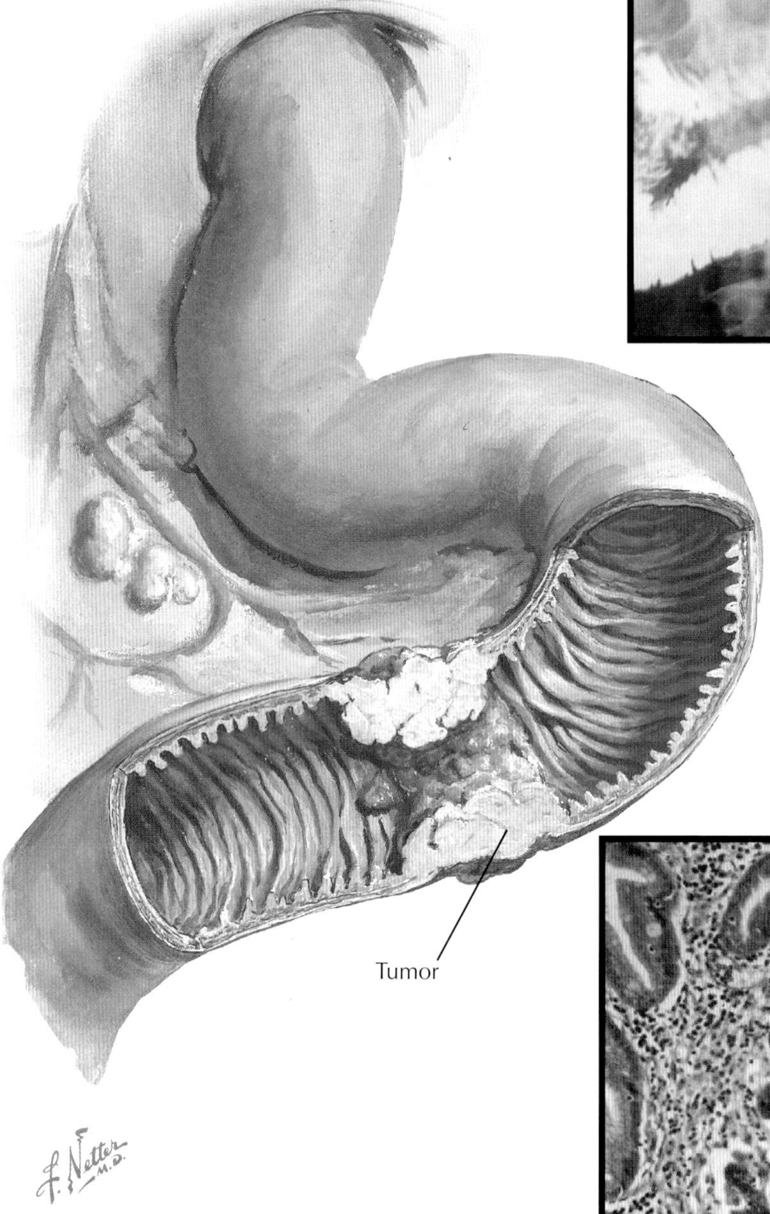

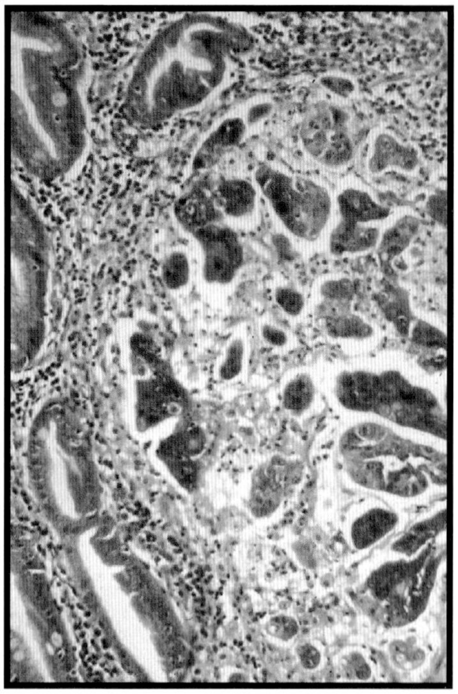

**Atypical tubular glands of adenocarcinoma.** Invading normal intestinal mucosa.

## Malignant Tumors of Small Intestine (Continued)

the highest distribution of lymphoid follicles. Conditions that can lead to the development of small intestine lymphoma include AIDS, Crohn's disease, irradiation complications, and use of long-standing immunosuppressive therapy. *Sarcomas* are malignant mesenchymal tumors that account for an estimated 10% of malignant small intestine tumors. GIST is the most common type of intestinal sarcoma. These tumors are most commonly found in the jejunum and ileum. The determination of whether a GIST will display aggressive behavior is based on its size and mitotic rate. Lesions are considered high risk if they are larger than 10 cm with any mitotic rate, any size with a mitotic rate of more than 10 per 50 HPF, or larger than 5 cm with a mitotic rate of more than 5 per 50 HPF. GISTs with more than 10 mitoses per 50 HPF have a 5-year survival rate of 5% and are metastatic 100% of the time. More GISTs are being reported; it is uncertain whether this is due to enhanced diagnostic tools or a true increase in incidence. Metastatic cancers can invade the small intestine through local invasion or hematogenous spread. Common lesions that metastasize to the small bowel through direct invasion are ovarian, colon, and gastric cancers. Melanoma, lung, breast, cervical, and colon cancers can metastasize to the small intestine via hematogenous spread.

Malignant tumors of the small intestine are indolent, and thus diagnosis is frequently delayed. These patients do not usually seek emergent evaluation because their symptoms are so nonspecific and persist over months. Patients may present with anemia, abdominal pain, or weight loss. If there is an infiltrating tumor, it may lead to malabsorption and intermittent abdominal cramps. Some patients may present with acute abdominal pain from obstruction or intussusception. Others may present with an acute, massive GI bleed. Imaging with barium studies, CT scanning (with or without enterography), magnetic resonance enterography, and video capsule endoscopy can identify and localize malignant lesions of the small intestine. Once lesions have been localized, endoscopic procedures such as push enteroscopy, single-balloon or double-balloon enteroscopy, or spiral enteroscopy can allow for tissue diagnosis. If the tumor cannot be accessed endoscopically, surgical intervention is needed for biopsy and diagnosis. The treatment of malignant tumors of the small intestine is contingent upon obtaining a histologic diagnosis. The cornerstone of therapy is endoscopic or surgical resection. Once the lesion has been resected, histologic analysis and depth of invasion will dictate what type of chemotherapy is needed. The 5-year survival rate for adenocarcinoma of the small bowel is 30%, and the median survival time is less than 20 months. Ampullary adenocarcinoma has a better prognosis, with a 5-year survival rate of 36% and an even better survival rate for patients who undergo early resection. The overall prognosis for lymphoma depends on the disease stage. In advanced stages, the 5-year survival rate generally ranges from 25% to 30%. However, with radical surgery and improving chemotherapeutic agents, the survival rate has increased to as high as 60% to 70%.

SECTION 3

# COLON

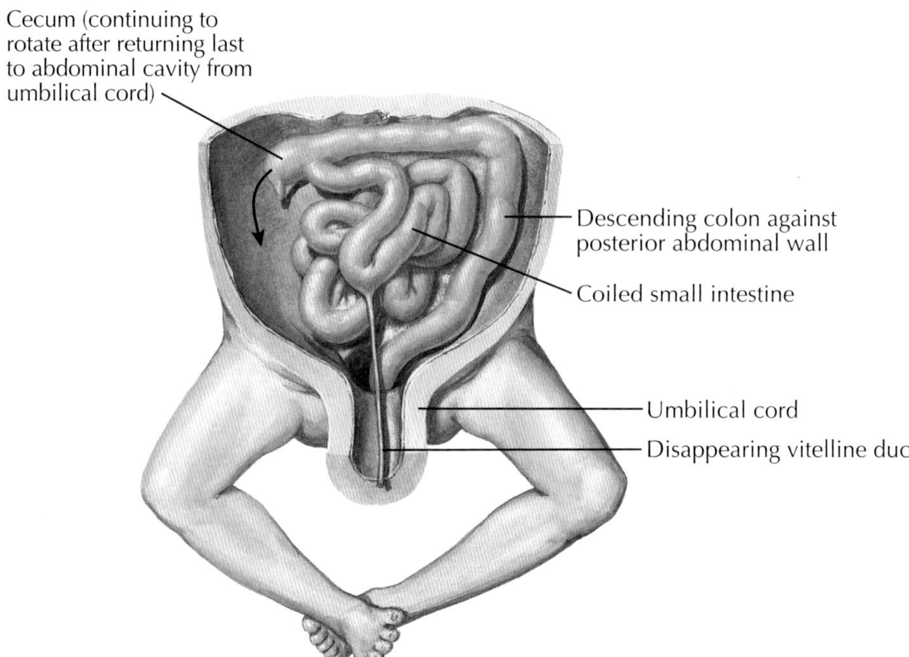


## Development of Large Intestine

The development of the large intestine is intimately tied to the development of other organs. The cecum, appendix, ascending colon, and transverse colon are part of the midgut and develop alongside the jejunum and ileum. The descending colon, sigmoid colon, and rectum are hindgut structures and develop in conjunction with the urogenital system. During normal development, the midgut elongates tremendously and herniates into the umbilical cord during the fifth week. The proximal limb of the midgut loop produces the jejunum and ileum, and the distal limb differentiates into the distal ileum, cecum, appendix, ascending colon, and transverse colon. The distal limb of the midgut loop rotates from the inferior side of the umbilical cord to the left, then superiorly, and finally to the right as the midgut returns to the abdominal cavity during the 11th week. This explains why these structures are typically on the right side of the abdomen.

The cecum appears as a dilated area on the distal limb of the midgut during the sixth week, while it is still in the umbilical cord. By the eighth week, the appendix has begun to form as a small diverticulum in the cecum wall. It elongates as the cecum continues migrating to the right inferior region of the abdomen during the fetal period between 4 and 5 months. The dorsal mesentery of the cecum and ascending colon fuse to the parietal peritoneum of the posterior abdominal wall after the appendix has developed, and because of this the appendix may be found in different locations relative to the cecum. In contrast with the retroperitoneal cecum and ascending colon, the transverse colon retains its mesentery and is an intraperitoneal structure. As the terminal end of the midgut, it travels from the right side of the abdomen across to the left, connecting with hindgut organs. In the process it passes anterior to the duodenum; this is one reason the dorsal mesentery of the duodenum is mostly fused with the parietal peritoneum. The descending colon, the first part of the hindgut, also loses its dorsal mesentery, fusing with the parietal peritoneum on the left side of the abdomen.

The hindgut is supplied by the inferior mesenteric artery and consists of the descending colon, sigmoid colon, and rectum. Although it does not take part in the physiologic herniation of the midgut, the hindgut must partition itself from the cloaca, separating the digestive system from the urogenital system. As described in the overview of development, the cloaca is divided into a urogenital sinus and rectum by a sheet of mesoderm, the urorectal septum. This also separates the cloacal membrane into a urogenital membrane and an anal membrane. The surface feature that marks the location of the urorectal septum is the perineal body, located anterior to the rectum, which serves as an important attachment site for the perineal and anal musculature.

4 to 5 months

Transverse colon
Duodenum
Right colic (hepatic) flexure
Left colic (splenic) flexure
Root of transverse mesocolon (right half)
Root of transverse mesocolon (left half)
Ascending colon
Duodenojejunal flexure
Triangular fusion of ascending mesocolon to dorsal wall
Descending colon
Root of mesentery of small intestine
Quadrangular fusion of descending mesocolon to dorsal wall
Cecum in final position of rotation
Vermiform appendix
Ileum
Cut edge of mesentery
Root of sigmoid mesocolon
Sigmoid colon
Rectum
Anus
F. Netter M.D.

The anal membrane separates the hindgut structures superior to it that are supplied by the inferior mesenteric vessels and inferior mesenteric plexus from the anal pit, a structure formed by involution of ectoderm and somatic mesoderm, which is supplied by branches of the internal iliac vessels and pudendal nerve. Once the anal membrane disappears, the rectum and anus form a continuous lumen, but the differences in their embryonic origin are evident from the differences in blood supply, innervation, and epithelial lining of the canal. The simple columnar epithelium lining the rectum contains many mucus-producing goblet cells and is derived from endoderm. At the *anocutaneous line,* there is a sudden transition from this epithelial lining to the stratified squamous epithelium of the anal region, which consists of epidermis that is derived from ectoderm. If the anal membrane fails to disappear or ruptures incompletely, the result is an *imperforate anus* or *anal stenosis.*

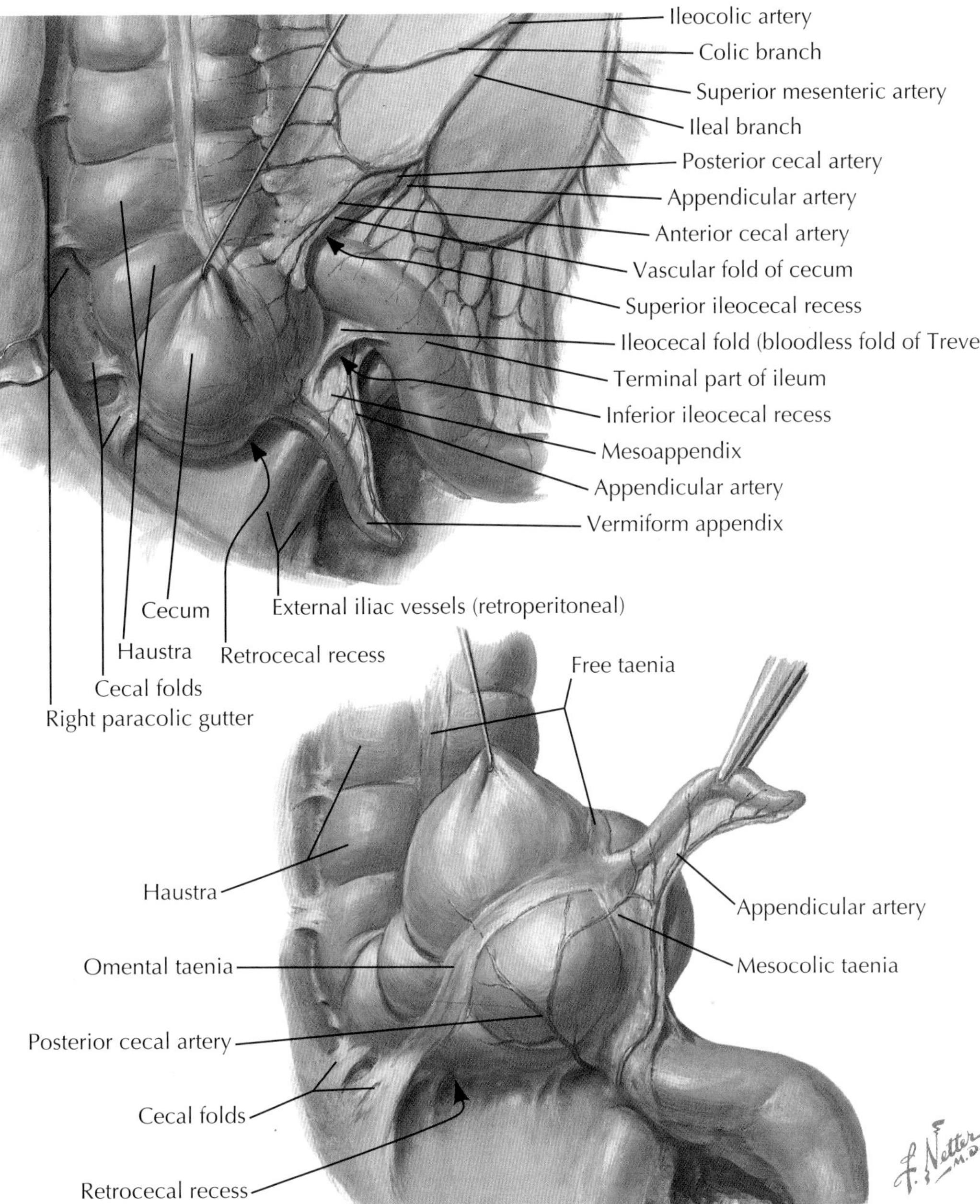


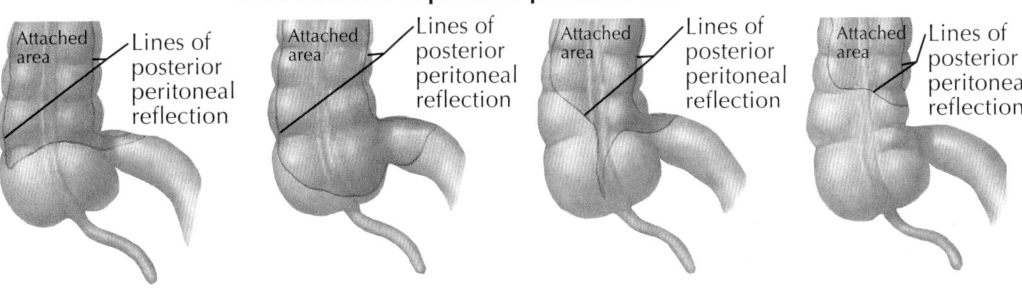


## Ileocecal Region

The final portion of the small intestine, the terminal ileum, lies in the pelvis anterior to the right iliac fossa. Typically the *ileal orifice* opens into the medial wall of the colon from the left. This opening has previously been called the *ileal valve, ileocolic valve,* or *ileocecal valve;* this nomenclature is no longer preferred, however, because the opening's method of closure is not strictly valve-like. From the ileal orifice, the *cecum,* a blind sac, extends inferiorly within the lower right quadrant and the large intestine extends superiorly as the *ascending colon.* Although its exact location can vary considerably between individuals, the ileal orifice usually resides deep to the surface feature called *McBurney's point.* This point can be found in the right lower abdominal quadrant by drawing a line connecting the anterior superior iliac spine with the umbilicus *(line of Monro)* and looking for the line's intersection with the lateral edge of the rectus abdominis muscle.

The cecum, which is the widest portion of the large intestine, extends inferiorly from the ileal orifice in the right ileac fossa. Medially, the cecum is typically in contact with loops of the ileum. Laterally and posteriorly it is in contact with the iliacus muscle. Anteriorly it is typically covered by coils of the small intestine and/or greater omentum, but when full or distended by intestinal gases, it may bulge and contact the anterior abdominal wall. In this case it is possible to elicit a distinct tympanic note by percussing the overlying abdominal wall. An enlarged cecum can extend inferiorly over the psoas major muscle and even into the true pelvis. It typically does not extend so far as the inguinal ligament, leaving room for loops of small intestine in this region.

The ileum is connected to the posterior body wall by a mesentery containing its blood vessels, lymphatic vessels, and nerve supply. The mesentery of the ileum also contains the blood vessels that supply the cecum. In the area where the ileum joins the large intestine, a peritoneal fold extends in almost all individuals from the terminal part of the ileal mesentery across the front of the ileum to the cecum and the lowermost part of the ascending colon. This fold is properly called the *vascular fold of the cecum* but may also be known as the *ileocolic fold* or *superior ileocecal fold.* It contains the anterior cecal artery, and it forms the anterior wall of a fossa, correspondingly termed the *superior ileocecal recess.* The posterior wall of this fossa is made up of the terminal ileum and its mesentery. Its mouth opens inferiorly and somewhat to the left.

Another fold known as the *ileocecal fold* is commonly encountered anterior to the mesoappendix, extending from the lower or right side of the terminal ileum to the cecum. It is also referred to as the *inferior ileocecal fold.* The ileocecal fold contains no important vessels, and its corresponding eponymic designation is the *bloodless fold of Treves.*

## ILEOCECAL REGION (Continued)

The third peritoneal extension, the *mesoappendix,* serves as the mesentery of the vermiform appendix. It stretches from the posterior leaf of the mesentery of the terminal ileum and actually travels posterior to the cecum to the left side of the cecum and then along the entire length of the appendix. It thus typically assumes a triangular shape, and it transmits between its two layers the vessels of the appendix, particularly the appendicular artery or one of its numerous variations. The *inferior ileocecal recess* is formed by the ileocecal fold anteriorly and the mesoappendix as the posterior wall.

In some individuals, one or more thin peritoneal folds spread from the parietal peritoneum of the posterolateral abdominal wall to the lateral (right) side of the cecum *(retrocecal folds)* and/or ascending colon *(retrocolic folds).* These folds create small, shallow recesses that in very rare instances are large enough to admit loops of the small intestine. Their apertures are normally too wide to permit an internal hernia to form.

The degree of mobility of the cecum depends on the level at which the posterior part of its visceral peritoneum is reflected to the parietal peritoneum of the posterior abdominal wall. The level and contour of the reflection vary considerably. Occasionally, the peritoneal reflection may be so inferior that the cecum and terminal ileum are both firmly fused to the posterior abdominal wall. Conversely, the reflection may also occur so far superiorly that the entire cecum, distal ileum, and parts of the ascending colon may be surrounded by visceral peritoneum and connected to the body wall by the mesentery of the ileum. In most cases, the reflection lies between these two extremes. The line of reflection may be straight, convex, or concave, or it may incline downward to the right or left or may be characterized by a narrow downward prolongation forming a sort of mesocecum.

As the terminal ileum enters the cecum, it is thrust through the wall of the cecum along with all of its layers except for the serosal layer. This creates an opening in the lumen that appears like a pair of lips, called the *ileal orifice* or *ileocolic valve.* When this opening is exposed in the cadaveric donor, it most frequently (60% of the time) appears to have transverse folds, the *frenula of the ileal orifice,* stretching away from either side of the ileal orifice. These folds resemble the crescent-shaped, *semilunar folds of the colon,* but they mark the place where contents of the ileum empty into the colon. The *superior frenulum* and *inferior frenulum* of the ileal orifice also mark the separation between the ascending colon above and the cecum below. For this reason, the superior frenulum is sometimes referred to as the *ileocolic lip* and the inferior frenulum as the *ileocecal lip.* Although the ileal orifice often has the two frenula, it can also protrude into the large intestine in the form of a round *ileal papilla,* the lumen of which looks like a star, or an asterisk, when closed. There is circular muscle within the papilla, and it may tonically contract to prevent retrograde motion of the colon contents but typically does not act as a true sphincter, selectively allowing contents from the ileum into the cecum. Some of the longitudinal smooth muscle fibers of the ileum are continuous with the mesocolic taeniae of the taeniae coli, and other longitudinal muscle fibers contribute to the ileal papilla. The muscle fibers of the ileum and large intestine meet at the papilla, with the circular muscle of the large intestine enveloping the circular muscle of the ileum. The two circular layers enclose the longitudinal fibers arising from the taeniae, except in the region close to the ostium, where the two circular layers meet.

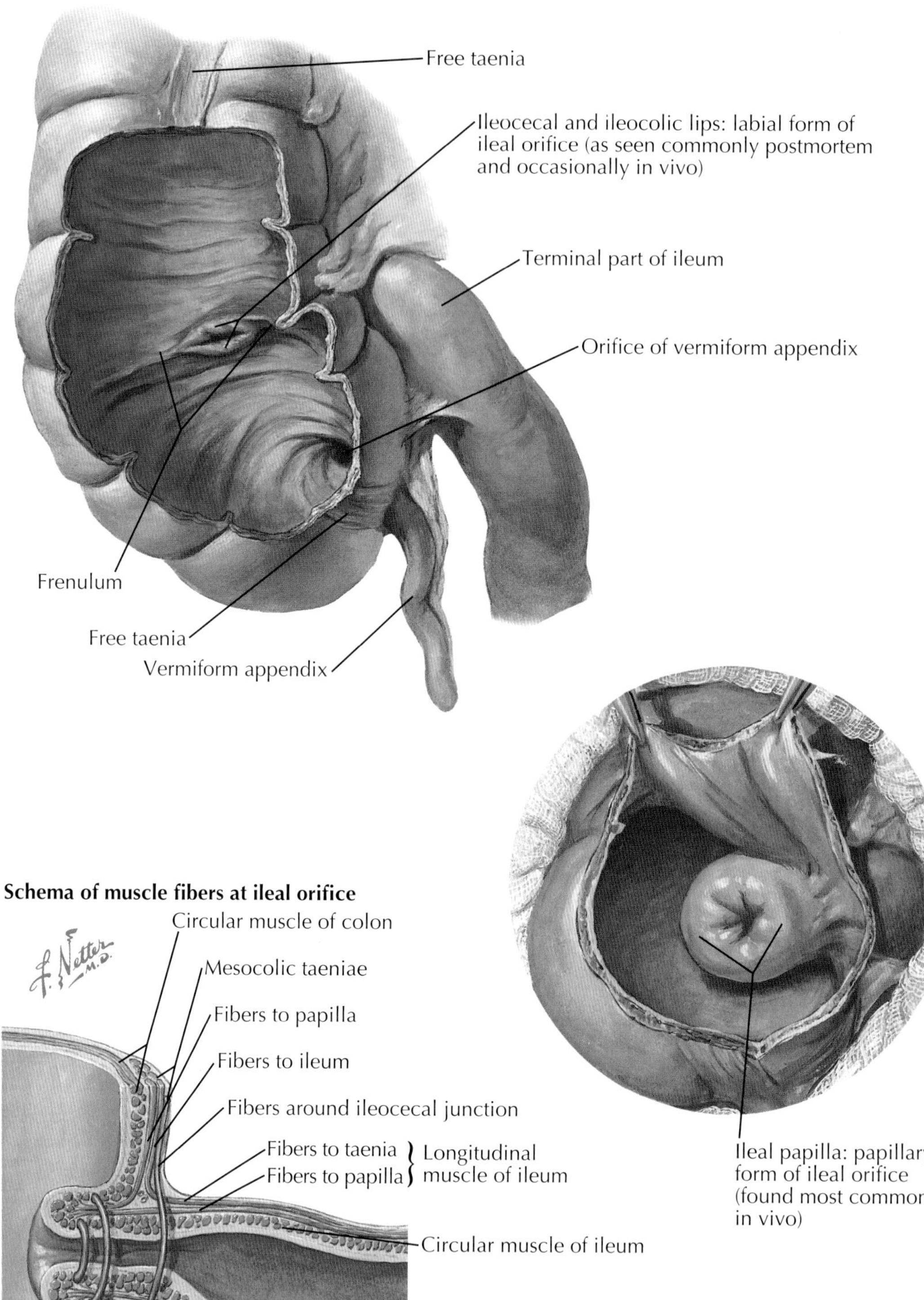

## VERMIFORM APPENDIX

One structure of the proximal colon with considerable clinical significance is the *vermiform appendix.* Its surface projection typically lies at the lateral third of an imaginary line drawn from the anterior superior iliac spine to the umbilicus *(McBurney's point).* In early fetal life the cecum extends caudally in the form of a cone, the tip of which grows more in length than in diameter, creating a vermiform (worm-like) process. Later, as a result of difference in the speed of growth of the cecal walls, the point where the appendix arises shifts from the distal end of the blind sac to a site on the posterior medial wall, where the three taeniae coli of the large intestine converge into one uniform coat of longitudinal muscle. In humans and apes, the appendix is a rather rudimentary, narrow, and thin (from 2.5 to 25 cm long; average, 6–9 cm) offshoot of the large intestine, which has no intestinal function (in contrast to the processus vermiformis of some birds and mammals, in which it may attain considerable length). However, it may serve as a reservoir for normal flora of the gut during diarrheal diseases or other dysfunctions related to the colon. The course and position of the appendix differ considerably between individuals and can also change over time in an individual. Variations in position of the vermiform appendix are largely the result of differences of the length and width of the *mesoappendix,* the peritoneal fold that represents the mesentery of the appendix. The mesoappendix and nearby *ileocecal fold* form the bookends of a space, the *inferior ileocecal recess.*

The mesoappendix allows the vermiform appendix some mobility. Typically it is suspended from above by its mesentery and hangs for a varying distance into the true pelvis and may actually come into contact with pelvic organs (e.g., the uterus and its adnexa or the bladder). Sometimes the appendix is mobile enough to be found within the sac of an indirect inguinal hernia or involved in a direct inguinal hernia. The vermiform appendix may also turn superiorly and extend anterior or posterior to the cecum or ileum. The appendix can sometimes be found in a *retrocecal* position, posterior to the cecum where it is "fixed" and relatively immobile. This fixation may have taken place as a result of inflammatory adhesions, or the appendix may have been trapped in the retrocecal position during fetal life at a time when the ascending colon fused to the posterior abdominal wall. Such a posteriorly fixed appendix may extend superiorly enough as to be more properly called *retrocolic* rather than retrocecal. In contrast to a fixed retrocecal appendix, in some instances the appendix may be capable of wandering into the retrocecal fossa and emerging thereafter.

The layers that make up the wall of the appendix are the same as those in other parts of the intestinal tract: mucosa, submucosa, muscularis externa, and serosa. The exterior of the appendix is enwrapped by the serous layer, or *visceral peritoneum,* except for a narrow line where the two layers of the mesoappendix attach to the appendix. Just deep to the serous layer, the *longitudinal layer of the muscularis externa* invests the entire circumference. The *circular layer of the muscularis externa* is well developed along the entire length of the appendix, though it may occasionally be deficient in one or two small regions, where the submucosal tissue becomes confluent with the serous coat. The appendix can be visualized in radiographic studies about 24 hours after the ingestion of barium. It usually fills uniformly, but the appearance of segments within the lumen is not to be interpreted as an expression of a pathologic process. The *submucosa* is endowed with lymphatic nodules as well as diffuse lymphatic tissue, the abundance of which is a characteristic of the appendix and explains one of its nicknames, "the intestinal tonsil." The structure of the *mucosa* is essentially the same as in the large intestine, with intestinal glands but no villi or plicae circulares. Occasional Paneth cells can be found within the epithelium of the pits.

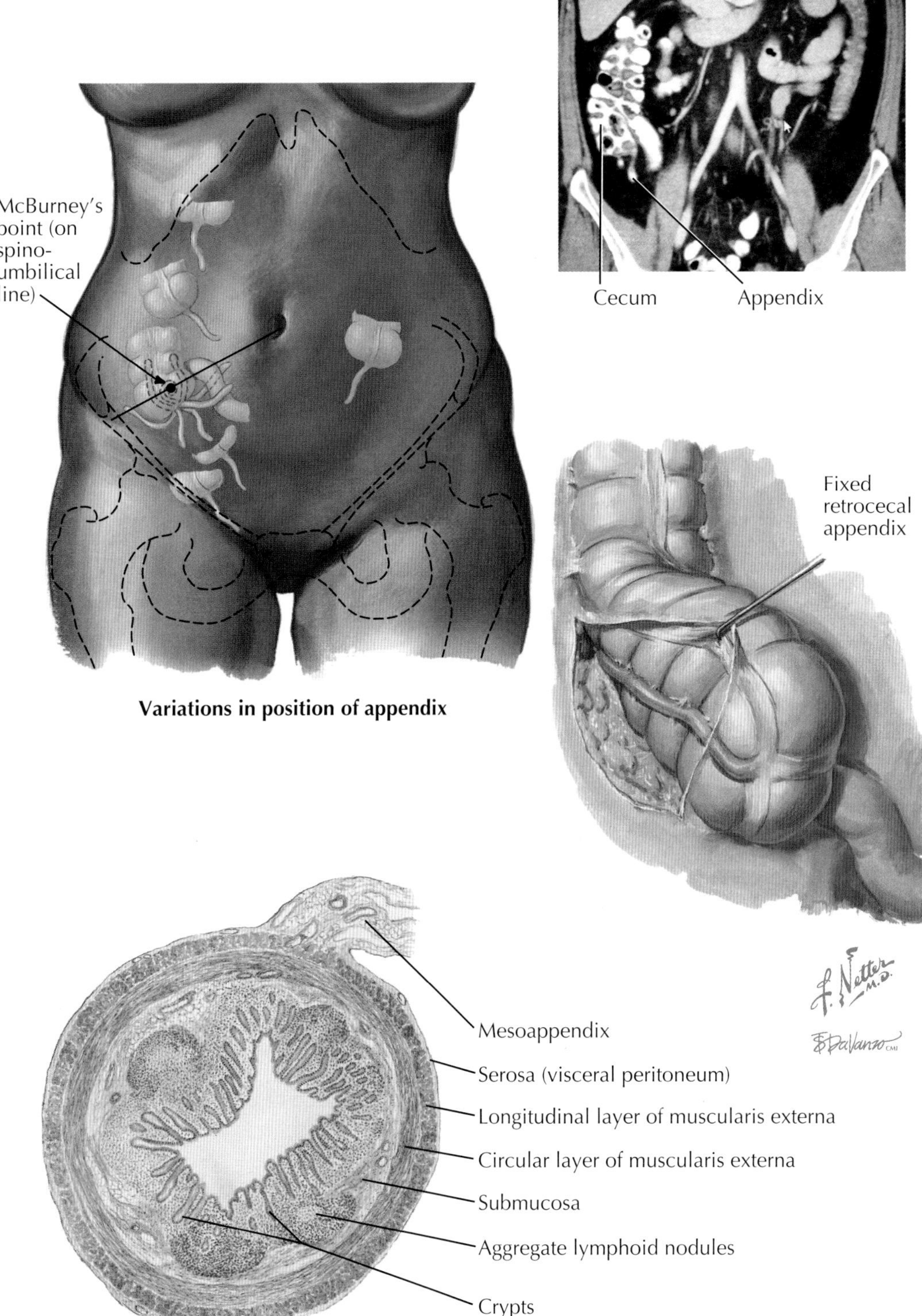

## Topography and Relations of Colon

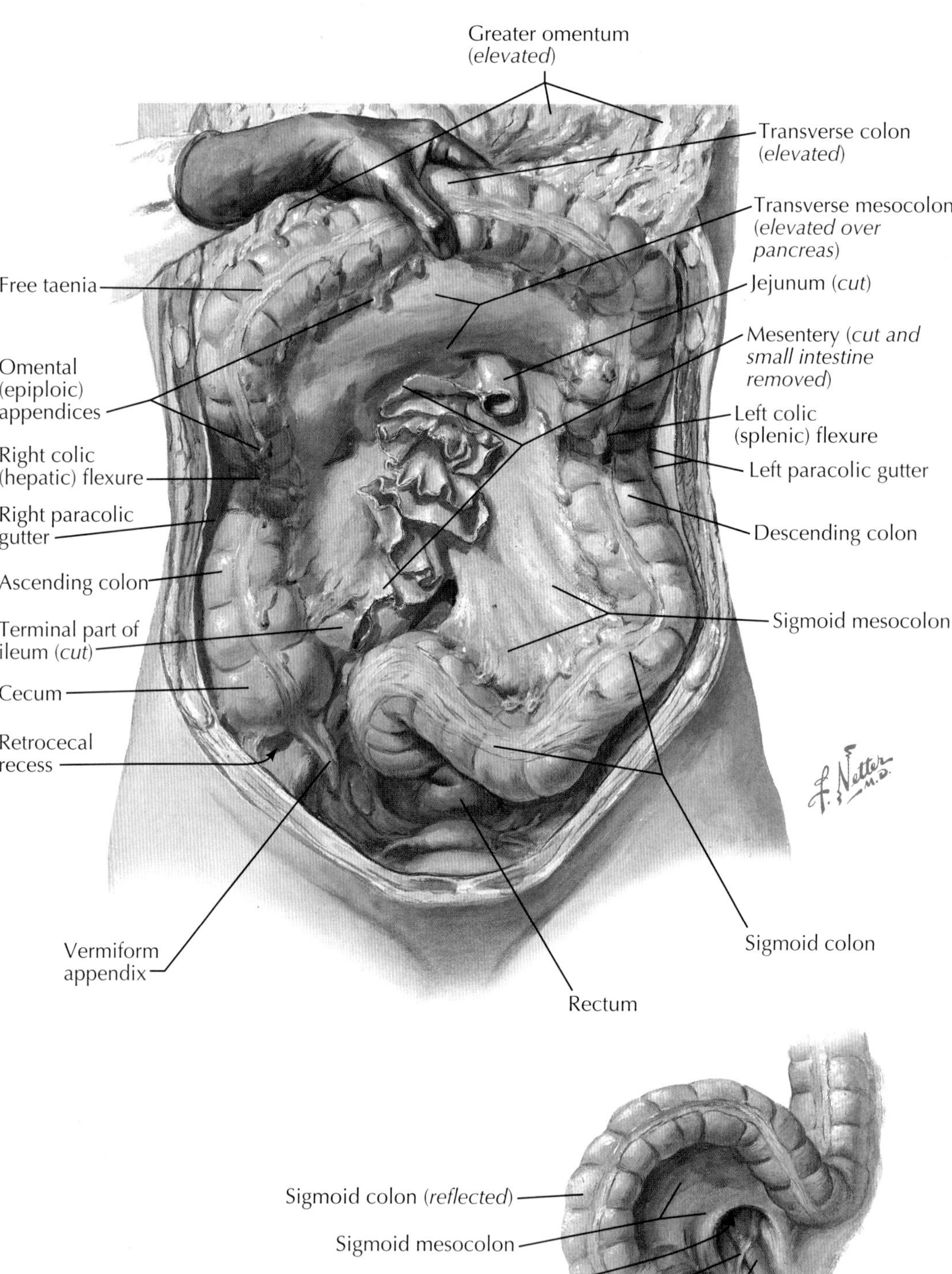


The lumen of the large intestine is generally greatest at the commencement of the large intestine (cecum) and narrows toward the rectum. However, the lumen of the large intestine varies considerably in caliber depending on its functional state. The *haustra* form sacculations separated by constricting furrows, so that the lumen bulges and contracts alternately during peristalsis. The total length of the large intestine is approximately 120 to 150 cm. From the cecum, the colon is subdivided into four segments: the ascending, transverse, descending, and sigmoid colon. The ascending colon and descending colon are *retroperitoneal structures,* fixed to the posterior body wall, and the transverse colon and sigmoid colon are *intraperitoneal structures,* loose but tethered to the posterior body wall by a mesentery. Viewed as a whole, the various parts of the large intestine describe an arch roughly in the shape of a horseshoe with the convex side directed superiorly. However, there is considerable variation in this appearance between individuals, largely due to differences in the length of the mesentery connecting the transverse colon and sigmoid colon to the posterior body wall.

The *ascending colon* averages about 15 to 20 cm in length and runs superiorly in a mostly straight course from the superior lip of the ileocolic valve to the right colic (or hepatic) flexure, where it passes into the transverse colon. Inferiorly, it starts in the right iliac fossa in contact with the iliacus muscles, and after crossing the iliac crest, it is positioned in the angle between the psoas major muscle and the quadratus lumborum and transversus abdominis muscles. The right colic flexure, responsible for the so-called *colic impression* on the undersurface of the right lobe of the liver, lies anterior to the right kidney, the two organs being linked together by loose connective tissue. The ascending colon is sometimes in contact with the anterior abdominal wall, depending on how distended its lumen may be as well as the degree to which it is overlapped by the loops of the small intestine. As the ascending colon turns leftward, becoming the transverse colon, it is related to the descending part of the duodenum and the medial surface of the right kidney.

The *transverse colon,* varying from 30 to 60 cm in length, continues from the *right colic (hepatic) flexure* to the slightly more superiorly situated *left colic (or splenic) flexure.* It is an intraperitoneal structure, attached to the posterior abdominal wall by a mesentery, specifically called the *transverse mesocolon,* which is very short in the region of the flexures and longest in the middle of the transverse colon. Because the transverse mesocolon is most pendulous in the middle, a long transverse colon may sag down some distance toward the pelvis. The line of attachment of the transverse mesocolon crosses first the descending part of the duodenum, then the pancreas, and, finally, the left kidney. At the lateral edge of the kidney near the lower pole of the spleen is situated the left (or splenic) flexure of the colon. The posterior surface of the greater omentum adheres to the superior surface of the transverse mesocolon and to the serosal coating on the anterior side of the transverse colon. The middle section of the transverse colon would lie directly adjacent to the anterior abdominal wall if the greater omentum were not draped anterior to it. Depending on the position and fullness of various organs, the transverse colon may be covered by the liver and gallbladder on the right and the stomach and spleen on the left.

The retroperitoneal *descending colon,* some 20 to 25 cm in length, extends inferiorly from the left colic flexure to the iliac crest or beyond it into the left iliac fossa. Depending on the distension of its lumen, it will

Typical Sigmoid Colon and Variations

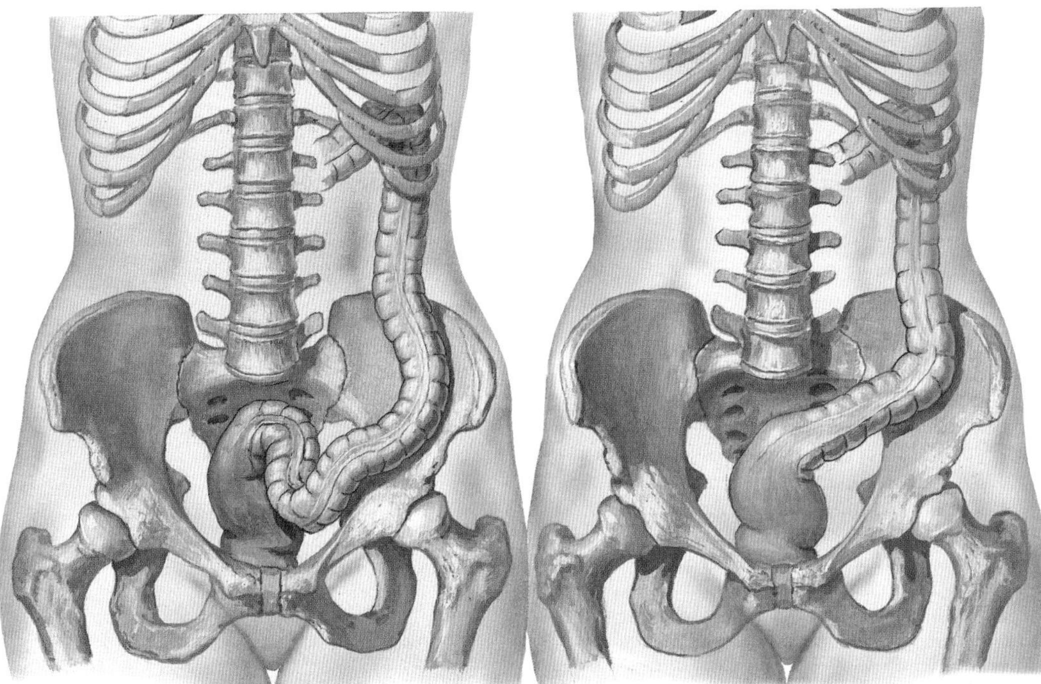

Typical

Short, straight, obliquely into pelvis

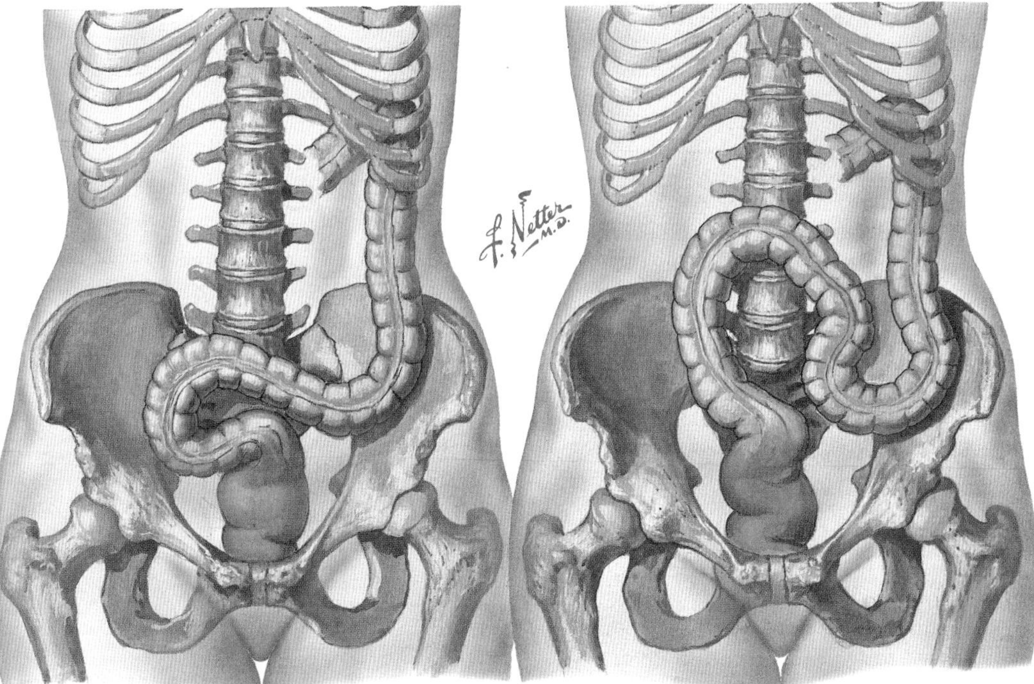

Looping to right side

Ascending high into abdomen

## Topography and Relations of Colon (Continued)

be in contact with loops of small intestine medially and anteriorly. After running first in the angle between the lateral edge of the kidney and the quadratus lumborum muscle and then over the iliacus muscle, it finally passes anterior to the psoas major. As it does so, it crosses the femoral and genitofemoral nerves and continues to become the sigmoid colon.

The exact point of transition between the descending colon and *sigmoid colon* is indefinite. The sigmoid is the segment of large bowel between the descending colon and the rectum, which is somewhat mobile as a result of its attachment to a mesentery, the *sigmoid mesocolon.* Because this mesentery is subject to great variations, the exact length of the sigmoid colon itself becomes variable. It has been described as beginning anywhere between the left iliac crest and the brim of the true pelvis. As a rule, the sigmoid colon assumes an omega-shaped flexure arching over the pelvic inlet toward the right side of the pelvis at the level of the first or second sacral vertebra. It finally joins the rectum at an acute angle at approximately the level of the third sacral vertebra. However, this typical shape of the sigmoid is not constant. The sigmoid colon may be short, in which case it will run straight and obliquely into the pelvis, or it may be so long that the loop extends far to the right or, in an extreme case, high into the abdomen. The sigmoid colon's average length is about 40 cm in adults and 18 cm in children, but with the variations already mentioned, it may reach a length of 84 cm or more. The root of its sigmoid mesocolon is variable but characteristically starts in the upper left iliac fossa, proceeds inferiorly a few inches, medially, and again superiorly to a point on the psoas muscle a little to the left of the fourth lumbar vertebra, where it turns inferiorly into the pelvis. The line of mesenteric attachment takes the shape of an irregular and blunt inverted V. Turning inferiorly after having reached its highest point, the attachment line of the sigmoid mesocolon crosses anteriorly to the left common iliac artery and vein just above the division of the artery. The length of the sigmoid mesocolon (i.e., the distance from its root to the bowel wall) is extremely variable. A small peritoneal fossa, the *intersigmoid recess,* is formed by the sigmoid mesocolon while it twists around its vascular pedicle. The loop of sigmoid colon in this region covers the external iliac vessels, making it a good landmark for identifying the vascular stalk to the sigmoid colon as well as the external iliac artery and vein. Rarely, loops of small bowel can become strangulated in this area, causing an intersigmoid hernia. The left ureter passes retroperitoneally posterior to the intersigmoid recess.

The arrangement of the circular and longitudinal muscle layers is practically identical to that of the corresponding structures of other parts of the colon, except for the most distal parts of the sigmoid colon, where the three flat longitudinal muscle bands, the *taeniae coli,* fan out to form a completely encircling longitudinal muscle layer at the rectosigmoid junction. In the same region the circular layer thickens as it approaches the rectosigmoid junction.

Throughout the course of the sigmoid colon, the *omental appendages* of the serous coat diminish gradually in number and size. These fatty appendages hang from the colon and are generally clinically silent unless they become twisted around their vascular pedicle; in such a case, the ischemia may mimic the pain of appendicitis or diverticulitis.

## Structure of Colon

The histologic appearance of the colon is a modification of the normal structure of the entire intestinal tract. Specifically, the colon, cecum, and appendix consist of a mucosa, submucosa, double-layered muscularis externa, and either a serosal or an adventitial layer. Despite having similar layers, the colon differs significantly from the small intestine, being larger in diameter and containing a wider lumen. The colon also differs from the small intestine because of the three structures that are typical of it: (1) the three taeniae coli, (2) the haustra, and (3) the omental appendages.

The *taeniae coli* are three longitudinal bands, each approximately 8 mm in width, running along the length of the colon. They are actually the external (outer) layer of the muscularis externa. This layer of smooth muscle typically runs longitudinally but, unlike elsewhere in the gastrointestinal (GI) tract, the taeniae do not form a uniform coat but condense into three distinct bands. The spaces between the taeniae coli consist of a thin longitudinal coating of smooth muscle. Each of the taeniae is named for its location on the transverse colon. The *mesocolic taenia* is located on the posterior aspect of the transverse colon between the two layers of the transverse mesocolon. It lies on the posteromedial surface of the ascending and descending colon. A second taenia, the *omental taenia,* is positioned along the attachment of the greater omentum as it lies across the anterosuperior surface of the transverse colon. It continues along the posterolateral aspect of the ascending and descending colon. The third taenia, called the *free taenia,* can frequently be noted without dissection on the inferior surface of the transverse colon and on the anterior aspect of both the ascending and descending colon. The three taeniae coli merge into a uniform longitudinal coat of smooth muscle where the appendix joins the cecum and as the sigmoid colon transitions to become the rectum. Generally, the posterolateral and anterior taeniae coalesce into a broad longitudinal band in the distal sigmoid colon. The external longitudinal muscular layer of the proximal rectum retains a slight trace of the taeniae because the layer is more strongly developed in its anterior and posterior parts than it is laterally.

A *haustrum* is a more or less prominent sacculation of the colon visible in the spaces between the taeniae coli. Individual haustra are separated from each other by constricting circular furrows of varying depth. The degree of their prominence depends on contraction of the taeniae; the more the taeniae contract, the more marked the haustra become. When the taeniae coli are relaxed, the haustra are almost completely absent. The *omental appendages* are subserous pockets filled with fat that are distributed in two rows along the length of the ascending and descending colon. In the transverse colon they form only one row along the line of the free taeniae. The size of each appendage varies according to the individual's state of nutrition or amount of overall body fat.

Within the lumen of the colon, the mucous membrane of the large intestine forms crescent-shaped transverse folds, known as *semilunar folds* or *plicae semilunares,* which correspond to furrows between haustra on the outer surface. Whereas the circular folds (plicae circulares, Kerckring folds) in the small intestine consist of only mucosa and submucosa, the semilunar folds of the colon include the circular layer of the muscularis externa.

One major difference in the microscopic appearance of the colon compared with the small intestine is that the mucosa of the large intestine has no villi. Like the small intestine, it does have deep *intestinal glands (crypts of Lieberkühn),* which increase in depth toward the rectum and can extend as far as the muscularis mucosae. In the submucosa, in addition to the usual blood vessels, lymphatics, and submucosal plexus, there are numerous solitary lymphatic nodules in the lamina propria that penetrate through the muscularis mucosae into the submucosa. The epithelial lining of the large intestine has one layer built up of tall columnar cells that replicate from a stem cell population in the lower third of the gland and move progressively toward the surface. Mucus-producing goblet cells are very numerous in the epithelium of the colon, especially at the base of the pits.

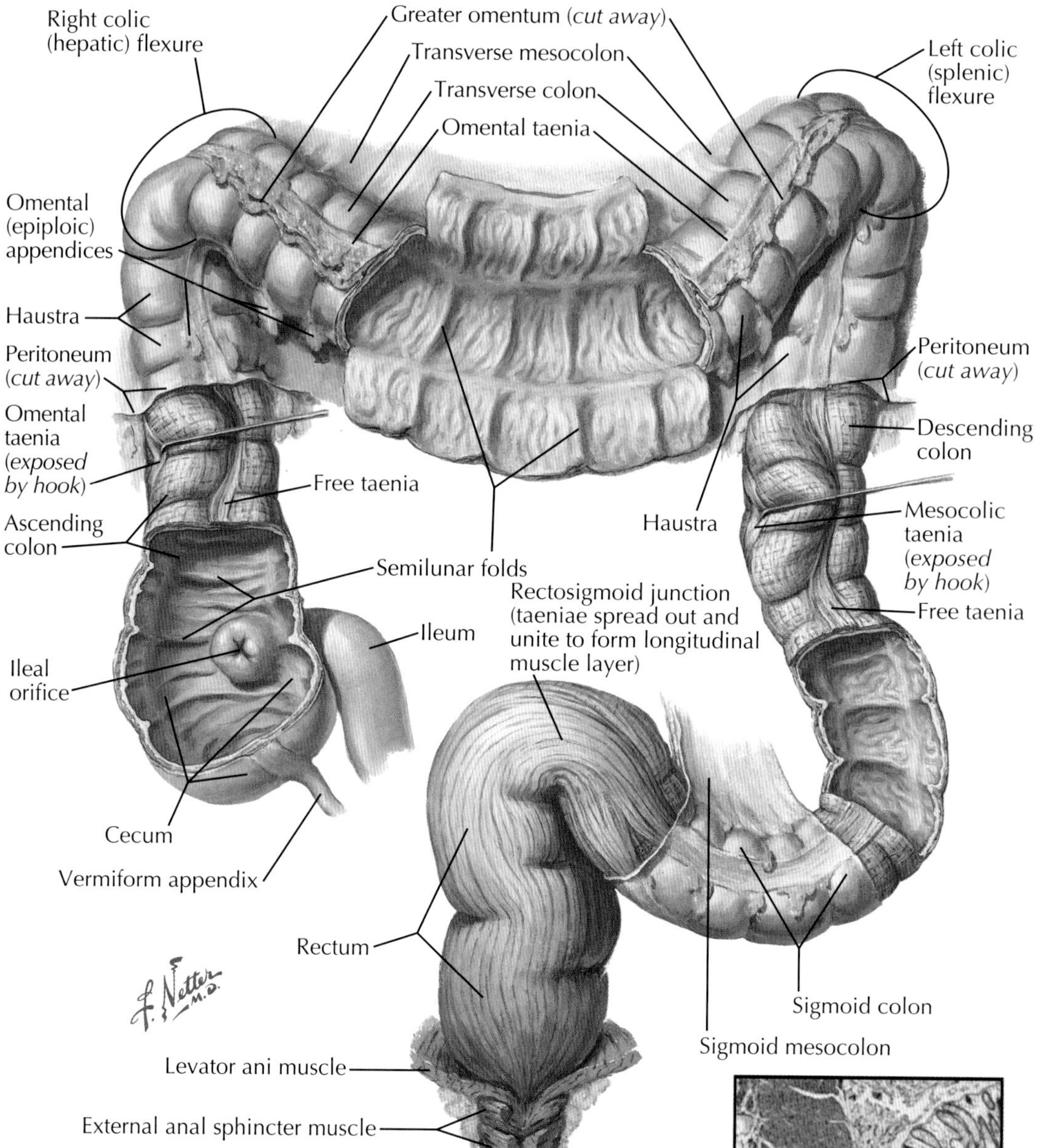

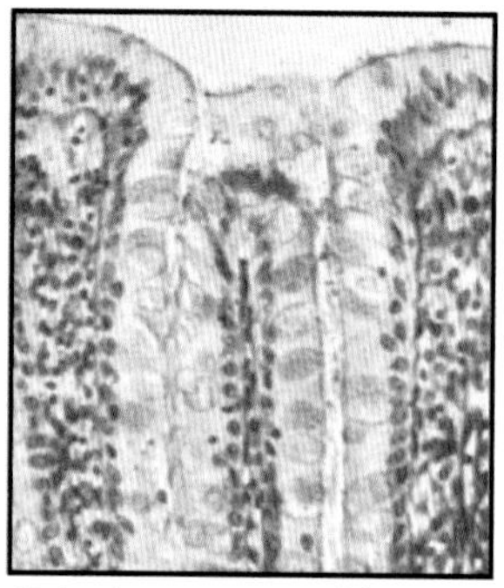

Colonic mucosa; goblet cells in crypts (Azan stain, ×160)

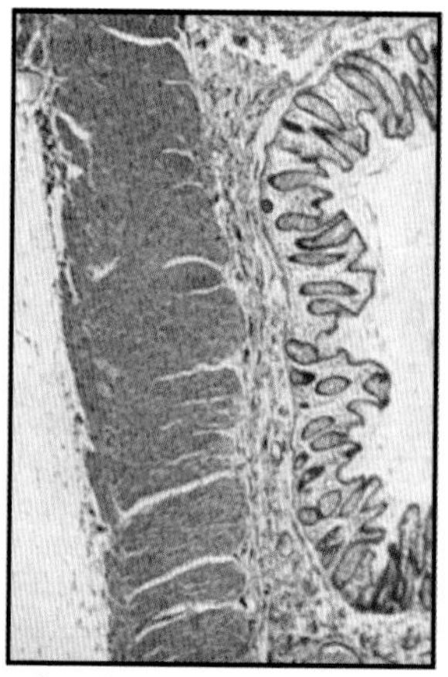

Colon: low-power longitudinal section through entire wall

## Rectum and Anal Canal

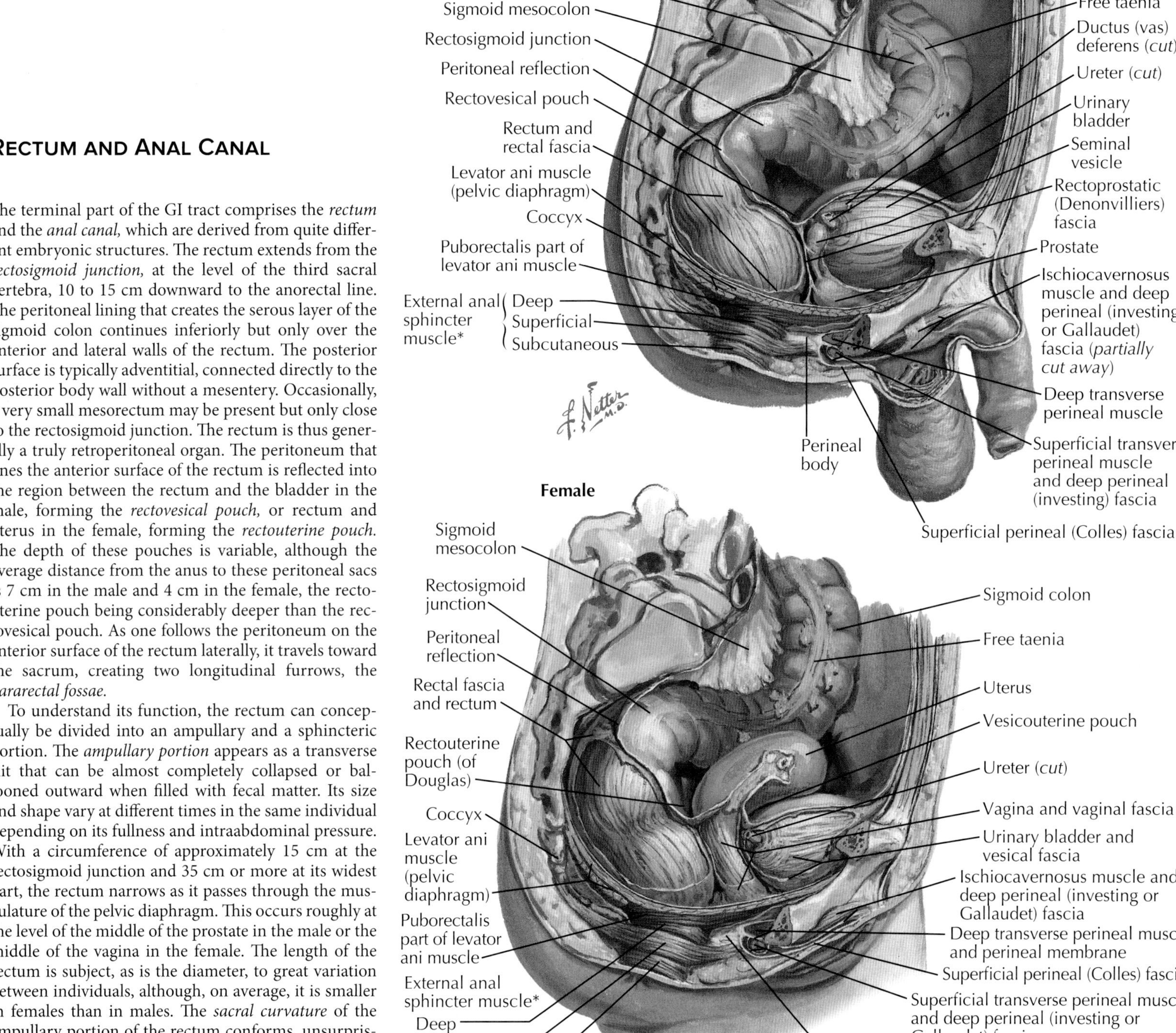


The terminal part of the GI tract comprises the *rectum* and the *anal canal,* which are derived from quite different embryonic structures. The rectum extends from the *rectosigmoid junction,* at the level of the third sacral vertebra, 10 to 15 cm downward to the anorectal line. The peritoneal lining that creates the serous layer of the sigmoid colon continues inferiorly but only over the anterior and lateral walls of the rectum. The posterior surface is typically adventitial, connected directly to the posterior body wall without a mesentery. Occasionally, a very small mesorectum may be present but only close to the rectosigmoid junction. The rectum is thus generally a truly retroperitoneal organ. The peritoneum that lines the anterior surface of the rectum is reflected into the region between the rectum and the bladder in the male, forming the *rectovesical pouch,* or rectum and uterus in the female, forming the *rectouterine pouch.* The depth of these pouches is variable, although the average distance from the anus to these peritoneal sacs is 7 cm in the male and 4 cm in the female, the rectouterine pouch being considerably deeper than the rectovesical pouch. As one follows the peritoneum on the anterior surface of the rectum laterally, it travels toward the sacrum, creating two longitudinal furrows, the *pararectal fossae.*

To understand its function, the rectum can conceptually be divided into an ampullary and a sphincteric portion. The *ampullary portion* appears as a transverse slit that can be almost completely collapsed or ballooned outward when filled with fecal matter. Its size and shape vary at different times in the same individual depending on its fullness and intraabdominal pressure. With a circumference of approximately 15 cm at the rectosigmoid junction and 35 cm or more at its widest part, the rectum narrows as it passes through the musculature of the pelvic diaphragm. This occurs roughly at the level of the middle of the prostate in the male or the middle of the vagina in the female. The length of the rectum is subject, as is the diameter, to great variation between individuals, although, on average, it is smaller in females than in males. The *sacral curvature* of the ampullary portion of the rectum conforms, unsurprisingly, to the anterior surface of the sacrum. The rectum's posterior wall continues to lie adjacent to the sacrum inferiorly to the level of the sacrococcygeal articulation, at which point it comes to lie more or less horizontally over the *levator ani muscle.* The anterior wall is comparatively straight and follows closely a line parallel to the posterior aspect of the vagina in the female or the urinary bladder in the male. In any event, the human rectum is not truly straight (the Latin term *rectus* ["straight"] is derived from the early anatomists' experience in dissecting mammals that do not walk upright).

The ampullary portion of the rectum typically has three *lateral flexures.* Of these, the superior lateral flexure is convex to the right, the intermediate lateral flexure is convex to the left, and the inferior lateral flexure is convex to the right. All three bends correspond to the indentations on the internal rectal wall on the concave side, which are produced by crescent-shaped infolding of the mucosa and submucosa that also includes the circular musculature but not the longitudinal layer of the muscularis externa. These more or less marked folds, known as *transverse folds of the rectum* (rectal valves, valves of Houston), encircle about one-third to one-half of the rectal circumference. The *superior* and *inferior transverse folds* are located on the left side, the former approximately 4 cm below the rectosigmoid junction and the latter about 2 to 3 cm above the pectinate line at a site where the ampullary portion of the rectum begins to narrow. The intermediate transverse fold typically lies on the right side at or slightly above the level of the peritoneal reflection, about 6 to 7 cm above the pectinate line. It is worth noting that this distance is about the limit to which a probing finger may reach during rectal digital examination. In most

## RECTUM AND ANAL CANAL (Continued)

instances the intermediate transverse fold is the largest of all three valves, but their size varies, as does their number. One or two additional folds or valves may be encountered, or only two may be present.

The *sphincteric portion* of the rectum, often considered to be the upper third of the *surgical anal canal,* begins at the palpable upper edge of the anorectal muscle ring, usually about 4 to 6 cm above the external opening of the anus, where the rectum narrows considerably. It extends down to the *pectinate line* (anatomic anorectal line, dentate line), an irregular, undulating demarcation in the rectal mucosa about 2 to 3 cm above the external anal opening. It has been assumed that this line marks the junction of the endodermal primitive gut with the ectodermal proctodeum; histologic evidence, however, has disclosed that this transition of the two fetal structures is not abrupt but spreads gradually over several centimeters. Nevertheless, the dentate line is visually recognizable, encircling the bowel, presenting from 6 to 12 superior extensions that are interrupted by an equal number of intervening inferior sinuses. The superior extensions of the pectinate line are generally related to and overlie longitudinal elevations in the anal mucosa, known as *anal columns,* or columns of Morgagni. These stretch 2 to 3 cm superiorly and blend into the anal/rectal mucosa. They contain a richer lymphatic and vascular bed than does the intervening tissue. The uneven nature of the pectinate line is partially due to the fact that it stretches along the length of the anal columns. The valley-like depressions between the anal columns are the *anal sinuses,* or sinuses of Morgagni. At their lower extremities (the pectinate line), the rectal columns are joined together by mucosal folds, the *anal valves.* These anal valves should not be confused with the transverse rectal folds, which are sometimes called *rectal valves.* Most, but not all, of the anal sinuses extend inferiorly to form pockets, designated as *anal crypts* (also known as *anal pockets, crypts of Morgagni,* and *saccules of Horne*), which may be 1 cm or more deep. The ducts of *anal glands* release mucus into the anal crypts, but the ducts and glands may extend for a variable distance into the adjacent tissues, even into the sphincter muscles; for this reason, they are sometimes referred to as "intramuscular glands." These glands and their ducts are sometimes foci for anorectal infections. Infection or inflammation can create perianal abscesses that extend to the skin surrounding the anus and rupture through the epidermis, creating a perianal fistula.

Occasionally, the anal columns form papillary projections into the rectal lumen, and the name *anal papillae* has been applied to these teat-like processes. In most instances these anal papillae are absent, but when they are present, they may hypertrophy and become prominent enough to appear as fibrous polyps that may even prolapse through the anal canal.

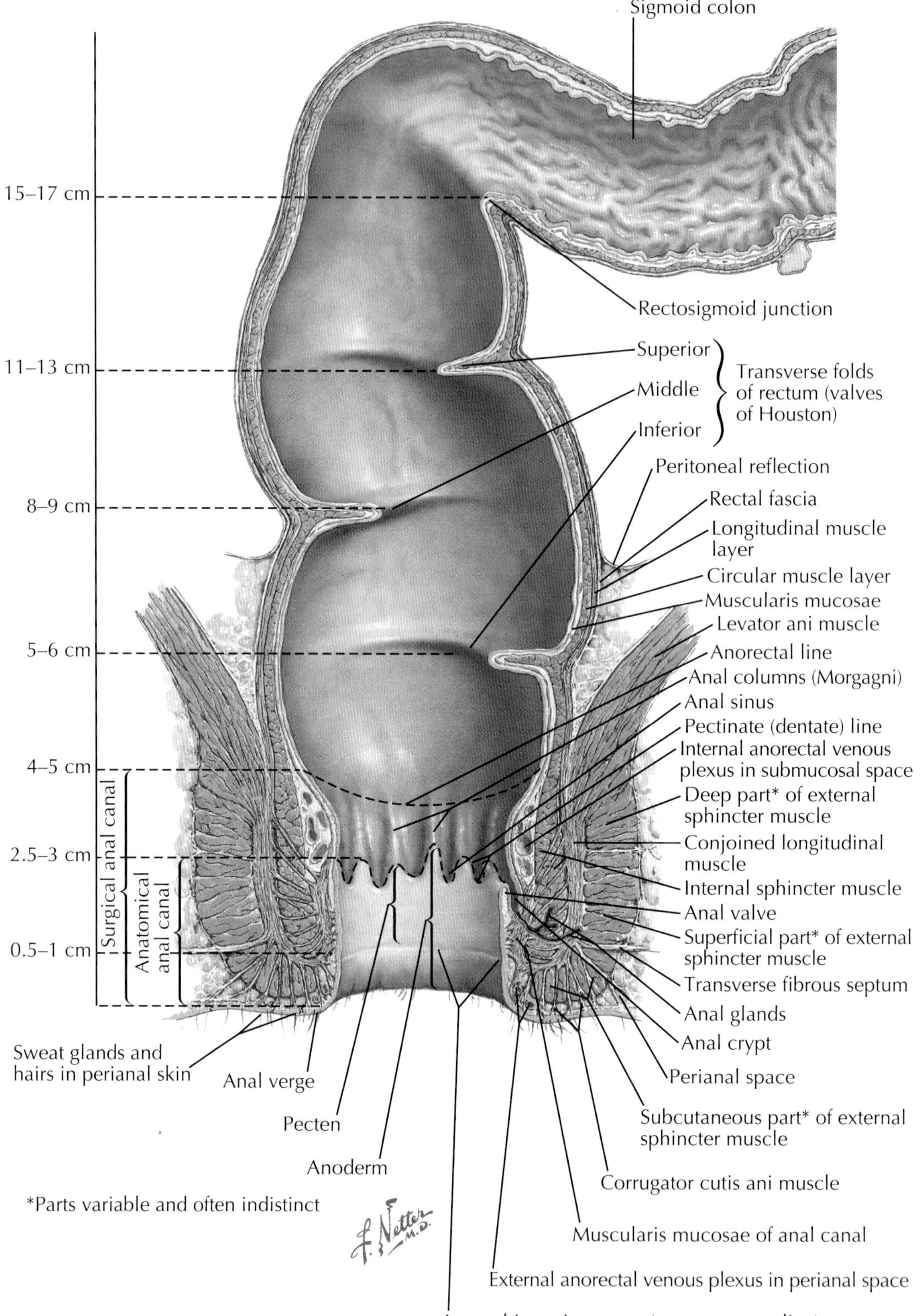


The section of the anus that forms the inferior two-thirds of the surgical anal canal is termed the *anatomic anal canal,* which starts at the pectinate line and extends to the external opening of the anus. The superior portion of the anatomic anal canal is called the *anal pecten* or just *pecten* (Latin for "comb") because of the comb-like appearance of the pectinate line. The pecten is made up of the mucocutaneous epithelial lining, sometimes called the *anoderm,* and the structures found within the subepithelial connective tissue. This region is important because it marks the transition between the visceral blood supply and innervation superiorly (rectum) and the somatic blood supply and innervation inferiorly (anus). Anastomoses between the portal venous system and branches of the internal iliac veins occur in this area, creating an *internal anorectal (venous) plexus* at the watershed areas between the two. Connections between the autonomic innervation of the rectum and the peripheral nerve supply of the anal canal, as well as the lymphatic drainage of both regions,

HISTOLOGY OF ANAL CANAL

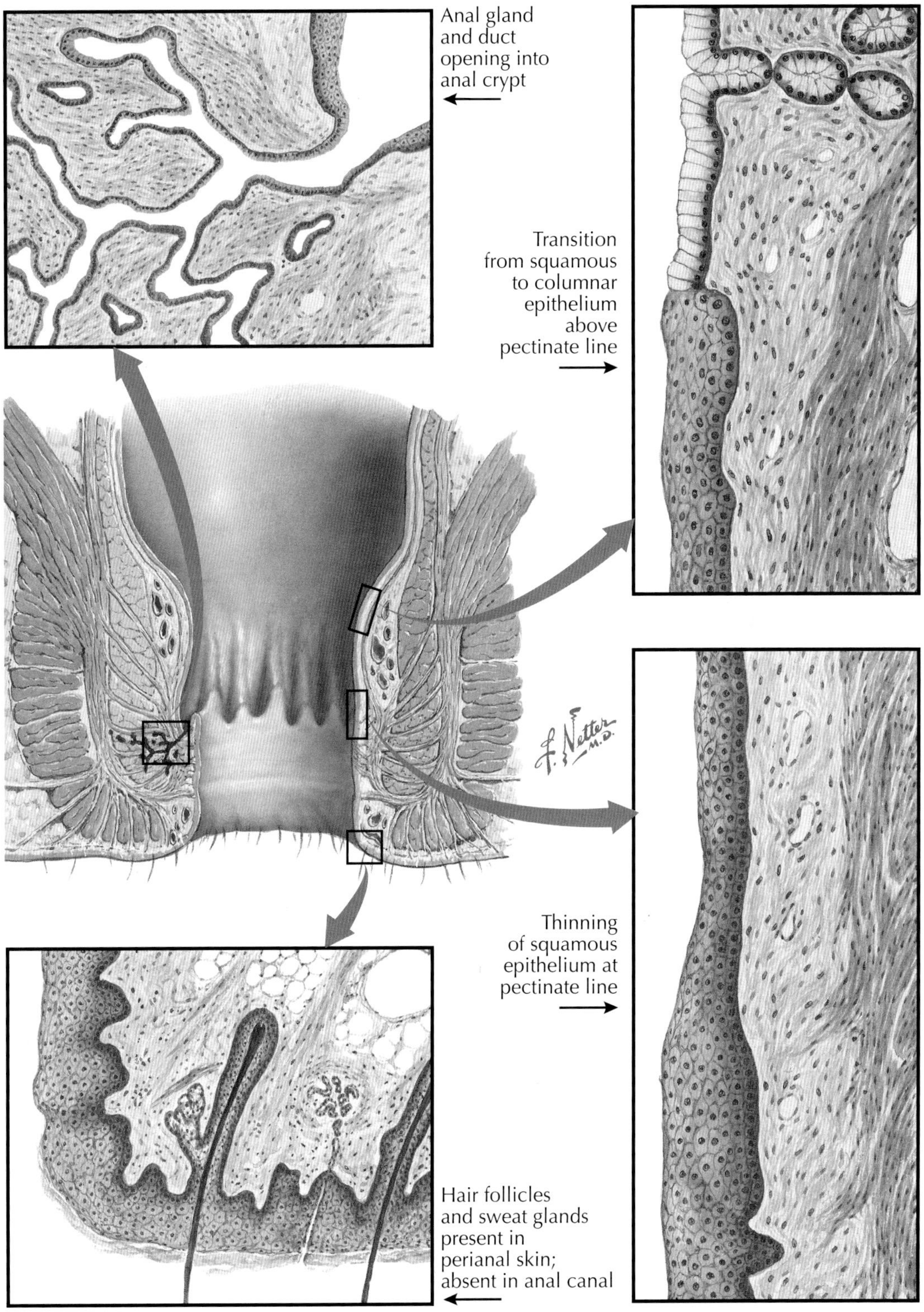

Anal gland and duct opening into anal crypt

Transition from squamous to columnar epithelium above pectinate line

Thinning of squamous epithelium at pectinate line

Hair follicles and sweat glands present in perianal skin; absent in anal canal

## RECTUM AND ANAL CANAL (Continued)

also occur in the region of the pecten. The pecten is surrounded by all of the muscles that constitute the anal muscular ring, extends inferiorly for a varying length of 1 to 1.5 cm to the pecten's inferior border, the *intersphincteric groove (white line of Hilton, intermuscular groove)*. The intersphincteric groove is a palpable landmark created by the attachment of the *conjoined longitudinal muscle* (combination of the levator ani and muscularis externa) to the anoderm at the level between the blunt lower margin of the internal anal sphincter and the subcutaneous portion of the external anal sphincter. The clinical significance of the pecten is indicated by its being the zone of predilection for anal fissures, fibrosis (pectenosis), and inflammatory processes. Inferior to the pecten, a ring of cutaneous tissue that is 1 cm broad begins at the intersphincteric groove and terminates at the external opening of the anal canal. The anoderm in this region of the anatomic anal canal contains the perianal space, the subcutaneous part of the external anal sphincter, and another portal/systemic venous watershed area, the *external anorectal (venous) plexus*.

The axis of the anal canal (anatomic as well as surgical) is, in adults, directed superiorly and anteriorly toward the umbilicus, in contrast to that of the rectum. In infants, both axes, that of the rectum and that of the anal canal, take the same direction because the child still lacks the adult rectal curves. This predisposes children to anal and rectal prolapse more frequently than adults.

Microscopically, the mucosa of the rectum is thicker than that of the nearby sigmoid colon. It also becomes increasingly redder and more richly vascularized as it approaches the surgical anal canal, until its lowermost portion assumes nearly a plum color. The extreme vascularity predisposes it to hemorrhagic disorders. The mobility of the rectal mucosa is also greater, and large folds, sometimes referred to as *pseudopolyps*, can form from it. The simple columnar epithelium of the rectum is similar to that of the colon, though the cells may appear more cuboidal toward the inferior end. Like the remainder of the colon, the rectum contains intestinal glands (crypts of Lieberkühn) that are particularly well developed and contain an abundance of goblet cells. The columnar epithelium of the rectum extends downward into the upper third of the surgical anal canal, where it changes into a stratified squamous epithelium at a point just *above* the pectinate line. This epithelium directly covers the internal anorectal (venous) plexus as well as the anal columns and anal sinuses. An *anal transitional zone* exists between the simple columnar epithelium of the rectum and the stratified squamous epithelium of the external anal and perineal areas. In this transitional zone, the epithelium appears blended, and it is possible to see simple columnar, simple cuboidal, stratified cuboidal, and stratified squamous cells in the region. This epithelial transition zone may extend far above the dentate line up to the region of the anorectal muscle ring but generally does not extend more inferiorly than the anal valves. It is therefore incorrect to refer to the pectinate line as being the "mucocutaneous junction."

The stratified squamous epithelium of the anoderm covers the rectal columns and sinuses and thickens as it approaches the intersphincteric groove. The anoderm itself is devoid of mucous, sebaceous, and sweat glands and is firmly attached to the muscular and fibrous tissues of the pecten, and it is separate from the perianal space located inferiorly. Below the intermuscular groove, the anoderm further thickens and continues as perianal skin with its usual cutaneous hair follicles, sebaceous glands, and eccrine sweat glands. The perianal skin also contains large apocrine glands, called *circumanal glands* (circumanal glands of Gay), in which perianal hidradenoma may occasionally be diagnosed.

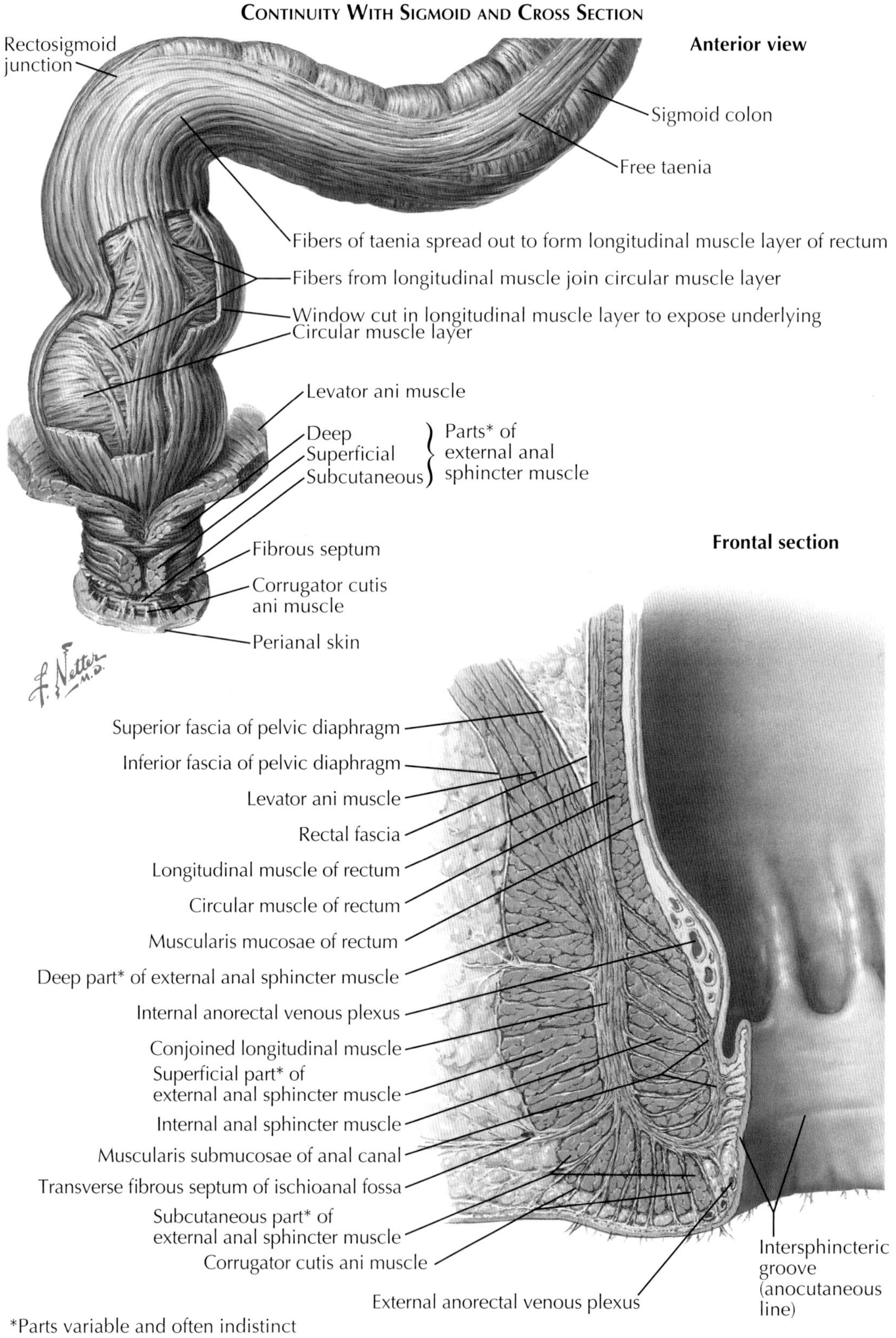

## ANORECTAL MUSCULATURE

Like the rest of the gut tube, the rectum has an inner circular and an outer longitudinal muscularis externa, which is made of smooth muscle. However, this simple organization becomes much more complex and quite peculiar as it integrates with the skeletal muscle fibers that make up the anal sphincters and levator ani muscles. In the rectum the longitudinal layer of the muscularis externa is formed by an expansion of the taeniae coli as they spread out in the region of the rectosigmoid junction to coat the rectum more uniformly. Similarly, the inner circular layer of the muscularis externa of the rectum is a continuation of the circular muscle of the sigmoid colon. The ampullary section of the rectum is characterized by frequent connections of longitudinal and circular fibers. Fan-like muscular bundles of the longitudinal musculature insert into the circular layer, particularly at the site of those indentations that correspond to the transverse folds. At the lower extremity of the rectum, the longitudinal smooth muscle fibers fuse with striated fibers from the *pubococcygeus* and *puborectalis portions* of the levator ani muscle as well as with fibers from the supraanal fascia to become a conjoined longitudinal muscle in the upper part of the surgical anal canal. At the same level, the inner circular layer of smooth muscle becomes thicker to constitute the *internal anal sphincter muscle.*

Thus the internal anal sphincter muscle, representing a gradual enlargement of the inner circular muscle of the rectum, is composed of smooth muscle fibers that are innervated by autonomic nerves via the intrinsic myenteric and submucosal plexuses. At the level of the intersphincteric groove (0.5–1 cm above the external opening of the anus), the internal anal sphincter, having a thickness of 0.6 to 0.8 cm and a length of 3 to 5 cm, ends with a sharply defined and readily palpable rounded lower margin, resulting from its strong fascial encasement and the recurrent arrangement of its more caudal muscle bundles.

The combined longitudinal muscle (from rectal longitudinal smooth muscle and skeletal muscle fibers of the levator ani) extends inferiorly, surrounding the internal anal sphincter, before itself becoming surrounded by the external anal sphincter. While continuing on its inferior course, the muscle gives off bundles of fibroelastic tissue interwoven with muscular fibrils, which penetrate the internal sphincter. These fascicles decrease successively in their obliquity as they pass through the internal sphincter, until the deepest fascicles actually ascend. Some of these penetrating fascicles fuse with the well-developed muscularis mucosae of the anal canal and were formerly designated as "sustentator mucosae of Kohlrausch" but are more properly referred to as *muscularis submucosae ani.* These fibers anchor the anoderm of the pecten to the underlying tissue and to the lower third of the internal anal sphincter. This fixation to the underlying fibromuscular structures supports the nearby *internal anorectal (venous) plexus* during defecation. It also helps the pecten resist eversion of the anal canal and prolapse of the rectum. When prolapse or procidentia does occur, it is also this fixation that is responsible for the formation of the intermuscular depression or groove. In its most inferior part, the conjoined longitudinal muscle gives off a fan-like series of fibromuscular septa, which pass through the circular fibers of the subcutaneous portion of the external sphincter ani to attach themselves to the perianal skin. Here, the muscular elements of these septa form (together with some extended fibers of the muscularis submucosae ani) the *corrugator cutis ani.*

Extensions from the conjoined longitudinal muscle pass outward through the external anal sphincter. The most important of these extensions are those that separate the subcutaneous and superficial portions of the sphincter and continue as the *transverse septum of the ischioanal fossae.* Anteriorly, extensions are also reflected to the urethra above the external sphincter,

CONTINUITY WITH SIGMOID AND CROSS SECTION

Anterior view

Rectosigmoid junction
Sigmoid colon
Free taenia
Fibers of taenia spread out to form longitudinal muscle layer of rectum
Fibers from longitudinal muscle join circular muscle layer
Window cut in longitudinal muscle layer to expose underlying Circular muscle layer
Levator ani muscle
Deep, Superficial, Subcutaneous: Parts* of external anal sphincter muscle
Fibrous septum
Corrugator cutis ani muscle
Perianal skin

F. Netter M.D.

Frontal section

Superior fascia of pelvic diaphragm
Inferior fascia of pelvic diaphragm
Levator ani muscle
Rectal fascia
Longitudinal muscle of rectum
Circular muscle of rectum
Muscularis mucosae of rectum
Deep part* of external anal sphincter muscle
Internal anorectal venous plexus
Conjoined longitudinal muscle
Superficial part* of external anal sphincter muscle
Internal anal sphincter muscle
Muscularis submucosae of anal canal
Transverse fibrous septum of ischioanal fossa
Subcutaneous part* of external anal sphincter muscle
Corrugator cutis ani muscle
External anorectal venous plexus
Intersphincteric groove (anocutaneous line)

*Parts variable and often indistinct

## ANORECTAL MUSCULATURE (Continued)

forming part of the rectovesicalis muscle and, posteriorly, to the coccyx as the anococcygeal ligament.

The significance of the conjoined longitudinal muscle for the physiologic study, pathologic study, and surgical procedures of the anal and rectal areas cannot be overemphasized. Together with the levator ani muscle, it exercises its levator and sphincteric actions on the entire length of the anal canal. By its extensions at the level of the intersphincteric groove and by its fascial frame in the upper third of the surgical anal canal, the muscle influences the spread of anorectal infections as well as the sites of the openings and main tracts of fistulas. From the surgeon's point of view, the terminal conjoined longitudinal muscle fibers are important because they permit the recognition of the lower border of the internal sphincter, which is a landmark during internal hemorrhoidectomy or hemorrhoidopexy.

The outermost and also most inferior muscular elements of the anal canal belong to the *external anal sphincter,* which is a trilaminar skeletal muscle. Its three parts, the *subcutaneous, superficial,* and *deep parts,* are more easily recognized surgically than in the cadaver. The subcutaneous portion, about 3 to 5 mm in diameter, surrounds the anal orifice directly above the anal margin and is readily palpable and often discernible as a distinct annular ridge. Separated from the internal anal sphincter by fibers of the conjoined longitudinal muscle at the level of the intersphincteric groove, the subcutaneous portion is situated inferior to and slightly lateral to the internal sphincter. Seen from below, the subcutaneous portion usually has an annular form, though its fibers may cross and branch in all directions and may extend posteriorly. In the male, anterior muscular extensions to the median raphe are not uncommon, and uncrossed posterior extensions of the subcutaneous external sphincter connecting with the coccyx may also be found. In the female, the subcutaneous portion is much more strongly developed, particularly anteriorly, where it forms a prominent annular band, frequently incised at episiotomy. The subcutaneous muscle is functionally integrated with the levator ani muscle through *extensions* of the conjoined longitudinal muscle that pass fan-like through it, to terminate as fibers of the corrugator cutis ani.

Just deep to the subcutaneous part of the external anal sphincter is the elliptically shaped *superficial portion,* which is the largest and strongest of the three parts. It is situated somewhat lateral to the subcutaneous portion and arises independently from the tip of the coccyx; this fact explains why it is sometimes referred to as the *coccygeal portion.* The fibers enclose, in a crescent-like fashion, the lower third or half of the internal sphincter and insert, in the male, at or around the *central point of the perineum* and the median fascial raphe of the *bulbospongiosus muscle.* In the female, however, only a few fibers of the superficial portion insert at the central point of the perineum; most merge with the bulbospongiosus muscle, and some may extend laterally as far as the *ischiopubic rami* and the *ischial tuberosities* in conjunction with, or independent of, the thin *superficial transverse perineal muscles.* It is not uncommon for fibers that pass around the anal canal on the left side to *cross over* to insert anteriorly or laterally on the right side, and vice versa, as they move anteriorly. Posteriorly, the superficial muscle forms the right and left muscular components of the *anococcygeal ligament.* Deep or superior to this ligament, the right and left ischioanal fossae are continuous through the deep postanal spaces, whereas the right and left perianal spaces communicate with each other through the superficial postanal space superficial or inferior to the anococcygeal ligament.

The *deep part of the external anal sphincter* is, for the most part, an annular muscle bundle that blends with the puborectalis muscle as it passes around the posterior end of the terminal rectum and does not usually

EXTERNAL ANAL SPHINCTER MUSCLE: PERINEAL VIEWS

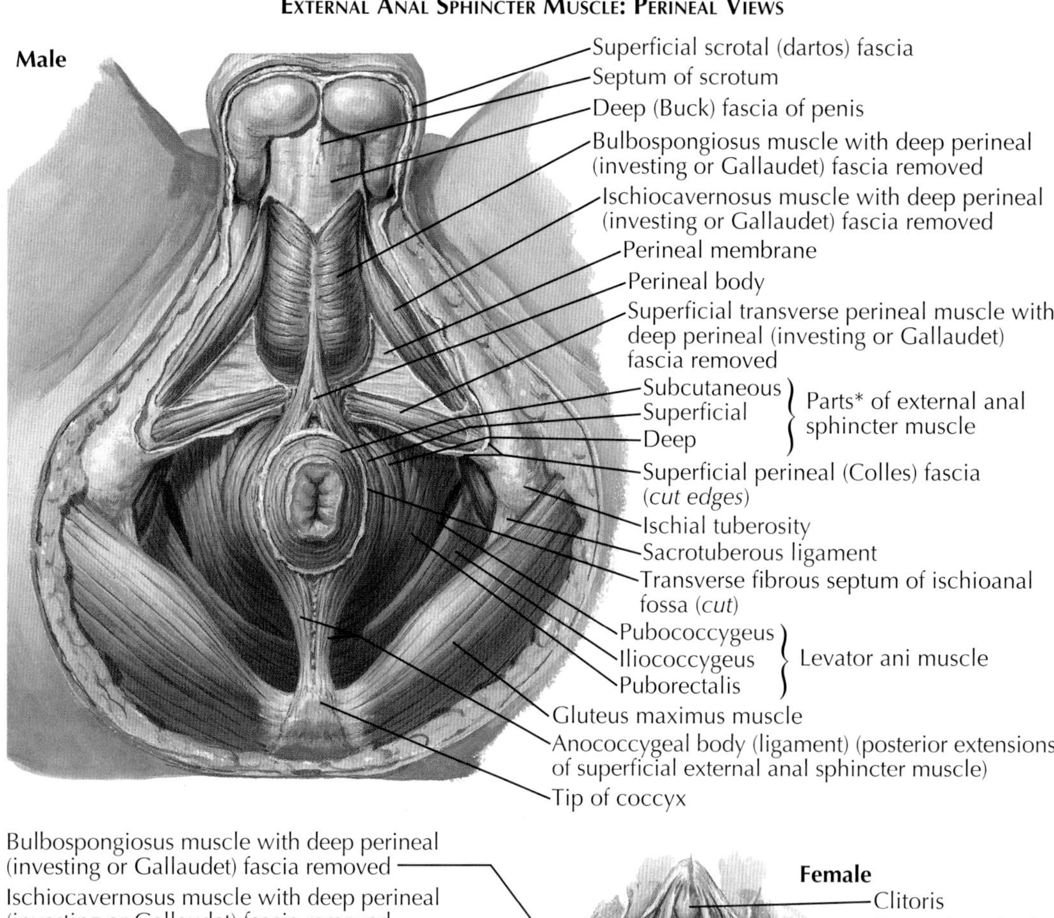


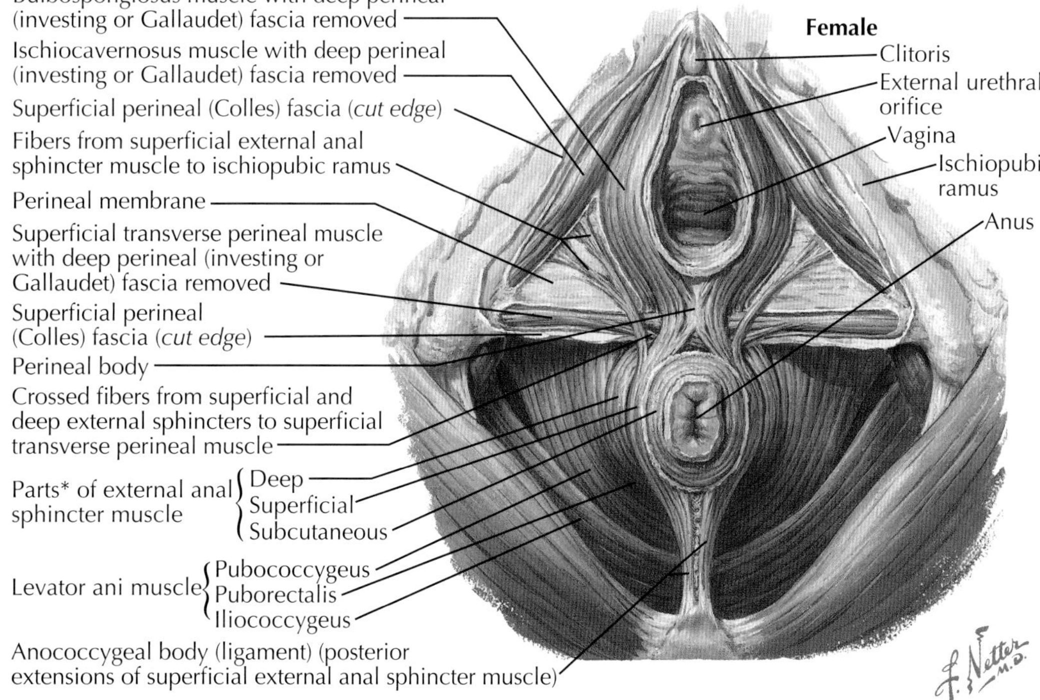


*Parts variable and often indistinct

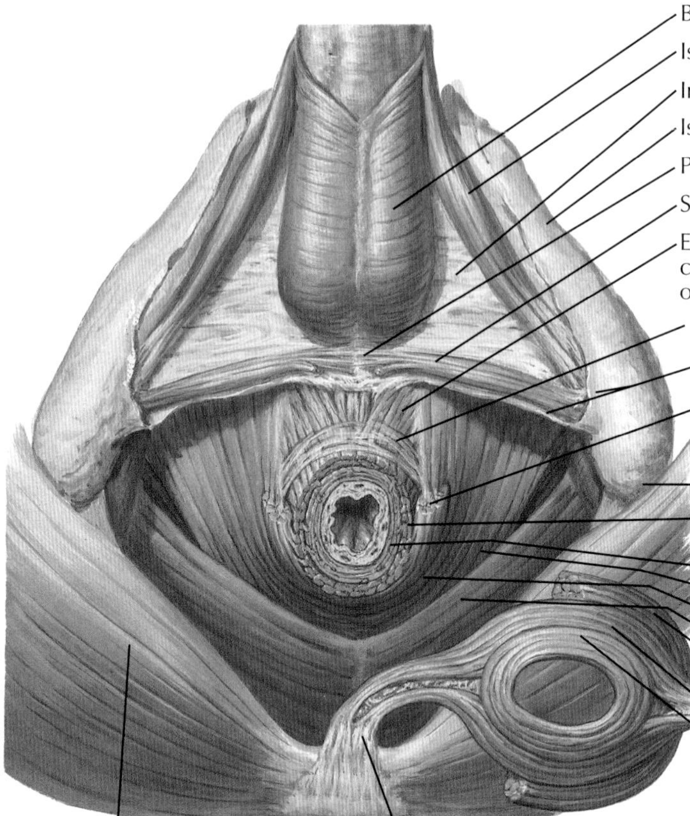

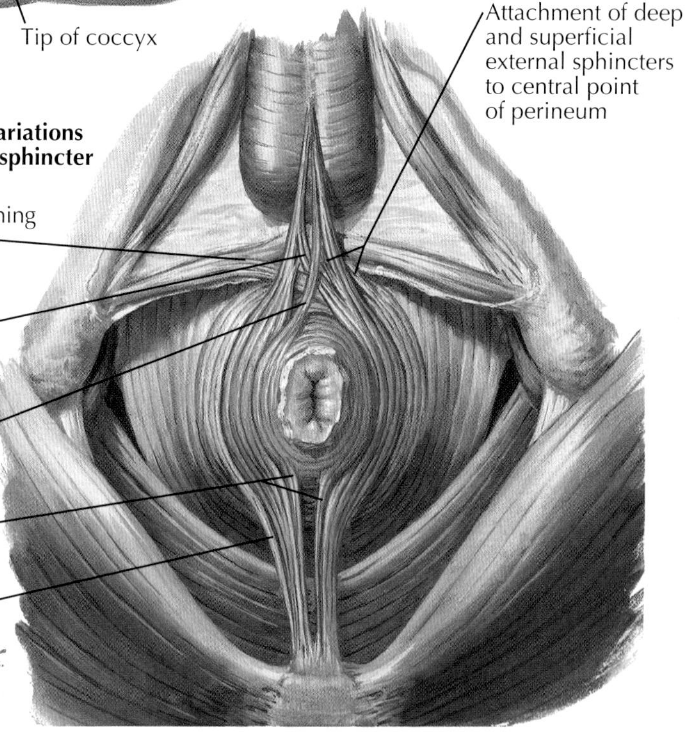

## ANORECTAL MUSCULATURE (Continued)

attach to the coccyx. The deep part of the external sphincter surrounds the upper third of the surgical anal canal and, with the prerectal muscle bundles of the levator ani, some fibers may attach themselves to the *perineal body* or, after crossing sides, may join the *superficial transverse perineal muscle* and extend as far as the ischium.

The muscles that form the pelvic diaphragm, in particular the *levator ani muscle,* keep the rectoanal canal in position. The levator ani is frequently subdivided into three individual components that form a nearly continuous sheet of skeletal muscle, namely, the *puborectalis, pubococcygeus,* and *iliococcygeus muscles.* Another way to view the levator ani is to conceptualize its component muscles as enclosing the pelvic outlets in two planes, a diaphragmatic and a subdiaphragmatic plane. The former is created by a broad, sweeping, muscular sheet of the pubococcygeus and iliococcygeus muscles, with the puborectalis muscles contributing a very small ventral muscle bundle. The subdiaphragmatic plane is formed by the inferior extensions of the pubococcygeus and puborectalis muscles into the nearby musculature of the visceral outlets, particularly of the anal canal. The subdiaphragmatic plane assumes a more vertical axis as its fibers funnel around the anorectal canal and urogenital outlets, whereas the diaphragmatic plane is oriented more horizontally.

The *puborectalis muscle* contributes only a small part to the diaphragmatic plane and lies almost entirely in the subdiaphragmatic plane. It is the most medial portion of the levator ani, taking its origin at the pubic bone just medial to the origin of the pubococcygeus muscle. Not readily recognizable as a distinct muscular structure in its region of origin, its fibers pass posteriorly and horizontally on either side of the pelvic aperture and gradually come to lie inferior and medial to the anal extensions of the nearby pubococcygeus muscle. In its course, the originally horizontal surface of the muscle becomes its inner surface and its originally medial edge its inferior margin. It then forms a sling around the posterior aspect of the rectum just superficial to the rectum's conjoined longitudinal muscle fibers. In conjunction with the deep part of the external anal sphincter, to which it is attached, this sling-like muscle band forms the posterior half of the proctologically important anorectal muscle ring. Although the fibers of the puborectalis muscle do not extend to the coccyx, the midline raphe sends fibrous bands posteriorly to the coccyx, fixing it posteriorly. Anterior to the rectum, the muscle also gives off fibromuscular extensions to the prostate or vagina and to the conjoined longitudinal muscle of the rectum. It is better developed and more readily visible in the female.

Just lateral to the puborectalis muscle origin is the origin of the *pubococcygeus muscle,* which arises from the posterior aspect of the pubic bone and superior pubic ramus and extends from a site near the pubic symphysis to a site just medial to the obturator foramen. It continues posteriorly, attaching to the anterior extremity of the arcus tendineus, formed from the thickened fascia of the obturator internus muscle. From this origin the muscle fibers stretch medially and posteriorly along the inner boundaries of the pelvic aperture, looping around the rectum, just superior to the puborectalis muscle. The fibers of both sides join in the midline, contributing to the muscular raphe that inserts into the anterior aspect of the coccyx, continuous with a contribution from the puborectalis muscle. Aponeurotic extensions from this raphe continue along the sacrum as *anterior sacrococcygeal ligaments.* The part of the pubococcygeus muscle that lies in the subdiaphragmatic plane consists of fibromuscular extensions to the prostate gland, urethra, and vagina as well as the rectum and anal canal. These extensions fuse with the longitudinal muscles and fascial collars of the visceral

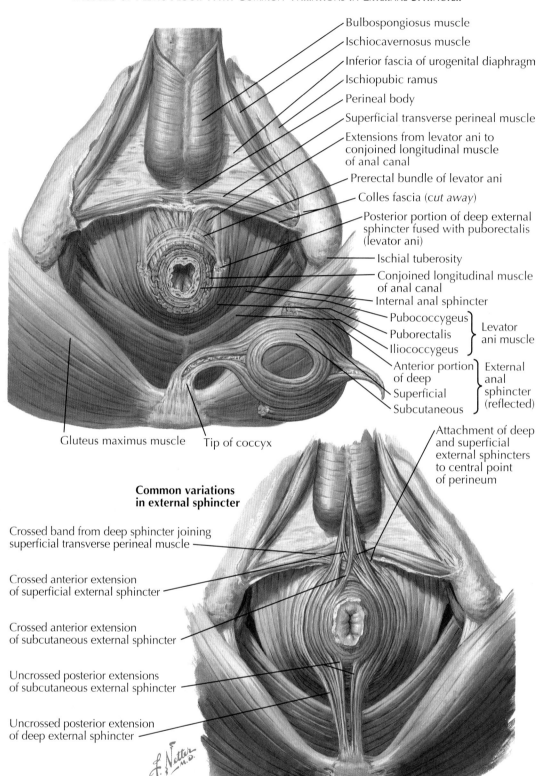

**MUSCLES OF PELVIC FLOOR WITH COMMON VARIATIONS IN EXTERNAL SPHINCTER**

Bulbospongiosus muscle
Ischiocavernosus muscle
Inferior fascia of urogenital diaphragm
Ischiopubic ramus
Perineal body
Superficial transverse perineal muscle
Extensions from levator ani to conjoined longitudinal muscle of anal canal
Prerectal bundle of levator ani
Colles fascia (*cut away*)
Posterior portion of deep external sphincter fused with puborectalis (levator ani)
Ischial tuberosity
Conjoined longitudinal muscle of anal canal
Internal anal sphincter
Pubococcygeus, Puborectalis, Iliococcygeus — Levator ani muscle
Anterior portion of deep, Superficial, Subcutaneous — External anal sphincter (reflected)
Gluteus maximus muscle
Tip of coccyx

**Common variations in external sphincter**

Attachment of deep and superficial external sphincters to central point of perineum
Crossed band from deep sphincter joining superficial transverse perineal muscle
Crossed anterior extension of superficial external sphincter
Crossed anterior extension of subcutaneous external sphincter
Uncrossed posterior extensions of subcutaneous external sphincter
Uncrossed posterior extension of deep external sphincter

F. Netter M.D.

## ANORECTAL MUSCULATURE (Continued)

outlets or bridge the interval between them. Some fibers from each side do interdigitate with those of the opposite side, and some cross from side to side as the *prerectal bundle.*

The *iliococcygeus muscle* arises almost entirely from the thickened medial fascia of the obturator internus muscle along a convex line, the *tendinous arch of the levator ani,* which begins posterior to the obturator foramen and extends posteriorly to attach just superior to the ischial spine. The muscle's fibers, directed medially, inferiorly, and slightly posteriorly, converge and contribute to the levator ani slightly inferior to the pubococcygeus muscle.

The muscular constituents of the levator ani muscle, when conceptualized together in the subdiaphragmatic and diaphragmatic planes, are shaped (from a superior view) like a funnel. The rims of the funnel attach to the pubic bone, arcus tendineus, and ischium, and the lowest point is marked by the hiatus for the anal canal. The levator ani thus fixes the pelvic floor and acts as a fulcrum against which increased abdominal pressure, as occurs in lifting, coughing, or defecation, may be resisted. Its pubococcygeal portion and the sling muscle of the puborectalis muscle have additional functions, insofar as they become integral parts of the anorectal muscle ring surrounding the inferior part of the rectal ampulla and the upper end of the surgical anal canal. The posterior half of this ring consists mainly of the puborectalis sling fibers, which also serve as a prominent, readily definable, proctologic landmark. The less prominent anterior half of the ring is composed of the internal anal sphincter, the thin muscular extensions from the pubococcygeus known as the *prerectal bundle* (Luschka fibers), and the conjoined longitudinal muscle surrounded by the deep portion of the external sphincter. In view of such integration between the skeletal (voluntary) musculature of the pelvic floor and the smooth (involuntary) or partly mixed muscles intrinsic to the terminal structures of the intestines, the role of the levator ani as supplement and synergist for the contraction and relaxation of the anorectal sphincter mechanism is evident. The posterior half of the anorectal muscle ring, in conjunction with the puborectalis muscle sling, contracts to pull the rectum toward the pubis (increasing the angulation in the anorectal tube), shortens and narrows the pelvic aperture, and elevates the anus and thus collaborates in closing the anal canal.

Posterior to the levator ani muscle, the remaining pelvic floor is formed by the *coccygeus muscle.* Together, the levator ani muscle and the coccygeus muscle are called the *pelvic diaphragm.* The levator ani and coccygeus muscles are innervated by special nerves derived from the anterior rami of the fourth (sometimes also third) sacral spinal nerve. These nerves course on the superior surface of the muscles until they penetrate them. The three laminae of the external sphincter muscle are supplied by the inferior anal and perineal nerves branching from the pudendal nerve.

### PELVIC DIAPHRAGM: MALE

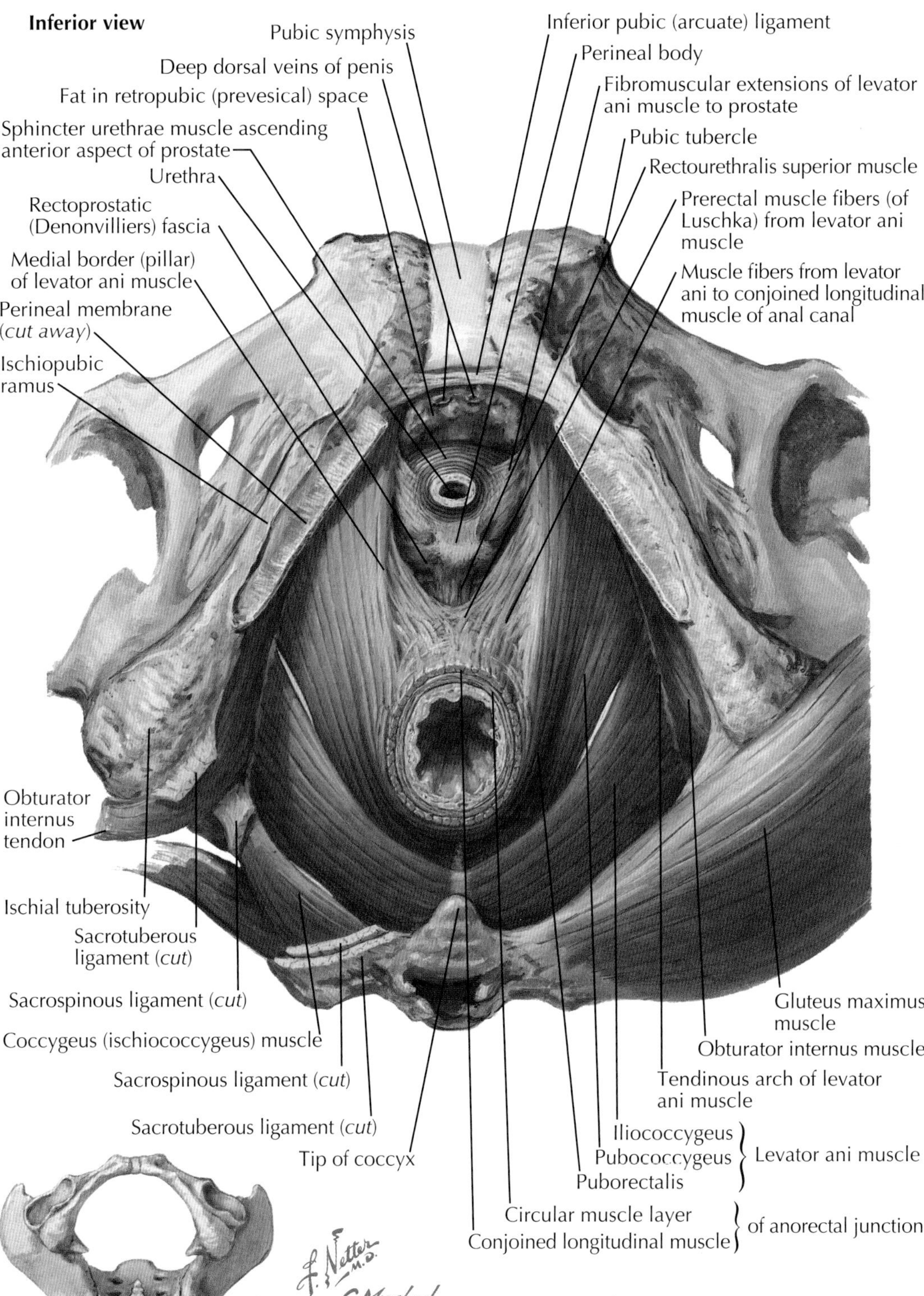


Clinical experience, especially in surgery of anterior anal fistulas, has shown that the greater portion of the anal musculature may be severed without materially interfering with anal continence, but some degree of incontinence is apt to follow as a result of a relatively greater retraction of the musculature, when the anorectal ring is divided through its entire thickness, particularly in its anterior and lateral aspects. A change in the anatomic relations of the anorectal musculature occurs under anesthesia, especially spinal anesthesia, a fact that is significant in anorectal surgery. All of the somatic components of the musculature relax, but the visceral components tend to retain or even increase their tone. As a result, the anal canal becomes foreshortened and the internal sphincter is displaced to a relatively lower level, becoming the principal presenting muscle surrounding the anal orifice. The subcutaneous portion of the sphincter flattens out and recedes laterally, so that the intermuscular depression may disappear and become less readily palpable.

VARIATIONS IN CECAL AND APPENDICULAR ARTERIES

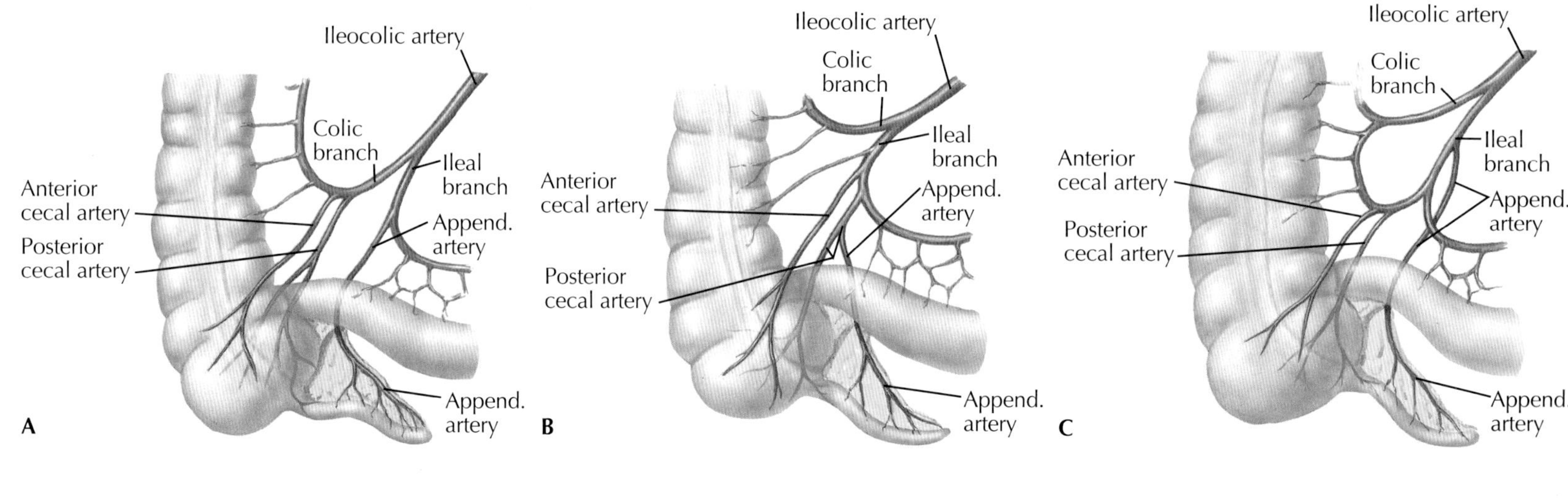


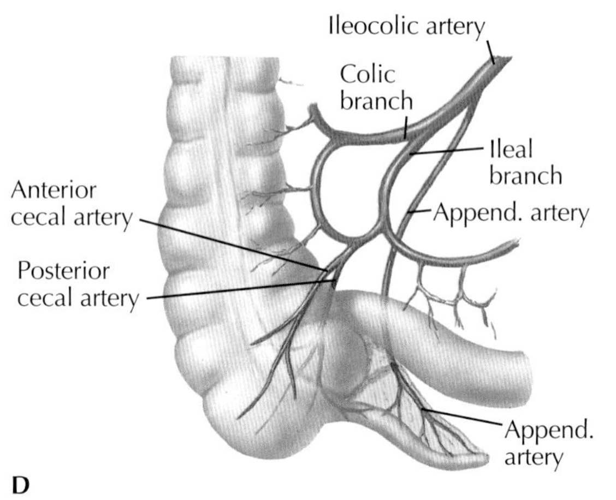


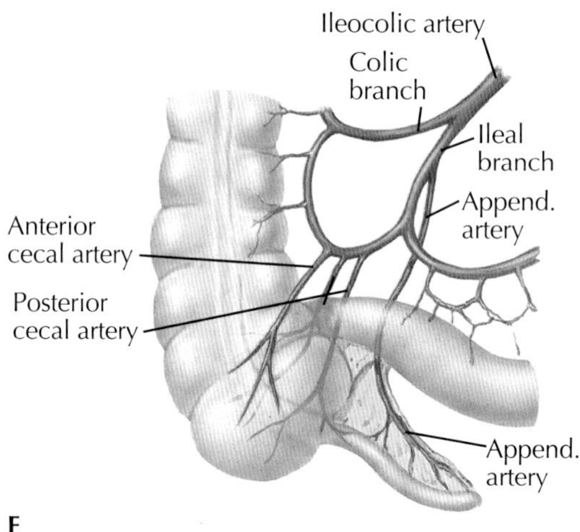


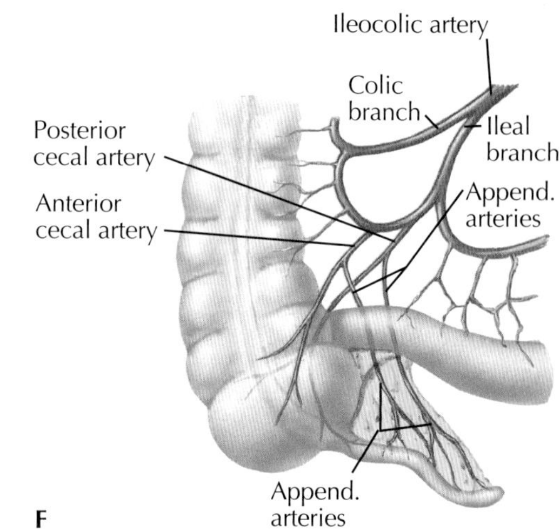


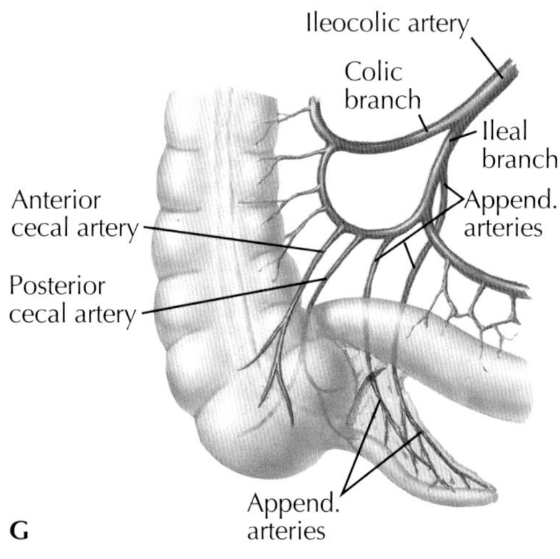


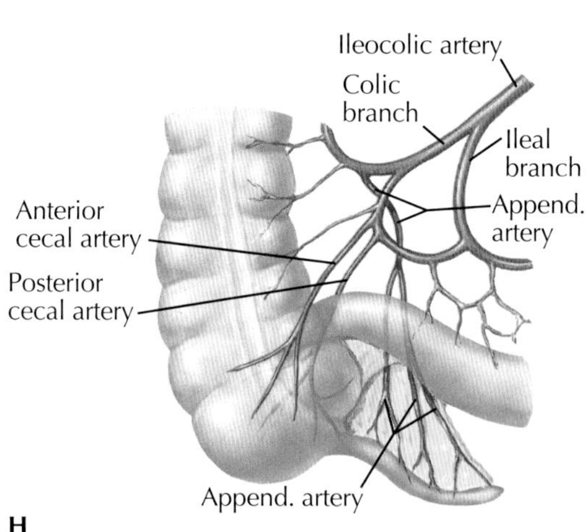


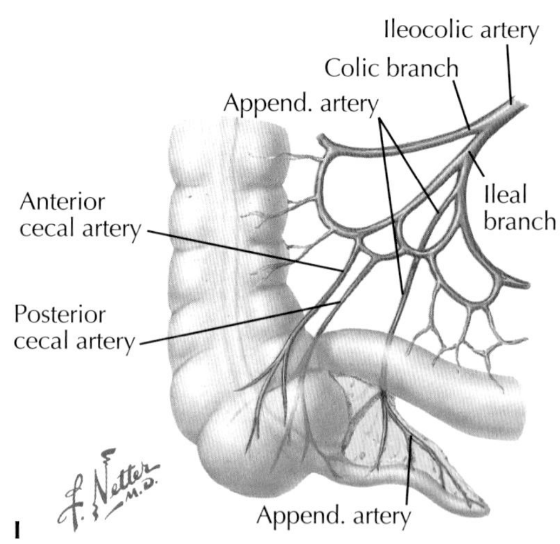


## BLOOD SUPPLY OF LARGE INTESTINE

For the typical pattern of arterial branching of the intestines, refer to Plates 1.1 and 1.2. This section describes the variations concerning the origin, course, anastomoses, and distribution of the vessels supplying the large intestine. These variations are so frequent that conventional textbook descriptions are inadequate for anyone attempting procedures in the area. Briefly, the typical pattern of branching of the arteries to the large intestine is as follows: The *ileocolic artery,* from the *superior mesenteric artery,* supplies the distal ileum and also gives off the *appendicular artery.* The cecum receives *anterior* and *posterior cecal arteries* from the ileocolic artery. Two other branches of the superior mesenteric artery, the *right* and *middle colic arteries,* supply the ascending and transverse colon, respectively. The *inferior mesenteric artery* splits into *left colic, sigmoid,* and *superior rectal arteries,* which supply the descending colon, sigmoid colon, and rectum, respectively. The right, middle, and left colic arteries all feed into the *marginal artery* (of Drummond), an artery that parallels the colon itself; it allows all of these vessels to anastomose and provides redundancy in blood supply. Many *straight arteries* leave the marginal artery and enter the colon itself.

## Variations in Colic Arteries

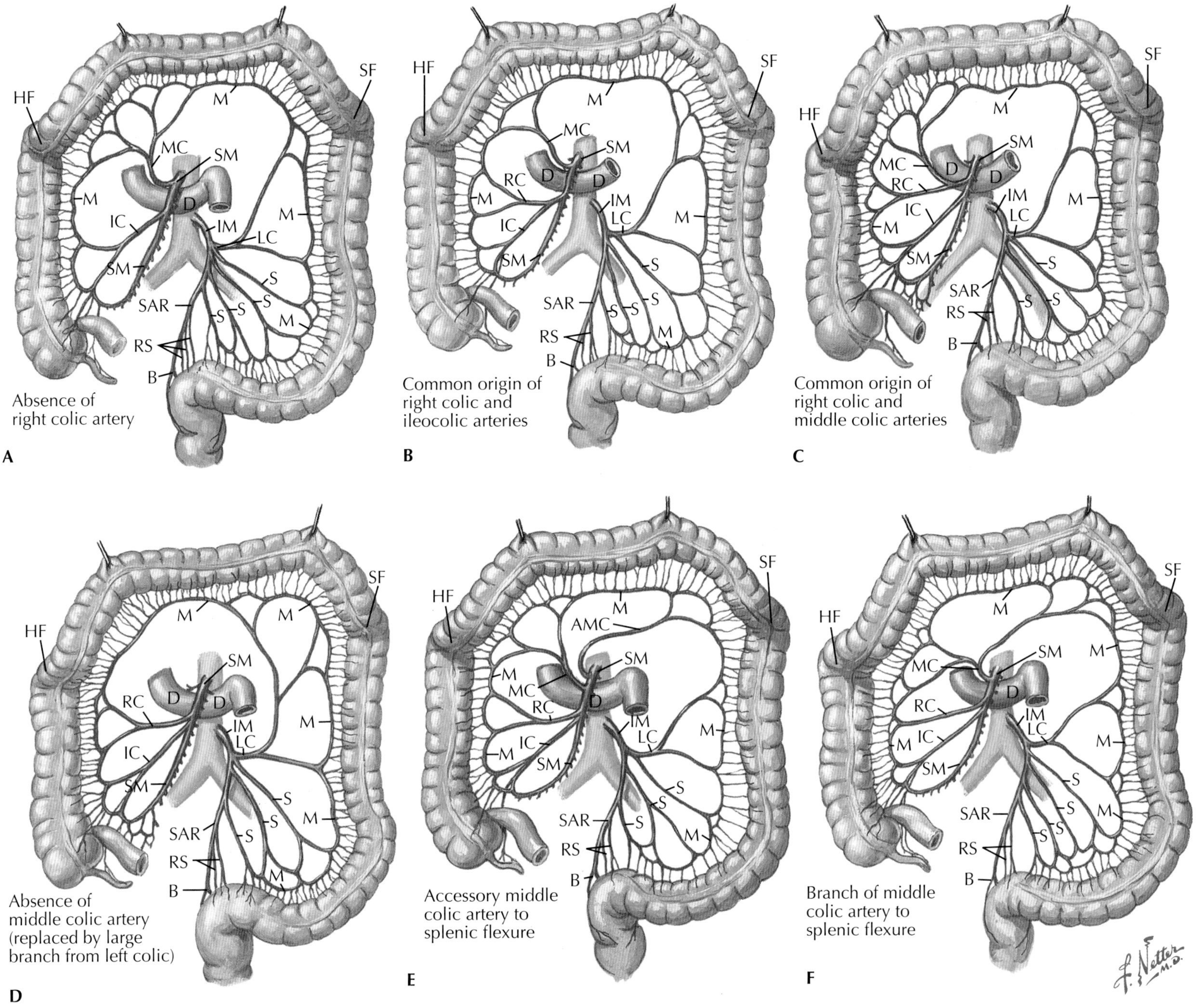

A Absence of right colic artery

B Common origin of right colic and ileocolic arteries

C Common origin of right colic and middle colic arteries

D Absence of middle colic artery (replaced by large branch from left colic)

E Accessory middle colic artery to splenic flexure

F Branch of middle colic artery to splenic flexure

**Key**

| | | | |
|---|---|---|---|
| AMC – Accessory middle colic artery | IC – Ileocolic artery | MC – Middle colic artery | SAR – Superior anorectal artery |
| B – Bifurcation of superior rectal artery | IM – Inferior mesenteric artery | RC – Right colic artery | SF – Splenic flexure of colon |
| D – Duodenum | LC – Left colic artery | RS – Rectosigmoid arteries | SM – Superior mesenteric artery |
| HF – Hepatic flexure of colon | M – Marginal artery | S – Sigmoid arteries | |

## Blood Supply of Large Intestine (Continued)

During an appendectomy, identifying and isolating the blood supply of the vermiform appendix are imperative, making familiarity with variations in the branching patterns of the distal ileocolic artery particularly important. The ileocolic artery usually splits into ileal and colic branches. The ileal branch anastomoses with the ileal arteries but also gives off the appendicular artery, which runs posterior to the ileal branch to reach the appendix. The colic branch of the ileocolic artery typically gives off the posterior and anterior cecal arteries. The appendicular artery may exit the ileal branch distally and not run posterior to it (Plate 3.15A). The anterior cecal, posterior cecal, and appendicular arteries may also branch from the ileal branch. In such a case, the appendicular artery may originate from the posterior cecal branch (Plate 3.15B). There may also be one or more arcades formed between the ileal branch and the colic branch of the ileocolic artery (Plate 3.15C to I). The anterior and posterior cecal branches may leave this arcade rather than the colic branch (Plate 3.15C), or they may leave as a common trunk and separate thereafter (Plate 3.15D). There may be two posterior cecal branches (Plate 3.15E), and the appendicular

### Variations in Colic Arteries (Continued)

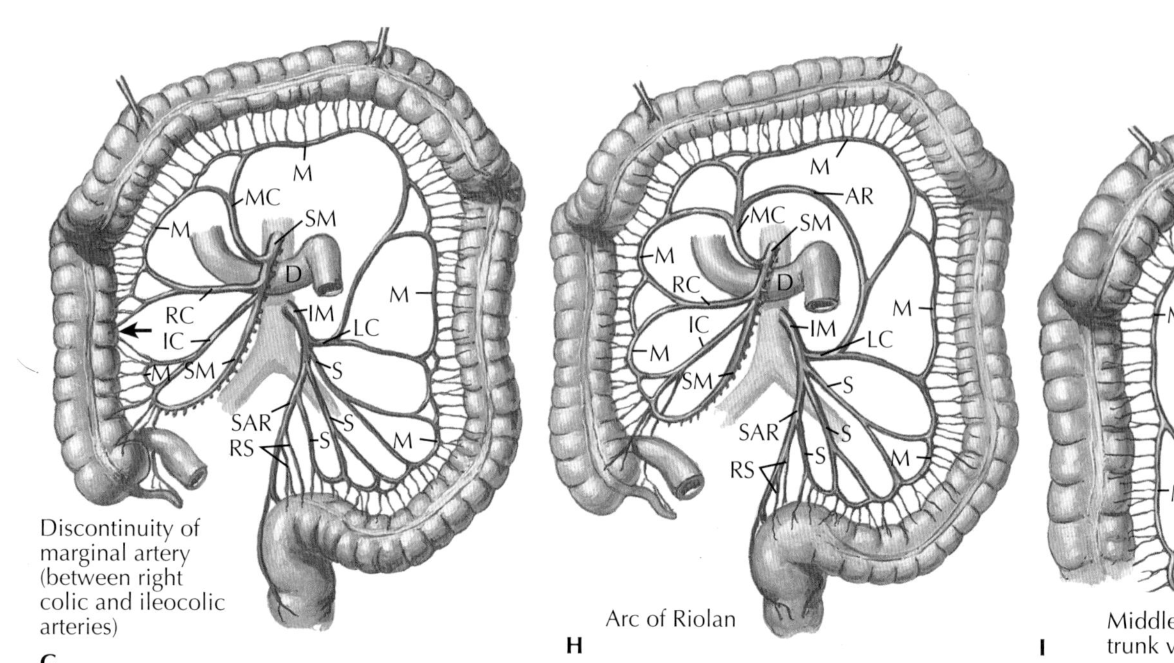


Discontinuity of marginal artery (between right colic and ileocolic arteries)

**G**

Arc of Riolan

**H**

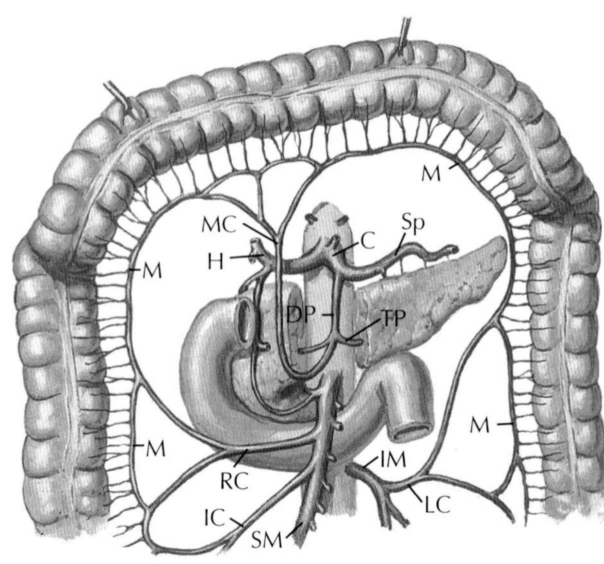


**I** Middle colic artery originates from celiac trunk via dorsal pancreatic artery

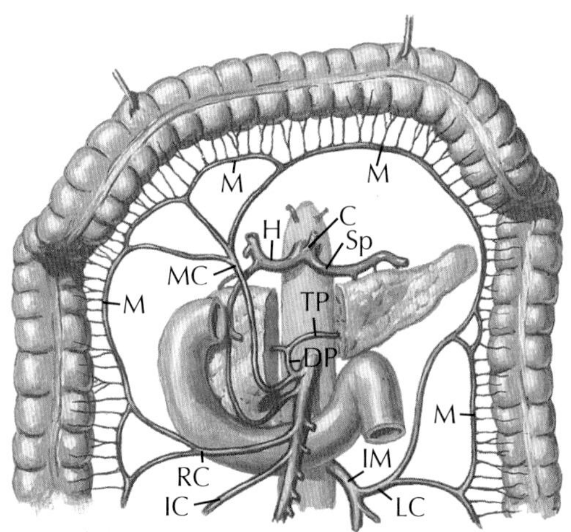


**J** Middle colic artery gives origin to dorsal pancreatic artery

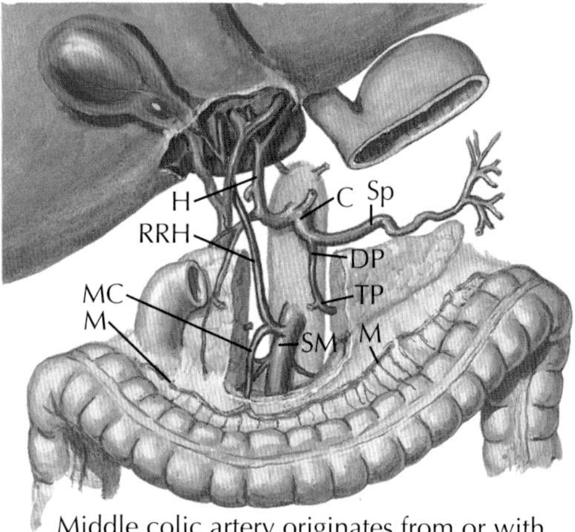


**K** Middle colic artery originates from or with replaced right hepatic artery (from sup. mesenteric a.)

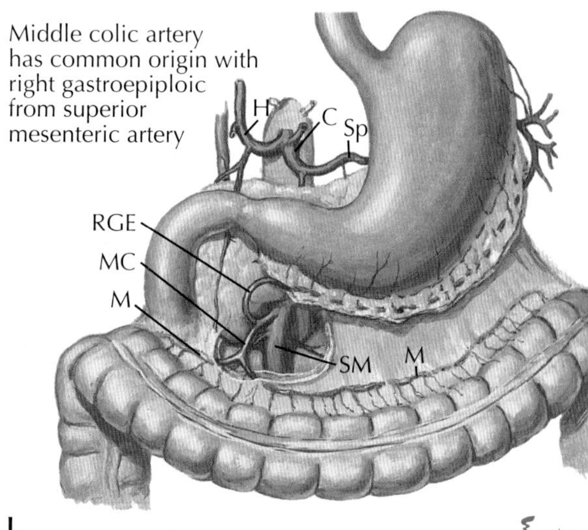


Middle colic artery has common origin with right gastroepiploic from superior mesenteric artery

**L**

**Key**

| | | | |
|---|---|---|---|
| AR – Arc of Riolan | IC – Ileocolic artery | RC – Right colic artery | SAR – Superior anorectal artery |
| C – Celiac trunk | IM – Inferior mesenteric artery | RGE – Right gastroepiploic artery | SM – Superior mesenteric artery |
| D – Duodenum | LC – Left colic artery | RRH – Replaced right hepatic artery | Sp – Splenic artery |
| DP – Dorsal pancreatic artery | M – Marginal artery | RS – Rectosigmoid arteries | TP – Transverse pancreatic artery |
| H – Hepatic artery | MC – Middle colic artery | S – Sigmoid arteries | |

## Blood Supply of Large Intestine (Continued)

artery may originate from the posterior cecal artery, or *both* the anterior and posterior cecal arteries can give rise to two appendicular arteries (Plate 3.15F). Multiple appendicular arteries may also arise from the arcade and ileal branch (Plate 3.15G), or, in some cases, the appendicular artery in its entirety may arise from the colic branch of the ileocolic artery (Plate 3.15H). There may be more than one arcade running between the ileal and colic branches, further complicating the possible variations (Plate 3.15I). With double appendicular arteries, both may supply the entire appendix or one may take care of the organ's base and the other, the tip.

In nearly one-fifth of the population, the right colic artery is absent. In such a case, the ascending colon is still supplied with blood from the ileocolic and middle colic arteries that perfuse the marginal artery (Plate 3.16A). At other times, the right colic artery may indeed exist but instead of leaving the superior mesenteric artery directly, it leaves the ileocolic artery (Plate 3.16B). As a separate branch of the superior mesenteric artery, the middle colic artery is frequently absent. In such instances the artery is often replaced by a common right middle colic trunk that gives off a middle colic branch

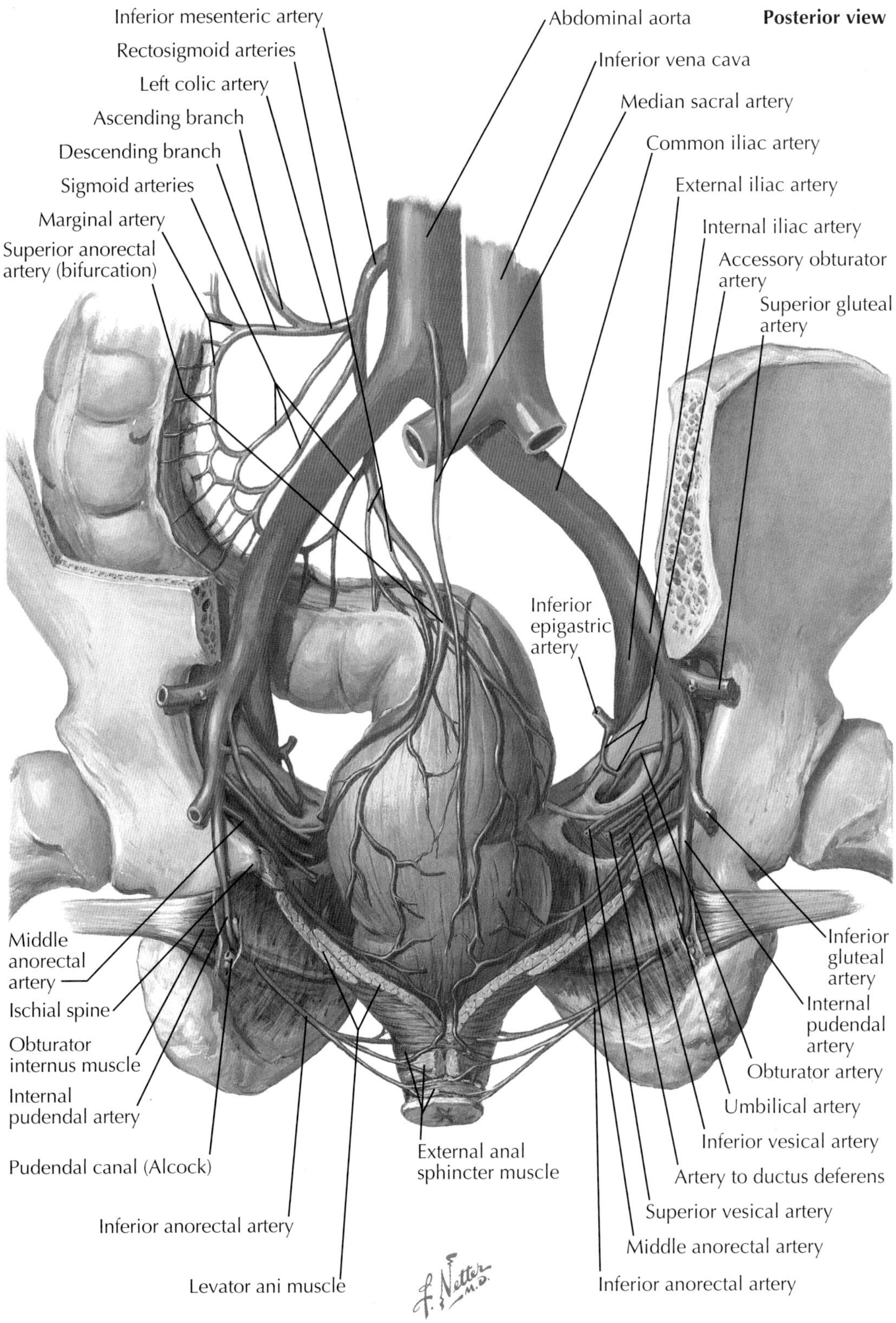

## BLOOD SUPPLY OF LARGE INTESTINE (Continued)

(Plate 3.16C) and occasionally by an enlarged branch of the left colic artery, the latter at times reaching the hepatic flexure (Plate 3.16D). An *accessory middle colic artery* may be present. It usually anastomoses with branches from the left colic artery in the left side of the transverse mesocolon (Plate 3.16E). This accessory middle colic artery may also arise from the trunk of the middle colic artery to serve the splenic flexure. At other times a single middle colic artery may give off two large trunks leading toward the hepatic and splenic flexures, where the ascending and descending colon meet the transverse colon (Plate 3.16F). The marginal artery, which parallels the ascending, transverse, and descending colon, typically allows significant anastomosis between the right, middle, and left colic arteries. It may be discontinuous, so that a region of the colon (Plate 3.17G shows the proximal ascending colon) has only one of the colic arteries contributing blood to the organ. Another variation is a large trunk running between the middle and left colic arteries, creating an additional anastomosis besides the marginal artery. This is referred to as the *arc of Riolan* (Plate 3.17H), and the additional vessel can be found in the transverse mesocolon between its two parent branches.

The middle colic artery also has the bizarre tendency to sometimes originate from branches of the celiac artery, which typically supplies only the foregut organs. This is strange because even though the transverse colon is located in close proximity to several foregut organs, it is near the end of the midgut; one would not therefore expect that it would have any blood supply in common with foregut organs. The middle colic artery may arise from the dorsal pancreatic artery in the vicinity of the transverse pancreatic artery before entering the transverse mesocolon to supply the transverse colon (Plate 3.17I). The situation may also be reversed, with the dorsal pancreatic artery originating from the middle colic artery (Plate 3.17J). Far less frequently, this situation may be more complex, with the middle colic artery originating directly from the celiac trunk or splenic artery before giving off the transverse pancreatic artery. Occasionally, the middle colic artery originates behind the head of the pancreas from an accessory right hepatic artery or from a common trunk, giving rise to both the right hepatic artery and middle colic artery (Plate 3.17K). The middle colic artery may also sometimes give off the right gastroomental artery (Plate 3.17L), which is typically a branch of the gastroduodenal artery, a tributary of the celiac trunk.

In all of these cases, an additional anastomosis between the celiac trunk and superior mesenteric artery is created within the body of the pancreas. Typically these two parent arteries anastomose via arteries originating from the superior pancreaticoduodenal branch (celiac trunk) and inferior pancreaticoduodenal branch (superior mesenteric artery), which supply the head of the pancreas and descending duodenum. The additional anastomosing arteries in the body of the pancreas are predominantly small (1 mm in diameter) but may enlarge, especially when connecting the superior mesenteric artery with the hepatic or right gastroomental artery, reaching a diameter of 2 to 3 mm.

## Lymph Drainage of Large Intestine

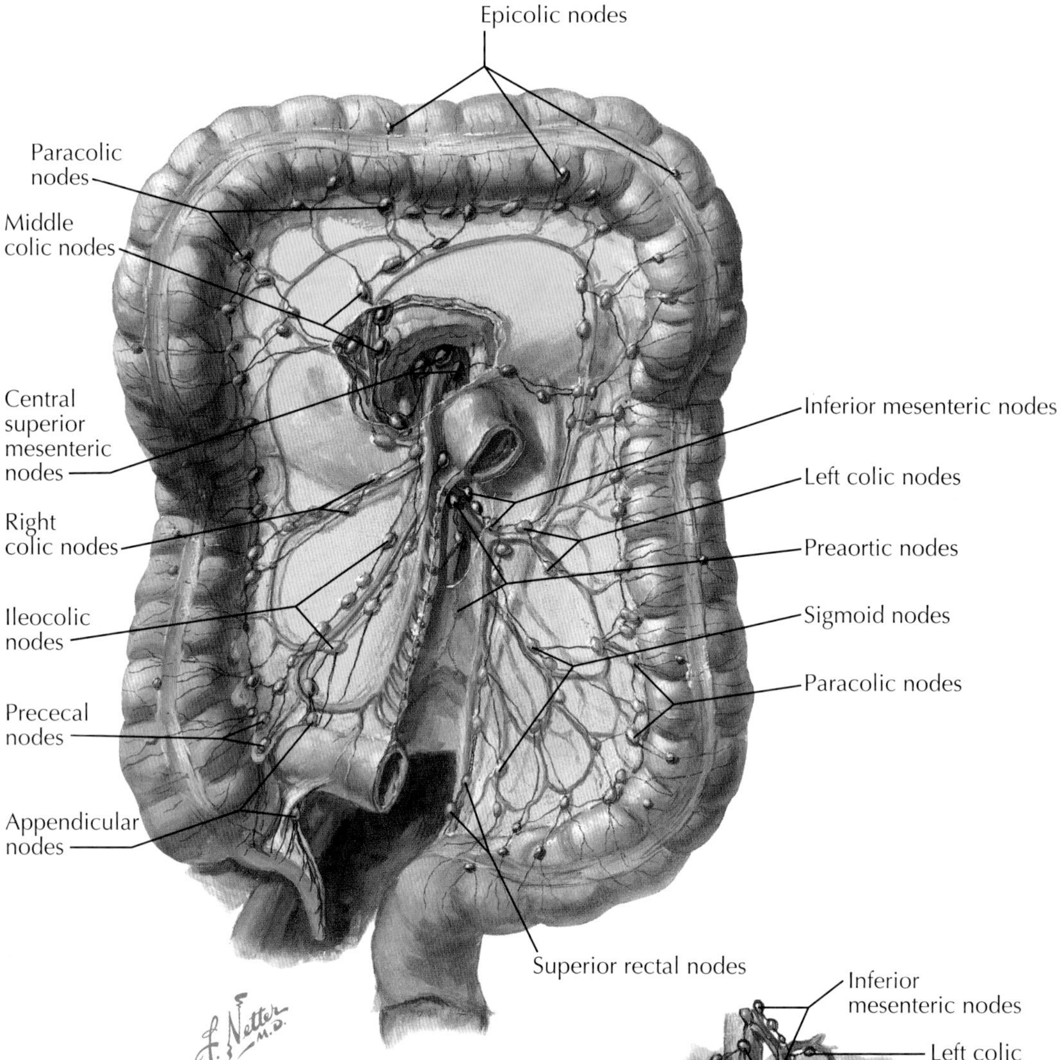

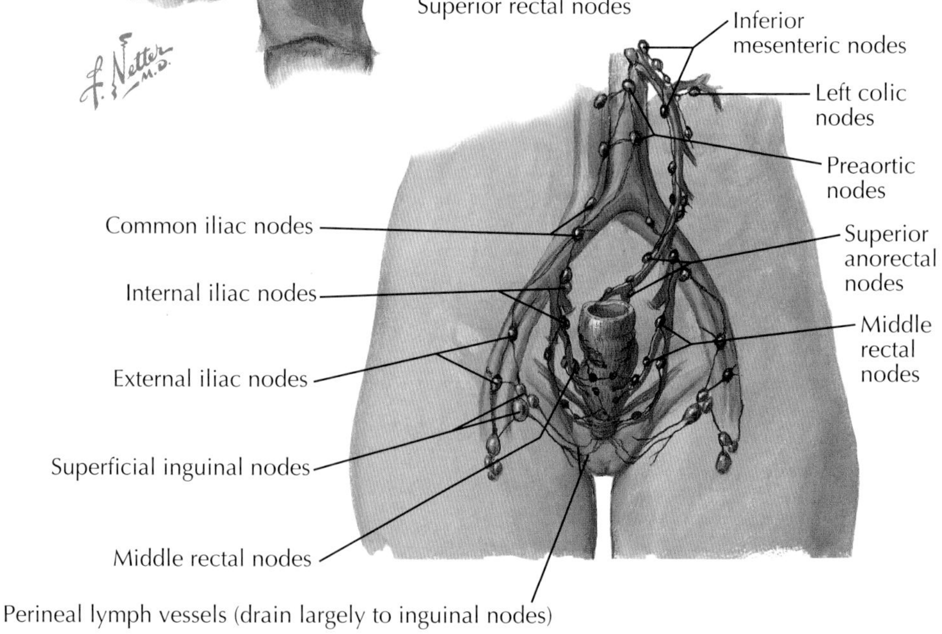

Lymphatic fluid from the large intestine might first encounter the diffuse *epicolic nodes,* which are situated immediately beneath the serous membrane on the intestinal wall. Because these are so few, much of the colon's lymphatic fluid likely bypasses these nodes. The first important regional lymph nodes are the *paracolic nodes,* located within the mesentery near its attachment to the ascending, transverse, descending, and sigmoid colon. These nodes send fluid through lymphatic ducts that parallel nearby vessels to reach regional lymph nodes: *ileocolic, right colic, middle colic,* and *left colic lymph nodes,* appertaining to the respective regions of the large intestine. The majority of the lymph nodes along the course of the ileocolic artery receive their lymph from the ileocecal region, including the appendix (prececal, retrocecal, ileocecal, and appendicular nodes). There are interconnections between the ileocecal and retroperitoneal lymphatics, including those that run near the spermatic vessels, accounting for the occasional migration of bacteria from the ileocecal zone into the superficial lymph nodes of the inguinal region. Similar interconnections occur on the left side of the body.

The ileocolic, right colic, and middle colic lymph nodes send fluid along the accompanying blood vessels to reach the *central superior mesenteric nodes* located at the base of the vessel. The lymph ducts from the descending colon, sigmoid colon, and superior rectum follow the branches of the inferior mesenteric vessels and lead to the *inferior mesenteric nodes.* The lymph from the region of the splenic flexure flows partly into the superior mesenteric lymph nodes and partly into the inferior mesenteric lymph nodes.

Some of the lymphatics emanating from the inferior mesenteric nodes follow the uppermost branches of the inferior mesenteric vessels, passing from left to right in a craniomedial direction around the duodenojejunal flexure to reach the central superior mesenteric nodes. Lymph ducts draining the lower parts of the colon on the left run to the *preaortic lymph nodes* and then into the *lumbar, central superior mesenteric,* and *celiac lymph nodes.* Lymphatic fluid in this region enters the *cisterna chyli,* a sac-like lymphatic vessel. The cisterna chyli receives much of the lymphatic fluid drained from the lower limbs, pelvic organs, hindgut, midgut, and foregut organs. From the cisterna chyli, lymph drains superiorly through the *thoracic duct.* This large lymphatic vessel has prominent valves in its wall and is found in the posterior mediastinum between the aorta and the esophagus. It travels posterior to the arch of the aorta to ultimately drain the lymphatic fluid into the venous system at the left subclavian vein near its junction with the left internal jugular vein.

Lymphatic vessels emanating from the *rectum* and *anal canal* run in two main directions. The upper part of the anal canal is drained cranially via various intermediary nodes to the *preaortic lumbar lymph nodes,* which project fluid to the *inferior mesenteric nodes.* From the lower part of the anal canal, lymph vessels pass over the perineum, alongside the scrotum or labia majora and inner margin of the thigh, to the *superficial inguinal lymph nodes.*

From the region of the surgical anal canal of the rectum, the lymphatic fluid passes into *anorectal nodes* lying immediately posterior to the lower portion of the ampulla and from there to *sacral nodes* situated behind and adjacent to the rectum in the concavity of the sacrum. From the area of the rectal ampulla and above, lymphatics run directly to the sacral nodes, and from the lateral parts of the inferior region of the rectum, lymphatics extend to the *pararectal nodes.* Lymph flows through vessels alongside the three anorectal arteries in a superior direction to the *internal iliac lymph nodes* and then via the *common iliac nodes* to the *preaortic* and *lumbar nodes.* This fluid follows the normal path to reach the cisterna chyli, thoracic duct, and left subclavian vein.

Abdominal physical examination

Digital rectal examination

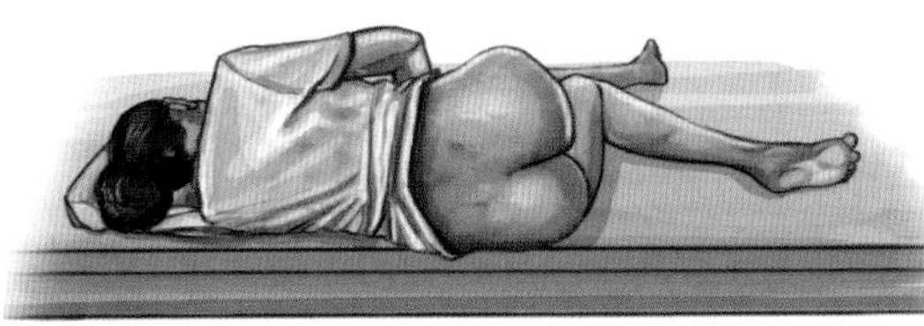


The physician's index finger is gently inserted in the patient's anus. The wall of the anal canal and lower rectum can be palpated.

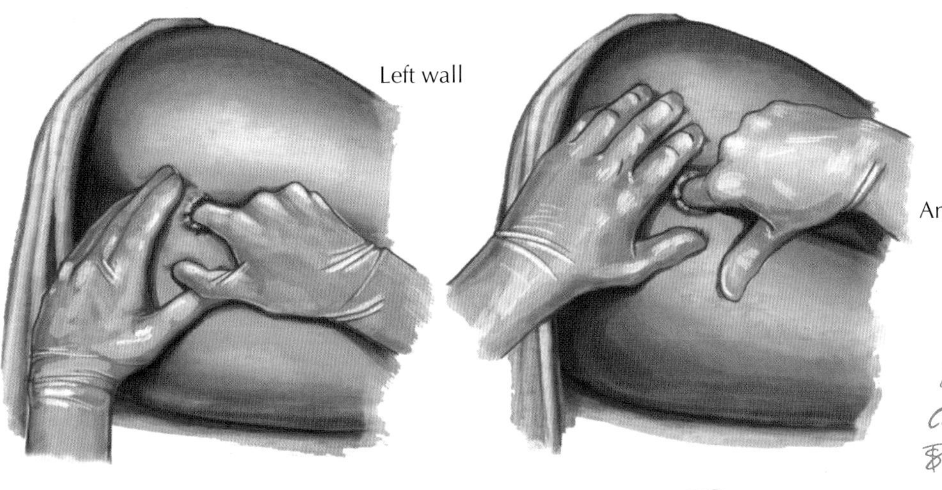


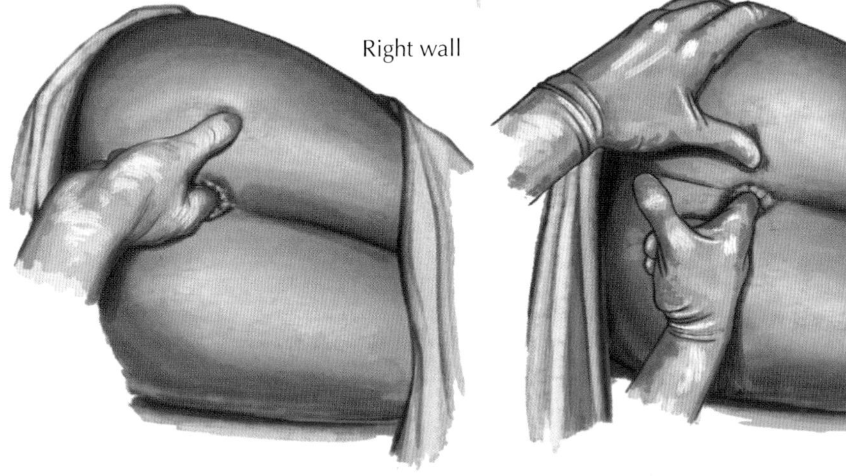


## Physical Examination

The physical examination is essential for determining the cause of a patient's primary symptoms and also guides further diagnostic testing and management. Gastrointestinal examinations have three general parts: inspection, auscultation, and palpation. The provider should first inspect the abdomen for asymmetry, protuberances, scarring, erythema, hernias, striae, or bruising. Inspection is best done by approaching the abdomen as four quadrants or nine segments, while keeping in mind each organ's anatomic position in the body.

Each of the four quadrants of the abdomen should be auscultated using a stethoscope. Auscultation should be performed before palpation to prevent disruption of the migrating motor complex of the intestines. Normal bowel sounds are heard at intervals of 5 to 10 seconds. Sounds heard at intervals of less than 5 seconds are considered hyperactive sounds, and sounds heard at intervals of anything over 10 seconds are considered hypoactive sounds. Hyperactive bowel sounds could be due to gastroenteritis, obstruction, irritable bowel syndrome (IBS), or bleeding. Hypoactive sounds could suggest obstruction, impaired motility, or perforation. It takes three full minutes of listening in one area to determine whether bowel sounds are absent. Borborygmus (plural, *borborygmi*) is the rumbling, growling, or gurgling sound produced by the movement of gastrointestinal contents by peristalsis.

The practitioner should conclude the abdominal examination with percussion and palpation of all four quadrants. Tympanic percussion may signify the presence of gas or free air, whereas dullness to percussion suggests the presence of a solid mass or excess fluid or stool. Palpation should start in a shallow manner; a second pass may become deep if tolerated by the patient. One should try to palpate the afflicted area last. Specialized maneuvers can also be done to rule in a specific pathologic condition. For example, a positive Murphy sign is elicited when a practitioner palpates the right upper quadrant and there is a pause in respiration from resultant pain. A positive Murphy sign would support a diagnosis of cholecystitis. Many practitioners are now being trained on point-of-care ultrasound (POCUS) to aid in the physical assessment. POCUS allows practitioners to evaluate organs such as the liver, gallbladder, spleen, and appendix as well as effectively identify for fluid in the abdominal cavity.

A digital rectal examination is indicated as part of a full physical examination and can be a focused component of a urologic, gynecologic, gastrointestinal, or neurologic complaint. A digital rectal examination may reveal a perianal pathologic condition, rectal bleeding, rectal pathologic condition, or prostate problems. There are many possible positions in which the rectal examination can be performed. The two most common are the dorsal lithotomy and the left lateral recumbent position where the knees are tucked toward the chest. It is important to explain each step to the patient when conducting the examination and refrain from using language that might make the patient uncomfortable or be misinterpreted. When beginning the examination, first inspect the external anal area for masses, hemorrhoids, skin tags, scars, fistulae, or fissures. The perianal area can be scratched first with a gloved finger or stick end of a cotton-tipped swab to determine the integrity of the anal wink, which is a sign of neurologic integrity. Next, the clinician should insert a lubricated, gloved finger into the rectum gently and assess the resting rectal tone. The entire circumference of the rectum should be assessed for masses, stool, decreased internal sphincter tone, and pain. The patient can be asked to squeeze the external anal sphincter to assess for tone if there are concerns for fecal incontinence. The prostate should be examined for hypertrophy or irregularities in male patients. A patient with the report of constipation could be asked to try to simulate defecation to determine whether the muscles perform correctly and to determine the degree of perineal descent. Failure of the muscles to perform correctly may indicate dyssynergia, but further testing is needed for confirmation because the patient may be embarrassed or feel inhibited during the examination and the examination may not be representative of true function. At the end of the examination, the gloved finger should be examined for blood, mucus, or abnormal stool.

## CT vs. MRI in Abdominal Studies

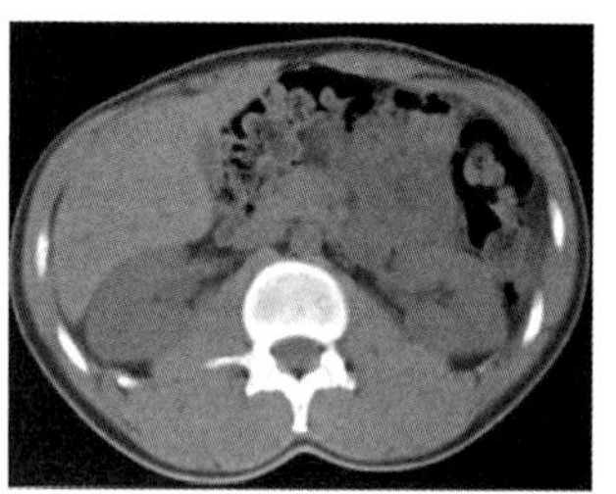
CT without contrast

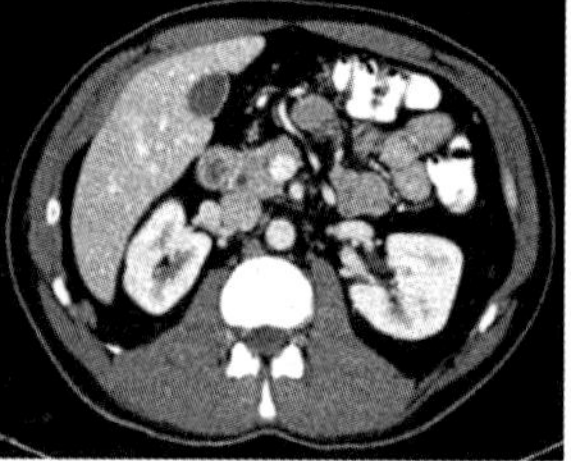
CT with oral and intravenous contrast

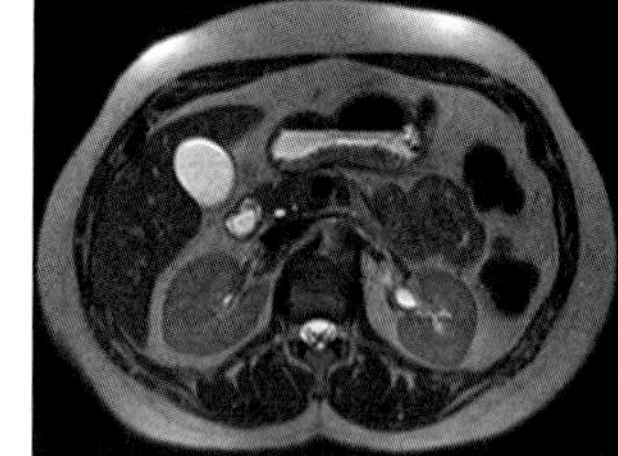
T2* MRI sequence without saturation of the fat signal (fat is light)

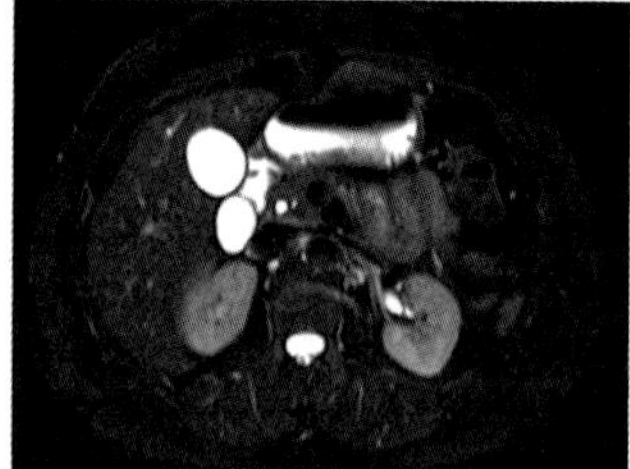
T2 MRI sequence with fat saturation (fat is dark)

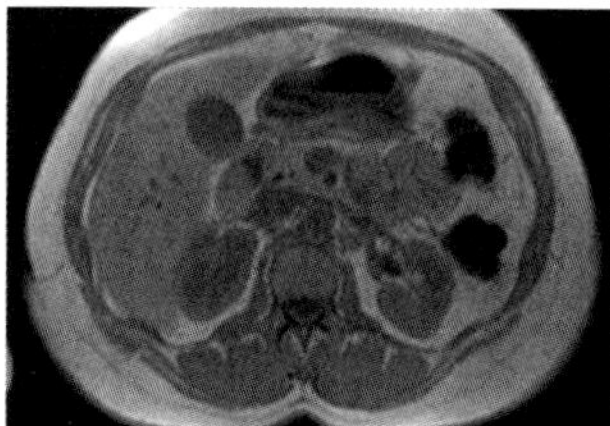
T1* MRI sequence without fat saturation

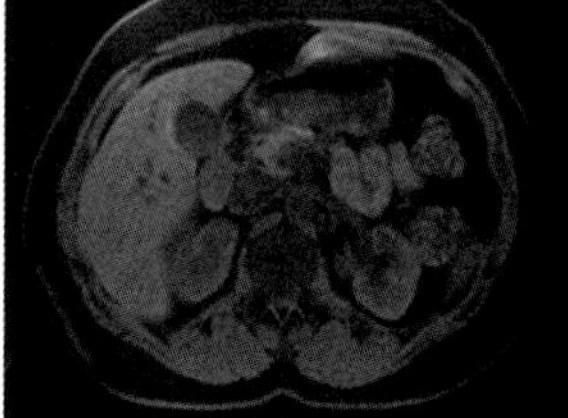
T1 MRI sequence with fat saturation

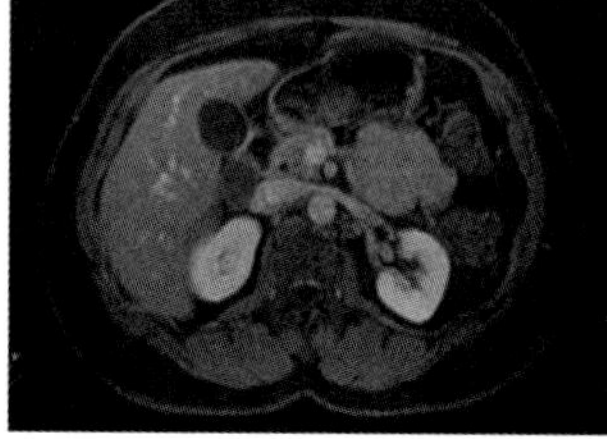
T1 MRI sequence with fat saturation and intravenous contrast

*T1 refers to longitudinal relaxation time and T2 to transverse relaxation time. Specific tissue characteristics affect signal intensity on T1 versus T2 images.

**CT**
Radiation
Fast (less than 5 minutes)
Good overall look at solid organs, fat planes
Best spatial resolution ("thinner" images, can "resolve" small things that are close to each other)
Excellent for calcification (i.e., small renal stones)
Good for overall look of pelvic organs, but with limited detail
Iodine-based intravenous (IV) contrast

**MRI**
No radiation
Not so fast (usually more than 20 minutes)
Good for characterization of lesions
Best tissue resolution (different tissues have different concentrations of hydrogen [water])
Not good for calcification (i.e., small renal stones)
Excellent for pelvic organs (uterus, ovaries, prostate, seminal vesicles)
Gadolinium-based IV contrast

*From Cochard LR, Goodhartz LA, Harmath CB, et al. Netter's Introduction to Imaging. Elsevier; 2012.*

| Common Diagnostic Tests | Indications |
|---|---|
| Abdominal x-ray | Evaluation of bowel perforation, bowel obstruction, urinary calculi, bowel ischemia, megacolon, and most forms of intestinal obstruction |
| Barium studies (Single or double contrast studies) | Used to diagnose IBD, strictures, obstruction, pseudoobstruction, diverticulosis, and neoplasms |
| Computed tomography (CT) | Best test for the evaluation of pancreatic, hepatic disease, staging of cancer. Useful for diverticulitis, colonic masses, and metastatic disease. NOTE: spiral CT uses helical movement pattern to improve resolution for conditions like colon cancer. |
| Computed tomographic angiography (CTA) | Evaluation of aortic dissection and aneurysm. Assessment of the kidneys, pancreas, and liver before and after surgery. Evaluation of hypertension secondary to renal artery disease. May have role in therapeutic cessation of bleeding. |
| CT Colonography or magnetic resonance colonography (virtual colonoscopy) | Can visualize disorders of the colon and is an alternative to the colonoscopy for screening for polyps and colon cancer |
| Defecography | Evaluation of pelvic floor dysfunction, rectocele, and other anatomical issues that result in problems with defecation |
| Functional magnetic resonance imaging | Can be useful in evaluating disorders of the pelvic floor |
| Magnetic resonance imaging (MRI) | Evaluation of the extent of Crohn disease and ulcerative colitis, infectious bowel disease and ischemic bowel disease, and malignancy and metastasis of the stomach and small and large intestines |
| Positron emission tomography (PET) scan | Used to evaluate extent and develop treatment plans for metastatic disease |
| Scintigraphy | Detection of metastatic disease, GI transit time, biliary pathology, and gastroesophageal reflux disease using radiolabeled materials |
| Ultrasound (endoscopic) | Used to visualize the alimentary canal and surrounding organs; option for staging of rectal cancer and identifying damaged or diseased mucosal tissue |
| Ultrasound (traditional) | Evaluation of solid organs (liver, pancreas, spleen, gallbladder, and biliary tract). Focused assessment with sonography in trauma (FAST) scan in emergency setting to rule out trauma. Guiding paracentesis for diagnostic evaluation of ascites or guiding large-volume therapeutic ascites. |

## Radiologic and Imaging Studies

Over the last century, radiologic imaging and other radiographic modalities have made significant advancements that allow practitioners to easily visualize, diagnose, and treat disease.

The best approach to ordering an imaging test is to choose one that best answers the clinical question at hand while limiting the cost and potential side effects. For example, a practitioner may choose to rule out perforation by ordering an upright abdominal radiography because it is faster to obtain, produces significantly less radiation, and costs less than a computed tomography (CT) scan. If the radiograph shows free air under the diaphragm, this is diagnostic of a viscous rupture. The clinician may still choose to get a CT scan to not only document but to also localize the area of perforation. The benefits of helping the surgeon characterize the perforation may be more important than limiting the expense or amount of radiation exposure. For example, a CT scan may show a localized perforation or inflammatory changes associated with diverticulitis. It should also be remembered that an erect posteroanterior radiograph may not be sensitive enough to rule out pneumoperitoneum in patients presenting with upper abdominal pain and perforation.

## Colonoscopy

Colonoscopy is a procedure in which a long flexible tube is inserted into the rectum and colon to detect diseases of the large intestine. The indications for colonoscopy can include screening to detect colorectal neoplasms or diagnostic intent for the investigation of blood in the stool, anemia, diarrhea, and other symptoms. Sigmoidoscopy is a procedure in which a shorter tube could be inserted up to 60 cm from the anal verge. Indications for sigmoidoscopy include colorectal cancer screening, preoperative evaluation prior to anorectal surgery, surveillance of a previously diagnosed lesion or hemostasis of a bleeding site within the range of the sigmoidoscope, local treatment of disorders such as radiation proctitis, removal of foreign bodies, biopsies for graft-versus-host disease or amyloidosis, and stent placement or balloon dilation of a stricture. The remainder of this section will focus on colonoscopy, although most information will also apply to sigmoidoscopy.

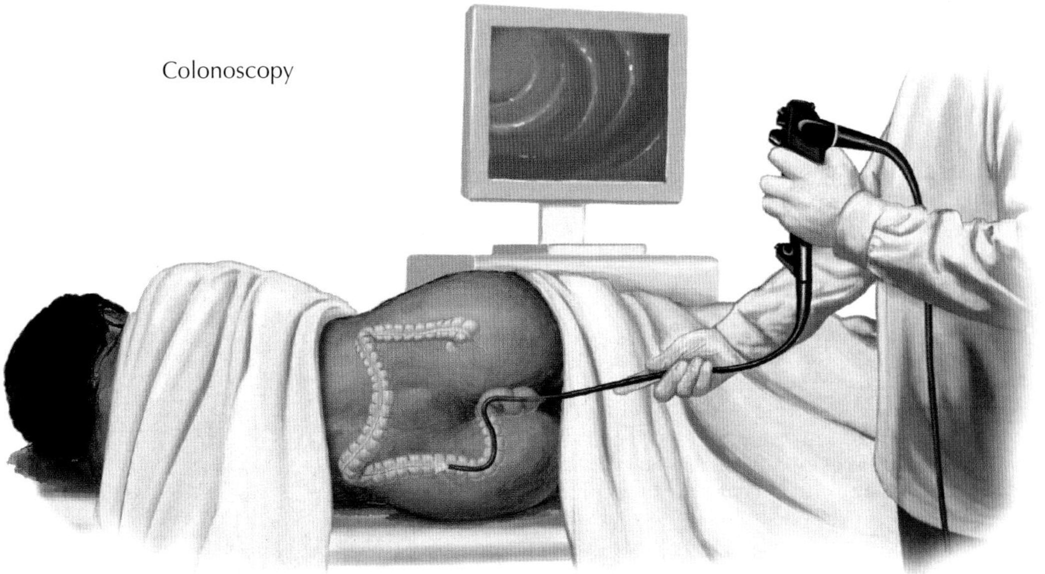

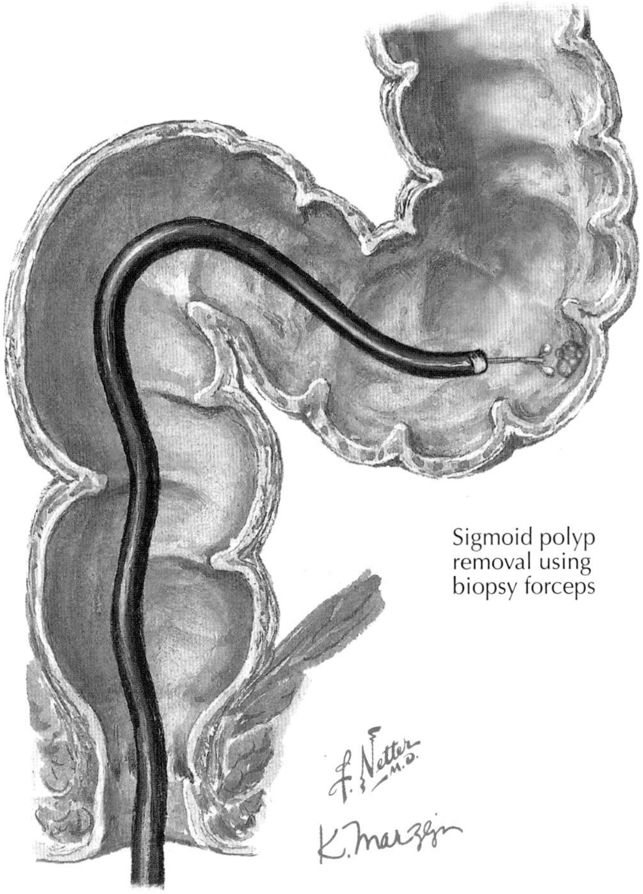

One must consider the indication for the procedure and if timing for the procedure is appropriate. For instance, colonoscopy would not be performed on a patient in the hospital with pneumonia who is noted to have iron deficiency anemia without evidence of active bleeding. The examiner should have adequate knowledge of the anatomy of the colon and the capabilities of the instrument and should be prepared to perform diagnostic and therapeutic procedures such as biopsy, control of bleeding, and polyp removal. Bowel cleansing in advance of a colonoscopy is required in most cases.

Sedation is indicated in most patients undergoing colonoscopy but may not be needed for sigmoidoscopy and can be accomplished with intravenous administration of short-acting hypnotic/amnestic agent such as propofol or with an opiate and benzodiazepine. The procedure can be carried out in the hospital or an outpatient endoscopy suite while the patient is placed in the left lateral position with knees bent. Digital rectal examination preceding the introduction of a colonoscope is obligatory to rule out any impediment to the free passage of the instrument and to inspect the anal area for any lesions.

The tip of the well-lubricated colonoscope (a long, flexible, narrow tube with a light and a small camera at the end) is inserted with steady pressure into the *anal ring* and slowly advanced into the rectum and entire colon while keeping the lumen in view. The scope enables the endoscopist to irrigate and suction the unwanted debris for better visualization.

Insufflation of the colon using air or preferably carbon dioxide ($CO_2$) or water is needed to open the opposed folds and have a better visualization during the procedure.

Complete colonoscopy requires the visualization of the cecum. This is documented by taking pictures from the appendiceal orifice and the ileocecal valve. The diagnostic value of intubating the ileum during colonoscopy depends on the indication for the procedure.

Not every patient requires a complete examination of the colon. For example, in acute severe ulcerative colitis (UC), the endoscopist may only need to evaluate the distal part of the colon and rectum because of a higher risk of complications with a complete examination. The examiner should not insist on advancing the scope if the bowel prep is prohibiting or a severe constricting lesion is encountered during the exam. In the absence of conditions of these types, however, every reasonable effort should be made to perform a complete examination. The endoscopist should avoid excessive looping and use torque steering and rotation of the scope to reach the cecum.

The mucosa is carefully evaluated as the instrument is withdrawn by viewing the display monitor. Colonoscopists with longer mean times for withdrawal of the colonoscope may have higher adenoma detection rates.

Like many other procedures, colonoscopy is not without risk, but mastering the required techniques will minimize the risk. The recognition and evaluation of pathologic conditions depend on a thorough acquaintance with the range of normal variation.

Trainees should develop technical and cognitive skills to be competent in performing colonoscopy. Although the Accreditation Council for Graduate Medical Education and the American Society for Gastrointestinal Endoscopy recommended a minimum number of 140 cases, trainees typically complete around 250 to 500 procedures to attain competency.

Colonoscopy

Colon polyps

Sigmoid polyp removal using biopsy forceps

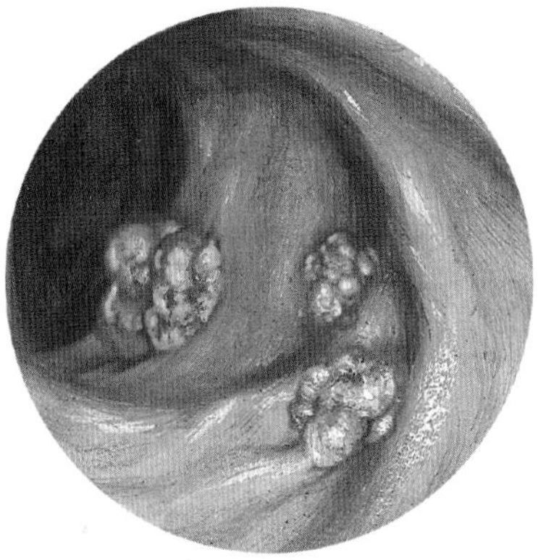

# Biopsy and Cytologic Studies

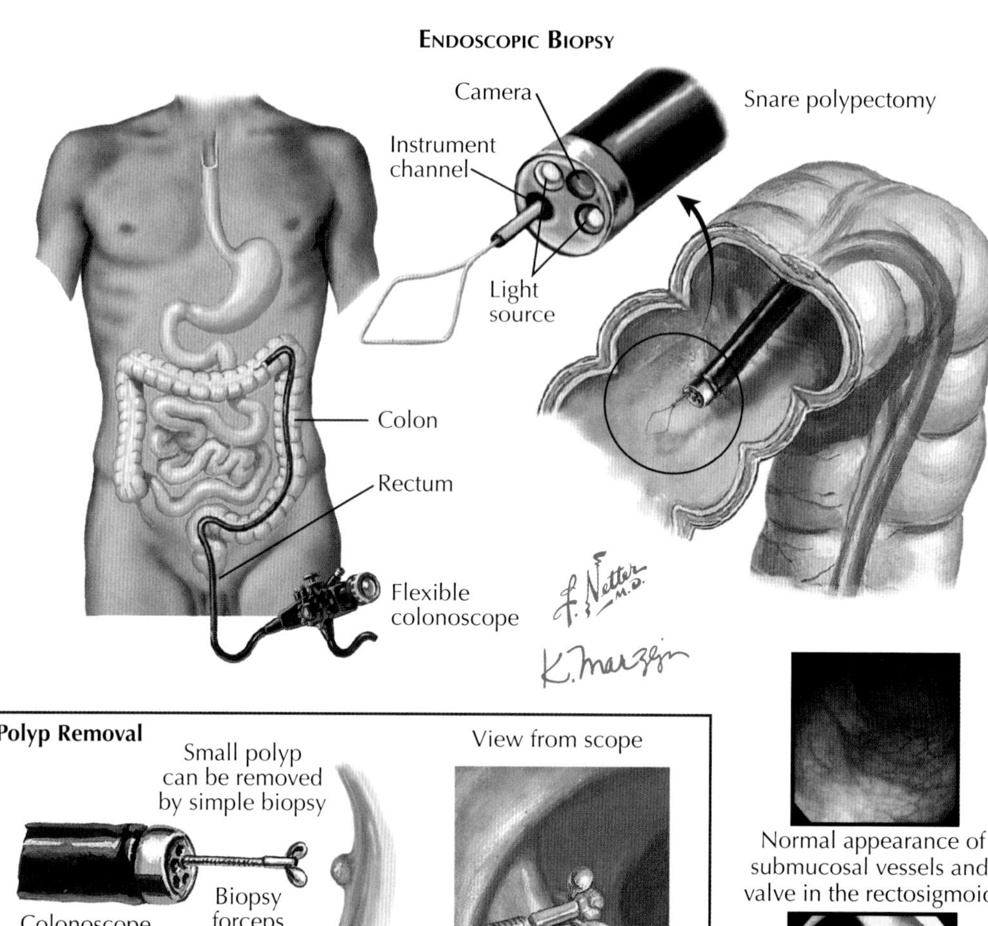


Polyp Removal

Small polyp can be removed by simple biopsy

Colonoscope

Biopsy forceps

View from scope

Normal appearance of submucosal vessels and valve in the rectosigmoid.

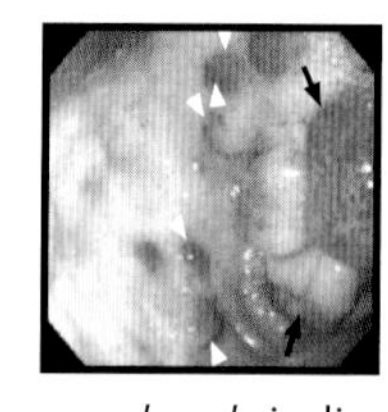

Normal appearance of haustra as the transverse colon is entered.

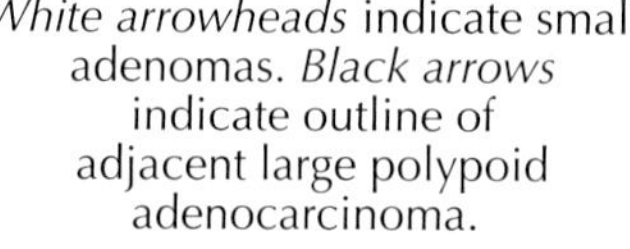

*White arrowheads* indicate small adenomas. *Black arrows* indicate outline of adjacent large polypoid adenocarcinoma.

Biopsy forceps with spike

Cytology brush

Pathologic specimens obtained through biopsy or cytologic studies provide critical information pertaining to a patient's illness. The following sections will discuss both biopsy and cytologic examination for the colon and rectum in greater detail.

## BIOPSY

Endoscopic biopsy is the most common technique used for tissue sampling of the colon and rectum. Biopsies are done using forceps with two cups varying in shape, size, and serration that allow for a single adequate grasp of tissue. Most forceps come with a needle-spike apparatus that acts as both a grip and an anchor for sampling. Endoscopic forceps are considered hot forceps when they can cauterize tissue and are generally used either to stop internal bleeding or for a polypectomy. Most procedures use cold forceps, or those that cannot cauterize tissue. Practitioners also have the choice to use either single-use or reusable forceps. Although using single-use forceps guarantees less sample contamination, reusable forceps are much more cost-effective and are sanitary if cleaned properly.

Biopsies are best used to confirm a diagnosis and help direct therapy. For example, in patients suspected of having colitis, a rectal biopsy can confirm the diagnosis before treatment is considered. How the biopsy is performed can vary considerably, as is seen with biopsy for ulcers, where the pathologist requires samples from the edge and the base to rule out different causes. Endoscopic biopsy is associated with a minimal risk of bleeding and perforation; however, biopsy is contraindicated when patients already are at high risk for bleeding or for colonic perforation. The following is a list of conditions that frequently warrant biopsy:

- **Chronic diarrhea:** To make the diagnosis of microscopic colitis (e.g., collagenous or lymphocytic colitis) and amyloidosis
- **Inflammatory bowel disease:** Diagnosis and evaluation of Crohn's disease (CD) and UC; screening for colon cancer
- **Polyps and colon cancer:** For initial diagnosis; follow-up for full removal of cancer
- **Infectious colitis:** Common causes being *Escherichia coli* O157:H7, *Salmonella*, *Shigella*, *Campylobacter*, and *Clostridium difficile*
- **Other conditions:** To confirm the diagnosis of Hirschsprung disease, anal cancers, lipomas, Peutz-Jeghers syndrome, Behçet disease, and any unexplained abnormalities of colonic tissue

## CYTOLOGIC STUDIES

Cytologic study is an alternative method to biopsy that can characterize infections and colonic growths, such as adenoma progressing to adenocarcinoma. As the name implies, in *brush cytologic study*, a flexible brush is rubbed across the area of interest in the colon. The act of brushing removes cells from the area that can later be studied with the use of a microscope. Although this technique has limited use for most diseases of the colon, brush cytologic study has been shown to be as accurate as endoscopic biopsy in diagnosing colorectal cancer, and it provides the best diagnostic yield when paired with biopsy results. Anorectal cytologic study is considered the diagnostic gold standard when screening for anal cancer.

## ANTICOAGULATION AND BIOPSY

There is a debate in the literature about holding anticoagulation agents (e.g., coumadin, heparin, and direct factor Xa inhibitors such as apixaban, edoxaban, rivaroxaban, and fondaparinux) and antiplatelet agents (e.g., aspirin and clopidogrel) when performing tissue sampling to reduce the risk of procedural bleeding. Holding these medications comes with the inherent risk of an adverse outcome from a thromboembolic event. The overall risk of bleeding for a cold biopsy is less than a 1%; the risk is higher with polypectomy and the use of hot forceps or a snare. The American Society for Gastrointestinal Endoscopy has created guidelines as to when these medications should be stopped based on both the risk associated with each procedure and the risk of an adverse event associated with each condition. Patients undergoing low-risk procedures should continue anticoagulation therapy and undergo the procedure as long as their international normalized ratio is therapeutic. Patients undergoing high-risk procedures should stop their anticoagulation medication 3 to 5 days before the procedure and restart it within 24 hours after the procedure or at the time judged best by the practitioner. Those with conditions that have a high risk of thromboembolic events should be started on intravenous heparin until a few hours before the procedure begins, whereas those with low-risk conditions do not need a heparin bridge. Conditions considered to have a high risk for thromboembolism are atrial fibrillation with a history of cerebrovascular accident or embolism with a mechanical valve, mechanical mitral valve, mechanical valves with a previous thromboembolic event, acute coronary syndrome, placement of a stent within the last year, and percutaneous intervention with no stent after a myocardial infarction.

IMPERFORATE ANUS

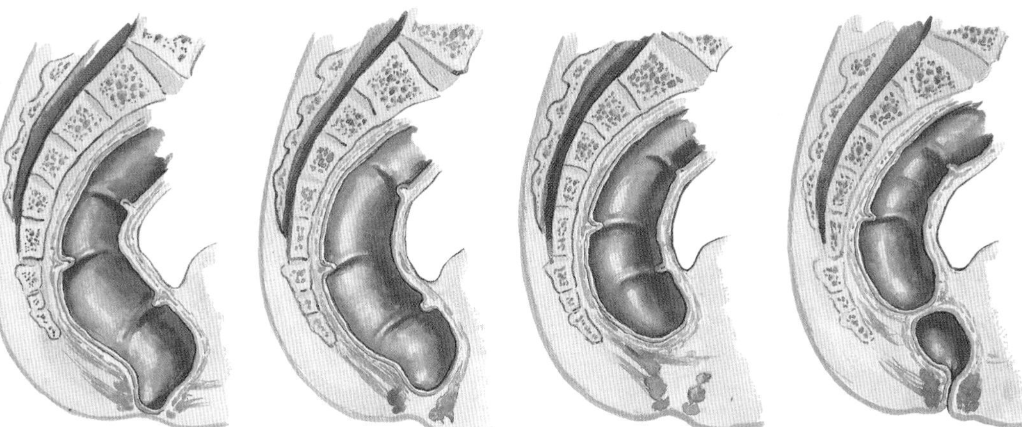


**Type 1.** Low anorectal malformation. **Type 2.** Intermediate malformation. **Type 3.** High malformation. **Type 4.** Atresia of the rectum with normal anus.

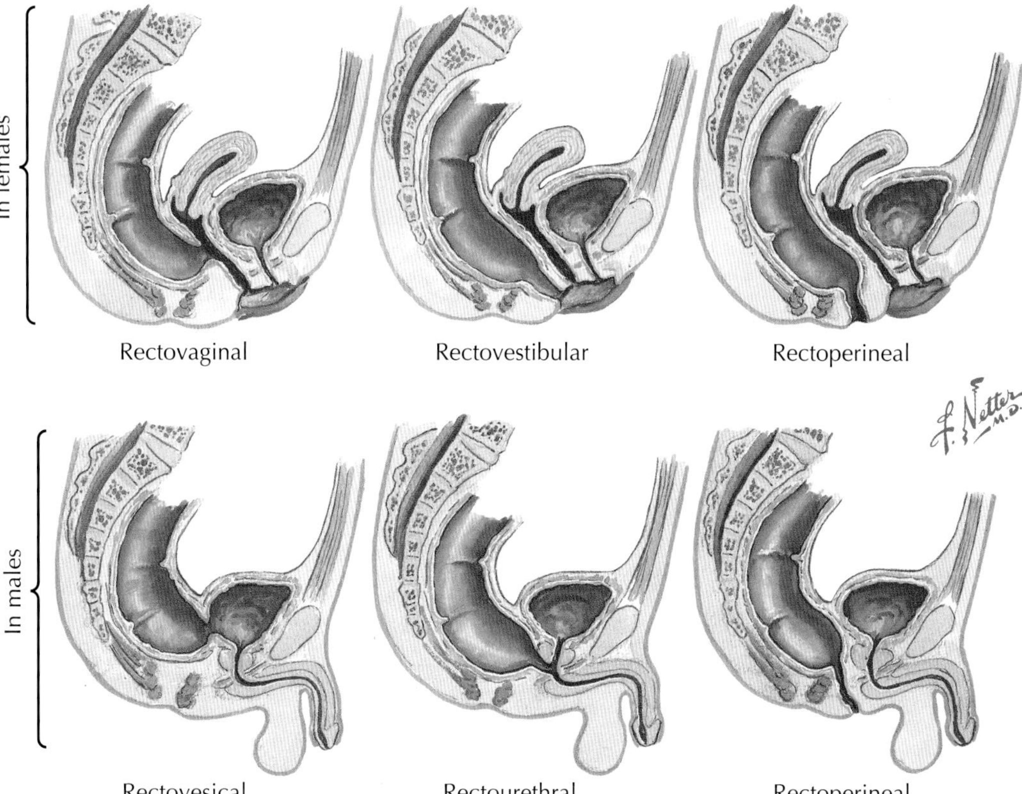


# CONGENITAL INTESTINAL OBSTRUCTION: ANORECTAL MALFORMATIONS

Normally, by the eighth week of embryonic life, the cloacal membrane, which separates the rectum and the anal invagination, is absorbed, so that the anus and rectum become one continuous canal. When this membrane fails to disintegrate, there is no opening where the anus should be, resulting in a condition known as *imperforate anus.* This is one of the most common congenital anomalies encountered in neonates (1:5000 live births) and is slightly more prevalent in males. Several variants of this condition have been observed. Traditionally, these defects have been classified as low, intermediate, or high based on anatomic criteria, including the position of the blind rectal pouch relative to the levator ani muscle complex and pelvic bony landmarks. Imperforate anus without fistula is rare (only 5% of anorectal malformations), and, of those, 95% occur in association with Down syndrome. Rarely, the anal canal develops normally but there is total atresia of the rectum. It is important to recognize the nature of the malformation because of the different surgical approaches used in the repair of these anomalies (see Plate 3.26).

Anorectal malformations are frequently accompanied by incomplete separation of the rectum and the urogenital sinus, so that most infants with an imperforate anus have a fistula between the rectum and the urinary tract or perineum in the male or between the rectum and the vagina or perineum in the female. In the male, the fistula may enter the bladder (rectovesical) or the prostatic or bulbar urethra (rectourethral) or may emerge in the skin of the scrotum or perineum (rectoperineal). Rectourethral fistular tracts are the most common in males, followed by rectoperineal fistulas. In the female, the fistula may open into the vagina (rectovaginal), the vestibule (rectovestibular), the posterior fourchette, or the perineum (rectoperineal). Rectovestibular fistulas are most common in females, followed by cutaneous rectoperineal fistulas. The next most common defect in females is that of persistent cloaca, in which there is a single opening formed by fusion of the rectum, vagina, and urethra.

Imperforate anus is usually diagnosed by careful inspection or discovered upon attempting to insert a rectal thermometer. If no meconium is seen within 24 hours, patency of the anus should be assessed to rule out the rare atresia of the rectal canal in the presence of a fully formed anus. When meconium is present, its source should be carefully identified. The presence of

PERINEAL APPROACH TO IMPERFORATE ANUS

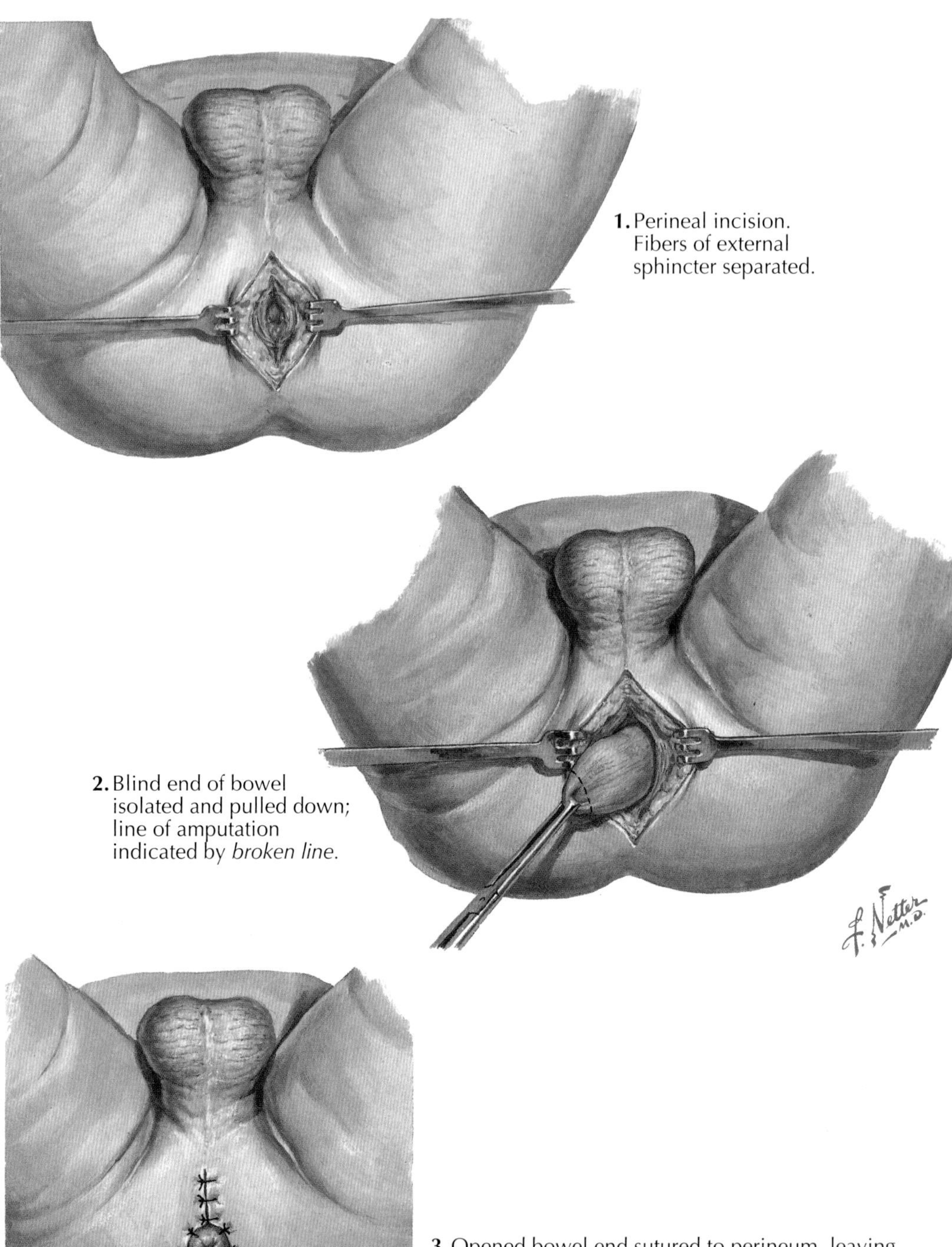

1. Perineal incision. Fibers of external sphincter separated.
2. Blind end of bowel isolated and pulled down; line of amputation indicated by *broken line*.
3. Opened bowel end sutured to perineum, leaving some redundancy; perineum sutured.


## CONGENITAL INTESTINAL OBSTRUCTION: ANORECTAL MALFORMATIONS (Continued)

a perineal fistula associated with a low anorectal malformation is sometimes missed when meconium has passed through the fistula rather than the anus. Inspection of the perineum also should be carried out to look for the presence of a rectoperineal fistula. A rectovestibular fistula is manifested as a third opening within the vestibule in addition to a normal urethral meatus and vagina. The presence of only a single perineal opening indicates a persistent cloaca. Other diagnostic signs depend on the size and location of the fistula. Meconium may appear at the urethral meatus, or flecks of it may be found in the urine on microscopic examination, but this typically takes 24 hours to occur. Air in the bladder, a rare demonstration by radiograph, indicates a communication between the intestinal and urinary tracts. If a fistulous opening is present in the perineum, introduction of contrast dye *(fistulography)* may reveal the origin and level of the fistulous connection. Alternatively, it may also be possible to outline the fistula by introducing contrast dye into the bladder *(cystourethrography)*. Newer radiologic techniques using magnetic resonance imaging (MRI) even in the fetal stage can be used to make the diagnosis.

If no clinical signs indicating the location of the anomaly become evident by 24 hours, the distance between a blind rectal pouch and the anal dimple can be assessed radiologically using anatomic criteria. Air taken into the GI tract and passed along by peristalsis toward the rectum during the first 24 hours is visualized on radiograph with the infant in an inverted position so that the air bubble reaches the lower limit of the rectal pouch. Its location relative to a radiopaque marker placed at the location of the anal dimple and relative to bony markers such as the pubococcygeal line and the ischial line are used to determine the distance between the rectal pouch and the anal dimple. This allows anorectal malformations to be broadly classified by location of the rectal pouch as high (supralevator), intermediate (partially translevator), or low (fully translevator).

## CONGENITAL INTESTINAL OBSTRUCTION: MANAGEMENT OF ANORECTAL MALFORMATIONS

The goal of surgery to repair anorectal malformations has evolved from a primarily lifesaving procedure to one that allows for as much preservation of gastrointestinal, urinary, and sexual function as possible. This is critical to allow affected children to have normal social interactions and to develop into healthy adults.

In the simplest case, an imperforate anus in which meconium can be seen behind a thin membrane over a properly located anus seldom needs major surgical management. Perforation of the membrane with a blunt instrument is simple, safe, and completely effective. For boys and girls with a low anorectal malformation, a definitive surgical repair can be undertaken using a perineal approach. The external sphincter is located using an electrical muscle stimulator. With the patient in the lithotomy position, any perineal fistula is dissected toward the rectum. A longitudinal incision in the perineum provides the best and safest exposure. Dissection in the operative area is kept close to the midline to avoid damaging the nerve and blood supply. The fibers of the external sphincter muscle appear as a rough horseshoe with the apex pointing posteriorly. The blind pouch of the rectum appears as a blue bulbous mass because it is filled with meconium. For the purpose of traction, the most distal portion of the rectal pouch is grasped (with a hemostat or silk sutures). Dissection is continued, keeping as close as possible to the bowel and avoiding disruption of adjacent structures, until sufficient length of colon has been mobilized to permit the apex of the pouch to be brought to the skin edge without tension. The pouch is opened and evacuated of meconium. A row of simple sutures approximates the full thickness of the open bowel with the skin of the opened anal dimple. The remaining anterior portion of the perineal incision is closed in layers.

In the case of intermediate and high anorectal malformations, the distance of the hindgut from the anus and the nature and location of a potential fistula may not be clear, necessitating additional anatomic studies. Because exploratory surgery from the perineum without knowledge of the anatomy carries the risk of iatrogenic injury, in such cases a decision may be made to create a divided stoma near the junction of the descending and sigmoid colon. The divided colostomy allows the passage of stool and is sufficiently proximal to allow further elucidation of the anatomy without impeding a subsequent surgical correction. Introduction of contrast dye through the mucous fistula with sufficient pressure can be used to delineate the location of a urinary fistula. Once the anatomy of the defect is fully appreciated, surgical repair can be undertaken.

The standard for surgical reconstruction in these cases, still frequently performed, is posterior sagittal anorectoplasty (PSARP), developed by Pena and colleagues. In this procedure, the patient is placed in a prone position with the pelvis elevated. A midline sagittal incision is made from the sacrum to the location of the anal dimple and the underlying muscle is divided. Muscle stimulation is used throughout the procedure to identify muscle layers, including the sphincter complex, which is usually poorly formed in these patients, and the levator ani. The posterior approach allows the hindgut to be safely accessed and the fistula to be dissected from associated structures of the urinary tract or vagina, for example. A sufficiently mobilized length of rectum is positioned within the sphincteric muscles, which are reconstructed and sutured to the rectum. Certain lesions, such as rectovesicular and rectoprostatic malformations, are so high in the pelvis that they cannot safely be reached by posterior sagittal anorectoplasty alone. These cases may require a concurrent laparoscopy or even laparotomy for successful division of the fistular connection and repositioning of the rectum. For maintenance and voluntary control of fecal continence, both afferent and efferent nerves must be carefully preserved. Despite these precautions, a significant percentage of patients with high anorectal malformations experience an increased incidence of fecal incontinence.

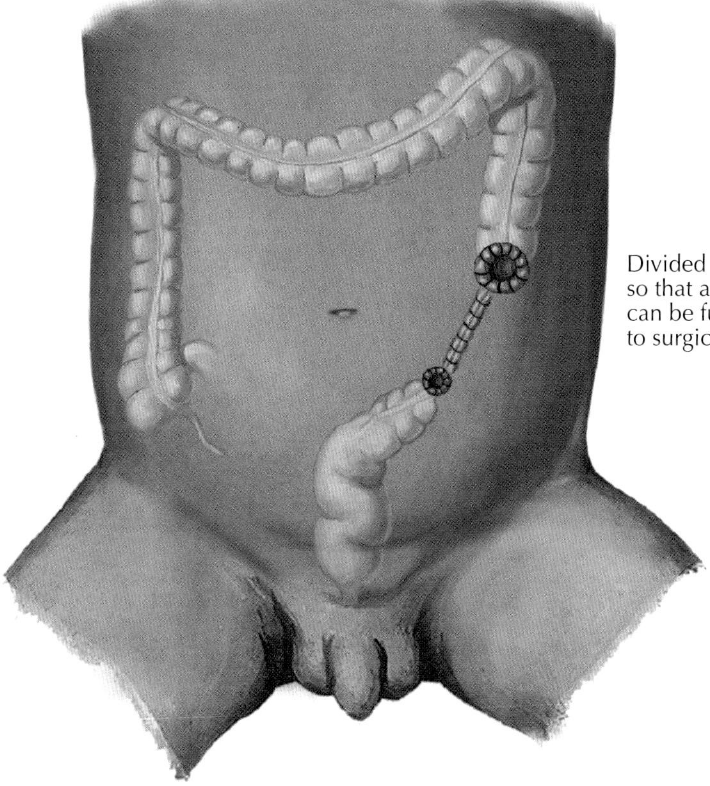

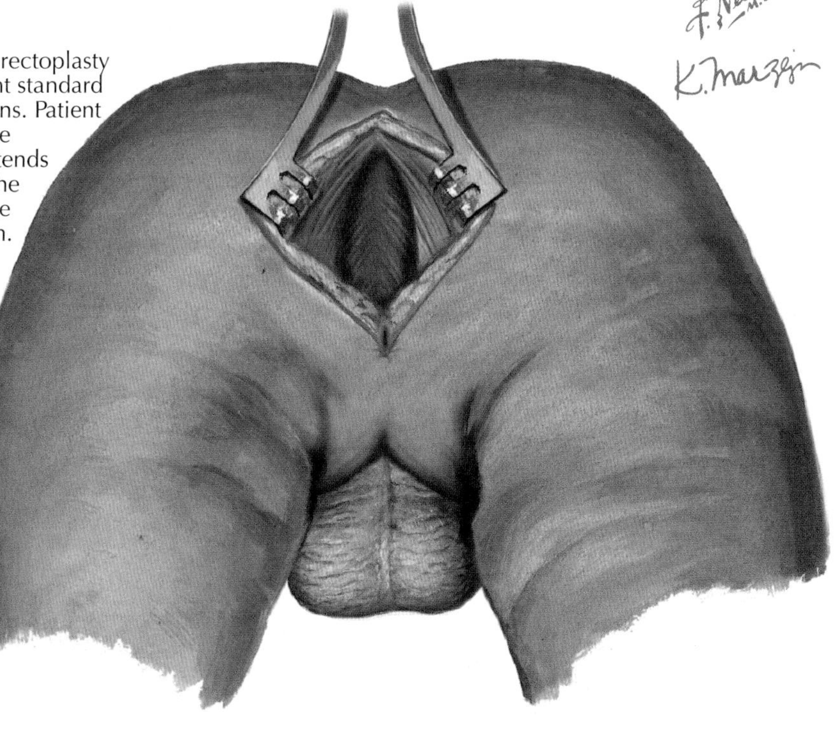

More recently, minimally invasive surgical therapies have been developed using a laparoscopy-assisted anorectal pull-through (LAARP) procedure, similar to laparoscopic pull-through techniques used in the treatment of Hirschsprung disease (see below). This approach is often indicated when the anatomic nature of the anorectal malformation requires entry into the abdomen.

Divided colostomy is performed so that anatomy of the defect can be fully assessed prior to surgical repair.

Posterior sagittal anorectoplasty (PSARP) is the current standard for high malformations. Patient is placed in the prone position. Incision extends from the sacrum to the anterior margin of the sphincter mechanism.

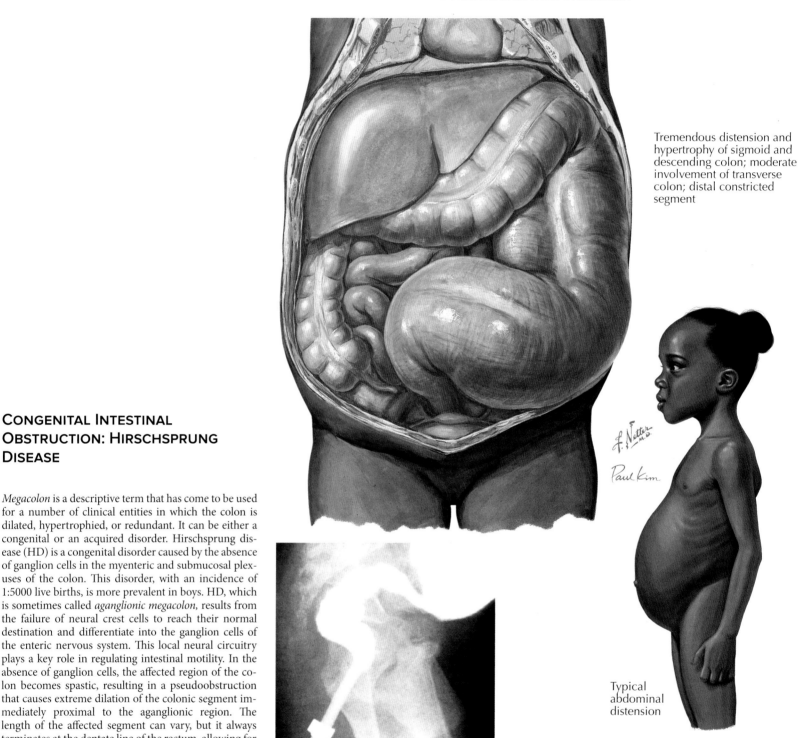

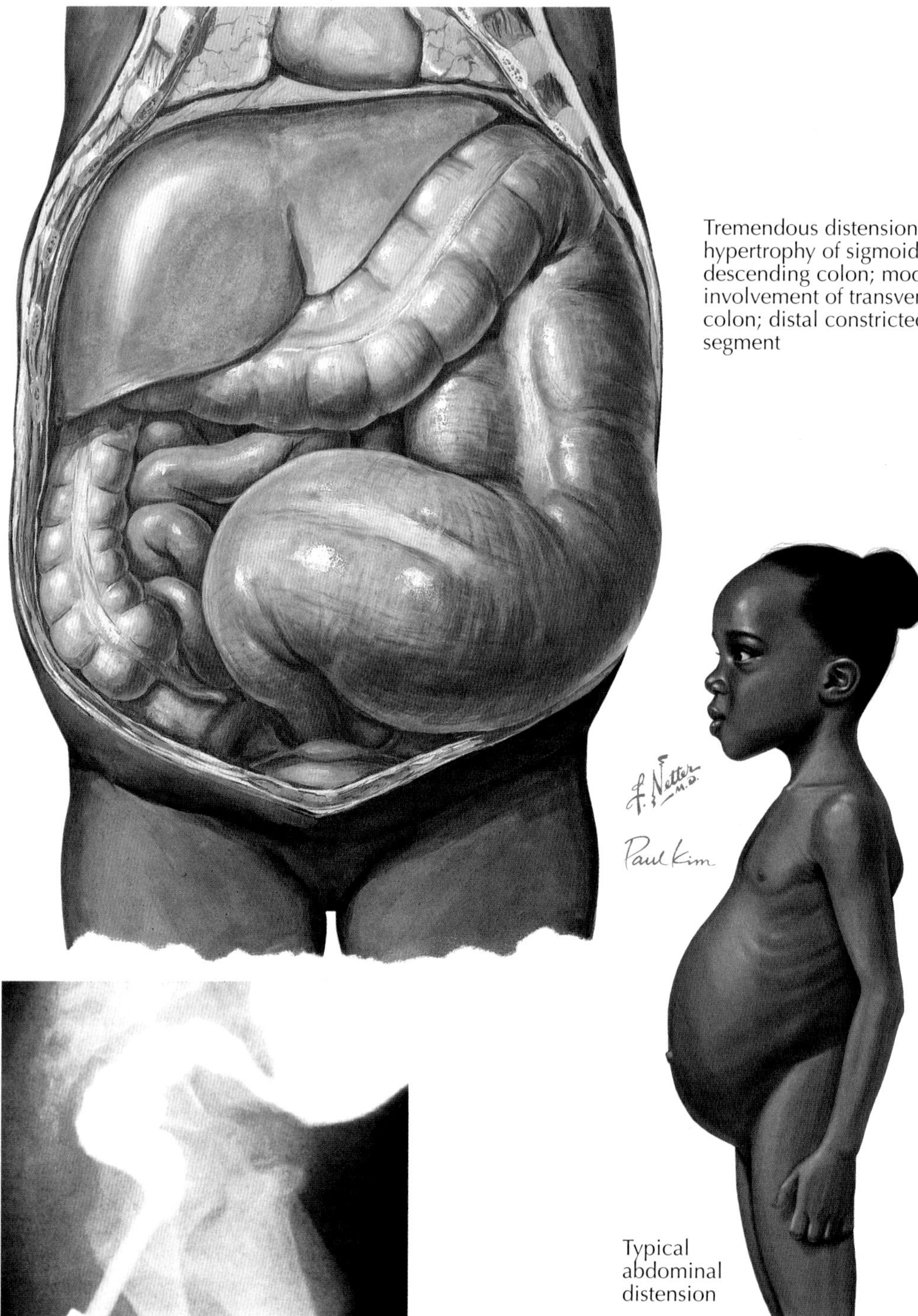

Typical Distension and Hypertrophy
Tremendous distension and hypertrophy of sigmoid and descending colon; moderate involvement of transverse colon; distal constricted segment
F. Netter M.D.
Paul Kim
Typical abdominal distension


Barium enema; characteristic distal constricted segment

## Congenital Intestinal Obstruction: Hirschsprung Disease

*Megacolon* is a descriptive term that has come to be used for a number of clinical entities in which the colon is dilated, hypertrophied, or redundant. It can be either a congenital or an acquired disorder. Hirschsprung disease (HD) is a congenital disorder caused by the absence of ganglion cells in the myenteric and submucosal plexuses of the colon. This disorder, with an incidence of 1:5000 live births, is more prevalent in boys. HD, which is sometimes called *aganglionic megacolon,* results from the failure of neural crest cells to reach their normal destination and differentiate into the ganglion cells of the enteric nervous system. This local neural circuitry plays a key role in regulating intestinal motility. In the absence of ganglion cells, the affected region of the colon becomes spastic, resulting in a pseudoobstruction that causes extreme dilation of the colonic segment immediately proximal to the aganglionic region. The length of the affected segment can vary, but it always terminates at the dentate line of the rectum, allowing for minimally invasive biopsies to be performed.

Diagnoses of HD are usually made in the neonatal period (>80%) in a child presenting with bilious emesis, abdominal distension, and a failure to pass meconium during the first 48 hours. In older children, constipation is the symptom that drives parents to seek medical advice. Severe functional constipation brings far more children to medical attention than does HD, and the differential diagnosis requires discrimination between these two conditions. Although great variations in clinical signs and symptoms are expected, the typical situations are readily categorized. The child with chronic functional constipation usually appears healthy and is reaching growth milestones, whereas the child with HD is more likely to be chronically ill, have a protuberant abdomen, and exhibit signs of malnutrition in growth and development. Children with HD often have a history of delayed passage of meconium (>36 hours) after birth. Frequently, the history includes a statement that the child has "never had a normal bowel movement." Enemas, laxatives, and other therapies are not effective. Occasionally, "diarrhea" has been noted, which is better described as liquid bowel content seeping around a fecal impaction. Unlike functional constipation, HD is never associated with passage of very large caliber stools.

On physical examination, the functionally constipated child has a relatively normal abdomen, in which firm fecal masses may be felt in the sigmoid colon. On rectal examination, the sphincter may be normal or loose, and feces are encountered at the sphincter or, if the bowel has recently been evacuated, the rectal ampulla may seem to have a large capacity. The child with

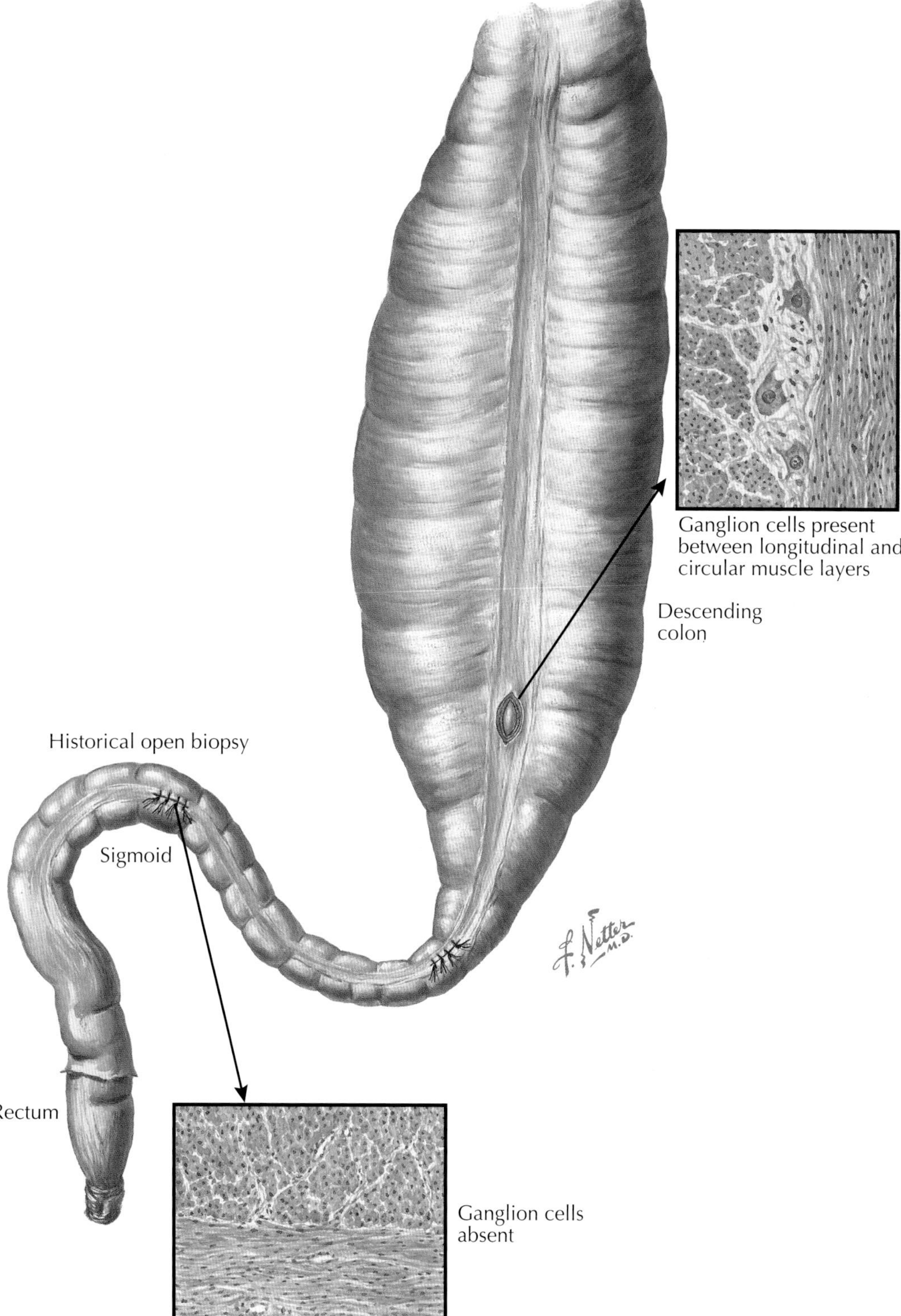


## Congenital Intestinal Obstruction: Hirschsprung Disease (Continued)

HD, on the other hand, has a large abdomen, and its musculature is somewhat lacking in tone. Tremendous fecal impaction of the bowel is palpable. Rectal examination reveals a tight sphincter; the rectal canal is often empty and of normal caliber, and if feces can be felt at all, they are typically encountered high up at the rectosigmoid/rectal ampulla junction.

On the basis of the history, signs, and symptoms, the diagnostician can distinguish most HD from chronic constipation. Plain radiograph and barium enema may be helpful. Contrast enema examinations will be normal in the first 3 months of life and can be normal in appearance with total colonic disease. In HD, the barium enters a colon of normal caliber and flows a short or long distance to a point where a sudden transition to an enlarged colon occurs. This transition is abrupt and may occur at any point in the large bowel. In the typical case, the aganglionic segment is distal and does not extend proximal to the splenic flexure. On attempted evacuation in the patient with HD, most of the barium remains behind, and the transition is prominent because peristalsis is normal to that point but absent distal to it.

Anorectal manometry can be performed; in HD, there will be an absence of the rectoanal inhibitory reflex. This reflex normally represents relaxation of the internal anal sphincter with air insufflation. Biopsy is diagnostic and, in contrast to the historical approach shown in Plate 3.28, should be performed at least 2 cm above the anal verge because the normal distal rectum may be physiologically hypoganglionic or aganglionic. This minimally invasive procedure can be performed without anesthesia because of the absence of somatic innervation in this region. The diagnosis of HD is confirmed by the absence of ganglion cells, the presence of thickened nerve fibers, and increased cholinesterase staining.

The only current treatment that alleviates the clinical syndrome of HD is surgery. There are several surgical approaches described in the literature. Recently there has been a trend toward performing a single-stage surgical repair in the neonatal period without the need for a colostomy. There are now three variations of this basic surgical procedure. In the original Swenson procedure, the bowel is dissected to the distended portion, and biopsies are examined by frozen section to identify ganglionic colon proximal to the transitional zone. The aganglionic segment is then pulled through, and

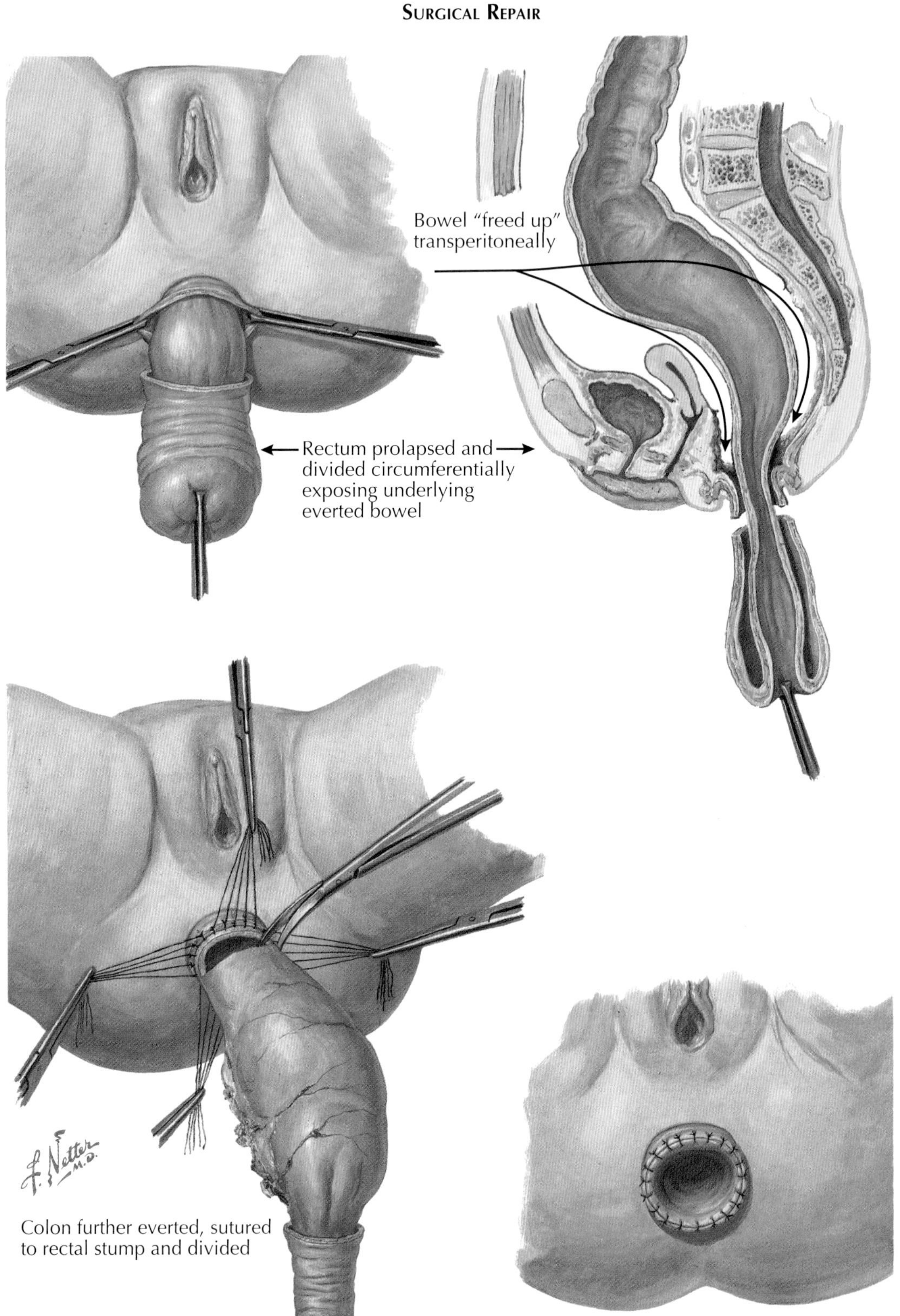
Surgical Repair
Bowel "freed up" transperitoneally
Rectum prolapsed and divided circumferentially exposing underlying everted bowel
Colon further everted, sutured to rectal stump and divided
Rectal and colonic mucosa approximated

## Congenital Intestinal Obstruction: Hirschsprung Disease (Continued)

healthy colon is anastomosed above the dentate line, after which the aganglionic segment is resected. In the Soave procedure, dissection is done in the plane between the submucosa and muscularis layers of the colon, leaving a cuff of muscle around the pull-through segment. The muscular cuff is transected to prevent spastic contraction. Lastly, in the Duhamel procedure, the ganglionic segment is dropped down and anastomosed posterior to the aganglionic native rectum, creating a pouch-like structure. Recent evidence suggests that Duhamel is the procedure of choice for long-segment HD (aganglionosis proximal to the descending-sigmoid colon junction) or total colonic HD. There remains controversy about the relative merits and shortcomings of these procedures. Proponents of the newer procedures believe that they are more likely to preserve sacral outflow and sphincter function, thereby preventing incontinence. Advocates of the Swenson procedure counter that there is little risk of iatrogenic injury if the plane of dissection is kept close to the rectum. Depending on the preference and experience of the surgeon, these procedures can either be performed with laparoscopic assistance or entirely via a transanal approach.

Although surgical repair of HD has markedly improved in recent years, there is still significant morbidity in these patients, depending on the length of the aganglionic segment and the surgical repair technique. These include fecal incontinence, constipation, and susceptibility to enterocolitis. As an alternative approach to surgery, there are a number of studies underway examining the ability of stem cells to reconstitute the enteric nervous system in an aganglionic segment of the colon. Sources of cells for transplant being studied include pluripotent stem cells derived from the central nervous system, neural crest, or enteric nervous system. Following transplantation, it has been demonstrated that stem cells can survive, proliferate, and differentiate into enteric neurons. Although considerable obstacles remain, these studies provide hope for the eventual development of stem cell therapies as a nonsurgical alternative in the treatment of HD.

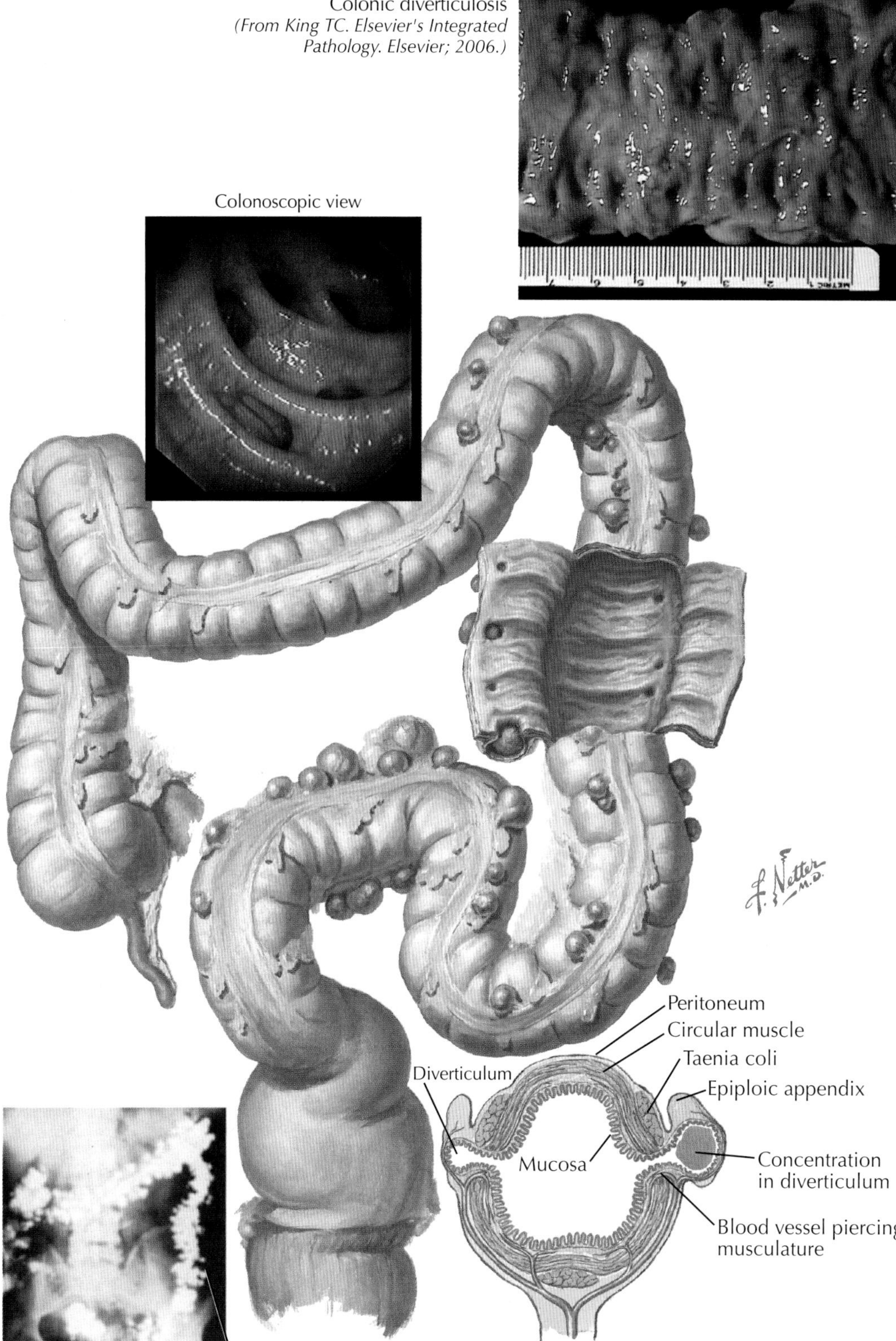


## Diverticulosis of Colon

Diverticulosis of the colon is an acquired condition that results from herniation of the mucosa through defects in the muscle coats. The defects are usually located at sites where the blood vessels pierce the muscular wall to gain access to the submucous plane. These vessels, the *long circular arteries,* enter at a very constant position just on the *mesenteric side of the two lateral taeniae coli,* so diverticula commonly occur in two parallel rows along the bowel. The *appendices epiploicae* are also situated in this part of the circumference; thus diverticula frequently enter the base of the appendices epiploicae.

Diverticula are thought to arise from weak areas in the wall of the colon and a differential in pressure between the lumen and the serosa. Localized areas of high pressure may be susceptible to their formation. A defect in cholinergic innervation may contribute as well. Obesity and constipation may be aggravating factors but are not the primary causes.

*Diverticula* do not occur in the rectum but may be found throughout the *whole length of the colon.* They are more common on the left side and most frequently affect the sigmoid colon. Diverticulosis is rare before age 40 years, but its incidence increases with age, and it occurs in about 10% of persons of middle age, being more common in males. After age 40 years, diverticula become more prevalent in females.

Diverticula of the colon are flask shaped, with a narrow neck through the muscle wall and a wider body. Because the wall lacks a muscular layer, diverticula are actually “pseudodiverticula”; they are unable to expel any fecal material that enters them, and the material tends to harden within the sacs into firm *concretions.* The mucosa of the diverticulum may become ulcerated or devascularized by the hard fecalith, and organisms may enter the tissues and cause infection, which leads to the various forms of diverticulitis.

The diagnosis of diverticulosis is commonly made by colonoscopy but may be demonstrated on CT scan or contrast study. Contrast studies are most useful in cases where there is concern for large bowel obstruction from a diverticular inflammatory stricture. Contrast studies help differentiate between complete and partial large bowel obstructions. Clinically, diverticulosis is a symptomless condition, with symptoms arising in about 10% to 20% of cases. No active treatment is usually recommended for the patient with incidentally discovered diverticulosis. The most common symptom to be aware of for diverticulosis is painless bleeding, as it is one of the most common causes of lower gastrointestinal bleeds.

## DIVERTICULITIS

Inflammation in and around the diverticula occurs in only a small percentage of patients with diverticulosis. The manner in which infection may arise is discussed in Plate 3.30. Once infection occurs around one or more diverticula, the subsequent course varies according to the virulence of the organism and the resistance of the patient. Acute inflammation, in which all structures of the intestinal wall participate, may follow and terminate in perforation, leading to general peritonitis; more commonly, a localized abscess forms, sealed off by the abdominal wall, omentum, epiploicae, and other viscera. A more usual course is that of a low-grade inflammatory process *(peridiverticulitis),* which leads to the formation of *fibrofatty tissue around the affected part* of the bowel, resulting in *narrowing* of its *lumen,* shortening of the loop, and adherence of the loop to nearby structures. This thickening may extend over several inches of bowel, giving rise to a firm, tender mass along the line of the colon. Within this thickened tissue, infection persists, and recurrent activity of inflammation may lead to the further extension of small *abscesses,* which may open into the organs walling off the infection. In this way, *fistulae* may form to *the anterior abdominal wall, the bladder, small bowel,* or female pelvic organs.

The complications that may follow diverticulitis are, therefore, obstruction of the colon, more usually partial and chronic than complete; free perforation and general peritonitis; abscess formation; and the occurrence of internal or external fistulae. The most common is the formation of a *vesicocolic fistula,* which gives rise to persistent infection of the urinary tract; it rarely occurs in females because of the interposition of the uterus.

Clinically, acute diverticulitis presents with pyrexia and pain in the left lower quadrant of the abdomen, and examination will reveal a tender mass in that area, the lower edge of which may also be palpable per rectum. Patients with chronic diverticulitis usually report dull or recurrent pain in the same region, often associated with some alteration of bowel habits, a sense of distension, and dyspepsia. Bleeding is unusual but is said to occur in about 10% of patients. Examination may reveal some tender enlargement of the sigmoid colon, and sigmoidoscopy may show rigidity and edema of the bowel above the rectosigmoid junction. Should a vesicocolic fistula form, the classic symptom is *pneumaturia,* often associated with pain on micturition and with frequency of urination. An enterocolic fistula may give rise to severe diarrhea. If the patient is stable, a CT scan is performed to determine the extent of the disease.

Diverticulitis is broken down into simple and complex disease. Simple diverticulitis includes peridiverticular inflammation, whereas complicated disease includes diverticular abscess, fistula, and purulent or feculent peritonitis. For simple disease, antibiotics do not improve the outcomes and are not recommended. Antibiotics are indicated in patients with complicated disease, signs of systemic inflammatory response, and significant comorbidities.

Complicated diverticulitis can be treated nonoperatively, but there is a high risk of recurrence and a discussion of an immediate or elective colectomy is necessary.

Treatment for a diverticular abscess requires antibiotics and source control of the infection with a drain placed by interventional radiologic or surgical means. There is a high treatment failure with antibiotics alone in abscesses greater than 3 cm in size. Once the initial infection has resolved, a colonoscopy is performed due to the concern for malignancy leading to the perforation as opposed to a perforated diverticulum. The incidence of malignancy found on colonoscopy done for complicated diverticulitis follow-up is 8% to 10%.

For frank perforation with diffuse peritonitis and pneumoperitoneum, an immediate colectomy is indicated. For purulent peritonitis, a colectomy with anastomosis and proximal diversion can be performed, but a colectomy with colostomy is also an acceptable alternative. For feculent peritonitis, often a Hartmann's procedure (colectomy, colostomy, and oversewing of distal stump) is indicated.

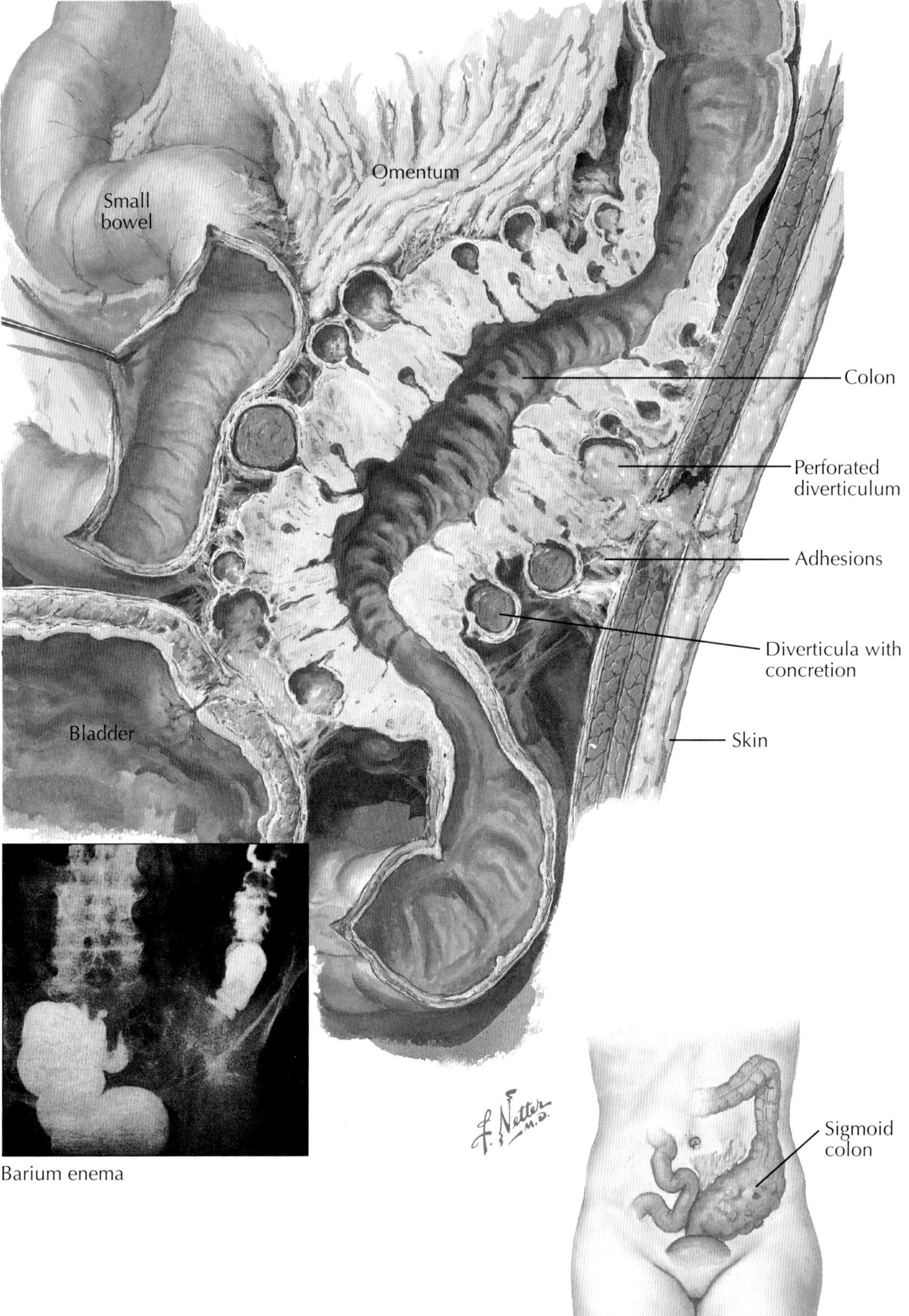


Barium enema

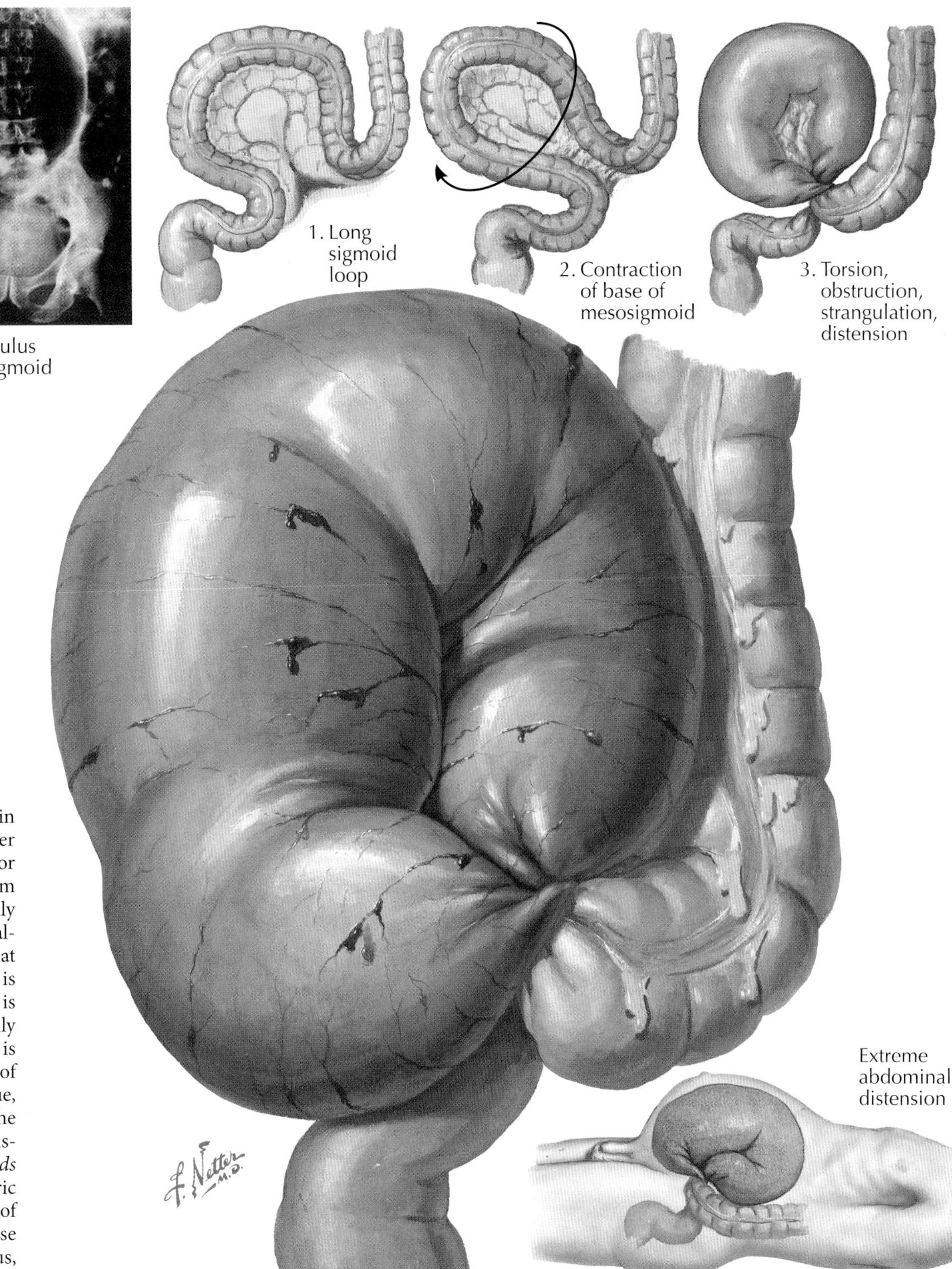


## VOLVULUS OF SIGMOID

Primary volvulus of the colon typically occurs only in the sigmoid colon and in the cecum, because the other parts of the large bowel are well fixed to the posterior abdominal wall. Volvulus is a comparatively rare form of intestinal obstruction in the Western world, usually occurring in patients who are elderly or institutionalized, commonly with neuropsychiatric disorders that predispose a patient to have larger stool burden. It is more common in Eastern Europe and Asia, and it is probable that the difference in incidence is due mainly to different dietary habits. A bulky vegetable diet is more common in less-developed and poorer parts of the world, and this diet results in a bigger fecal residue, which leads to a persistently loaded colon. In time, the loaded *sigmoid colon* may become chronically distended and *elongated,* and, as it elongates, its *two ends* tend to *approximate,* resulting in a narrower mesenteric attachment. Some fibrosis often occurs in the base of the mesosigmoid, accentuating the *narrow base.* These are the essential predisposing features of a volvulus, and, once they exist, the actual precipitating cause is often trivial, such as straining or coughing.

In its early stages a volvulus produces a "check-valve" effect, allowing flatus and some fluid feces to enter the loop but not allowing them to leave it. In this way, great and rapid distension is produced. If the twist becomes tighter, a complete "closed-loop" obstruction develops, and pressure on the vessels in the mesentery may lead to impairment of blood supply and *gangrene of the bowel.*

Clinically, the onset of the symptoms and signs of a sigmoid volvulus is usually sudden, with lower abdominal pain; constipation is absolute, but sometimes tenesmus with passage of a little mucus may occur. Vomiting is unusual. The general condition is commonly well maintained unless infarction and gangrene of the loop have started, in which case blood and fluid loss soon lead to shock. Distension occurs early, progresses rapidly, and is always a dominant part of the clinical picture; within a few hours it may be extreme, and no other features may be observed on abdominal examination.

The most valuable aid to diagnosis is plain radiograph of the abdomen, with the patient in both the erect and supine positions. A single, enormous, gas-filled loop containing a little fluid is usually revealed, giving a characteristic picture known as the *coffee bean sign.* Contrast enema may reveal a *bird's beak deformity* at the point of the volvulus and may also be therapeutic. CT scan may demonstrate a mesenteric whirl.

## Volvulus of Cecum

Volvulus of the cecum is an infrequent condition in the Western part of the world, accounting for only about 1% of the cases of intestinal obstruction. Like volvulus of the sigmoid colon, it appears to be more common in those parts of the world in which vegetables and roughage form a greater part of the diet, and it is thought that persistent loading of the bowel with a heavy fecal burden may also play a part in causing this condition. Cecal volvulus is also seen more commonly in patients with a history of chronic constipation, use of cathartics, pregnancy, or prior surgery. This problem occurs more commonly in females but can occur in any age group, with a mean age of presentation in the fourth decade.

The predisposing factor is *inadequate fixation of the cecum* and ascending colon to the posterior abdominal wall. Normally, in the third stage of intestinal rotation, the cecum descends from the subhepatic region to lie in the right iliac fossa, and the ascending colon and most of the cecum become fixed to the posterior abdominal wall. If this last process is not fully completed, the cecum, a few inches of ascending colon, and a few inches of terminal ileum may be attached by a mesentery with a relatively short base and may then be free to rotate around this axis. Should a twist occur, all of these parts of the intestine are involved, and the condition should really be called *volvulus of the ileocecal segment*.

As in volvulus of the sigmoid, the twist may not be tight at first and may untwist spontaneously. At this stage, the *check-valve effect* will tend to lead to rapid distension of the cecum. If the twist becomes tighter, complete closed-loop obstruction is produced, and, finally, strangulation of the vessels will result in *gangrene of the bowel,* which is likely to occur more rapidly with a volvulus of the cecum than with that of the sigmoid.

The onset is sudden, with severe central abdominal pain, and vomiting soon follows. The pain is constant, but intermittent "griping" pains also occur. Examination reveals some general abdominal distension as a result of an obstruction in the lower part of the small intestine, and in most cases the distended cecum may be distinguished as a palpable tympanitic swelling in the central part of the abdomen. On palpation a feeling of emptiness in the right iliac fossa may be encountered. The most valuable aid to diagnosis is the plain radiograph. If the radiograph has been taken with the patient in an erect position, the greatly distended kidney bean–shaped area, with perhaps a fluid level within it, is very conspicuous; distension of loops of ileum above the point of obstruction may also be recognizable. CT scan may show a whirl of the mesentery as in sigmoid volvulus. In the case of cecal volvulus, contrast enema can be performed to rule out a distal obstructing lesion but is contraindicated for reduction.

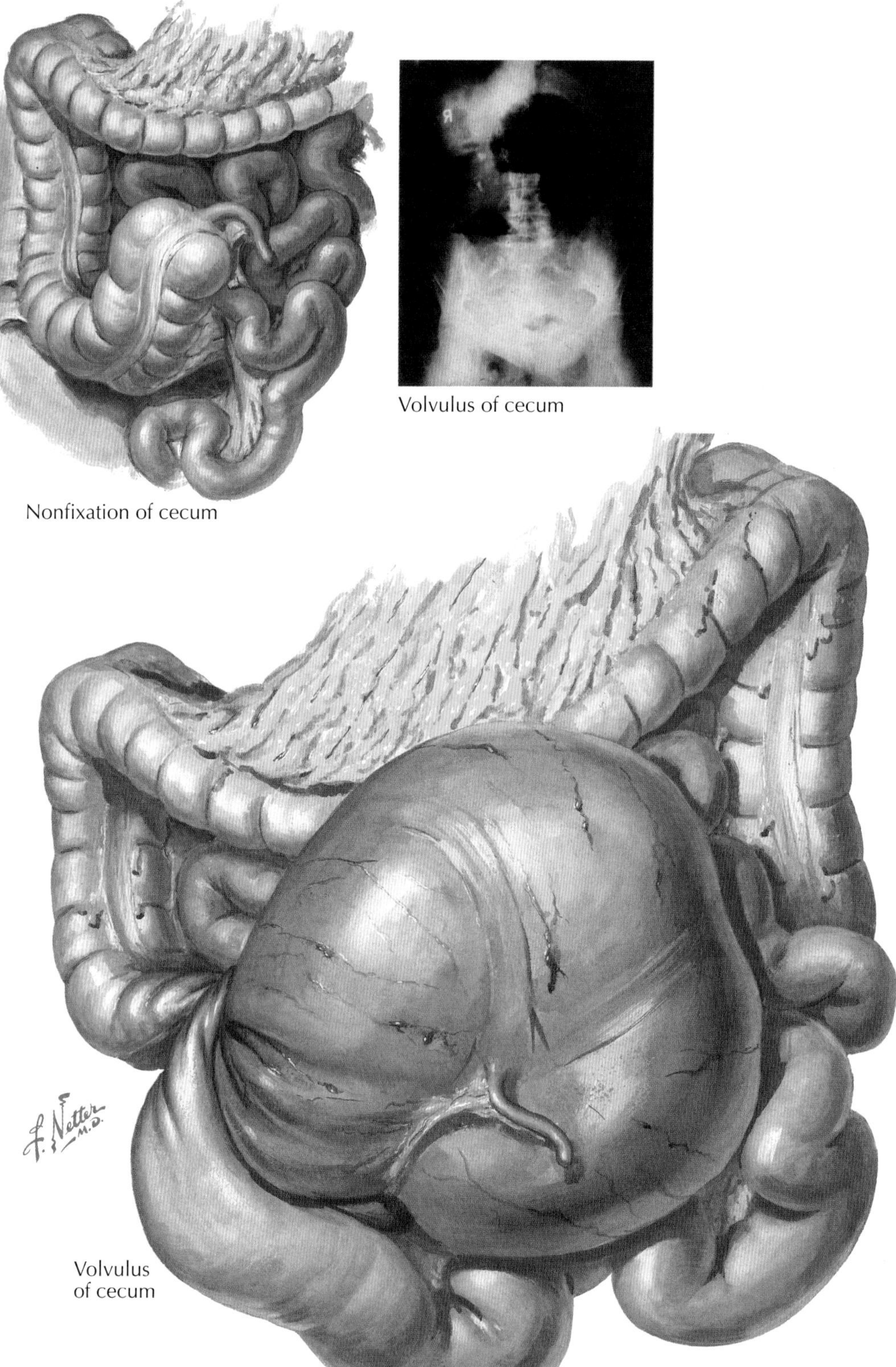

Nonfixation of cecum

Volvulus of cecum

Volvulus of cecum

Nonoperative management of cecal volvulus is much less successful than sigmoid volvulus. Less than 30% of patients have successful colonoscopic decompression. There should also be concern about insufflating gas into the obstructed segment, which may cause the ischemia to worsen. As soon as the diagnosis of cecal volvulus is made, a laparotomy is typically indicated. If possible, the bowel should be untwisted. Given the high recurrence rate of 30% to 40% with suturing the cecum to the abdominal wall, a resection of the involved bowel with anastomosis is the wiser course. If the patient has many comorbidities with high risk for severe complications, an ileostomy and mucous fistula are performed.

Cases of partial volvulus with spontaneous untwisting occur, giving rise to recurrent attacks of lower abdominal pain. In such instances, the diagnosis may be difficult, but the cause of the repeated attacks usually becomes apparent if laparotomy is undertaken; resection of the cecum will prevent further attacks.

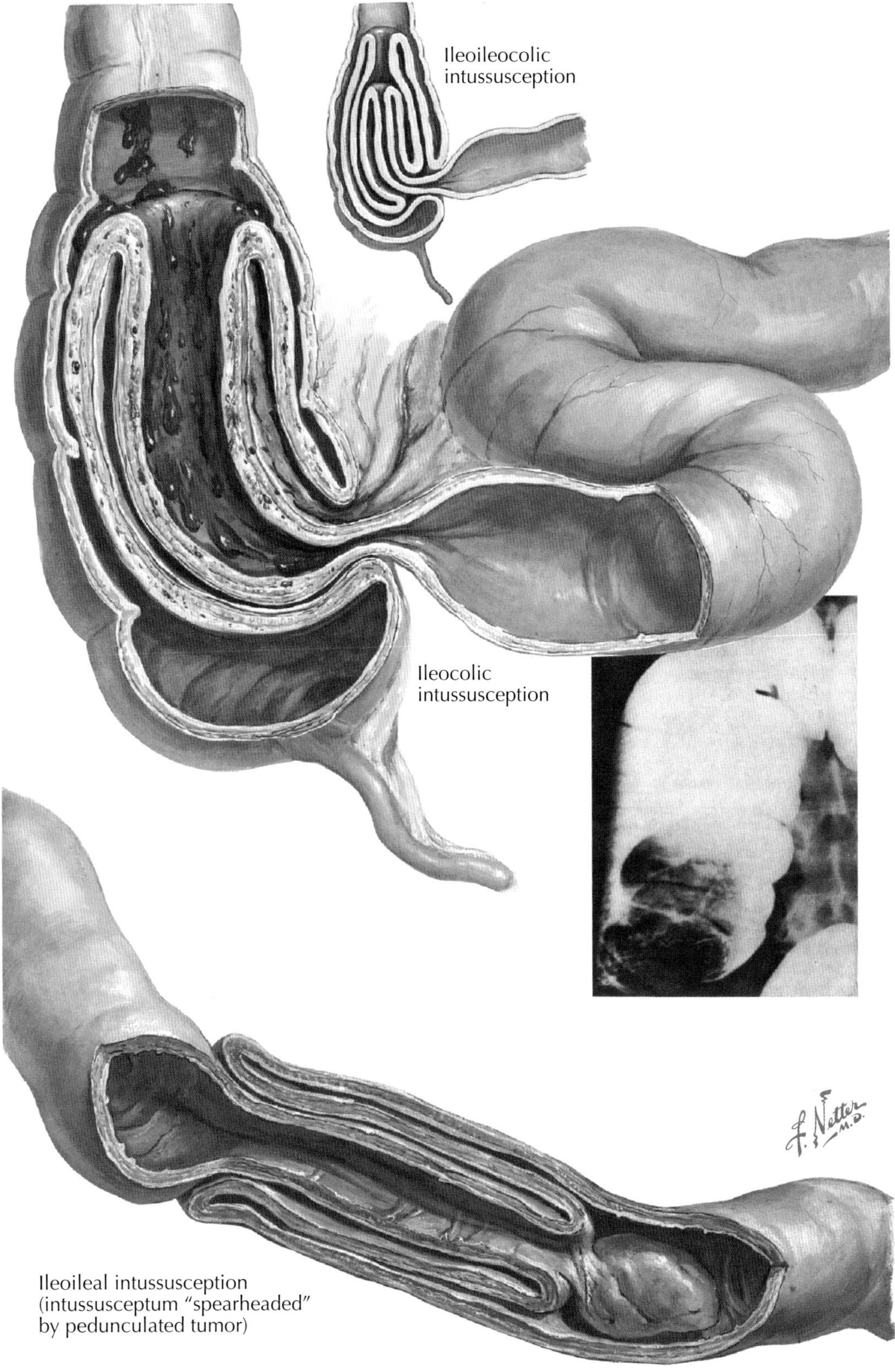


## INTUSSUSCEPTION

Intussusception is, by definition, the invagination of a portion of the intestine into the contiguous distal segment of the enteric tube. Much has been speculated about the cause of this condition. The fact that intussusception occurs more frequently at 4 to 10 months of age suggests that the change from a pure milk diet to a more solid one plays a role by altering intestinal peristalsis in such a way that the intussusception is initiated. Acute enteritis, allergic reactions, and intestinal spasms—in short, any condition with hypermotility—may result in an invagination. In older individuals it may be a lead point, such as a *polyp,* a malignancy, an enlarged Peyer's patch, or Meckel diverticulum that may mark the site at which the wall of the proximal segment turns and intrudes into its neighboring distal part. Whatever the etiologic factor may be, it remains undiscovered in more than 90% of cases.

Intussusceptions are described according to the part of the digestive tube that telescopes the intussusceptum into the intussuscipiens; that is, the receiving part. Thus one may encounter an *ileoileal invagination,* jejunoileal invagination, and so on. *Ileocolic (ileocecal) intussusception* is the most frequent location in the pediatric population. A kind of double invagination or an intussusception within an intussusception (e.g., *ileoileocolic intussusception*) may also occur. How far the intussusceptum enters the intussuscipiens depends on the length and motility of its mesentery, which, furthermore, is easily compressed and then causes the development of edema, peritoneal exudation, vascular strangulation, and, finally, intestinal gangrene.

The clinical manifestations of the disease are almost always alarming and usually begin rather suddenly in children who are generally normal, well developed, and well nourished. Colicky abdominal pains recur, as a rule, at intervals of 15 to 20 minutes and are accompanied by signs of acute shock, with the child becoming extremely pallid. During the intervals, the patient seems to recover, relaxes, and behaves as if nothing had happened. In about 85% of cases, a movable mass may be palpated in the abdomen. In the more advanced stage of the disease, bloody stools are found, the sudden appearance of which may be considered pathognomonic. In children, diagnosis can be made with ultrasound. An air contrast enema is then often performed if there is no peritonitis, which is usually successful at reducing the intussusception. No further intervention is required if the condition resolves.

In adults, the presentation is variable, and the classic signs seen in children of bloody diarrhea, mass, and pain are not typically seen. Many will present with symptoms of a partial bowel obstruction, often with recurrent attacks. Barium enema may show a lesion, but CT scan is the most accurate method of diagnosis. The classic target sign or sausage-like mass is characteristically seen. Surgical resection is necessary given the concern for a malignant tumor acting as the lead point. Primary anastomosis is typically feasible with minimal complications. Resection is typically performed in those patients who have a spontaneous reduction of their intussusception preoperatively. Intraoperative reduction may facilitate a limited resection, particularly when the lesion is known to be benign preoperatively.

In general, the prognosis of this disease is favorable. The mortality rates after laparotomy and resection have decreased significantly in recent decades and will improve further with the ability to arrive at an early diagnosis and with increasing knowledge of supportive therapy.

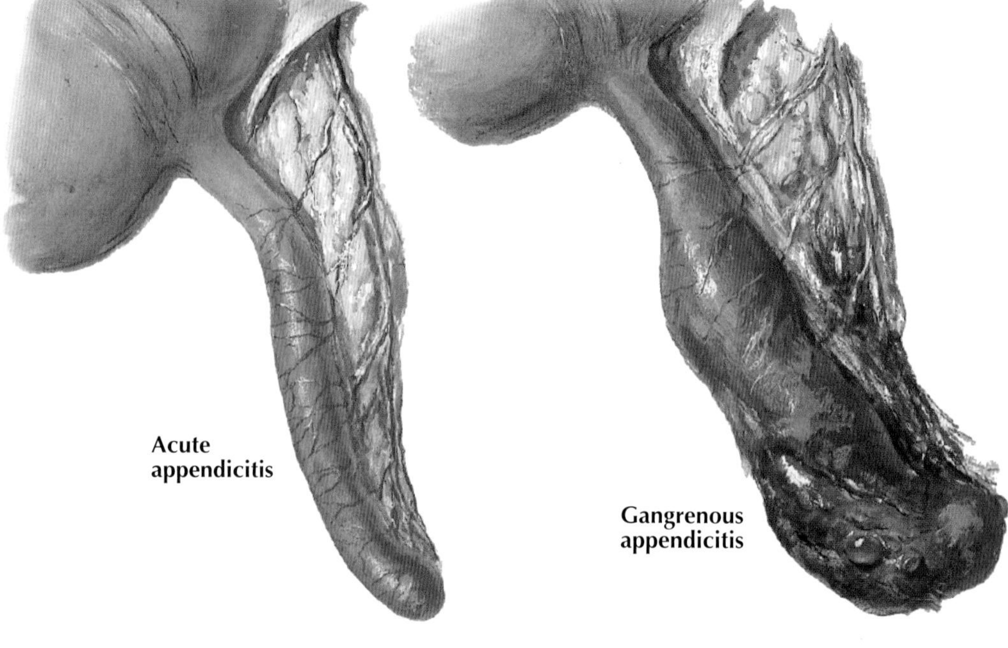


# Diseases of Appendix

## ACUTE APPENDICITIS

Acute appendicitis is a common surgical emergency and a frequent cause of an acute abdomen.

The vermiform appendix is located near the ileocecal valve and at the base of the cecum. Although the base of the appendix is always attached to the cecum, its tip may migrate to different positions. These variations can complicate the clinical presentation of appendicitis with regard to pain location.

Acute appendicitis starts with inflammation of the lining of the vermiform appendix and can progress with inflammation of the submucosa and the other layers. The appendix appears thickened and enlarged, and the lumen is filled with mucopurulent material. Abscess formation and perforation with peritonitis may follow.

The incidence is highest in the second and third decades of life. It is also higher in males than females.

Infection and obstruction are the most important inciting factors. Obstruction of the appendiceal lumen has been proposed as the initial step in the pathogenesis of appendicitis. This can increase the intraluminal pressure, with subsequent occlusion of the small vessels, leading to ischemia and necrosis of the appendix. Inflammation, followed by ischemia, perforation with subsequent development of an abscess, or generalized peritonitis, may follow.

The classic presentation consists of anorexia, periumbilical abdominal pain that subsequently migrates to the right lower quadrant (pain location may vary), nausea, and vomiting. A change in bowel habits can be seen in some patients. Fever, abdominal tenderness, rebound tenderness, guarding, and rigidity are some of the physical examination findings.

Although there is no specific laboratory test for appendicitis, the following can help confirm the diagnosis or exclude other possible diagnoses: complete blood count, C-reactive protein, urinalysis (to differentiate from urinary tract infection), and liver and pancreas chemistry tests. In females of childbearing age, a pregnancy test should be considered, with recognition that acute appendicitis is one of the most common surgical emergencies in pregnancy.

Urologic and gynecologic conditions, CD, acute infectious ileitis, and diverticulitis should be considered in the differential diagnosis of patients presenting with the symptoms of acute appendicitis.

Imaging studies play a major role in the diagnosis of acute appendicitis. Ultrasonography is a safe imaging modality to confirm the diagnosis of appendicitis. A healthy appendix cannot usually be seen with ultrasound, and an appendiceal diameter of more than 6 mm is an accurate finding for acute appendicitis. If ultrasound imaging is negative or inconclusive, a CT scan is usually obtained. CT scanning is the most important imaging test in the evaluation of patients with atypical presentations. MRI can also be considered in the evaluation of suspected appendicitis in pregnant females.

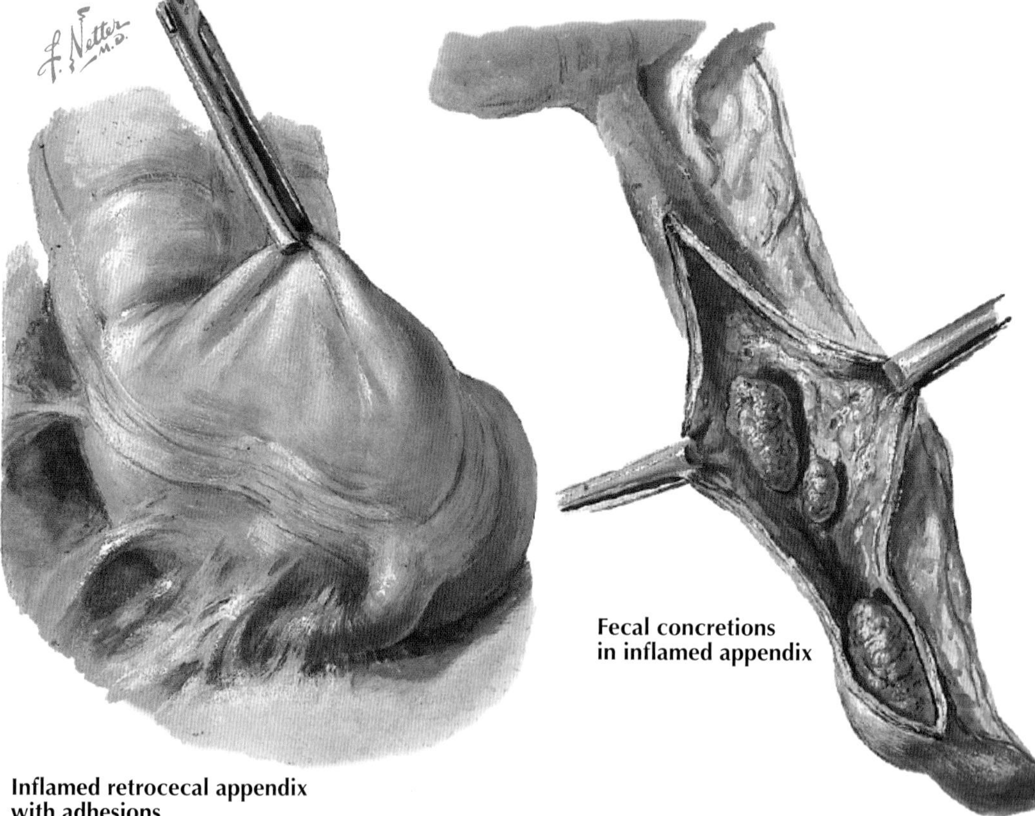


Treatment of appendicitis includes supportive management with intravenous hydration, analgesia, antibiotics, and evaluation to determine the need for, and timing of, any surgical intervention. Patients with nonperforated appendicitis can be considered for nonoperative management with antibiotics, initially intravenous for 1 to 3 days followed by a 7- to 10-day course of

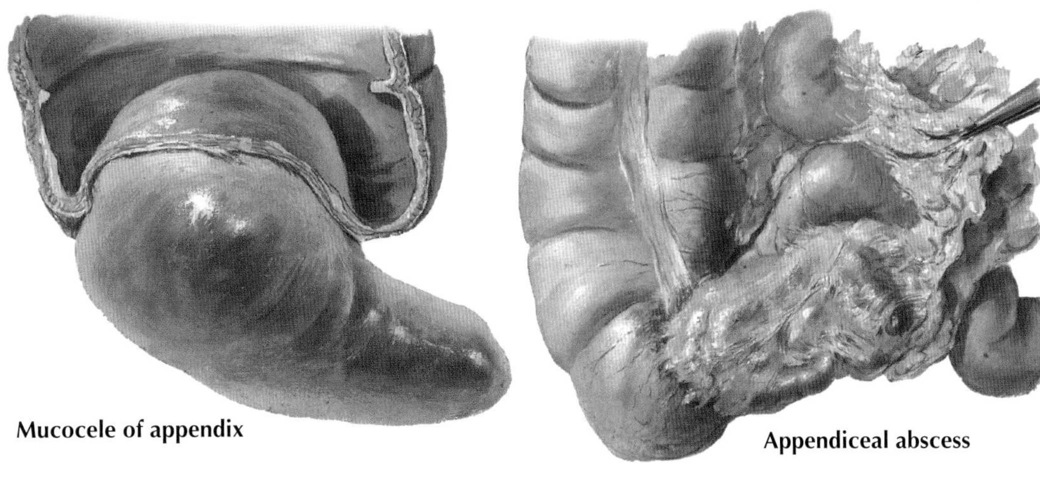

Mucocele of appendix

Appendiceal abscess

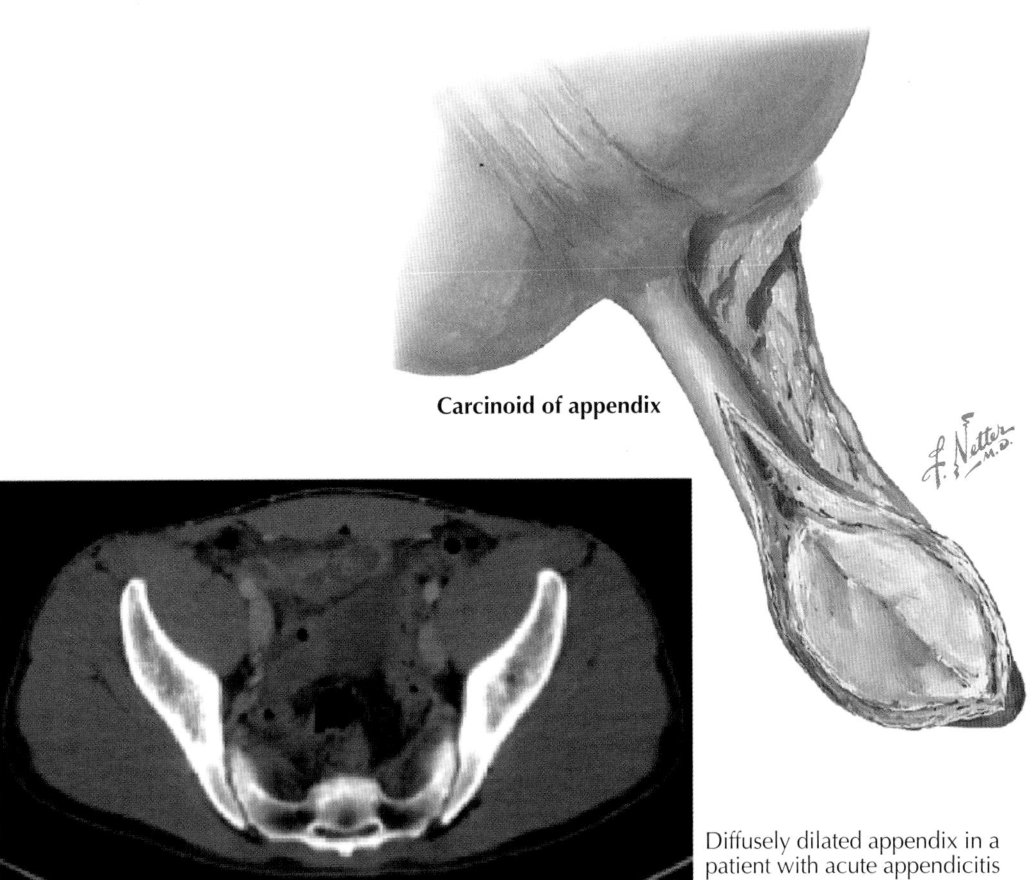

Carcinoid of appendix

Diffusely dilated appendix in a patient with acute appendicitis

## DISEASES OF APPENDIX (Continued)

oral antibiotics. Contraindications to the nonoperative approach include patients with diffuse peritonitis, hemodynamic instability or severe sepsis, pregnancy, immunocompromise, or history of inflammatory bowel disease (IBD) because this approach has not been well studied in these groups. Relative contraindications to nonoperative management are age >45 and presence of appendicolith. Nonoperative treatment has about a 70% 1-year success rate to avoid surgery. Appendectomy is the surgical treatment for appendicitis and is still the most common option. Appendectomy can be performed by either laparoscopy or open laparotomy; the decision is based on the surgeon's experience, patient's body habitus and age, and severity of the disease, among other factors. Percutaneous drainage of an abscess followed by appendectomy in 6 to 8 weeks is needed in some cases.

### CHRONIC APPENDICITIS

Patients with chronic appendicitis have prolonged (>7 days) symptoms. The white blood cell count is usually normal. Appendectomy resolves the pain in most patients.

### APPENDICEAL NEOPLASMS

The incidence of appendiceal tumors in appendectomy specimens is approximately 1%. The most common tumors include carcinoid tumors, cystic neoplasms, and adenocarcinoma but, rarely, nonepithelial tumors (neuroma, lipoma, leiomyoma, lymphoma, and others) can be seen in the appendix.

### CARCINOID TUMOR

Carcinoid tumors, which are neuroendocrine tumors, are the most common appendiceal tumors. Some secrete serotonin or other vasoactive substances, which can play a role in the associated clinical symptoms. Appendectomy is the standard treatment in most cases; hemicolectomy is indicated if the lesion is larger than 2 cm or in cases of nodal involvement.

### CYSTIC NEOPLASMS

Mucoceles are characterized by a mucus-filled, distended appendix and can be benign or malignant. Surgical resection should be considered because of the possibility of harboring cystadenocarcinoma. Pseudomyxoma peritonei is a clinical syndrome resulting from mucin deposits within the peritoneal cavity. Repeated debulking surgeries are the standard treatment in most symptomatic patients.

### PRIMARY ADENOCARCINOMA

Although a minority of patients with acute appendicitis have adenocarcinoma, the majority of patients with adenocarcinoma present with acute appendicitis. Right hemicolectomy is usually the standard of care.

## Abdominal Wounds: Colon

Injuries to the colon are commonly iatrogenic or traumatic. Patients receiving certain medications may be more susceptible to spontaneous perforations of the colon. Other procedures, such as endoscopy, may be potential causes of perforation.

Angiogenesis, epidermal growth factor, phosphoinositide 3-kinase, and MEK inhibitors have been shown to be complicated by acute perforation of the GI tract. Deconditioning from malignancy with a lack of overt symptoms early and a resulting delay in treatment lead to high mortality rates when perforation occurs.

Colonoscopic polypectomy has a low rate of associated complications, with the majority of these being minor in severity. Perforation of the colon may occur because of maneuvering the colonoscope or from polypectomy. Often these perforations will become sealed off and can be managed nonoperatively in stable patients because these injuries occur in a mechanically clean bowel. Patients are initially managed with bowel rest, systemic antibiotics, and fluid resuscitation and are monitored clinically. If they have continued symptoms that do not respond to these measures, they will require surgical intervention. Typically, simple closure can be performed, but occasionally, segmental resection with primary anastomosis, with or without fecal diversion, is needed. Outcomes are best when the perforation is recognized within 24 hours. Overall, the mortality rate ranges from 2.9% to 25% in these cases. Laparoscopic and endoscopic repairs have also been performed for these complications.

Traumatic injuries to the colon can be blunt or penetrating. Blunt injuries to the colon are rare and are typically the result of motor vehicle collisions, assaults, or falls. Often, these injuries are diagnosed at the time of laparotomy for other injuries. The right colon is typically the most commonly injured segment. Penetrating trauma to the colon can occur in the civilian setting, typically the result of stabbings or gunshot wounds. Colonic injury is identified in approximately half of patients with penetrating hollow viscus injuries, and the transverse colon is the most commonly injured segment. Penetrating colonic injury can also occur in the setting of war. Mortality from these injuries has fallen significantly from the time of the American Civil War of 90% to approximately less than 5% in recent conflicts.

In patients who are victims of penetrating or blunt trauma with unrecognized colorectal injuries, the injuries can be significant causes of death. Being able to quickly identify an acute abdomen or pathologic condition that requires operative intervention is key to reducing the mortality rate in this patient population. Even in intubated patients, physical examination findings such as guarding or rebound should be apparent. Injuries of the colon vary from isolated bruised areas to large perforations or extensive, ragged tears, with infarction. In contrast to the small bowel, wounds of the colon are less likely to be multiple. Isolated bruised areas are occasionally found remote from the tract of the

**Exteriorization of Sigmoid Wound**

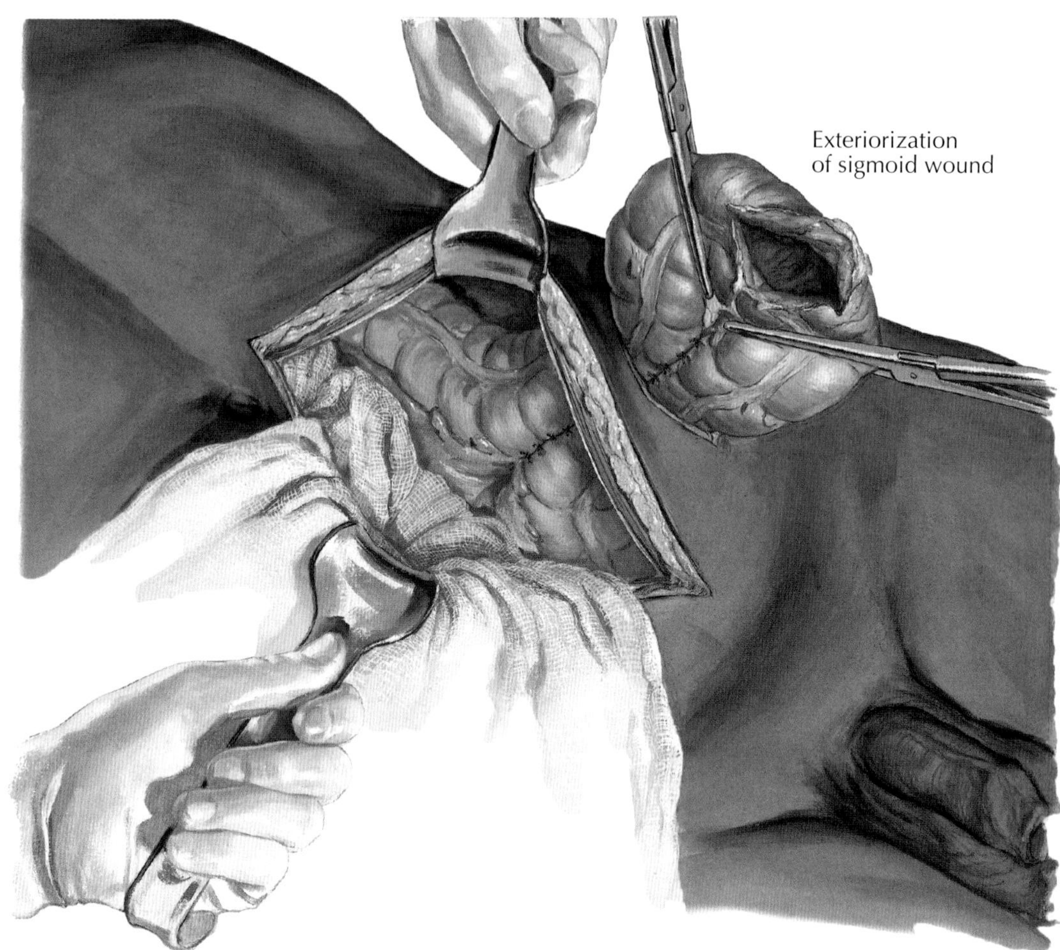


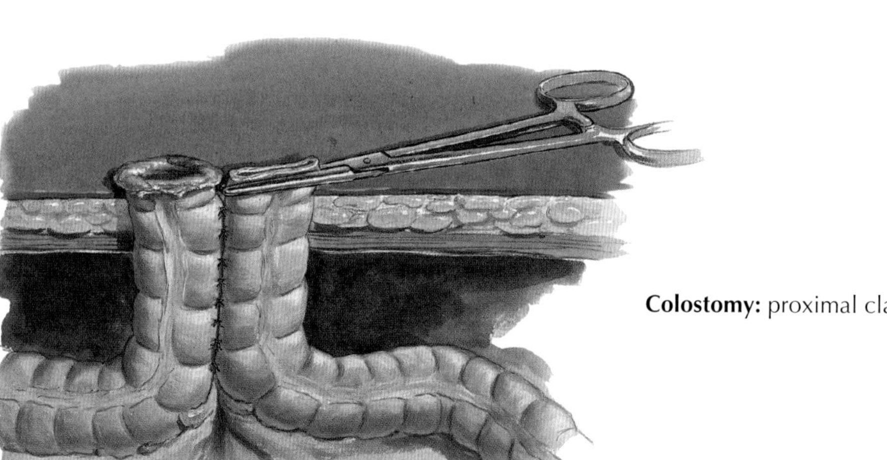

**Colostomy:** proximal clamp removed

Wound of Hepatic Flexure

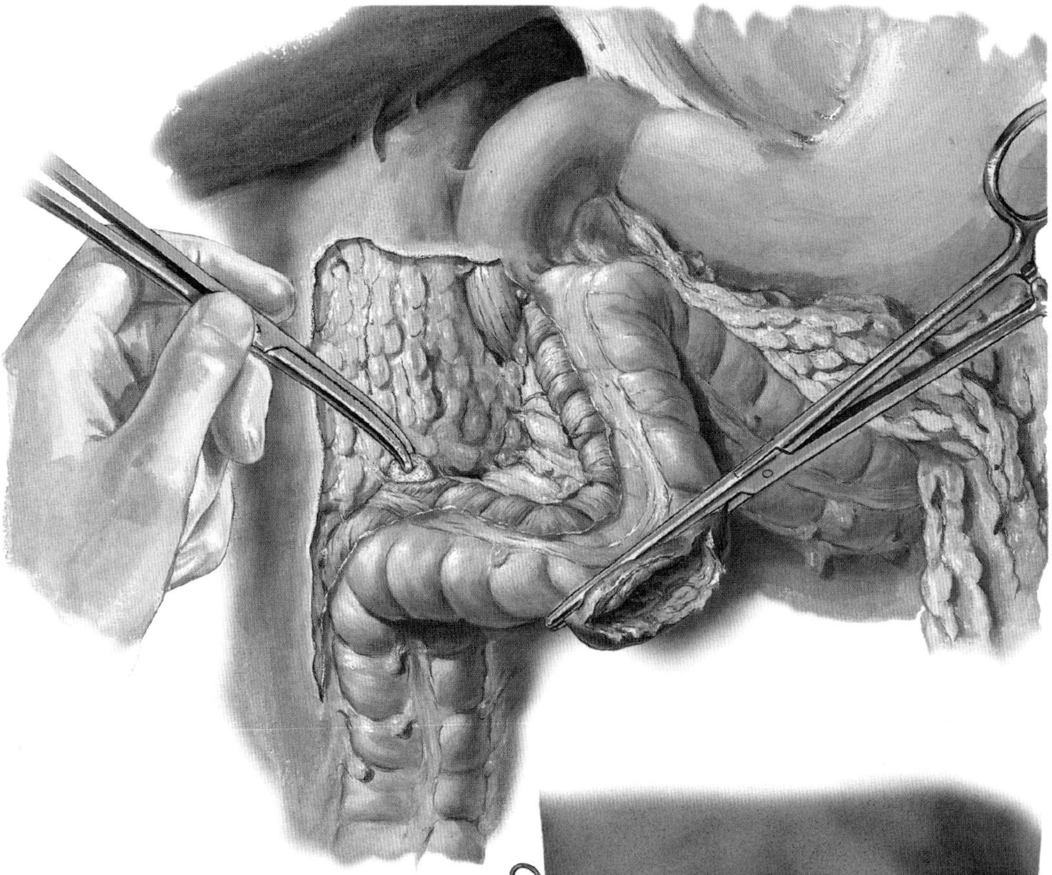

Wound of hepatic flexure: mobilization

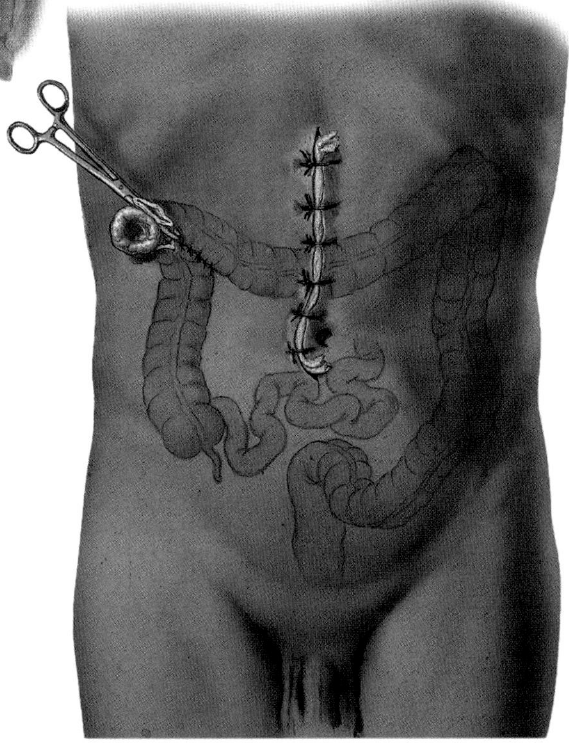

Colostomy after exteriorization

## Abdominal Wounds: Colon (Continued)

inflicting agent, and in some cases, the outer layer of the bowel wall will be found ruptured and stripped back from the intact mucosal layer. Multiple lesions, when present, usually involve the flexures and redundant colon within the pelvis. Small lesions involving the ascending and descending portions of the colon may be intraperitoneal or extraperitoneal and are particularly grave, because they may be easily overlooked and because of the vulnerability of the retroperitoneal tissues to anaerobic infection. Wounds of the colon are frequently associated with injuries to other viscera in the injured region.

The clinical symptoms of wounds of the colon and those of the small bowel are practically the same. Uncomplicated wounds and small perforations, especially if they are extraperitoneal, may cause few early symptoms, so that thorough exploration of a suspected area is essential. Shock is usually apparent if the wound is a large one.

In small, uncomplicated wounds involving the more distal part of the bowel, the prognosis is more favorable if spillage of semisolid fecal material is slight and if surgery is performed early.

If there is concern for an intraabdominal injury, broad-spectrum antibiotics should be given. Patients found to have pelvic fractures should elicit concern for associated colorectal injury. A digital rectal examination is essential for every patient with trauma to assess for a colorectal injury as well. For hemodynamically stable patients, CT scanning will provide a thorough assessment of the abdomen. Focused abdominal sonogram for trauma examination is a reliable assessment for patients who cannot undergo CT scanning because of instability, or it may be used in conjunction with CT scanning for a thorough evaluation. The incidence of a colorectal injury with blunt trauma is approximately 0.3%. Diagnosis is often made at laparotomy for another cause.

Damage control techniques for dealing with traumatic injuries have significantly improved the mortality rates after laparotomy. In these procedures, packing is performed for nonsurgical bleeding, with selective ligation of vessels and bowel resection without anastomosis or stoma formation to terminate a procedure quickly. Once coagulopathy begins, the procedure should be terminated with the intent to return after resuscitation and control of the coagulopathy.

Operative intervention should be performed via a midline laparotomy. The primary intent should be to stabilize or stop ongoing blood loss. Then attention can be turned to detection and management of other injuries. Treatment options for colonic injury may include proximal diversion and repair, exteriorization of the wound as a colostomy, simple suture repair, or resection with anastomosis. Judgment must be exercised to determine the best course of action given the mechanism of injury.

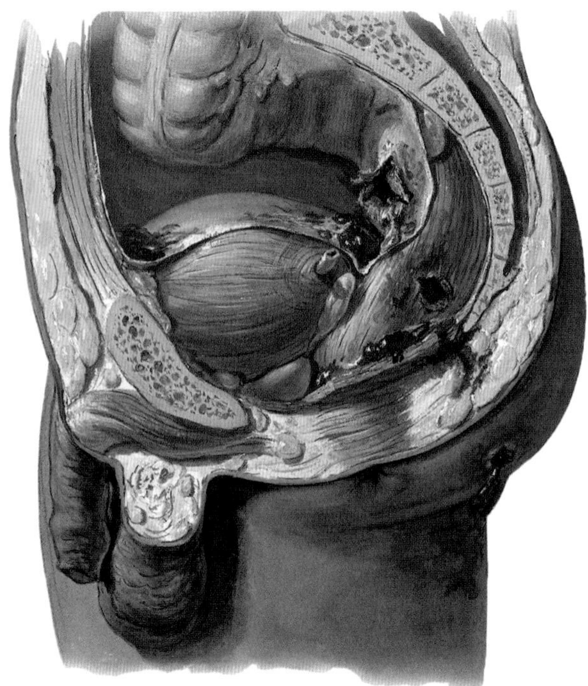

Intraperitoneal and extraperitoneal lesions

## Abdominal Wounds: Rectum

Injuries of the rectum occur less frequently than those of other abdominal viscera but are particularly important because of their gravity. In World War I they made up 2.4% of all abdominal injuries. In World War II the incidence of rectal injuries among abdominal injuries was 3.7%. Rectal trauma is often associated with lesions of the bladder, the pelvic colon, and the small intestine. Other causes of penetrating rectal trauma include stab wounds, accidental (e.g., all-terrain vehicle accident) or intentional impalement, foreign bodies, or iatrogenic causes.

Wounds of the rectum vary in type and extent. They may be extraperitoneal or intraperitoneal, or both. The lesion often consists of a small perforation, produced by a small missile or a fragment of pelvic bone, or an extensive laceration produced by shell fragments of high explosives or land mines. The entrance wound in such injuries frequently is located posteriorly or posterolaterally in the thigh or buttocks and may deceptively suggest that the bowel has been missed. In some cases, damage to tissues externally is extensive, with tearing and laceration of the gluteal region and destruction of the anus and lower rectum. In others, the anal region remains intact, the injury being limited to the lower portion of the rectum. These cases are particularly dangerous because of infection in the extraperitoneal perirectal region. Rectal injuries are especially prone to anaerobic infection. The intraperitoneal portion of the rectum can also be injured in cases in which the missile has entered from behind or from the side. Such wounds are not infrequently associated with fracture of the bones of the pelvis. These cases are commonly accompanied by injury of the bladder or small bowel. In addition to peritonitis, danger of infection in the presacral areolar tissue is associated.

Intraperitoneal rectal injuries are diagnosed and treated in a fashion similar to colonic injuries. If an injury is in the extraperitoneal rectum, it may be difficult to diagnose. Such injuries usually become apparent after signs of infection develop, typically over the next 24 hours. Patients should be managed with intravenous broad-spectrum antibiotics, and diagnosis should be confirmed with an examination or imaging. Sigmoidoscopy should be performed in the operating room if there is blood in the rectum on digital rectal examination or if there is a bladder, urethral, vaginal, or pelvic injury that causes concern for an associated rectal injury.

The treatment of rectal injuries can be broken down by two factors, location and tissue destruction. If there is minimal destruction of tissue and an intraperitoneal lesion, treatment consists essentially of repairing the bowel if possible. If there is significant tissue destruction to the bowel, a resection with primary anastomosis is performed. Concerns for breakdown of the repair and consideration of diversion or resection with end colostomy should occur with significant comorbid conditions, blood transfusion of more than 6 units, shock, delay in operation, and significant fecal contamination. Extraperitoneal rectal injuries with little tissue, such as penetrating rectal injuries from bone fragments or low-velocity missiles, can often be treated with a diverting colostomy alone. Extraperitoneal rectal injuries with little tissue damage, such as penetrating rectal injuries from bone fragments or low-velocity missiles, can often be treated with a diverting colostomy alone. Significant tissue destruction and extraperitoneal injury can occur from high-velocity missiles, blast injuries, and exposure of the perineum to the water jet from jet skis. If there is significant destruction to the perineal tissues (>25%), distal washout of the involved tissues, direct repair of the injury, diverting colostomy, and presacral drainage are the mainstays of treatment.

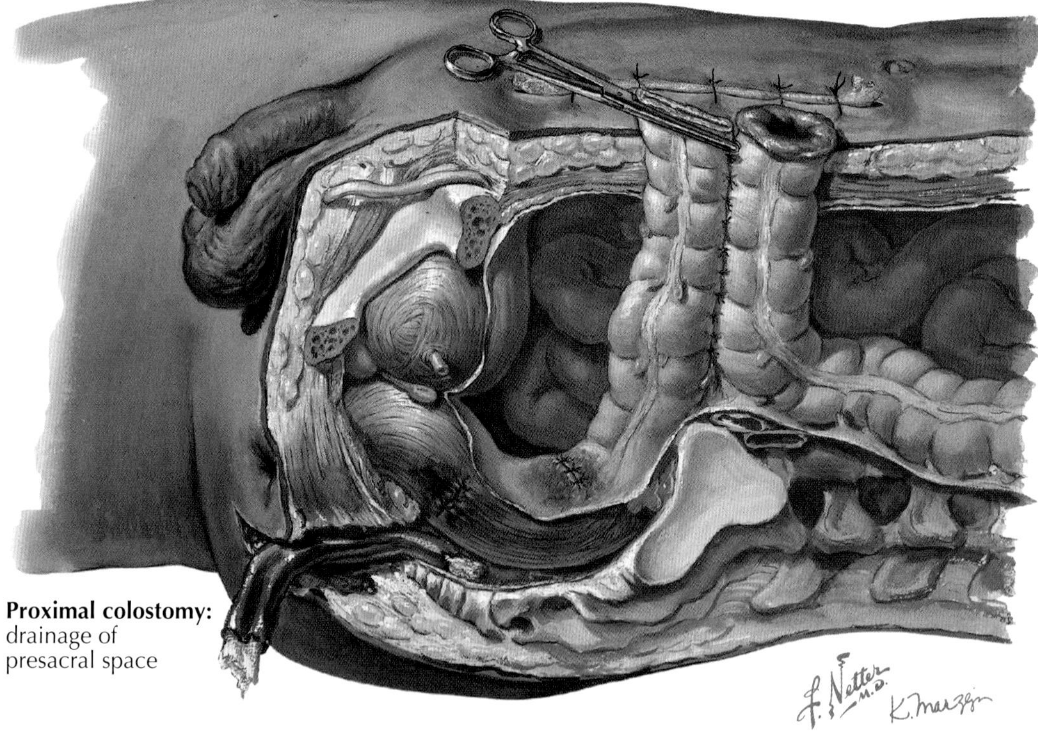

**Proximal colostomy:** drainage of presacral space

# Anorectal Melanoma, Radiation Injury, and Typhlitis

## ANORECTAL MELANOMA

Anorectal melanoma is the most common gastrointestinal primary melanoma and typically has a poorer prognosis than cutaneous melanomas. These comprise 0.4% to 1.6% of all melanomas. Seventy to 80% are located within the anal canal or anal verge. Its varied presentations may involve a mass, pain, or bleeding. It may be incidentally discovered on examination or upon resection of another lesion such as a hemorrhoid, particularly if it is the amelanotic type, which occurs in approximately 25% of cases. Only 375 new cases were documented in the National Cancer Database between 1973 and 2011. The median age at diagnosis is 60 years, and the disease is more commonly seen in females, with metastatic disease often present at the time of diagnosis.

The overall prognosis is poor, with 5-year survival rates ranging from 6% to 22% if the disease is metastatic or locally contained. Treatment requires an R0 resection (complete removal of the tumor, with microscopic evaluation of the margins showing no tumor cells), which often will require an abdominoperineal resection, but local excision may be adequate for many patients. Better 5-year survival rates are seen if negative margins are obtained with surgery. Sentinel lymph node biopsy has not been shown to be effective in the staging of anorectal melanoma. Use of adjuvant chemotherapy and irradiation is unproven, but case reports have shown greater regional control after radiation therapy when complete excision can be performed. Given the rarity of the disease, little data exist regarding the efficacy of immunotherapy in the treatment of anorectal melanoma.

## RADIATION INJURY

Given the rapid turnover of intestinal epithelia, the colon and small intestine are at significant risk for radiation injury. Radiation therapy results in mucosal atrophy, with decreased crypt height in the colon and rectum. Mucosal injury also occurs in the areas that lie within the field of radiation. Diarrhea and hematochezia often occur because of resultant colitis or proctitis.

Effects of irradiation can be delayed in onset and occur months or years after exposure. Fibrosis, strictures, fistulas, and telangiectasias may occur. Imaging with barium enema may help identify the extent of strictures. Bacterial overgrowth may occur, necessitating the use of antibiotics. Dilation of strictures may also be necessary. Surgery should be reserved for refractory strictures or fistulas because the associated morbidity is significant; it may lead to difficulty in healing due to impaired blood supply.

## TYPHLITIS

Typhlitis, also known as *neutropenic enterocolitis,* is a complication that occurs in patients receiving cytotoxic chemotherapy; it may be life-threatening. It may also occur in patients with aplastic anemia, cyclic neutropenia, or after autologous stem cell transplantation, but it is felt to be most commonly associated with treatment for leukemia and lymphoma. Typically, it occurs in the cecum, ascending colon, and terminal ileum. A spectrum of mucosal and submucosal necrosis with hemorrhage and ulceration may be seen.

Clinically, patients present with fever, abdominal pain, and diarrhea in the presence of neutropenia. Patients may also experience nausea, vomiting, hematochezia, and abdominal distension. Symptoms typically begin about 7 to 9 days after the onset of neutropenia. Other diagnoses that need to be considered in the differential diagnosis include any other cause of acute abdominal pain, including appendicitis, diverticulitis, and ischemic colitis.

Laboratory studies are typically not helpful in making the diagnosis, but polymicrobial infection may be revealed on blood culture. A paucity of gas may be seen in the right lower quadrant on abdominal radiograph, with dilated small bowel loops, thumbprinting, pneumatosis intestinalis, and free air, or the films may appear normal. Ultrasound and CT scan are typically more sensitive and may show bowel wall thickening; a fluid-filled, dilated cecum; ascites; phlegmon; pericolic fluid; or pneumatosis or free air in severe cases.

Treatment usually consists of aggressive medical therapy, including bowel rest, hydration, and nasogastric suction. Early broad-spectrum antibiotic coverage with β-lactam monotherapy or combined with aminoglycoside is essential because mortality rates increase for each hour they are not given. Patients should be observed closely for clinical signs of deterioration. Surgery is recommended for patients who have perforation, persistent bleeding, or clinical deterioration suggestive of uncontrolled sepsis. Typically, resection with proximal ostomy is performed. Often, clinical improvement is not seen until there is recovery of the neutrophil count. This can be hastened with the use of recombinant granulocyte colony-stimulating factor. Chemotherapy can be resumed when patients have completely recovered.

**Anal melanoma**

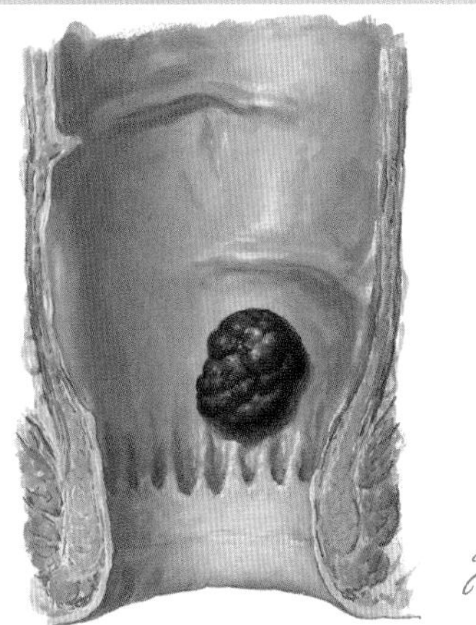


**Radiation injury**

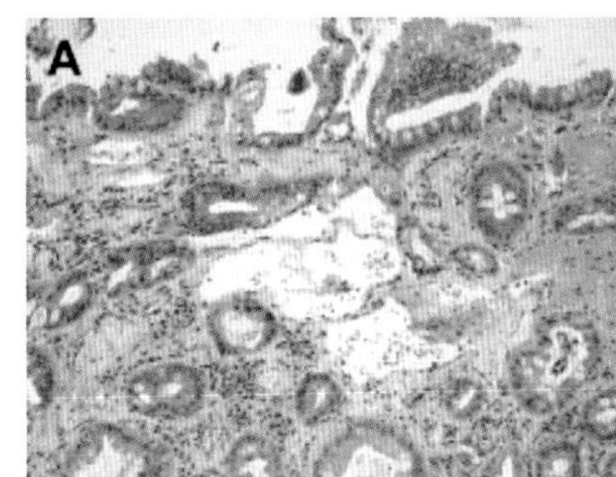


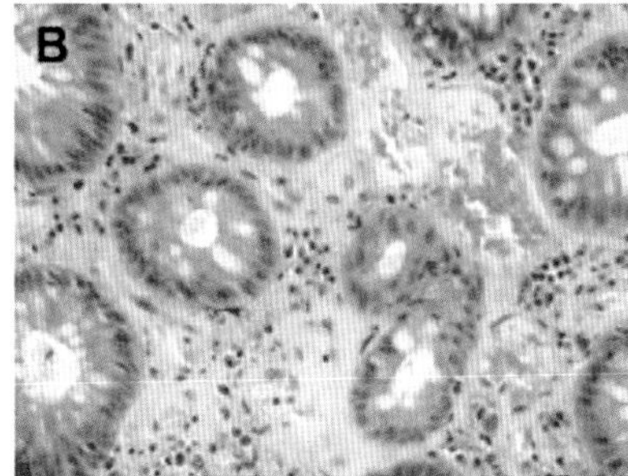


Radiation proctitis. **A**, Magnification x20; **B**, magnification x40. *(From Sarin A, Safar B. Management of radiation proctitis. Gastroenterol Clin North Am. 2013;42:913–925.)*

**Typhlitis**

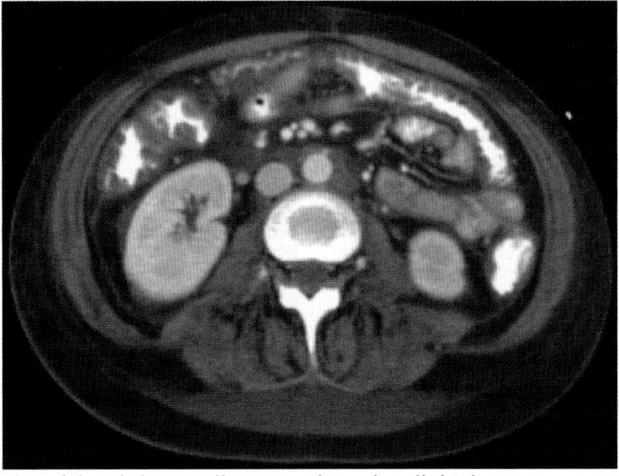

Computed tomography of the abdomen illustrating bowel wall thickening associated with neutropenic enterocolitis. This is most notable in the upper portions of the image surrounded by intraluminal contrast. *(From Cloutier RL. Neutropenic enterocolitis. Emerg Clin North Am. 2009;27:415–422.)*

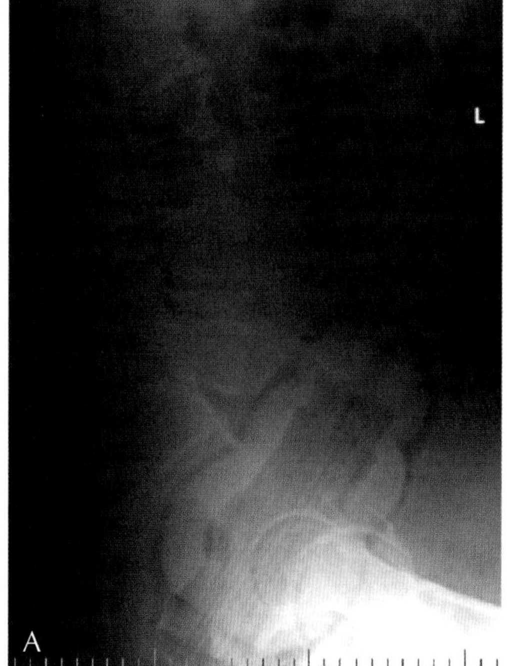


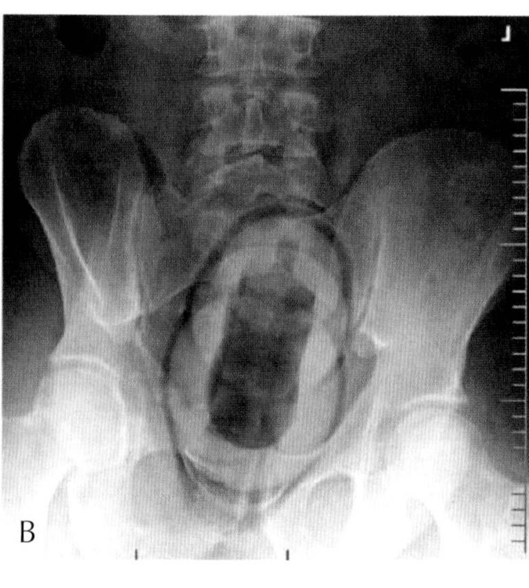


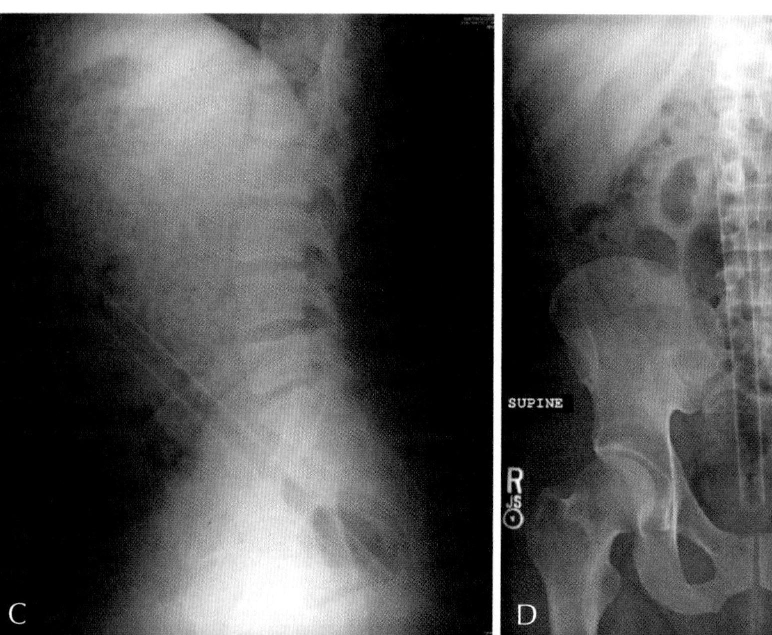


Lateral (**A** and **C**) and supine (**B** and **D**) radiographs demonstrating retained rectal foreign body.

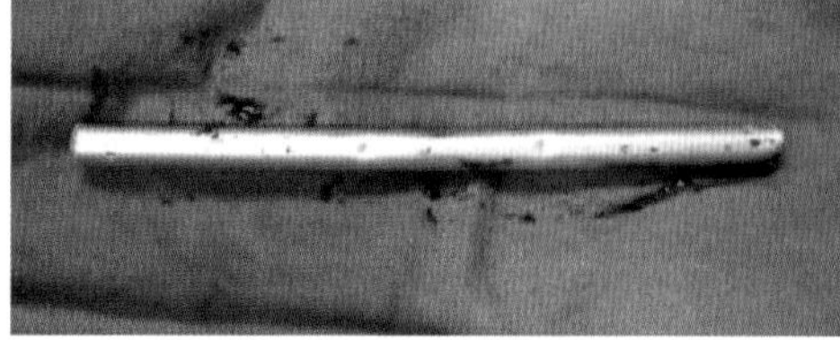

Foreign body after removal.

## Foreign Bodies in Anus and Colon

Patients with anorectal foreign bodies are often reluctant to present to known physicians and so will present to the emergency room after some delay. These foreign bodies may have been placed transanally for therapeutic or for sexual purposes. Rectal foreign bodies can also be a result of oral ingestion as seen in body packing. The most commonly reported items are cylindrically shaped, but items such as balls, vibrators, foods (fruits and vegetables), and bottles have been removed. Rarely, rectal thermometers have accidentally broken with a retained portion beyond the anal canal. Patients will usually have tried to remove the object prior to presentation to the emergency room and may fabricate stories to explain what happened. Suspicion for abuse or assault should be triggered. A systematic approach to diagnosis and management is essential due to the varied nature of foreign bodies and outcomes. Concern should remain for delayed perforation or significant bleeding even after extraction. The majority of patients are males 30 to 40 years of age.

First, determination should be made as to whether perforation has occurred. If a patient is unstable, resuscitation and broad-spectrum antibiotics should be immediately initiated prior to surgical exploration. If the patient is stable, a CT scan can be performed to determine whether a perforation has been sustained. Perforations may occur into the extraperitoneal space below the peritoneal reflection, so care should be taken to make the diagnosis.

For extraction, patient relaxation with a perianal nerve block, spinal anesthetic, and/or conscious sedation should be undertaken. With the patient in the lithotomy position, a rectal examination can be performed with downward abdominal pressure to facilitate extraction if needed. A plain film should be taken after the extraction to ensure that no perforation developed as a result. Proctosigmoidoscopy should be performed after removal to determine whether there is any damage to the mucosa of the colon or rectum.

If transanal extraction is not possible even with general anesthesia, exploration via laparotomy is indicated. Attempts may be made to push the object distally and extract it transanally. If this is unsuccessful, a colostomy can be performed to remove the object with a primary closure. If a perforation is identified, proximal diversion may be necessary. Traumatic disruption to the anal sphincter may result in fecal incontinence. Surgical intervention for this should be delayed until adequate time has passed to allow a full evaluation of clinical symptoms.

## Proctologic Conditions: Hemorrhoids

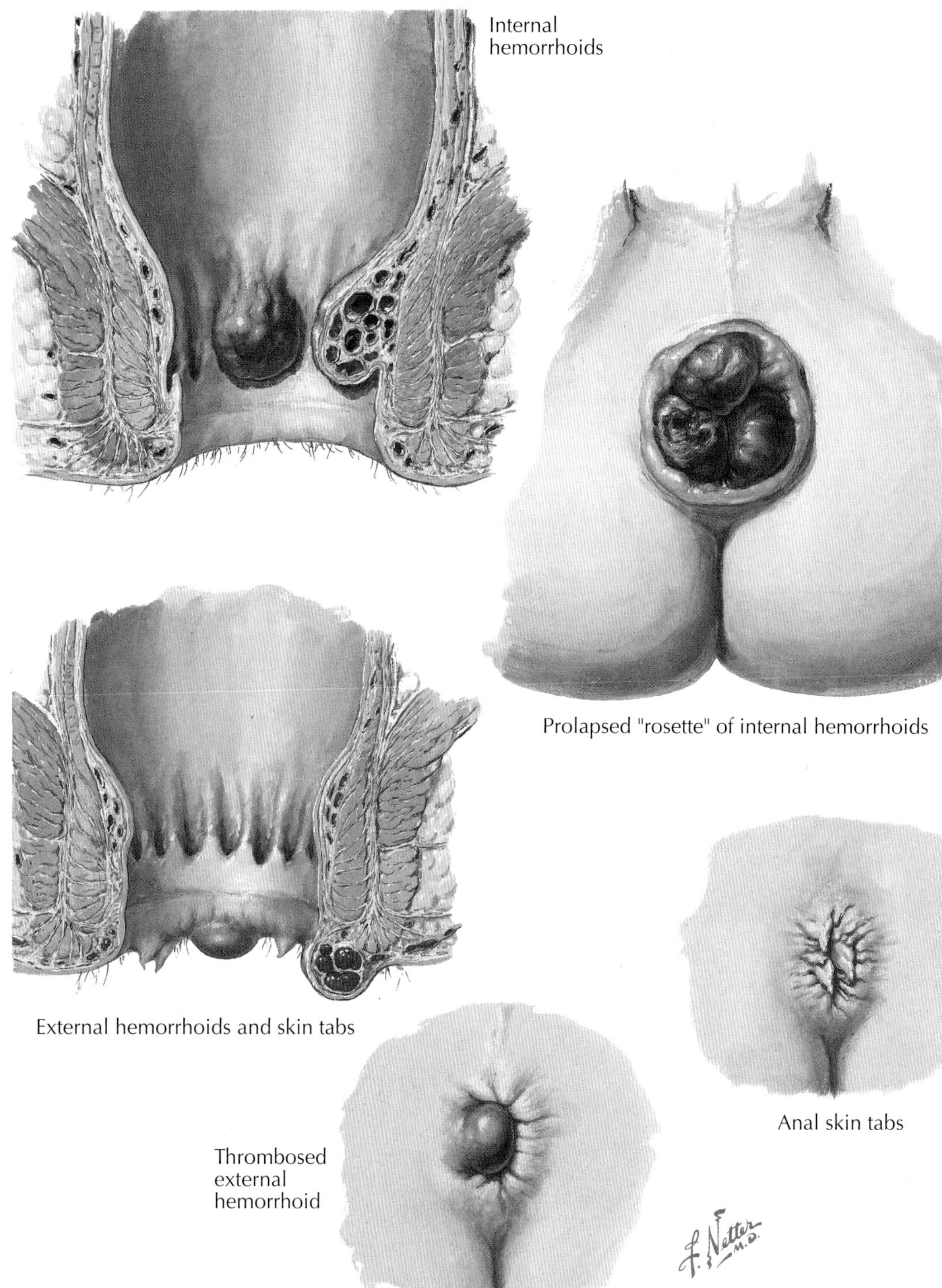


Hemorrhoids are varicose dilations of the radicles of the hemorrhoidal (rectal) veins, in either the superior or the inferior plexuses or both, accompanied in varying degrees by hypertrophy and round cell infiltration of the perivascular connective tissue. Hemorrhoids are present in about 35% of the population. They usually occur between the ages of 25 and 55 years and only seldom under the age of 15 years. Both sexes are affected equally.

To explain the formation of hemorrhoids, a great variety of factors have been considered. A hereditary predisposition seems to play a role in some individuals. Erect posture, the absence of valves in the portal venous system, the arrangement of the collecting veins in the rectal submucosal space with the veins being susceptible to compression in passing through the anorectal musculature, and other biologic and anatomic conditions are contributory elements. More direct causes are all of the various events that produce transient or constant increased pressure or stasis within the rectal venous plexuses, such as straining at stools because of constipation or diarrhea, tumors or strictures of the rectum, pregnancy, tumors and retroversion of the uterus, hypertrophy and tumors of the prostate, and portal hypertension.

External and internal hemorrhoids must be differentiated by anatomic location. Varicosities of the inferior hemorrhoidal plexus present as *external hemorrhoids,* situated below the pectinate line and covered by the modified skin of the anus. Thrombotic external hemorrhoids are an acute variety of external hemorrhoids, resulting from the formation of a thrombus within a vein or, more frequently, from the rupture of a vein with extravasation of blood into the cellular tissue, constituting, strictly speaking, a hematoma. The *thrombotic variety* usually occurs as the result of strain. The patient complains of a sudden painful lump at the anus, and inspection reveals a rounded, bluish, tender swelling. Thrombosed external hemorrhoids finally result in so-called *skin tags,* consisting of one or more folds of the anal skin and composed of connective tissue and a few blood vessels. Skin tags may form also by imperfect healing of the skin after hemorrhoidectomy or as a consequence of an inflammatory process in the anal region.

*Internal hemorrhoids* are varicose enlargements of the veins of the superior hemorrhoidal plexus. In the early stage (first degree), they do not protrude through the anal canal and can be detected only by proctoscopy, where they appear as globular, reddish swellings. Because the superior rectal veins are fairly constantly distributed, internal hemorrhoids are usually located in the right and left posterior and right anterior quadrants. Histologically, the walls of the dilated veins are atrophic and surrounded by a perivascular inflammatory infiltrate. In a later stage, internal hemorrhoids may protrude through the anal canal. Initially, the protrusion may occur only at defecation, receding afterward spontaneously (second degree); in time, the protrusion becomes more pronounced, occurring with exertion and receding only by manual reduction (third degree). Finally, the *hemorrhoids* may become permanently *prolapsed,* in which case the mucosal surface of the hemorrhoids is constantly subjected to trauma and may become ulcerated. Increased mucoid discharge may also cause irritation of the perianal skin, producing burning and itching.

The earliest symptom of internal hemorrhoids is usually intermittent bleeding, occurring during or following defecation. Pain is not a characteristic symptom, being present only in cases with complications (thrombosis, strangulation) or other concomitant conditions (fissure, abscess).

The so-called *strangulated hemorrhoids* constitute the most common and also the most painful complication of internal hemorrhoids. This complication occurs when the prolapsed hemorrhoids cannot be reduced because of sphincteric contractions and because of the blockage of the thrombosed internal varices by the simultaneously or subsequently thrombosed inferior hemorrhoidal veins.

Patients should be examined with anoscopy and proctosigmoidoscopy to determine the extent of hemorrhoidal tissue. The degree of prolapse can be evaluated by asking the patient to strain on the toilet. More proximal evaluation may be deemed necessary with further endoscopy.

For most, conservative management with fiber supplementation is the first-line treatment, to relieve constipation and the need for straining. Various over-the-counter ointments can be used as well to help with symptoms. Patients with advanced disease that does not respond to this conservative management may benefit from other interventions such as sclerotherapy, diathermy, or band ligation. Excisional hemorrhoidectomy should be reserved for patients who have not responded to more conservative measures and have significant symptoms or have difficulty with anal hygiene. For some patients with prolapsing hemorrhoids, a pexy procedure using a device to place a purse-string suture transanally may be an alternative to surgical hemorrhoidectomy.

## Proctologic Conditions: Prolapse and Procidentia

Prolapse

Prolapse; only rectal mucosa involved

Key
Outline of peritoneum
Outline of rectal mucosa
Anorectal musculature

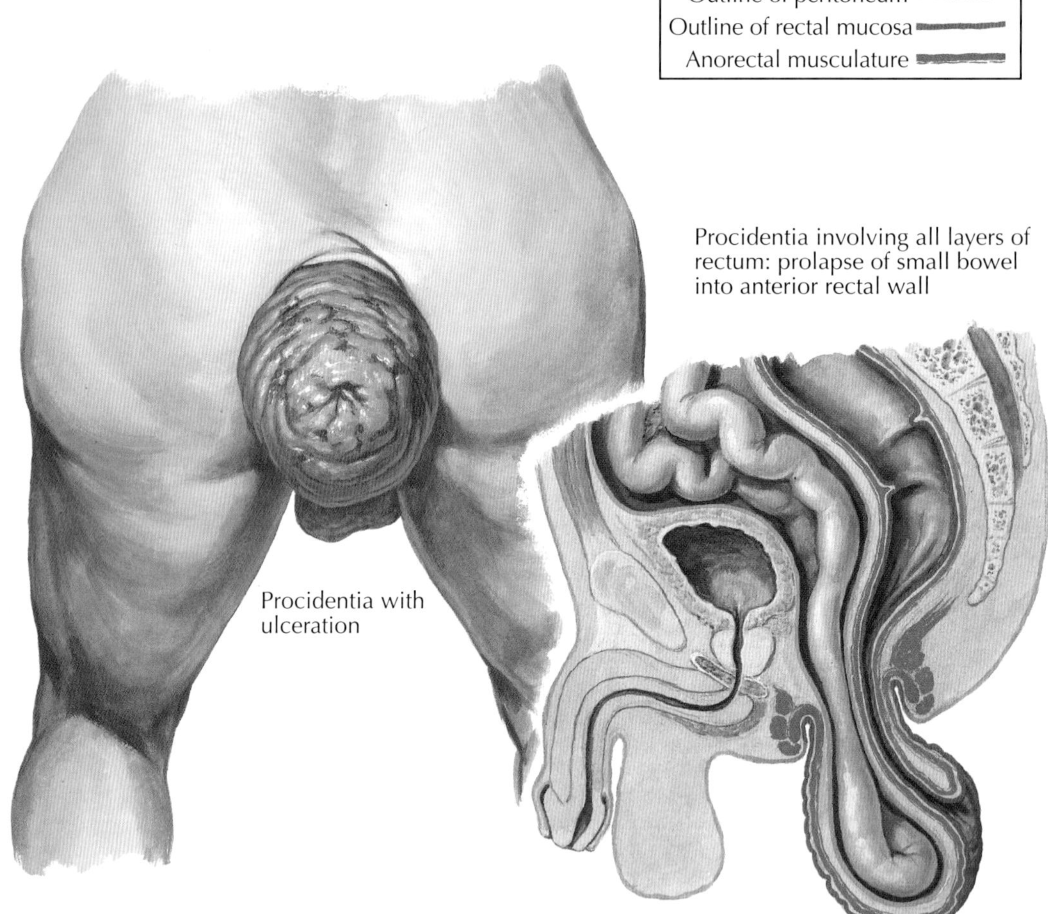

Procidentia involving all layers of rectum: prolapse of small bowel into anterior rectal wall
Procidentia with ulceration


Prolapse of the rectum, as ordinarily understood, is a condition in which one or more layers of the rectum and/or the anal canal protrude through the anal orifice. A prolapse can be partial or complete. In partial prolapse (usually called simply *prolapse*), only the mucosa is involved; it extends usually not more than 0.5 to 1 inch. In total prolapse (called *procidentia*), all of the layers of the rectum are involved; it presents as a larger, bulbous mass, which may eventually contain a hernia sac of peritoneum with a segment of bowel in its interior.

In procidentia, in addition to the descent of the rectal tissues, an eversion of the lining of the anal canal takes place, so that the covering of the displaced tissues becomes continuous at approximately a right angle with the perianal skin. When only the rectal tissues descend while the anal structures remain in their normal position, a sulcus will surround the protruded rectum.

Sigmoidorectal intussusception (concealed or protruded) has been previously described as a procidentia, but this is, in fact, a different entity. The confusion arises when the intussusception protrudes through the anal orifice. However, digital examination will easily differentiate this condition from rectal procidentia. In the former the finger will pass into the rectal ampulla. In the latter the finger will meet a blind end in the anal canal, or the displaced tissue is continuous with the perianal skin.

The cause of prolapse and procidentia is unknown. A defect in one or more of the supporting structures of the anorectum seems to be the chief predisposing factor; it is not likely that increased abdominal pressure, in the absence of alterations in the supporting structures of the anorectum, will result in prolapse or procidentia.

Prolapse occurs most frequently in childhood and in old age. In children, most cases occur at 1 to 4 years of age, and a shallow sacral curve and reduction of the supporting fat, as may occur in wasting diseases, are the chief predisposing causes. In patients who are older or who are debilitated, the prolapse is usually due to the loss of sphincter tone. It is obvious that some lesions within the bowel that drag down the mucosa, such as polyps, hemorrhoids, and tumors, and anatomic or neurologic disturbances of the sphincters may favor the occurrence of prolapse.

Procidentia may occur at any age, but it is uncommon in children. It is now commonly accepted that the disorder is, in reality, a sliding hernia of the pouch of Douglas through a weakened or damaged pelvic fascia and levator muscles, the occurrence of which is possibly favored by an abnormally mobile rectum. Attention has been called to the importance of some neurologic and rectal sensory factors related to the defecation mechanism. Faulty rectal sensation either as a result of poor interpretation of the normal stimulus or as a result of a neuromuscular abnormality with associated hypoexcitability may lead to a lack of coordination between the appreciation of the full-rectum stimulus and defecation.

The most common report in patients with prolapse or procidentia is the protrusion of a mass from the anus during defecation or walking, which will become increasingly difficult to reduce. Other symptoms are a sensation of fullness, soiling, incontinence, diarrhea, and bleeding.

The examination is best carried out with the patient in a standing or squatting position; the patient should be asked to strain so that the full extent of the protrusion can be observed. In prolapse the inspection reveals a relatively small mass with *radially* arranged folds. In procidentia the protruded mass is bulky, showing a congested, eventually *ulcerated* mucosa with folds arranged in a *concentric* pattern.

# Proctologic Conditions: Papillitis, Cryptitis, Adenomatous Polyps, Villous Tumor, Fissure, and Pruritus Ani

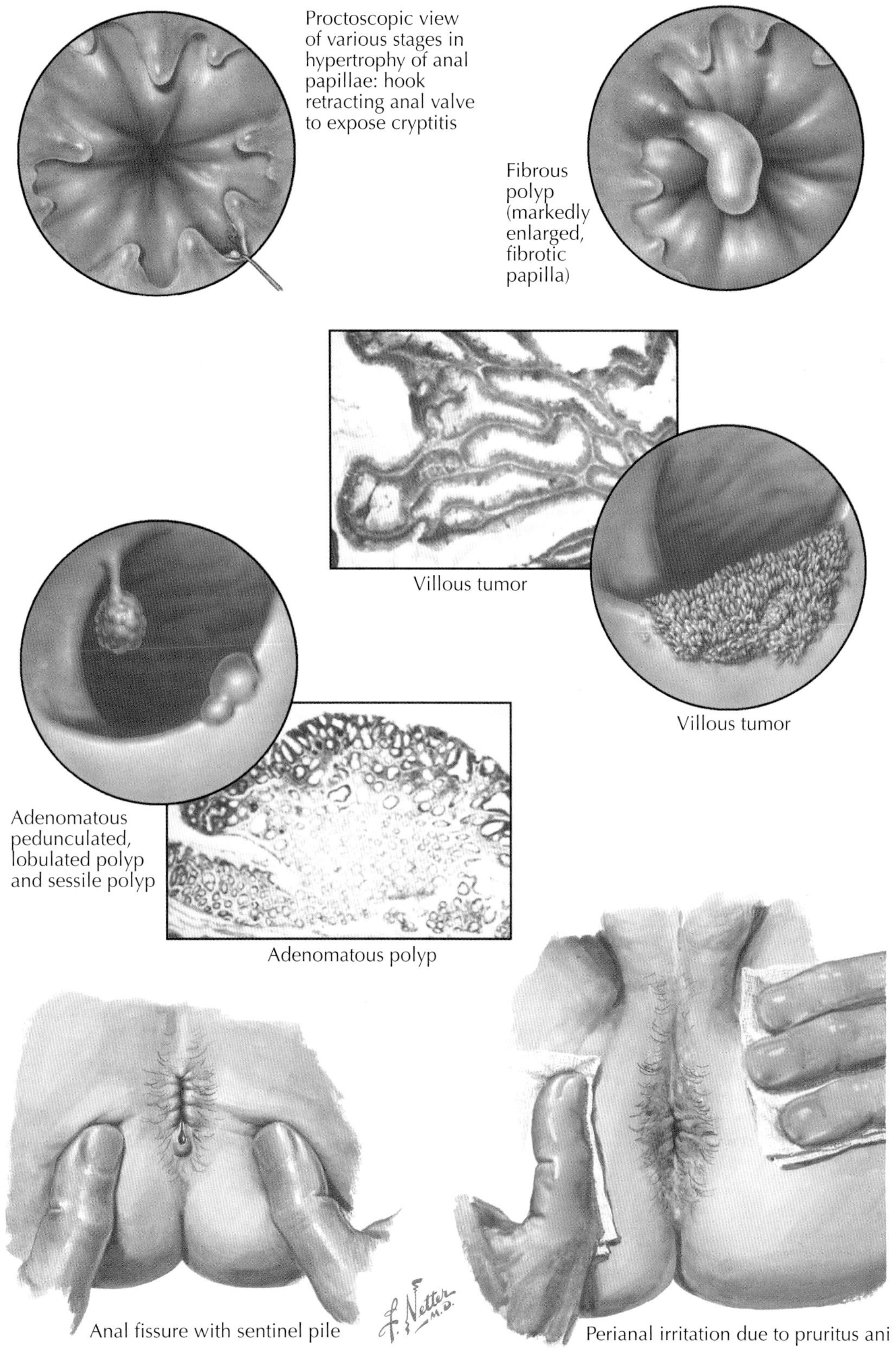

Proctoscopic view of various stages in hypertrophy of anal papillae: hook retracting anal valve to expose cryptitis

Fibrous polyp (markedly enlarged, fibrotic papilla)

Villous tumor

Villous tumor

Adenomatous pedunculated, lobulated polyp and sessile polyp

Adenomatous polyp

Anal fissure with sentinel pile

Perianal irritation due to pruritus ani

Inflammatory processes of the papillae, which usually start in one of the crypts, give rise to extreme pain (and tenesmus) out of all proportion to the size and severity of the lesion. In *acute papillitis,* the structure is *swollen, edematous,* and *congested,* later becoming, in the chronic stage of the papillitis, *fibrosed* and *hypertrophied.* Gradually, the hypertrophic papilla may develop a stalk and may change into a so-called *fibrous polyp,* which may produce the sensation of a foreign body in the anal canal, a dissatisfied feeling after defecation, itching, and objective signs of irritation.

The crypts of Morgagni, in which fecal material can collect and which are continuously exposed to trauma, become easily involved in infectious inflammatory processes. The *cryptitis* may remain restricted to circumscribed reactions in and around the crypts or may spread to the surrounding tissues, inducing the formation of abscesses and fistulae. The symptoms of cryptitis (sometimes resembling those of a fissure *[phantom fissure]*) are anal formication, itching, and radiating pain, which are aggravated by defecation and ambulation. Anoscopy, under anesthesia, permits recognition of the affected crypt, a purulent discharge or granulation tissue, and enlargement of the related papilla.

Benign tumors of epithelial origin occur in the rectum in two varieties, the simple adenomatous polyp and the villous tumor (also termed *papilloma, papillary tumor, papillary adenoma, papillary polyp, villous polyp,* and *villoma*). The usually lobulated *adenomatous polyps* may be sessile or pedunculated; they may vary in size from a few millimeters up to about 2 cm in diameter, only rarely becoming larger. The less common *villous tumor* is mostly attached to the mucosa by means of numerous papillary stalks and is soft and velvety to the touch. Both of these benign epithelial tumors tend to undergo malignant degeneration and may manifest themselves by bleeding, mucous discharge, diarrhea, tenesmus, and protrusion through the anal canal.

An *anal fissure* is a crack or slit-like ulcer of the anal canal lining below the pectinate line, extending often as far as the anal verge. It starts rather suddenly, and the lesion is usually associated with severe pain. If untreated, it tends to run a course of exacerbations and remissions. Fissures occur at all ages, particularly in middle life, and somewhat more frequently in females. When single, an anal fissure is most commonly located at the posterior commissure. Multiple fissures, also more frequent in females, usually involve the anterior and posterior commissures and only rarely the lateral margins. Mechanical traumatic factors (overdistension of the anal canal at defecation) and anal infection are the most frequent pathogenic causes. The typical anal fissure is racket shaped and has sharply defined edges; at the lower, wider, rounded end, the skin frequently forms an edematous tab *(sentinel pile);* the upper end, quite close to the anal valves, is often guarded by one or two hypertrophied papillae. Pain related to defecation is the main symptom; occurring during passage of the stools or shortly thereafter, it may be extremely severe and may persist for some time. The diagnosis can be made by simple inspection of the anus.

*Pruritus ani* is a symptom that may accompany every known anorectal disease as well as other organic or systemic affections. Most commonly, however, no evident primary cause is found. Perianal itching without any apparent cause (by some authors believed to be a neurodermatitis, by others simply designated as "cryptogenetic") is usually more intense at night in bed and during warm weather. The perianal skin is hyperemic and will show superficial abrasions from scratching. In more chronic cases, a whitish discoloration of the skin, accentuation of the folds, rhagades, lichenification, hyperkeratosis, and patchy parakeratosis are characteristic.

## Proctologic Conditions: Anorectal Abscess and Fistula

A localized infection with collection of pus in the anorectal area is designated as *anorectal abscess.* It usually results from the invasion of the normal rectal flora (*Bacillus coli, Bacillus proteus, Bacillus subtilis,* staphylococci, and streptococci) into the perirectal or perianal tissues. The pathologic process seems to start, as a rule, with an inflammation of one or more crypts (cryptitis). From the crypt (portal of entry), the infection may spread to the anal ducts and anal glands and from there submucously, subcutaneously, or transsphincterally to the surrounding tissue. This sequence of events closes with a spontaneous rupture of the abscess, either into the anorectal canal or through the perianal skin, if the abscess has not been drained surgically. Once the abscess has perforated, the cavity, as well as its outlet, shrinks, leaving a tube-like structure, an *anorectal fistula.* An anorectal fistula is invariably the result of an abscess.

Anorectal abscesses and fistula are identified per Park's classification based on their anatomic location and noted as intersphincteric (type I), transsphincteric (type II), suprasphincteric (type III), and extrasphincteric (type IV). By position, *supralevator abscesses* are the least common type; they extend from the intersphincteric plane through the puborectalis muscle and exit via the skin after passing through the levator ani. Because the surrounding affected tissues have a visceral rather than a somatic sensory nerve supply, a sensation of discomfort and pressure rather than pain is perceived in the anorectal region. These abscesses may be palpated by digital examination or observed through the proctoscope as swellings encroaching on the rectal lumen. In contrast to the infralevator abscesses, they may produce signs of toxemia and extreme prostration. The retrorectal and, more so, the pelvirectal abscesses, in most instances, originate from infectious processes in other pelvic organs and are thus not anorectal lesions in the strict sense, though they usually rupture into the rectum or anal canal or sometimes through the levator ani.

The course of a fistula, which will eventually remain as the end phase of abscess formation, evacuation, and healing, will essentially depend on the original localization and point of drainage of the abscess. A *fistula* is called *complete* when both openings, the primary (cryptic) and the secondary openings, can be detected and are accessible. Complete fistulae usually connect the rectal lumen with the anal or perianal skin. If only one opening can be identified, either the primary opening or, as is more often the case, the secondary opening, one deals with a *blind fistula,* also designated as a *sinus,* which may discharge either into the lumen of the bowel (internal sinus) or through the perianal skin (external sinus). The former comes into existence when the abscess has drained spontaneously through the crypt from which the infectious process started. The external sinuses are, in principle, always complete fistulae, despite the fact that the primary (cryptic) opening cannot be demonstrated. Applying *Goodsall's rule,* one may obtain a rough idea of the course of the fistulous tract and the probable location of its primary opening. This rule proposes that by drawing an imaginary transverse line across the center of the anus, one may expect a curved tract and the primary opening posterior to the midline when the secondary opening is situated posteriorly to this line, whereas a straight tract and an anteriorly located primary opening may be expected when the secondary opening is anterior to this proposed line.

Complicated fistulas are difficult to treat and are considered Parks type II to IV. A branched fistulous tract with several openings is also considered complex. The different tracts include the *transsphincteric fistula* (Parks type II), which passes through the musculature. An *intrasphincteric fistula* (Parks type I) runs between the internal and external sphincter. Finally a *subcutaneous fistula* passes submucosally, leaving the sphincter intact. A curved tract partially encircling the anus is known as a *horseshoe fistula.*

Simple fistulas can be treated with fistulotomies in patients without threatened continence. Patients with complex fistulas or threatened continence should have a seton placed through the tract to allow for drainage and control of infection.

Types of abscesses in anorectal region

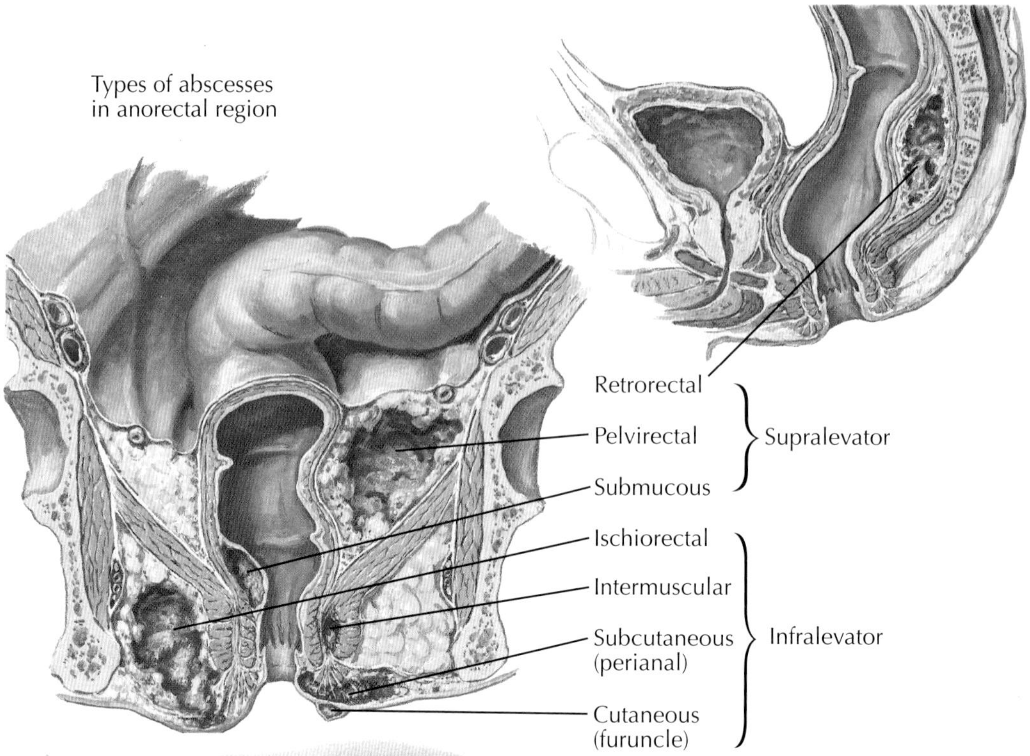

Retroretal / Pelvirectal / Submucous — Supralevator

Ischiorectal / Intermuscular / Subcutaneous (perianal) / Cutaneous (furuncle) — Infralevator

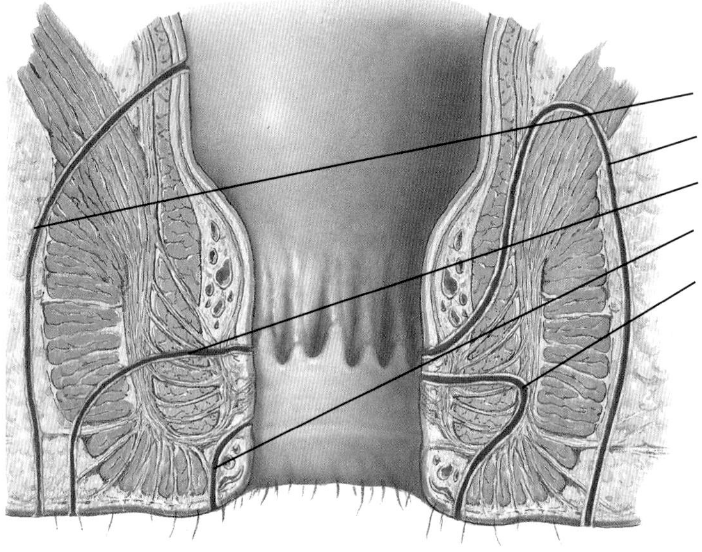

Extrasphincteric (Parks type IV)
Suprasphincteric (Parks type III)
Transsphincteric (Parks type II)
Superficial
Intersphincteric (Parks type I)

Types of anal fistulas

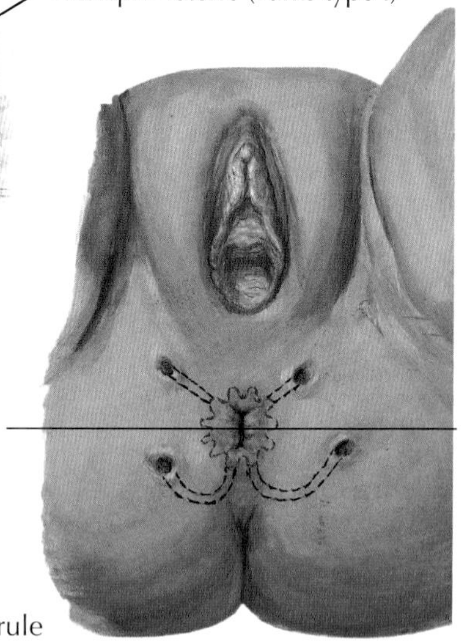

Goodsall rule

## Proctologic Conditions: Sexually Transmitted Diseases

Lymphogranuloma venereum, caused by the L serovars of *Chlamydia trachomatis,* may produce lesions in the genital tract, inguinal region, and/or anorectal-colonic tissues. A primary papule or ulcer, usually not noticed, appears at the site of inoculation. This is usually located on the glans penis or prepuce in the male and on the fourchette, posterior vaginal wall, or posterior lip of the cervix in the female. Subsequent disease is due to local extension and spread to draining lymph nodes. Inguinal adenitis (bubo) marks the second stage, because the lymphatic drainage of the external genitalia, the common site of the initial lesion, is by way of the inguinal nodes. Local extension may lead to elephantiasis of the penis and scrotum. In females, the site of the primary lesion is commonly vaginal or cervical, and invasion of the perirectum and rectal wall is much easier. Thus the second-stage manifestations are more apt to be rectal stricture, abscesses, and fistulae. Anovulval esthiomene (elephantiasis) may be seen from local extension. Rectal strictures in men who have sex with men may be seen owing to primary rectal infection. Rectal symptoms may include anal pain, rectal discharge, constipation, fever, and tenesmus.

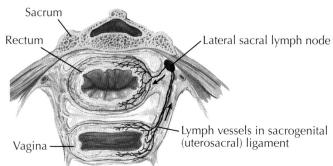

The characteristic pathologic changes in the rectum are those of an ulcerative inflammatory process with an extensive production of contracting connective tissue in the mucosa and deeper layers of the bowel. When the entire intestinal wall and the perirectal tissues become involved, the affected segment is transformed into a firm, fixed, narrowed canal. Multiple blind sinuses and perirectal abscesses may form, which can perforate into the vagina, bladder, or perianal skin. Occasionally, other segments of the large intestine (particularly left-sided colon) may also be involved by the disease.

Genital *Chlamydia trachomatis* is a common cause of proctitis in men who have sex with men. *C. trachomatis* has three human biovars, and when seen in proctitis, serovars D to K are usually involved. Infection may result from direct inoculation of the rectum or through the local spread of infected cervical secretions in females. Infection is superficial, and symptoms may include anal pruritis and a mucoid discharge.

Infection with *Treponema pallidum* may lead to syphilitic manifestations of the anorectum in all stages of the disease. In adults, the primary lesion consists of a painless and indurated chancre that is usually present at a genital location (penis or labial posterior commissure) but may also be seen perianally or within the anal canal or rectum itself. The diagnosis can be readily established by dark-field examination of the lesion that reveals the presence of spirochetes. The manifestations of secondary syphilis occur usually as perianal condylomata lata (flat warts), which have a flat surface rather than the pedicle and cauliflower lobulations of human papillomavirus (HPV)-related condylomata acuminata. *Treponema pallidum* may be demonstrated in the former. Serologic tests are generally positive at this stage of the disease. In late syphilis, ulcerated gummas may occur in the anus and rectum. In infants, multiple superficial fissures may indicate congenital syphilis.

*Neisseria gonorrhoeae* may cause proctitis after direct inoculation from sexual activity. Disease is characterized by a friable mucosa that may lead to abscess or fistula formation. Symptoms characteristically include purulent anal discharge, anal pain, and tenesmus.

**Lymphogranuloma venereum**

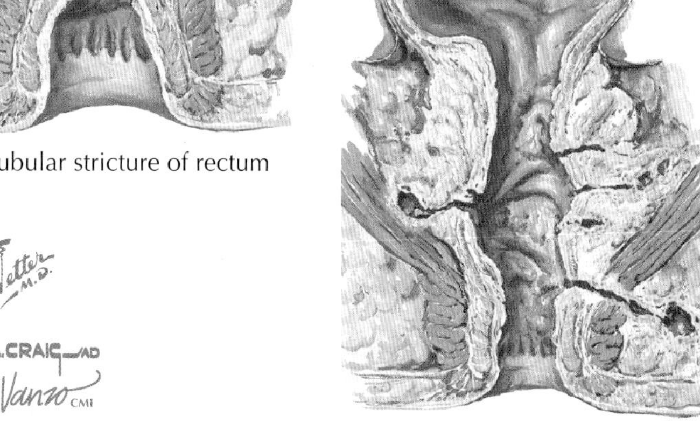


Pathway of spread of lymphogranuloma venereum from upper vagina and/or cervix uteri to rectum via lymph vessels

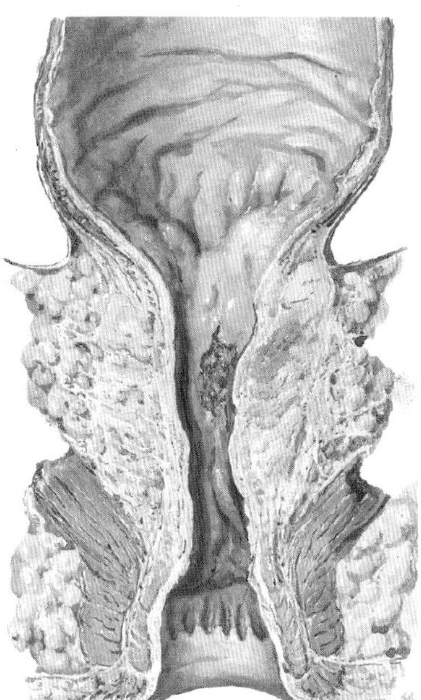

Long tubular stricture of rectum

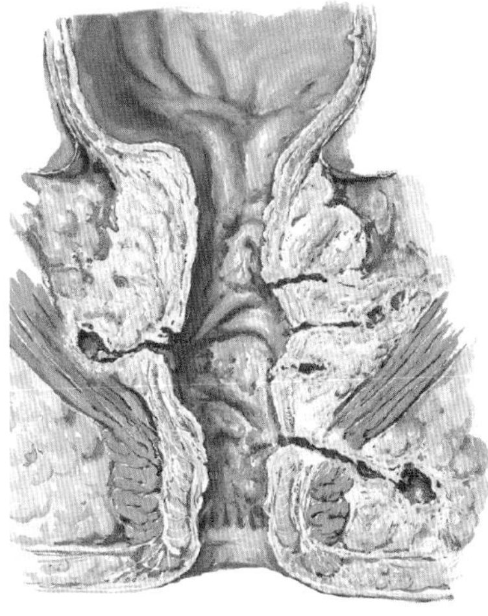

Stricture of rectum with multiple blind sinuses

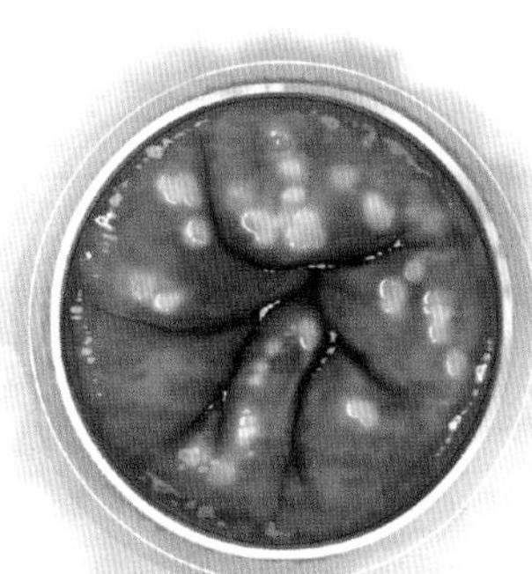

Anal intraepithelial neoplasia due to HPV

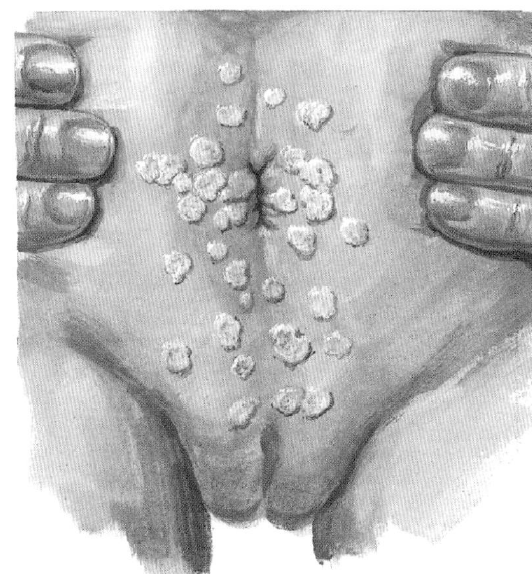

Condylomata lata (secondary syphilis)

Herpes simplex virus type I or II may lead to proctitis and perianal infections. Infection is usually associated with rectal intercourse but may also be seen with reactivation of disease from a prior genital infection and is associated with anorectal pain, tenesmus, constipation, and discharge. Ulcerative lesions may be seen on proctoscopy or colonoscopy.

HPV is associated with 80% to 85% of anal cancers worldwide. High-risk HPV serotypes include 16, 18, 31, 33, 39, 45, 51, 52, 56, 58, and 59. Infection of anorectal tissues may result from direct inoculation through sexual activity or autoinoculation of infected secretions from a primary genital site. Similar to cervical carcinoma, HPV-related anorectal malignancies evolve from metaplastic activity induced by viral transformation of anal epithelial tissues. High-risk patients, such as those with HIV with a history of receptive anal intercourse or other documented HPV-related disease, may benefit from screening by anal cytology and/or high-resolution anoscopic examination of the anal canal to identify precancerous lesions.

### Gut Microbiome

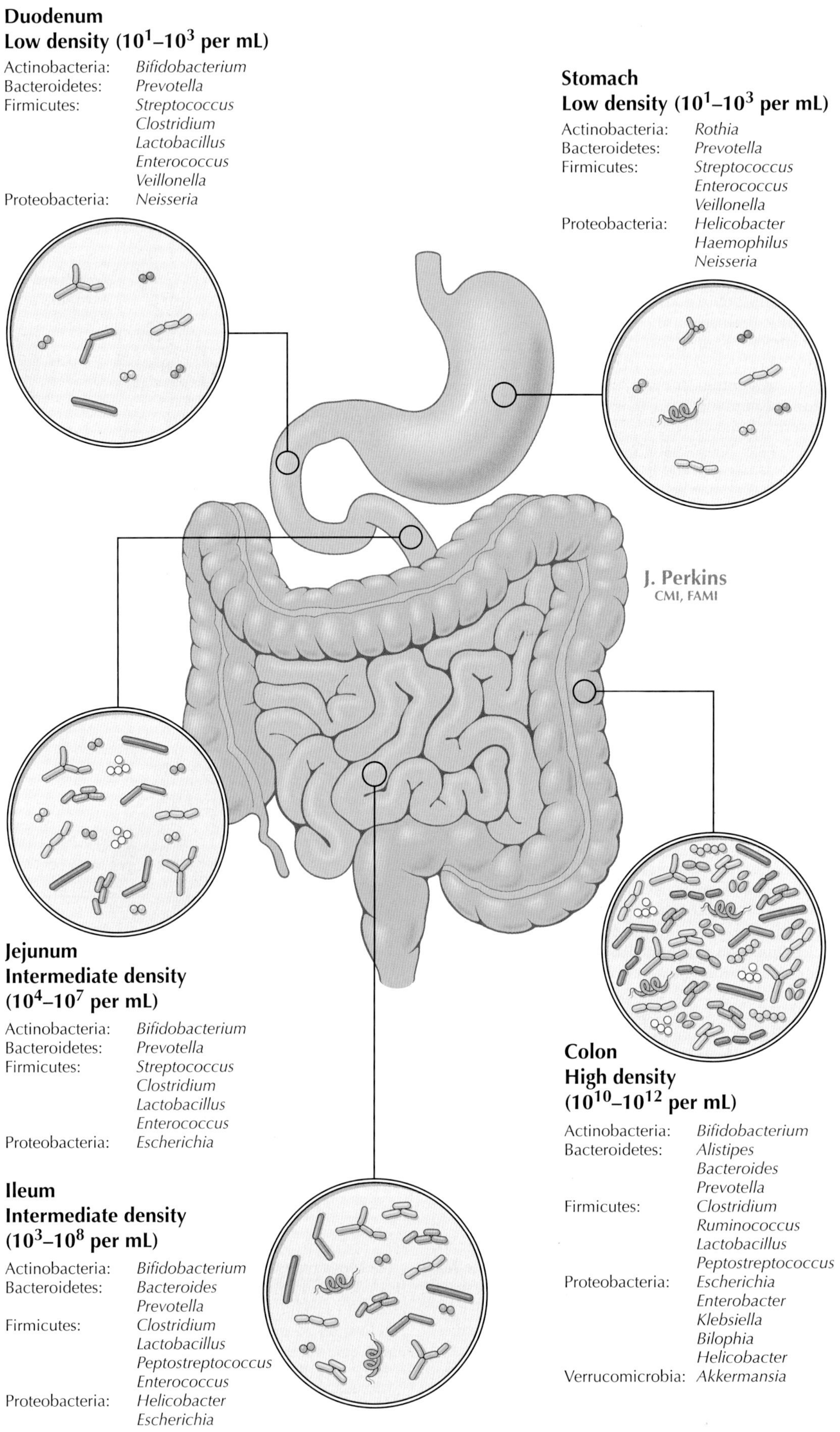

**Duodenum**
**Low density ($10^1$–$10^3$ per mL)**

Actinobacteria: *Bifidobacterium*
Bacteroidetes: *Prevotella*
Firmicutes: *Streptococcus*, *Clostridium*, *Lactobacillus*, *Enterococcus*, *Veillonella*
Proteobacteria: *Neisseria*

**Stomach**
**Low density ($10^1$–$10^3$ per mL)**

Actinobacteria: *Rothia*
Bacteroidetes: *Prevotella*
Firmicutes: *Streptococcus*, *Enterococcus*, *Veillonella*
Proteobacteria: *Helicobacter*, *Haemophilus*, *Neisseria*

J. Perkins
CMI, FAMI

**Jejunum**
**Intermediate density ($10^4$–$10^7$ per mL)**

Actinobacteria: *Bifidobacterium*
Bacteroidetes: *Prevotella*
Firmicutes: *Streptococcus*, *Clostridium*, *Lactobacillus*, *Enterococcus*
Proteobacteria: *Escherichia*

**Ileum**
**Intermediate density ($10^3$–$10^8$ per mL)**

Actinobacteria: *Bifidobacterium*
Bacteroidetes: *Bacteroides*, *Prevotella*
Firmicutes: *Clostridium*, *Lactobacillus*, *Peptostreptococcus*, *Enterococcus*
Proteobacteria: *Helicobacter*, *Escherichia*

**Colon**
**High density ($10^{10}$–$10^{12}$ per mL)**

Actinobacteria: *Bifidobacterium*
Bacteroidetes: *Alistipes*, *Bacteroides*, *Prevotella*
Firmicutes: *Clostridium*, *Ruminococcus*, *Lactobacillus*, *Peptostreptococcus*
Proteobacteria: *Escherichia*, *Enterobacter*, *Klebsiella*, *Bilophia*, *Helicobacter*
Verrucomicrobia: *Akkermansia*

## GUT MICROBIOME

The human body is colonized by a diverse group of microorganisms including bacteria, archaea, viruses, bacteriophages, parasites, and fungi that influence human physiology, immune function, metabolism, and nutrition. Although every anatomic site may be characterized by a unique density and pattern of microbial organisms, the GI tract harbors more than 100 trillion microorganisms, representing 95% of the body's microbiome. Changes in microbiome composition and character may lead to significant beneficial or harmful health consequences. Gut microbiota may be commensal, conferring neither harm nor benefit, or symbiotic, where both host and organism derive benefit from the association.

The gut microbiome includes more than 1000 different bacterial species, primarily of the phyla Bacteroidetes, Firmicutes, Actinobacteria, and Proteobacteria. Only 10% to 50% of gut bacteria are amenable to standard culture techniques, hindering the ability to grow these organisms in in vitro cultures. 16S rRNA gene and DNA sequencing methods may further identify nonculturable species. Metagenomic sequencing characterizes the genetic content of the entire sample bacterial community, assessing functional attributes of the bacterial population as a whole. Metabolites, small molecular substrates, and proteins produced by the microbiome affect human health, homeostasis, and disease. These microbiome derivatives may be analyzed through metabolomics and proteomic methods.

Changes in the balance of microbiota that occur from elements such as age, genetics, diet, infection, antimicrobial therapy, and other factors are implicated in a multitude of human diseases. Microbes use diverse mechanisms to compete with other members in the ecology of the gut. Properties such as antibiotic production, bacteriocins, adhesiveness, toxic effector proteins, and signaling molecules may determine the unique gut microbiota profile for any individual. This profile differs by anatomic location and may change over time and with differing exposures and stimuli.

A diverse and healthy gut ecology prevents colonization and proliferation of potentially pathogenic organisms by competing for unique etiologic conditions such

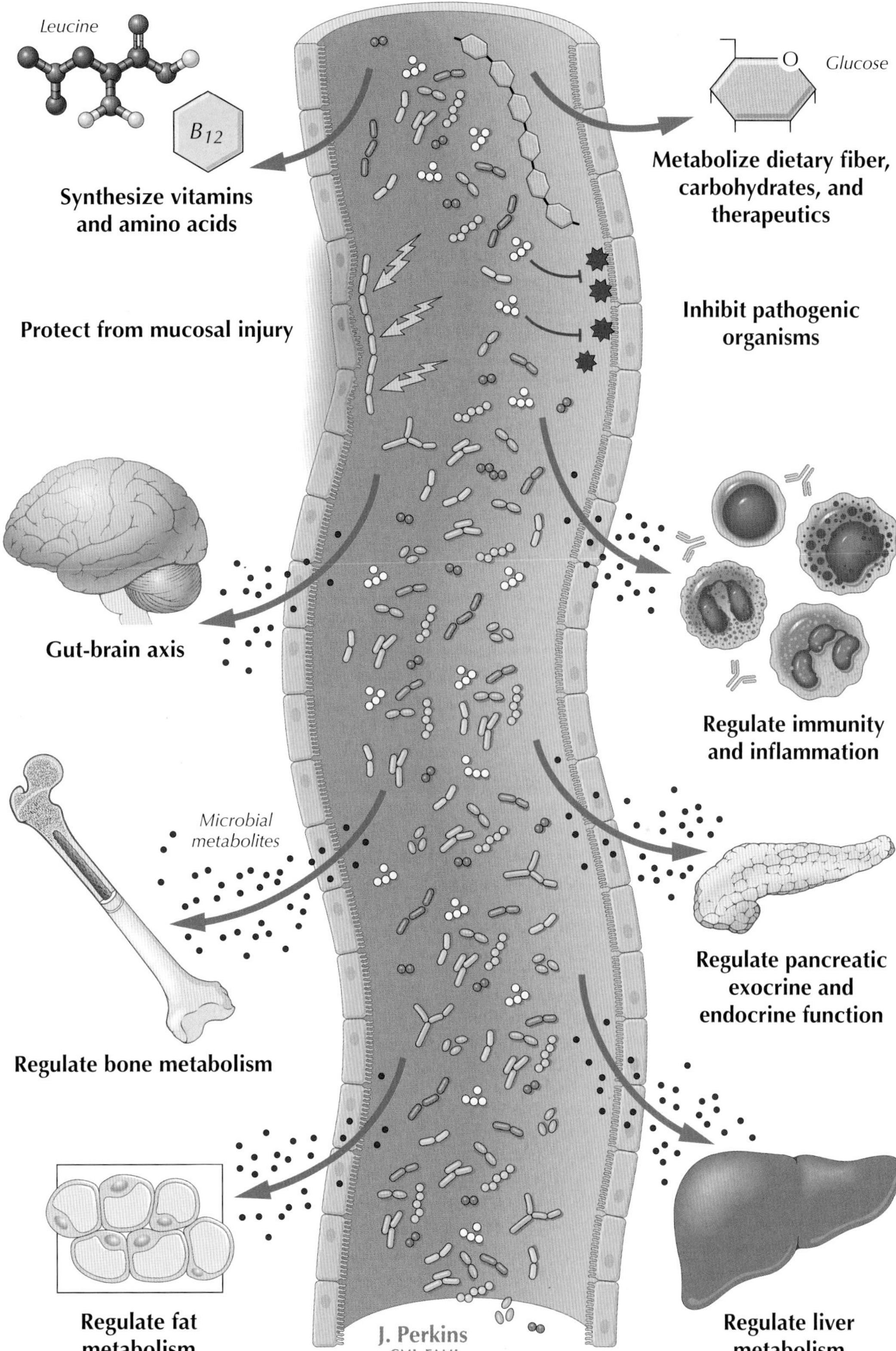


## GUT MICROBIOME (Continued)

as nutrition, adherence sites, and other resources necessary for pathogenic bacteria to expand in the gut. A loss of this homeostasis may progress toward illness. For instance, loss of the normal microbiome diversity and density through the use of broad-spectrum antibiotics allows overgrowth of *C. difficile* with resultant toxin production and clinical illness. IBS may be associated with microbiota alterations that promote low-grade intestinal inflammation and adherence of pathogenic bacteria to the bowel wall. IBDs including CD and UC, have been linked to reduced bacteriologic diversity, microbiome-related inflammatory dysregulation, and specific metabolic microbial derivatives. Certain microbial species or their metabolic by-products may have direct cytotoxic effect to the intestinal epithelium, leading to disproportionate proinflammatory signaling at the GI tract mucosa. This may result in increased sloughing and repair of the intestinal epithelium, leading to increased risk for colorectal neoplasia.

Beyond the GI tract, the gut microbiome has been associated with a wide variety of medical conditions. Microbiome-related effects on systemic metabolism, inflammation, and immune regulation have been implicated in neurologic conditions such as autism, Parkinson disease, Alzheimer disease, and multiple sclerosis; cardiovascular diseases including hypertension and atherosclerosis; metabolic diseases including obesity, nonalcoholic fatty liver disease, and diabetes; allergic disorders including asthma and food allergies; pancreatitis; and fibromyalgia.

Therapeutic manipulation of the gut microbiome through use of probiotics and prebiotics may treat or prevent disease conditions by restoring gut homeostasis. Prebiotics are indigestible dietary fibers and carbohydrates that can only be metabolized and fermented by microbial enzymes, resulting in production of simple sugars and short-chain fatty acids. The resulting lower pH affects the microbial ecology and inhibits pathologic species such as *C. difficile,* stimulates immune cell activity and regulates metabolic homeostasis. Probiotics are live microorganisms, typically bacteria and yeast derived from culture, designed to replace or enhance deficient microbiota. In extreme cases, fecal microbiota transfer, also known as *fecal transplantation* or *bacteriotherapy,* from a healthy donor may be used to treat *C. difficile*–associated colitis.

## PARASITIC DISEASES: ENTEROBIASIS

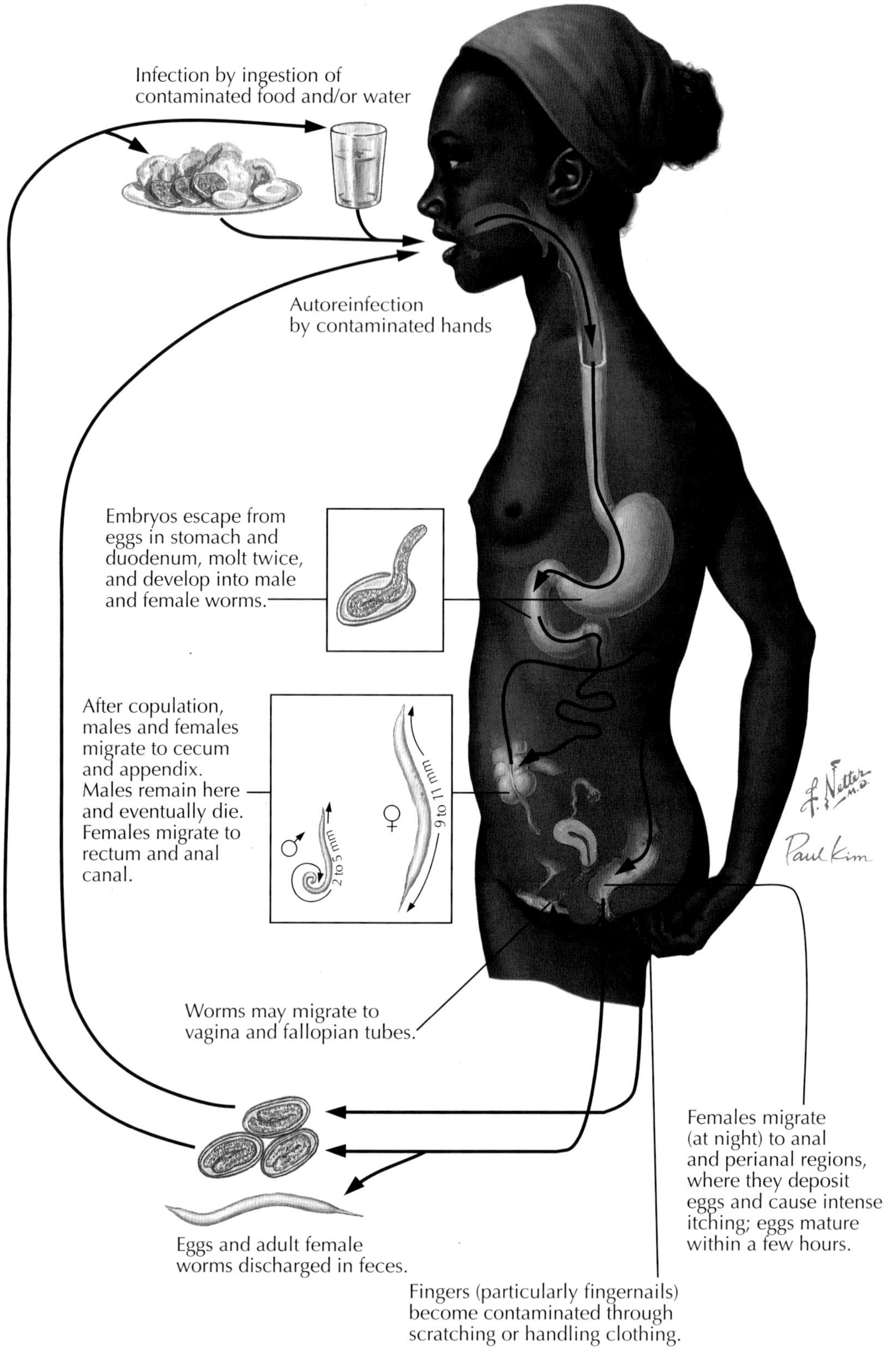

*Enterobius vermicularis* (the human pinworm) is found worldwide in both tropical and temperate climates. It is common in children, institutional settings, and households and is not associated with socioeconomic status. The small, spindle-shaped, round adult worms inhabit the cecum, appendix, and adjacent portions of the large and small intestine, with their heads attached to the intestinal mucosa. The male worm measures 2 to 5 mm in length and 0.1 to 0.2 mm at its greatest diameter and has a sharply curved and blunted posterior end. The female worm, 8 to 13 mm in length and 0.3 to 0.5 mm at its greatest diameter, has a sharply pointed tail. The female produces eggs in its ovary and releases them into a reservoir, the "uterus," where fecundation takes place. When the reservoir is filled, the worm detaches itself from the bowel wall and migrates down the colon to the rectum, and from there through the anal canal to perianal and perineal regions. Some of the parasites are expelled from the host's rectum passively with the feces. Migration beyond the anal sphincter occurs at night; the female worm, while crawling on the skin, deposits eggs in the perianal and genitocrural folds. The average number of eggs deposited by a single female has been found to be about 11,000. At the time of laying, the eggs are already embryonated and, within a few hours, develop into the infective vermiform stage. The embryonated eggs measure 50 to 60 μm by 20 to 30 μm and are flattened on one side. They have a translucent shell that consists of an outer, albuminous covering and an inner, embryonic, lipoidal membrane. The eggs require no intermediate host for their subsequent development; they become infective within a few hours after being laid and may remain viable for weeks or months. From the perianal region the ova are transferred to clothes and bed linens. The hands of the patient, particularly the fingernails, may become contaminated through scratching the perianal regions or handling clothing. The ova may be transferred to the same or another host either by hand to mouth or indirectly through food and drink. The eggs from bed linens and clothes may also be blown into the air and get indirectly into the mouth or be inhaled and swallowed. Female parasites that are expelled in the feces empty their "uteri" outside the host; part of the discharged ova become infective and may be ingested with contaminated food or water. Eggs lose viability after a few days in the environment, with most becoming nonviable within 2 weeks. When eggs containing infective larvae are ingested and reach the stomach and duodenum, the digestive secretions soften the eggs' walls and the larvae released. These larvae pass down the small bowel, molt twice, and develop into mature male and female worms. After copulation the female becomes "gravid" and a new cycle begins. The duration of the cycle from the ingestion of the ovum to the development of a mature worm is from 2 to 6 weeks.

*Enterobius vermicularis* is a relatively innocuous parasite that only seldom produces significant local pathology. Attachment of the worms may produce a mild inflammation of the intestinal mucosa from mechanical irritation. Occasionally, migration of adult worms may lead to disease outside the GI tract. The most common and most disturbing symptom of enterobiasis is pruritus ani, which can vary in degree from mild to extreme and is most troublesome at night. Affected individuals, particularly children, may experience sleep disturbances, restlessness, and insomnia. Scratching of the irritated region may lead to excoriation, dermatitis, and folliculitis. In female patients the parasites may migrate to produce vulvitis and vaginitis. Rarely, female worms may migrate to the fallopian tubes and became encysted there or migrate out into the peritoneal cavity, leading to pelvic, cervical, vulvar, or peritoneal granulomas. Infection of the bladder may occur. The psychological impact of infection for both the patient and the affected family may be significant. The diagnosis of enterobiasis is made by identification of the worms on perianal skin or the vagina of persons who are infected. Eggs may be identified in feces or by microscopic examination of transparent tape that has been applied several times to the perianal skin to capture eggs deposited by gravid females (see Plate 3.58).

Infection by ingestion of contaminated food and/or water
Autoreinfection by contaminated hands
Embryos escape from eggs in stomach and duodenum, molt twice, and develop into male and female worms.
After copulation, males and females migrate to cecum and appendix. Males remain here and eventually die. Females migrate to rectum and anal canal.
♂ 2 to 5 mm
♀ 9 to 11 mm
Worms may migrate to vagina and fallopian tubes.
Females migrate (at night) to anal and perianal regions, where they deposit eggs and cause intense itching; eggs mature within a few hours.
Eggs and adult female worms discharged in feces.
Fingers (particularly fingernails) become contaminated through scratching or handling clothing.
F. Netter M.D.
Paul Kim

## Parasitic Diseases: Trichuriasis

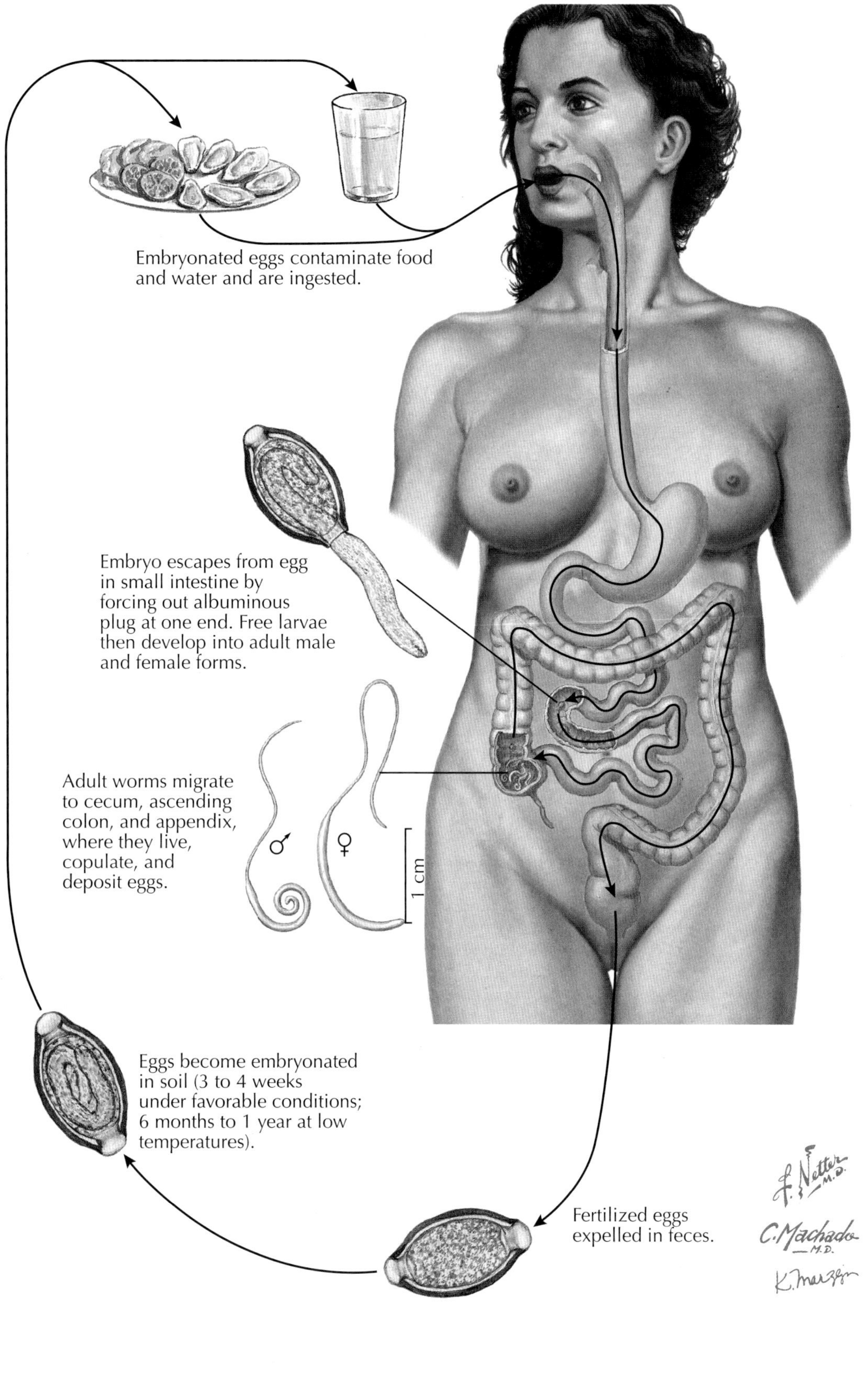

Trichuriasis is parasitism produced by the worm *Trichuris trichiura* (human whipworm). This worm is cosmopolitan in distribution but is common in temperate zones and humid tropical environments. Humans seem to be the only host, although whipworms obtained from pigs and monkeys are morphologically similar. The male worm measures 30 to 45 mm in length and the female measures 35 to 50 mm. In both sexes the pinkish body of the parasite shows two portions: the cephalic portion, which is longer and attenuated (whiplike), containing the esophagus, and the caudal portion, which is shorter and thicker, containing the intestine and sex organs. The posterior end of the male is coiled, whereas that of the female is comma shaped.

The adult parasites live predominately in the cecum and ascending colon, but infection may extend to the transverse colon, descending colon, or rectum. After fertilization the female lays eggs, which are expelled in the feces. Each worm may produce 3000 to 20,000 eggs daily. The eggs are barrel shaped and measure approximately 50 to 55 μm in length and 22 to 24 μm in diameter. They have a double shell, which is perforated at the poles, with the polar orifices closed by prominent, colorless, refractive albuminous plugs. At oviposition, the fertilized ova show unsegmented granular contents. Embryonic development takes place outside the host, in the soil. Under favorable conditions with warm moist soil, the ova reach the motile embryo stage in about 3 to 4 weeks and may survive in the environment for years. Human beings become infected by swallowing fully embryonated eggs obtained directly or indirectly from the soil. Food (especially uncooked vegetables), water, and hands may become contaminated directly by infected soil or indirectly by domestic animals, flies, and other insects. The ingested embryonated egg reaches the intestine, where it encounters digestive enzymes that allow the embryo to excyst through one of the two albuminous plugs at the poles. The adult worms attach to the intestinal wall with the thin anterior portion embedded in the mucosa, where they develop into mature adult worms, copulate, and release fertilized eggs that are then released into the environment via the feces. About 3 months is required for maturation and oviposition from the time of ingestion of the embryonated eggs. In most cases the infection is not very intense, with fewer than 20 worms. Clinical disease is usually associated with more than 200 worms. Occasionally, however, a patient may harbor a thousand or more worms in the large intestine.

The pathologic effects of whipworm infection are usually mild, if at all present, and are chiefly due to trauma of the intestinal mucosa and to toxic substances produced by large numbers of parasites. The anterior portion of the worm is buried in the intestinal mucosa, which may result in minor local inflammation. At the site of the worm's penetration into the mucosa, however, a secondary invasion by intestinal bacteria may occur and may give rise to inflammatory reactions, including acute appendicitis in rare circumstances. Significant worm burdens may result in a friable and edematous bowel wall, which may bleed, leading to anemia in patients with limited iron intake. The worm itself does not actively suck blood.

The clinical signs of trichuriasis vary with the intensity of infection, extent of intestinal penetration, and secondary bacterial infection. In most instances no noticeable or only vague digestive disturbances occur. Pronounced symptoms are associated with massive infection or bacterial invasion. This may include diarrhea, dysenteric syndrome, constipation, abdominal pain, abdominal distension, weakness, weight loss, and anemia. Chronic inflammation of the rectal mucosa may lead to tenesmus and rectal prolapse. Adult worms may be seen in the prolapsed rectal tissue. The diagnosis is made by identifying the characteristic eggs on stool examination or the adult worms on prolapsed rectal tissue or at colonoscopy.

Embryonated eggs contaminate food and water and are ingested.
Embryo escapes from egg in small intestine by forcing out albuminous plug at one end. Free larvae then develop into adult male and female forms.
Adult worms migrate to cecum, ascending colon, and appendix, where they live, copulate, and deposit eggs.
♂
♀
1 cm
Eggs become embryonated in soil (3 to 4 weeks under favorable conditions; 6 months to 1 year at low temperatures).
Fertilized eggs expelled in feces.
F. Netter M.D.
C. Machado M.D.

## Parasitic Diseases: Ascariasis

*Ascaris lumbricoides* (the large intestinal roundworm) is the most common helminthic infection of humans. This worm is cosmopolitan in distribution but is common in temperate zones and humid tropical environments. The white or pinkish adult worms are elongated nematodes, tapering anteriorly and posteriorly to conical ends. Their smooth cuticle is finely striated, and two faint whitish streaks run along either side of the entire body length. The adult male (15–30 cm by 2–4 mm) is smaller than the female (25–35 cm by 3–6 mm) and is characterized by a ventral curvature of its posterior extremity. Specimens of both sexes, however, sometimes may reach a considerably larger size. The adult worms live, as a rule, in the lumen of the small bowel, obtaining their nourishment from the semidigested food of the host. A mature female worm produces about 200,000 eggs a day. The fertilized ova, measuring from 45 to 70 μm in length and 35 to 50 μm in breadth, contain a mass of coarse lecithin granules. Fertilized eggs demonstrate an outer coarsely mammillated, albuminous covering and a thick, hyaline shell composed of several layers. The unfertilized ova are larger, can have bizarre shapes, may lack one or more layer of the normal shell layers, and have disorganized, globular internal contents. In both fertilized and unfertilized eggs the albuminous covering is easily broken or may be absent. The ova are expelled with the feces and must undergo a process of maturation before becoming infective. Under favorable conditions (moist, shady soil and a temperature of about 25°C) the embryo molts into a second-stage infective larva. This phase may take from 10 days to 6 weeks depending on temperature. If the conditions are unfavorable, the ova may remain dormant for several years and develop with the return of a favorable environment.

Human infection occurs by swallowing mature ova, which are conveyed to the mouth by contaminated fingers, water, vegetables, or other food. In the small intestine the larvae are liberated, penetrate the intestinal wall, and pass into the portal circulation; via the liver and heart they reach the lungs, penetrate the capillaries, and enter the alveoli. From the alveoli, the worms, now 1.5 mm in length, ascend the bronchi and trachea to the glottis, are swallowed, and pass down to the small intestine, where they develop into adult male or female worms.

In the lungs the larvae give rise to local inflammation and hypersensitivity. A marked eosinophilia may be present in peripheral blood. Allergic manifestations of ascariasis can include reactive airway disease or episodes of urticaria. An extensive alveolar exudation of red blood cells, neutrophils, eosinophils, and fibrin may evolve, resulting in a lobular pneumonia. Eventually, an entire lobe may become consolidated (*Ascaris* pneumonitis). Sensitive individuals react to the larvae with an allergic edema and eosinophilic infiltration of the lungs (Löffler syndrome).

Infection with a few adult worms in the intestinal lumen is usually asymptomatic. Heavier infections may cause local mechanical disturbance and impair the nutritional status of children, especially in regions where other coexisting intestinal infections may be present. In most cases the symptoms consist of abdominal discomfort, pain, loss of appetite, nausea, and diarrhea or constipation. Occasionally, masses of worms may obstruct the intestinal lumen, often at the terminal ilium, especially in children. Adult worms may migrate up or down the intestinal tract and be passed by the anus or emerge from the mouth or nose or, sometimes, may penetrate into the appendix, diverticula, bile ducts, gallbladder, pancreatic duct, peritoneal cavity (especially after gastrointestinal surgery), pharynx, or middle ear, giving rise to serious local complications. The diagnosis is usually made by recovery of the characteristic eggs in the feces; demonstration of the adult worm passed through the mouth, anus, or nose; or the identification of adult worms on colonoscopy. Radiographs may demonstrate Ascaris worms in gas-filled loops of bowel, or, following a radiopaque meal or barium enema, may reveal adult worms as characteristic filling defects. Worms may also be demonstrated by CT or ultrasound studies.

1. Ova contaminate food and are ingested with it.
2. Larvae emerge from eggs in small intestine.
3. Larvae penetrate gut wall and pass to heart via portal vein, liver, and inferior vena cava.
4. Larvae reach lung by way of pulmonary artery, penetrate alveoli, and enter bronchi.
5. Larvae ascend trachea to larynx and are swallowed.
6. Larvae molt and develop into adult worms in small intestine. Worms are harbored here and may pass to other organs (biliary tract, lung, heart) or emerge from anus, mouth, or nose.
7. Ova expelled in feces
8. Fertilized eggs become embryonated in 10 days to 6 weeks.

15 to 25 cm

20 to 35 cm

Male

Female

Fertilized

Unfertilized

(Outer covering lost owing to pressure of cover glass)

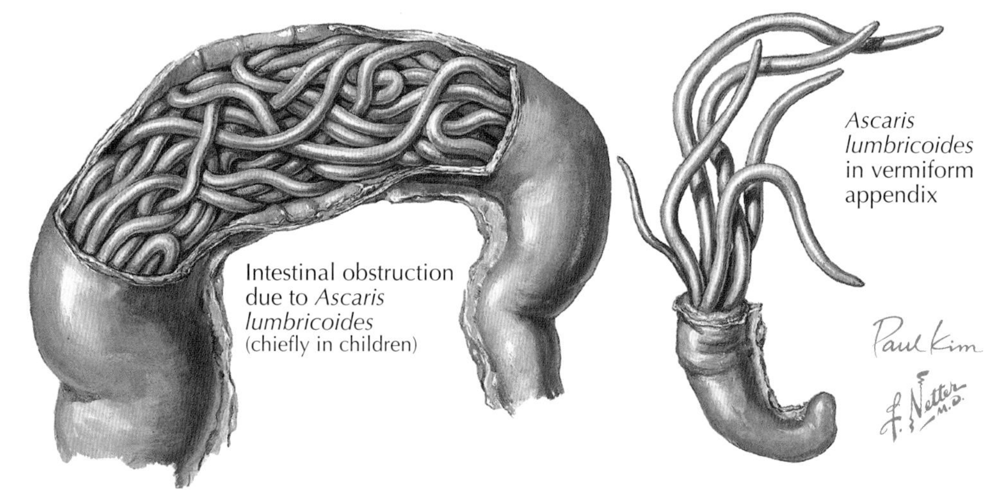

Intestinal obstruction due to *Ascaris lumbricoides* (chiefly in children)
*Ascaris lumbricoides* in vermiform appendix
Paul Kim
F. Netter M.D.

## PARASITIC DISEASES: NECATORIASIS AND ANCYLOSTOMIASIS

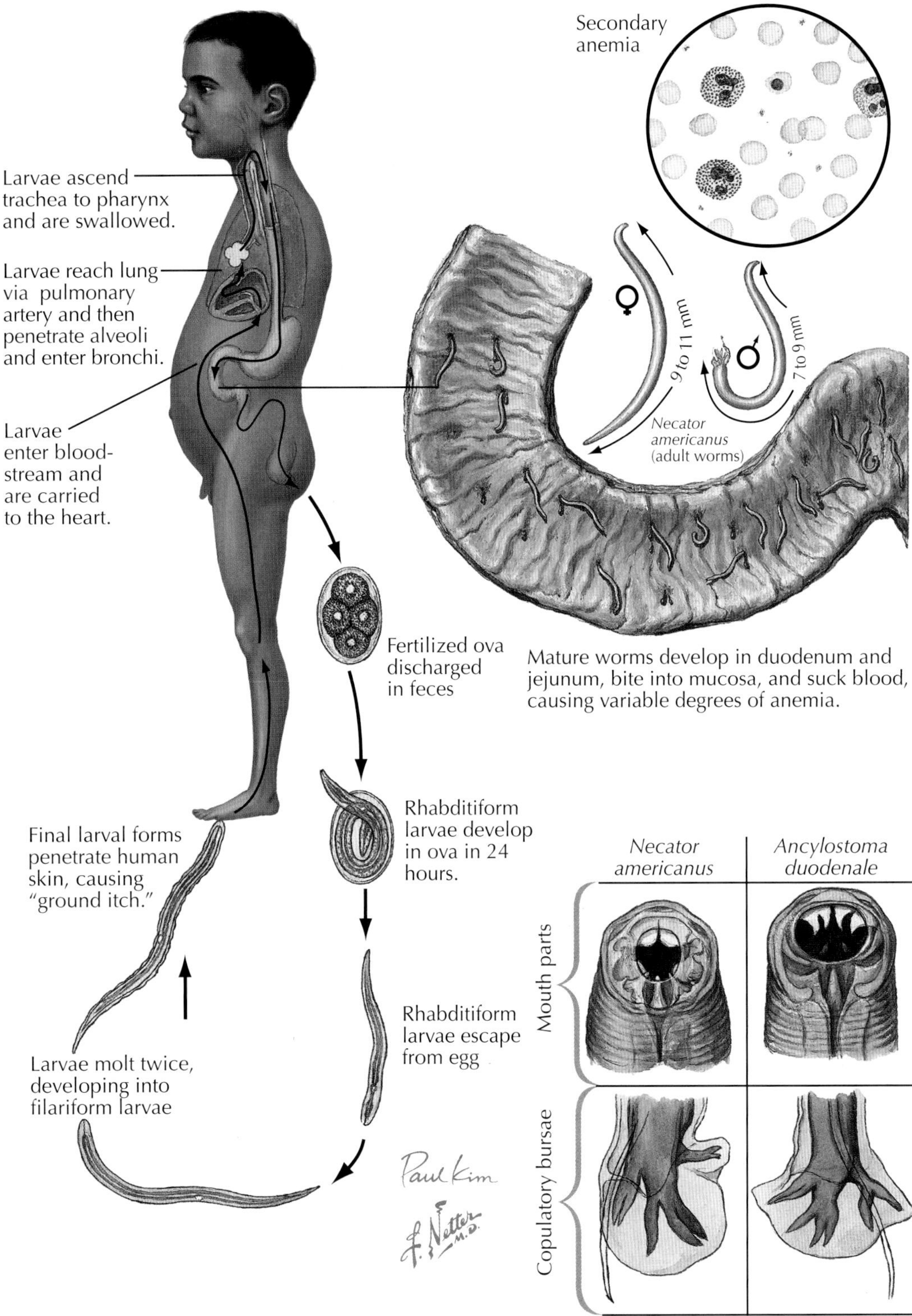
Secondary anemia
Larvae ascend trachea to pharynx and are swallowed.
Larvae reach lung via pulmonary artery and then penetrate alveoli and enter bronchi.
Larvae enter bloodstream and are carried to the heart.
9 to 11 mm
7 to 9 mm
Necator americanus (adult worms)
Fertilized ova discharged in feces
Mature worms develop in duodenum and jejunum, bite into mucosa, and suck blood, causing variable degrees of anemia.
Rhabditiform larvae develop in ova in 24 hours.
Final larval forms penetrate human skin, causing "ground itch."
Rhabditiform larvae escape from egg
Larvae molt twice, developing into filariform larvae
Necator americanus
Ancylostoma duodenale
Mouth parts
Copulatory bursae
Paul Kim
F. Netter M.D.

*Necator americanus* and *Ancylostoma duodenale* are nematodes that produce the human hookworm disease. *N. americanus* is the species that predominates in the Western Hemisphere, Central and South Africa, South Asia, the East Indies, Polynesia, Micronesia, and Australia, whereas *A. duodenale* is the predominant species in coastal North Africa, the Mediterranean, Southern Europe, northern India, northern China, and Japan. *N. americanus* is a cylindrical, fusiform worm, grayish-yellow or reddish in color; the adult male measures 5 to 9 mm in length by 0.3 mm in breadth, and the female measures 9 to 11 mm in length by 0.35 mm in breadth. The posterior end of the male is extended into a bell-shaped bursa, whereas that of the female is cone shaped. *Ancylostoma* is slightly larger, with the female measuring 10 to 13 mm in length and 0.6 mm in breadth. The morphology assumed by *N. americanus* is very characteristic: the body forms an arc, with the ventral surface on the inner side, while the anterior extremity curves sharply backward over the body. The chief morphologic characteristics differentiating *N. americanus* and *A. duodenale* are the mouth parts and copulatory bursae. The buccal capsule of *N. americanus* is located on the upper (ventral) side with two semilunar cutting plates, whereas that of *A. duodenale* exhibits two pairs of teeth. The male copulatory bursae, functioning to hold the female during copulation, show morphologic differences, including differing muscular digitations and copulatory spicules between species.

The life cycles of *N. americanus* and *A. duodenale* are essentially the same. The adult worms live in the small intestine, where they attach themselves to the mucosa by their buccal capsules and feed on the blood and lymph of their host. The fertilized female lays 10,000 to 25,000 eggs daily. The eggs, ovoid in shape, measuring 60 to 70 μm in length and having a thin shell, are usually passed in the feces in the two- to eight-cell stage of segmentation. Under favorable conditions of aerated soil, moderate moisture, and an optimal temperature, rhabditiform larvae hatch from the eggs within 24 hours. They grow while feeding on fecal material for about 3 to 5 days, molt twice, and develop into infective filariform larvae. When the human host comes in contact with contaminated soil, the filariform larvae penetrate skin. They then enter the lymphatics or venules and are carried in the blood through the heart to the lungs, where they pass from the capillaries into the alveoli, ascend the respiratory tree, pass to the pharynx, are swallowed, and reach the duodenum and jejunum, where they mature into adult male and female worms.

The clinical manifestations caused by *N. americanus* and *A. duodenale* are also similar. Penetration of the larvae into the skin may occasionally give rise to a local pruritic dermatitis ("ground itch"), with edema, erythema, and a papular or vesicular eruption. Non-human-adapted hookworm species, *A. braziliense* and *A. caninum,* may penetrate the skin, creating local inflammatory tracks and erythema (creeping eruption), but do not progress beyond this stage. The blood-lung migration of the larvae causes minute hemorrhages and cellular infiltration in the alveolar tissues. Lung involvement usually remains subclinical unless large numbers of larvae are migrating simultaneously. In the intestinal phase, the adult worms may eventually provoke hyperperistalsis with cramps and diarrhea. By sucking blood and producing small erosions in the mucosa, the parasites may be responsible for development of hypochromic, microcytic anemia. Blood loss is 0.03 mL/day per *A. duodenale* worm and 0.15 to 0.26 mL/day per *N. americanus* worm. Thus a severe anemia is likely to occur only in cases of heavy worm burden when food intake is deficient in iron and protein. At times, a single massive infection may induce acute symptoms that include headache, nausea, prostration, pulmonary and circulatory disturbances, severe abdominal pain, and dysentery. Eosinophilia is commonly seen in peripheral blood smear. Chronic infection has been associated with impaired physical and intellectual health of children and diminished work capacity and productivity of adults in endemic regions. The diagnosis of hookworm disease is made by recovery of characteristic eggs in the feces.

## Parasitic Diseases: Strongyloidiasis

*Strongyloides stercoralis* is a cosmopolitan nematode parasite but is encountered mostly in the tropics and subtropics. The adult female, a delicate, filiform worm measuring about 2.2 mm in length and 0.03 to 0.075 mm in diameter, lives within the mucosa of the small intestine, laying several dozens of embryonated eggs a day, from which rhabditiform larvae (indirect, sexual, or heterogonic life cycle) hatch. These are expelled in the feces. Under favorable conditions of a warm, moist climate the rhabditiform larvae may develop in the soil into free-living, sexually mature rhabditiform males and females measuring about 0.7 and 1 mm in length, respectively. The fertilized, free-living female discharges eggs, from which a second generation of rhabditiform larvae hatch. With favorable environmental conditions, the second rhabditiform larvae may develop into free-living adults, reproduce sexually, and create successive generations of rhabditiform larvae. Rhabditiform larvae expelled with the feces or generated from free-living environmental larvae may also metamorphose directly into infective filariform larvae (direct, or asexual, homogonic life cycle). When in contact with human skin, the infective filariform larvae penetrate the cutaneous blood vessels and are carried to the capillaries of the lungs, where they break through the alveoli, ascend the respiratory tree to the pharynx, are swallowed, and reach the intestine. During this migration the filariform larvae change into the adolescent stage and may copulate (heterogonic development). The mature parasitic females burrow into the mucosa of the duodenum and jejunum, but occasionally also in the ileum, appendix, and colon, and start oviposition after fertilization or by parthenogenesis (asexual reproduction). Eggs are typically oval and thin-shelled but are usually not identified because they rapidly hatch within the host to release rhabditiform larvae, which are passed into the environment to complete the cycle. The males, not being tissue parasites, are voided in the feces after a brief stay in the intestine. Time from infection to shedding of larvae is typically 3 to 5 weeks. Rhabditiform larvae may, in lieu of passage into the environment, reinfect the host through the intestinal mucosa or perianal skin, leading to autoinfection and successive generations of organisms.

Penetration of the larvae into the skin is usually asymptomatic, but in hypersensitive individuals it may cause a pruritic eruption at the site of penetration (larva currens) and is most notable on the buttock of patients with significant autoinoculation. The migration of the larvae through the lungs may occasionally lead to local inflammation and hemorrhage manifesting as pulmonary infiltrates with reactive airway disease and peripheral eosinophilia (Löffler syndrome). Occasionally, bronchial congestion may prevent the escape of larvae from the lungs, so that some of them may develop at this site into adult worms, causing more pulmonary damage and, eventually, invasion of the pleural and pericardial cavities. In the intestine, the reaction of the intestinal mucosa varies from a light inflammatory cellular infiltration to patchy necrosis, with sloughing, followed by fibroblastic repair or the development of granulomatous masses. Accordingly, the clinical manifestations vary also from an asymptomatic course to pronounced dysentery, with alternate diarrhea and constipation prevailing in moderate infections. Alterations of host responses resulting from hematologic malignancies, organ transplantation, HIV/AIDS, human T-lymphotropic virus type 1 infection, hypogammaglobulinemia, corticosteroid use, and anti–tumor necrosis factor therapies may result in acceleration and augmentation of the autoinoculation cycle to a hyperinfection syndrome. The most common manifestation of hyperinfection syndrome is pulmonary disease with focal or diffuse infiltrates and bronchospasm. Erratic migration of larvae may occur as well with seeding of many tissues via the bloodstream, including myocardium, liver, gallbladder, meninges, brain, pancreas, thyroid, kidney, spleen, and lymph nodes. Bacteremia resulting from larval invasion of the bowel wall may lead to gram-negative meningitis. The diagnosis of strongyloidiasis rests upon recognition of the characteristic rhabditiform larvae in the feces or duodenal contents. An enzyme-linked immunosorbent assay is available for serologic diagnosis. Patients with hyperinfection syndrome may have larvae identified from pulmonary secretions.

Larvae ascend trachea to pharynx and are swallowed.

Filariform larvae migrate via bloodstream, passing through heart and pulmonary artery to lungs.

In lungs, larvae may cause hemorrhage or infiltration.

Parasitic adult females develop in duodenum, penetrate duodenal or jejunal mucosa, and deposit embryonated eggs.

Rhabditiform larvae are hatched from eggs, find way to intestinal lumen, and are expelled in feces.

Rhabditiform larvae discharged in feces

Indirect (long, sexual) cycle

Direct (short, asexual) cycle

Rhabditiform larvae discharged in feces

In soil, larvae develop (within 36 hours) into sexually mature, free-living rhabditiform males and females.

Rhabditiform larvae may again differentiate into males and females and repeatedly originate new free-living generations.

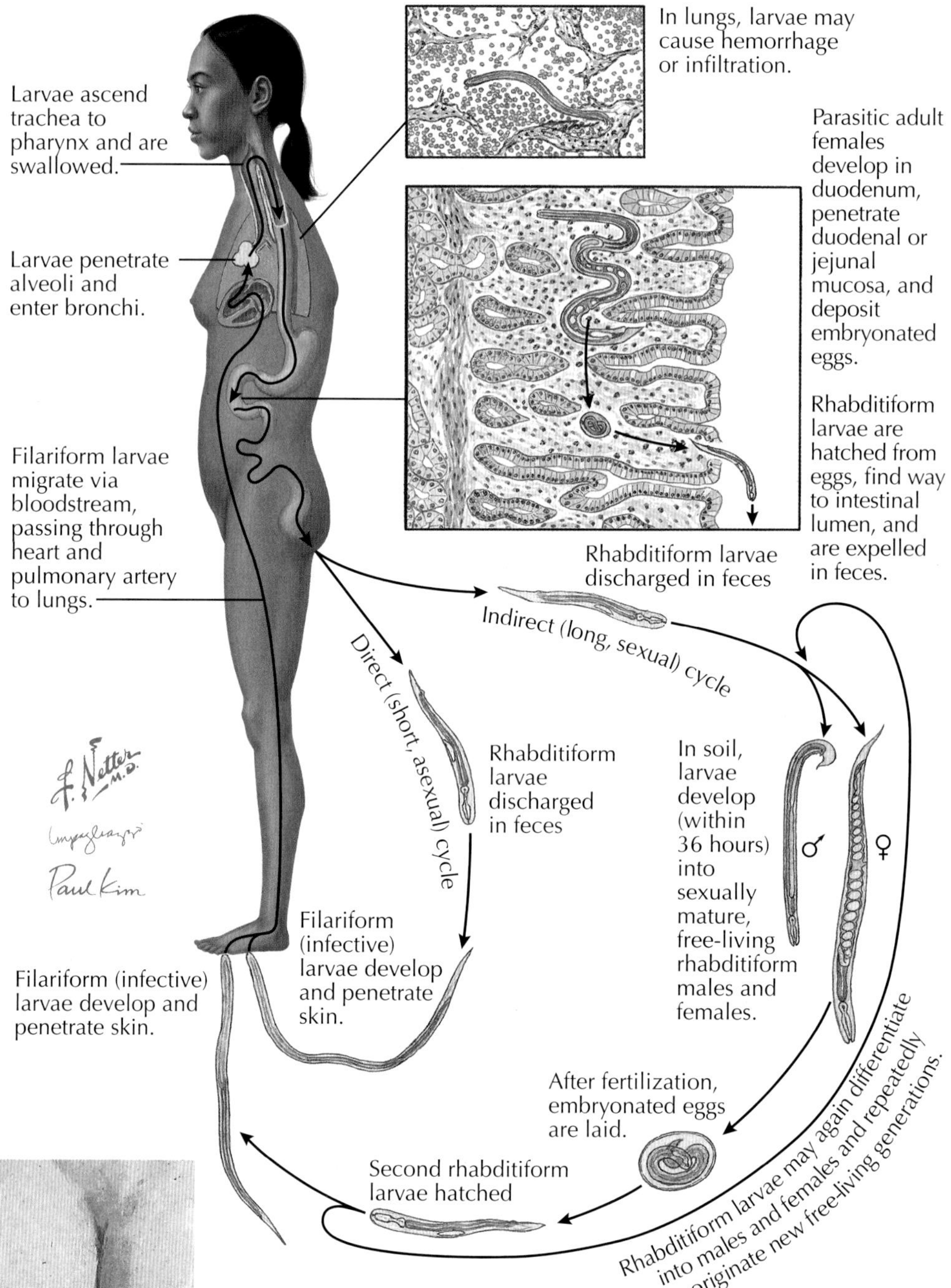

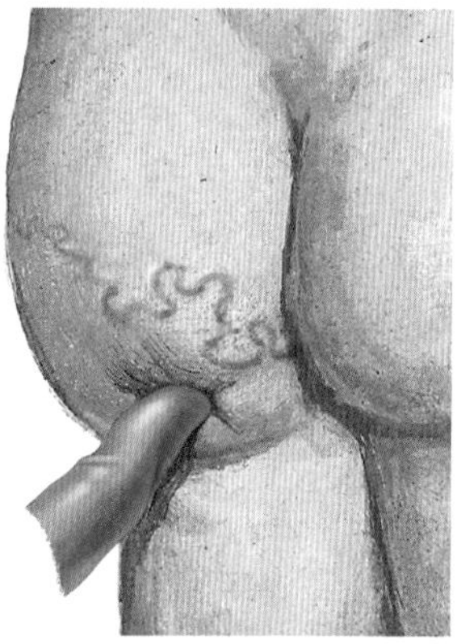

A serpiginous skin rash (lava currens) caused by filariform larvae migrating subcutaneously may develop on the buttocks or thighs.

## PARASITIC DISEASES: *TAENIASIS SAGINATA*

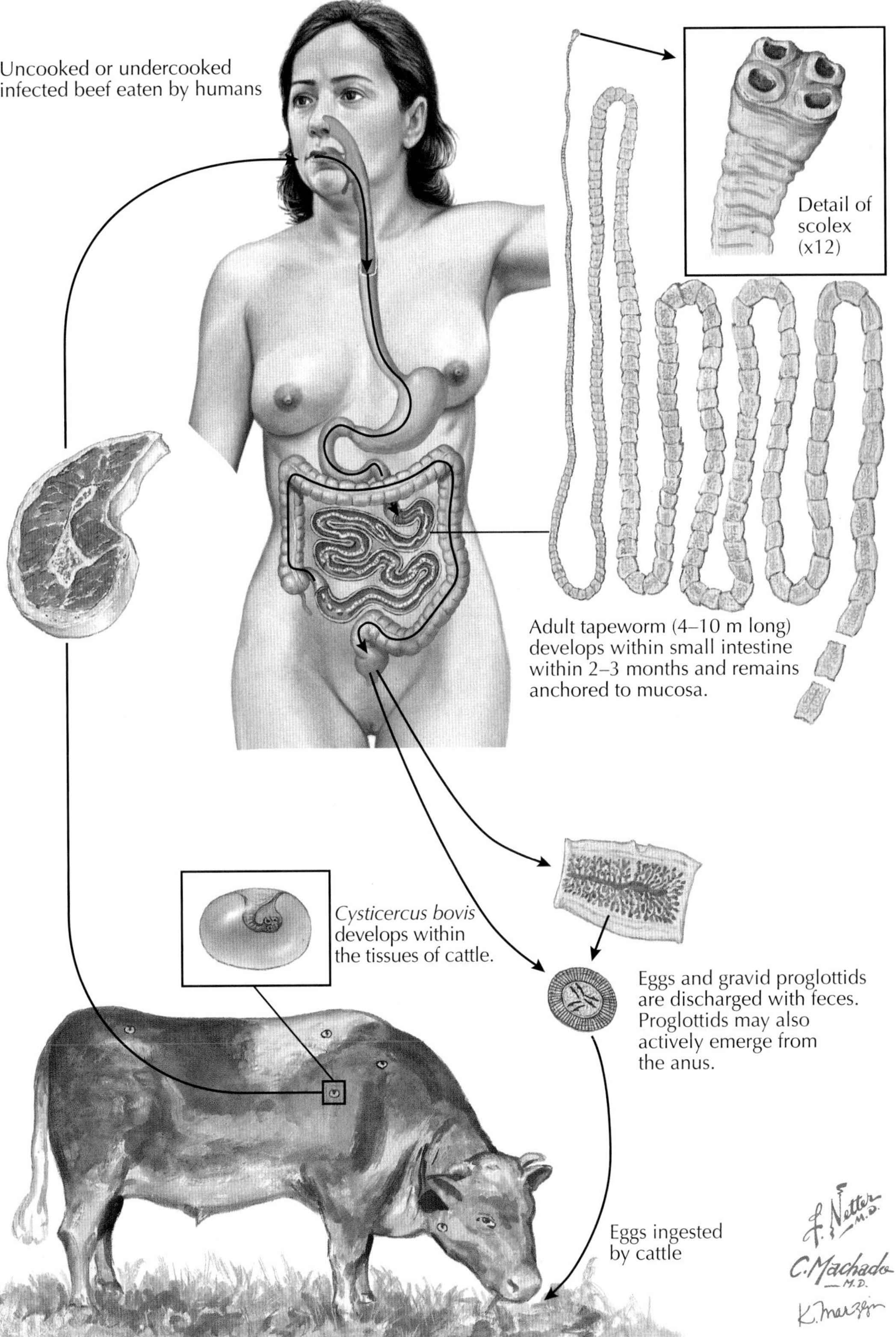

Uncooked or undercooked infected beef eaten by humans
Detail of scolex (x12)
Adult tapeworm (4–10 m long) develops within small intestine within 2–3 months and remains anchored to mucosa.
*Cysticercus bovis* develops within the tissues of cattle.
Eggs and gravid proglottids are discharged with feces. Proglottids may also actively emerge from the anus.
Eggs ingested by cattle
F. Netter M.D.
C. Machado M.D.
K. Marzejon


*Taeniasis saginata* is a parasitosis produced by *Taenia saginata* (beef tapeworm), a cestode of the phylum Platyhelminthes. The definitive host of this is the human, who harbors the adult worm, and the major intermediate host is cattle, which harbor the larval form called *Cysticercus bovis*. This parasite is found throughout the world, and associated infections usually occur with those who work with cattle or consume the meat. The adult worm measures from 4 to 10 m in length, but it may be even longer. It inhabits the small intestine, attached to the mucosa of the jejunum by means of the scolex. Usually, only one parasite is harbored by the host, but on rare occasions two or even more may be present. The small, elongate, and quadrangular scolex, measuring 1 to 2 mm in diameter and having four hemispherical suckers, is connected by a short and narrow neck to up to 1000 to 2000 proglottids. The genital organs are not yet developed in the short and wide immature proglottids that lie behind the neck. Gradually, the proglottids increase in breadth and width up to 20 mm by 7 mm. At this stage they are mature, containing functioning male and female organs. In mature proglottids, ovules are produced and fertilized hermaphroditically. Still more distally the proglottids become elongated and slightly narrowed; they contain a uterus that has 15 to 20 lateral branches and is crowded with eggs. Gravid proglottids become detached successively from the parent worm, pass through the colon into the sigmoid and rectum, and are either expelled passively in the feces or emerge by means of their own motility through the anus. Outside the intestine, but eventually also inside, the gravid proglottids rupture to release eggs. Eggs are of spherical shape and are indistinguishable from other cestodes. They measure 30 to 40 μm in diameter and have a thick, radially striated shell that contains the embryo (oncosphere), which has three pairs of delicate, lancet-shaped hooklets. The eggs are originally enclosed in a thin, easily detachable hyaline membrane. When gravid proglottids or eggs, dropped on pasture or grazing land, are ingested by cattle, the hexacanth embryos hatch in their intestines, bore into the venules and lymphatics, and are carried to the skeletal muscles, heart, tongue, diaphragm, adipose tissues, and other regions, where they develop in 2 to 2.5 months into the cysticercus stage. *Cysticercus bovis* (bladder worm) measures 7.5 to 10 mm in length and has a miniature head like that of the adult worm, invaginated into the fluid-filled vesicle. The larvae remain viable in cattle for about a year, after which they become calcified. When uncooked or undercooked contaminated beef is eaten by humans, the membranes of cysticerci are digested. The embryos evaginate their heads, attach themselves to the mucosa of the small intestine, and grow into adult worms in about 2 to 3 months.

The infection with *T. saginata* is frequently asymptomatic. Patients may report only the inconvenience resulting from gravid proglottids spontaneously discharged from the anus to be found in clothing or perineal areas. Some patients, however, experience vague abdominal discomfort, loss of appetite, nausea, indigestion, diarrhea or constipation, pruritus ani, and nervous disturbances, including headache, dizziness, and irritability. Proglottids lodged in the lumen of the appendix may sometimes produce symptoms of appendicitis. A rare but serious complication may evolve when a mass of tangled proglottids leads to intestinal obstruction. Immunologic reactions may be experienced, including urticaria, pruritus, skin disorders, and peripheral eosinophilia with elevated immunoglobulin E (IgE) levels. The diagnosis of *T. saginata* is confirmed by recognition of gravid proglottids in the feces. Examined under low-power magnification, they can be differentiated from those of *T. solium* by the number of main lateral arms of the uterus (15–20 on each side). Less frequently, the diagnosis is made by recovery of eggs in the feces. Eggs of *T. saginata*, however, are morphologically indistinguishable from those of *T. solium*.

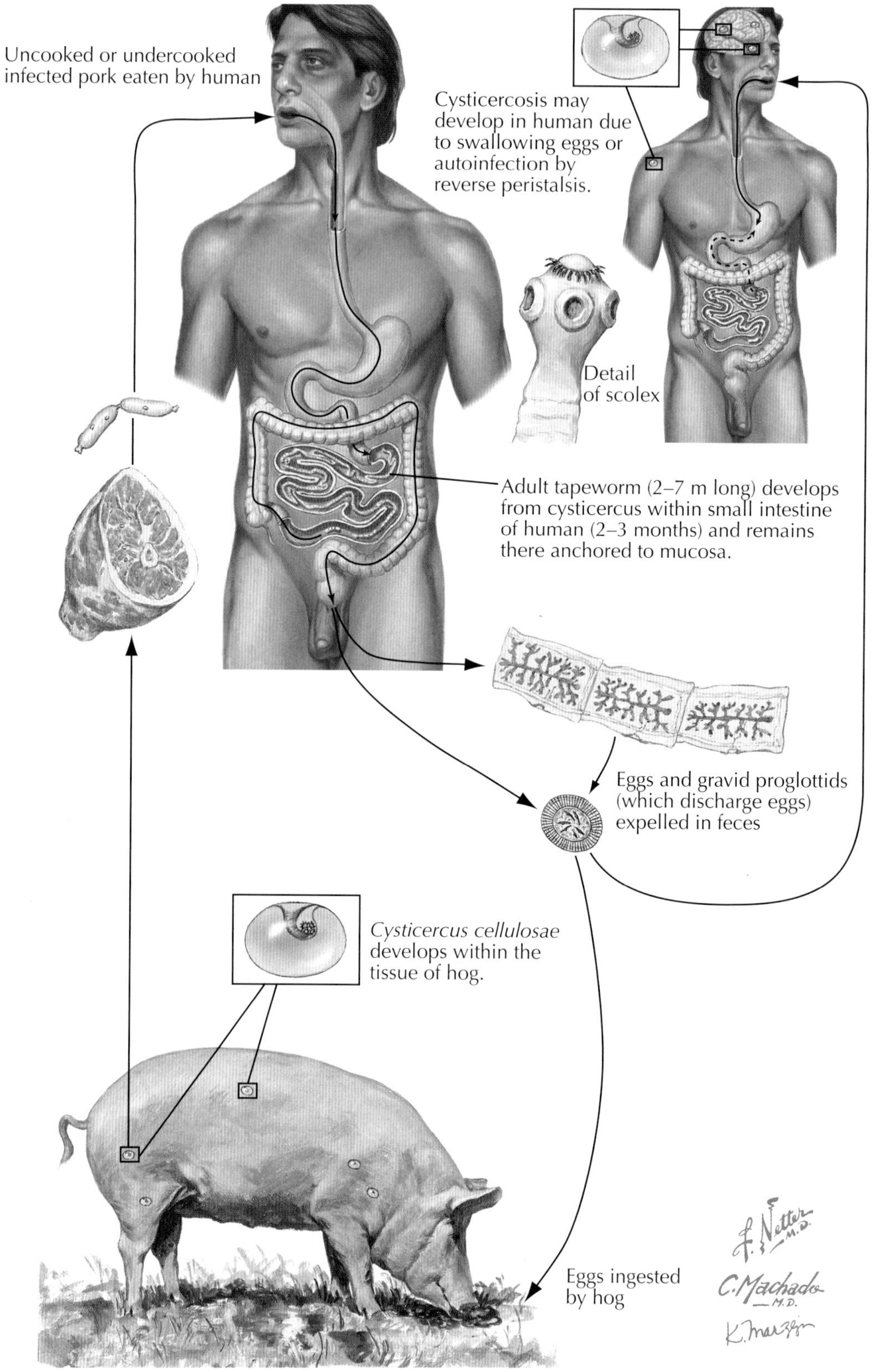

Uncooked or undercooked infected pork eaten by human

Cysticercosis may develop in human due to swallowing eggs or autoinfection by reverse peristalsis.

Detail of scolex

Adult tapeworm (2–7 m long) develops from cysticercus within small intestine of human (2–3 months) and remains there anchored to mucosa.

Eggs and gravid proglottids (which discharge eggs) expelled in feces

*Cysticercus cellulosae* develops within the tissue of hog.

Eggs ingested by hog

F. Netter M.D.

C. Machado M.D.

K. Marzejon

## PARASITIC DISEASES: *TAENIASIS SOLIUM (CYSTICERCOSIS CELLULOSAE)*

*Taenia solium* (pork tapeworm) is a cestode parasite occurring in countries where raw or inadequately processed pork is consumed. The adult worm, living in the small intestine of the human, usually attains a length of 2 to 7 m, rarely more. The globular scolex, measuring about 1 mm in diameter, has four cup-shaped suckers and a rostellum carrying a double row of 22 to 32 large and small hooklets, arranged alternately. As in *T. saginata,* a long chain of immature, mature, and terminal gravid proglottids follows the scolex. These may be expelled, singly or in short chains, in the feces. Unlike those of *T. saginata,* however, proglottids of *T. solium* are not motile. The ova, consisting of a hexacanth embryo surrounded by a spherical, radially striated shell, 30 to 40 μm in diameter, are indistinguishable from those of *T. saginata* and are liberated by the rupture of the proglottids before or after leaving the host in the feces. When the eggs are ingested by hogs, the hexacanth embryos hatch in the intestine, penetrate into blood or lymph vessels, and are disseminated to different parts of the body. They typically lodge in the skeletal muscles, tongue, and heart, where they develop in about 2 to 3 months into cysticerci (bladder worms). *Cysticercus cellulosae,* as this larval form is called, measures about 5 by 10 mm and consists of an ellipsoidal, fluid-filled vesicle and an invaginated scolex bearing four suckers and an apical crown of hooklets. When uncooked or undercooked pork containing viable cysticerci is eaten by humans, the cysticerci are digested, and the heads evaginate from the vesicle and themselves to the mucosa of the small intestine and grow into adult worms within about 2 to 3 months. The adult *T. solium* in the small intestine produces the same clinical manifestations as *T. saginata.* Because of the shorter length of the chain of proglottids, however, it is less likely to cause intestinal obstruction. The diagnosis of *T. solium* is made by the identification of gravid proglottids in the feces, which can be readily differentiated from those of *T. saginata* because the uterus they contain has only 5 to 10 main lateral arms on each side of the longitudinal stem. The eggs, morphologically indistinguishable from those of *T. saginata,* may also be found in the feces.

*T. solium* may give rise to another much more dangerous condition, resulting from the development of larval forms of this parasite in humans. Human cysticercosis, like that of the hog, results from ingestion of mature eggs. This may occur by swallowing eggs passed by another infected person, by the transmission of eggs from anus to mouth by the individual who is harboring *T. solium,* or by internal autoinfection when the ova or gravid proglottids reach the stomach by reverse peristalsis. Cysticerci may develop in any tissue or organ of the body but do so most commonly in the subcutaneous tissues, brain, eyes, and muscles. Around the larvae a cellular reaction takes place that leads to the formation of a fibrous capsule; later, the center of the lesion, including the larvae, may caseate or calcify. The symptomatology of cysticercosis varies according to the location and number of parasites. Subcutaneous lesions may be palpated as smooth, firm nodules the size of a pea or larger. Involvement of the brain, particularly after the death of larvae, may induce a local inflammatory reaction. The symptoms, which may simulate those of brain tumor, meningitis, general paralysis, and other nervous diseases, include severe headache, epileptiform seizures, motor and sensory disturbances, visual disturbances, deafness, aphasia, and psychiatric manifestations. Serology may help establish a diagnosis of cysticercosis but may be falsely elevated in patients infected with other cestodes because of cross-reacting antibodies.

A definitive diagnosis is made by the excision and microscopic examination of a larva. CT or MRI typically demonstrates cysticerci in soft tissues, including the brain and muscles; plain roentgenograms may identify lesions after calcification of the larvae has occurred.

## PARASITIC DISEASES: *HYMENOLEPIS NANA*

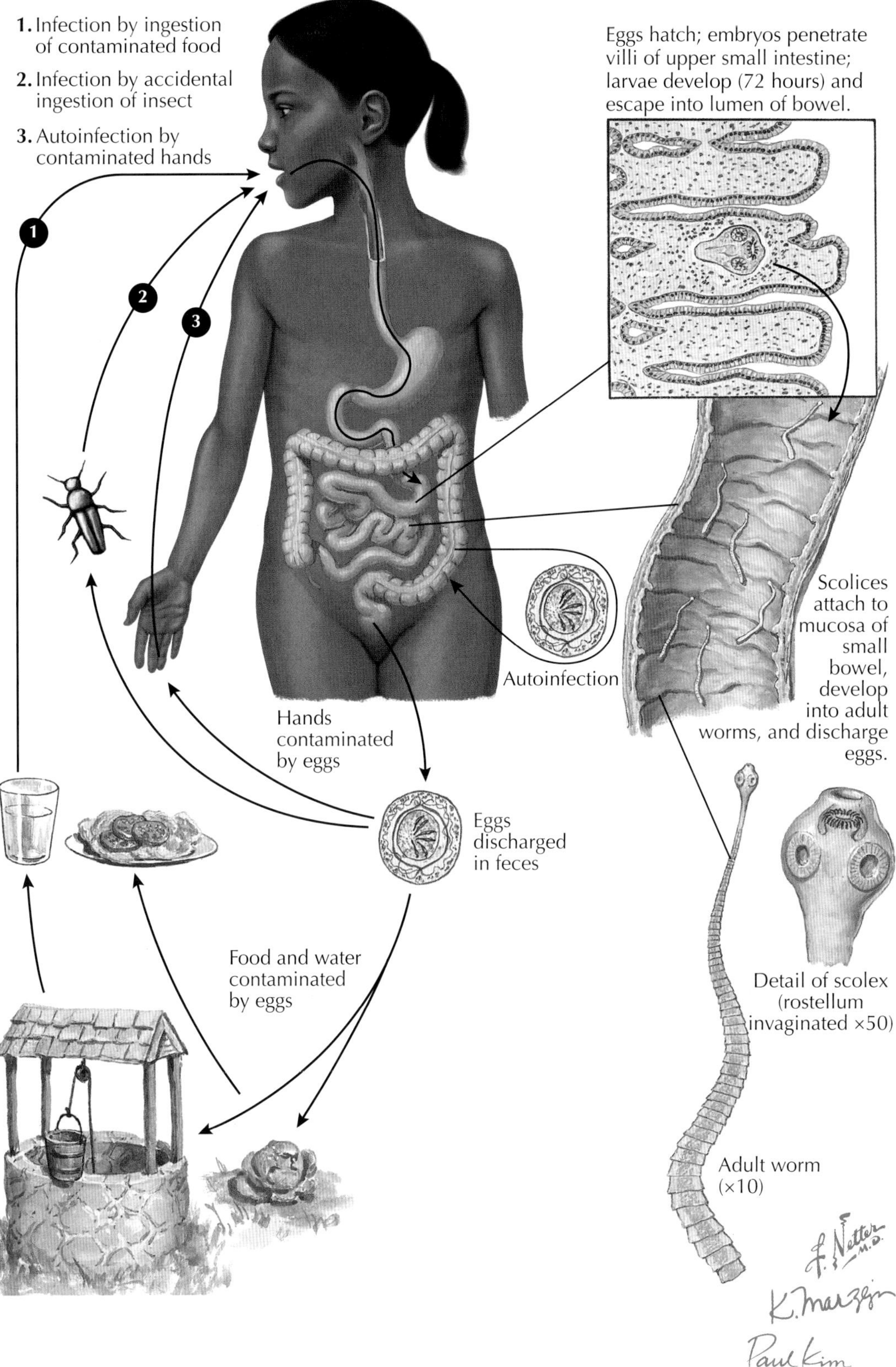
1. Infection by ingestion of contaminated food
2. Infection by accidental ingestion of insect
3. Autoinfection by contaminated hands
Eggs hatch; embryos penetrate villi of upper small intestine; larvae develop (72 hours) and escape into lumen of bowel.
Autoinfection
Scolices attach to mucosa of small bowel, develop into adult worms, and discharge eggs.
Hands contaminated by eggs
Eggs discharged in feces
Food and water contaminated by eggs
Detail of scolex (rostellum invaginated ×50)
Adult worm (×10)

*Hymenolepis nana* (dwarf tapeworm) is the most common tapeworm in humans. It is cosmopolitan in its distribution but is encountered in warm climates more frequently than in cold ones. The adult worm, measuring from 25 to 40 mm in length and from 0.8 to 1 mm in breadth, inhabits the small intestine, where it is attached to the mucosa by means of the scolex. The minute globular *scolex,* about 0.3 mm in diameter, bears four cup-shaped suckers and a short rostellum armed with a single ring of 20 to 30 hooklets. A long and slender neck connects the scolex to a chain of about 200 or more immature, mature, and gravid proglottids, which are more broad than long. The most distal gravid proglottids disintegrate gradually and release eggs. The spherical or subspherical, hyaline eggs, measuring 30 to 50 μm in diameter, have an outer and an inner envelope; the inner envelope (embryophore) has two polar thickenings, from each of which arise from four to eight thin, wavy, polar filaments that lie in the space between the two membranes. The embryophore encloses the embryo that has three pairs of lancet-shaped hooklets. These eggs are passed in the feces and are immediately infective for the same or another person. In the small intestine the ingested embryo is liberated and penetrates a villus, where, in about 3 to 4 days, it develops into a cysticercoid larva. This larva then migrates into the intestinal lumen and becomes attached by its scolex to the mucosa farther down in the small intestine, where, in the course of 2 weeks or more, it grows into an adult worm. No intermediate host is required for the completion of the life cycle. Infection occurs by ingestion of food or water contaminated by eggs, through autoinfection through contaminated hands resulting in fecal-oral inoculation, or through auto- or hyperinfection whereby ova released in the small intestine may penetrate a villus to complete the life cycle without being released into the environment. Individual worms may live 1 year, but the infection may persist for many years due to a cycle of autoinfection. Infection with *H. nana* may be intense; the presence of several hundred worms is not unusual. Infection with several thousand specimens has been described. Heavy worm burdens may be due to internal autoinfection as a result of immune suppression. The majority of those with *H. nana* infection have no clinical manifestations. Symptoms usually occur only in the presence of a large number of parasites. Irritation of the intestinal mucosa may result in diarrhea and cramps. The absorption of the metabolic wastes of the worms, particularly in children, may give rise to headache, dizziness, insomnia, and, rarely, epileptiform seizures. A slight to intense eosinophilia may be present. The diagnosis of hymenolepiasis nana is made by the recovery of the characteristic eggs from the feces.

Nonhuman animals may play a role in the life cycle of *H. nana* as well. Strains of *H. nana* may be adapted to nonhuman hosts. Rodents, especially rats and mice, may also serve as a definitive host, and certain insects (arthropods, fleas, mealworms) may allow cysticercoids to develop after ingestion of eggs that have been released into the environment. Rodents may thus play a role in shedding eggs into the environment. Accidental ingestion of infected insects may also contribute to *H. nana* infection in both rodents and humans.

A related cestode, *Hymenolepis diminuta,* may occasionally infect humans as well. *H. diminuta* is a common tapeworm of rats and mice and has various arthropods as intermediate hosts. The eggs of this cestode are passed in the feces and are morphologically similar to those of *H. nana.* They can be distinguished, however, by their greater size (70–80 μm × 60–80 μm) and the absence of polar filaments compared with *H. nana.*

## Parasitic Diseases: Diphyllobothriasis

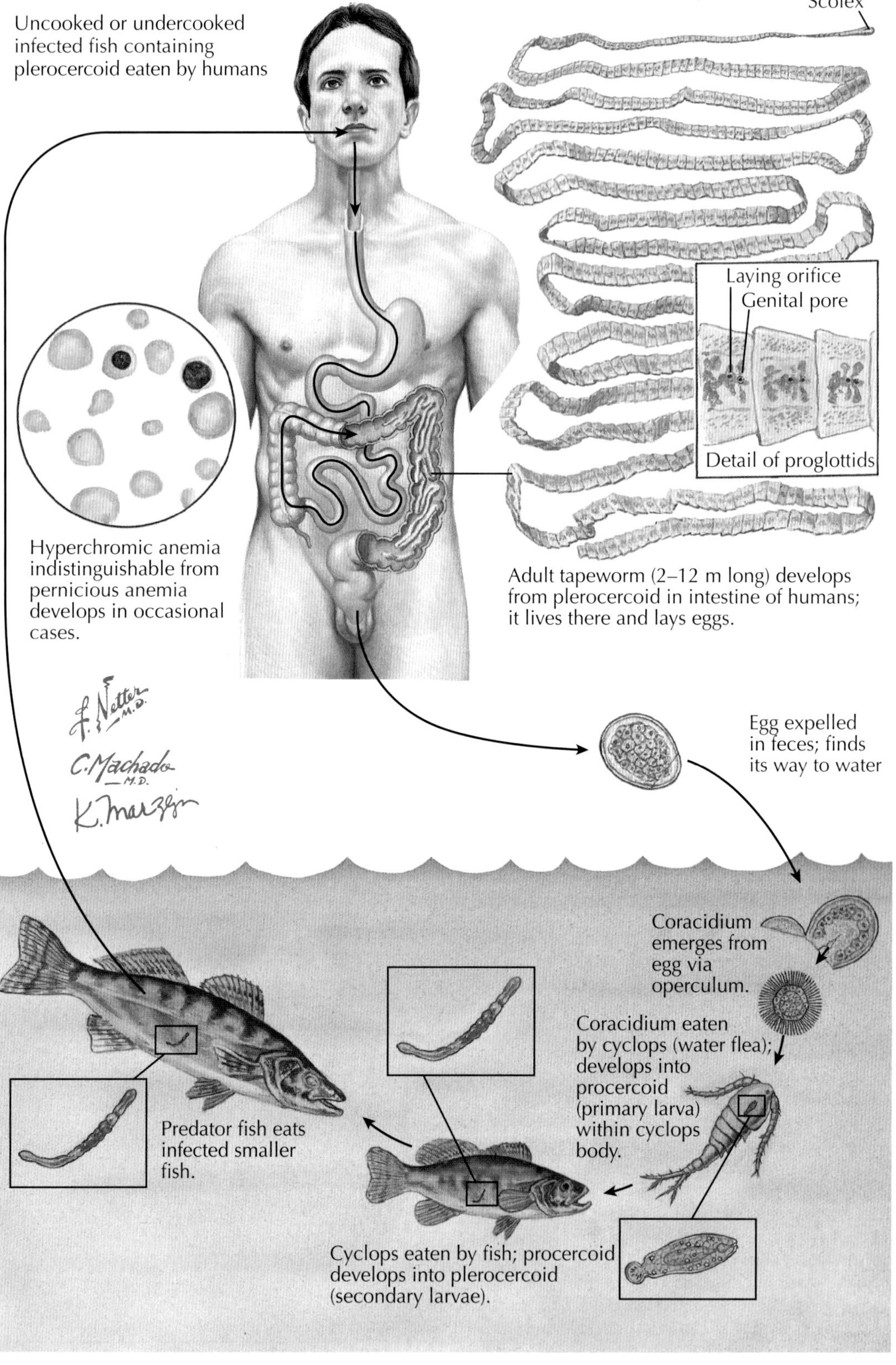


Diphyllobothriasis is parasitism produced by the adult form of the cestode *Diphyllobothrium latum* (fish or broad tapeworm). This parasite is found chiefly in the northern temperate regions where freshwater fish constitute a major portion of the diet of the population. In Europe, the most important foci are situated in the Baltic countries; in the region of the alpine lakes of Switzerland, France, Italy, and Germany; and in the delta of the Danube River and lower Volga River basin. In Asia, this tapeworm is found throughout extensive areas in Siberia, northeastern China, and Japan. In North America, several foci are known, particularly in the Great Lakes region, Alaska, and Canada. Other endemic foci exist worldwide, including Chile and Uganda. The adult worm ranges in length from 2 to 12 m. The elongated, almond-shaped scolex, which attaches to the mucosa of the small intestine, measures from 2 to 3 mm in length by 1 mm in breadth and is provided with a dorsal and a ventral sucking groove (bothrium). An attenuated neck, several times the length of the scolex, is followed by a chain of more than 3000 proglottids. The distal part of the strobila is formed by mature proglottids that contain minute spherical testes, a bilobate ovary, and a coiled rosette-like uterus provided with an opening (laying orifice or birth pore) in the midventral line just behind the genital pore. Fertilized eggs are evacuated periodically through the laying orifice. A single worm may discharge as many as 1 million eggs daily. The gravid proglottids normally do not separate from the parent worm; they are sloughed off only after completing their reproductive function. The ovoid eggs, 70 by 45 μm in diameter, have a single shell with an inconspicuous operculum at one end and contain immature embryos. After being discharged into water, the eggs mature at a favorable temperature in about 2 weeks. The free-swimming embryo (coracidium) then escapes through the opercular opening. If it is to develop further, it must be swallowed by a suitable first intermediate host, usually a crustacean of the genus *Cyclops* or *Diaptomus*. The coracidium metamorphoses in these crustaceans within 2 to 3 weeks into a procercoid larva, which is spindle shaped, is about 500 μm in size, and has a cephalic invagination and a posterior spherical appendage provided with hooklets. When the infected crustacean is ingested by a suitable species of plankton-eating freshwater fish, the procercoid larva penetrates the viscera, muscles, and connective tissues and develops within 1 to 4 weeks into an elongated, worm-like plerocercoid or sparganum larva, measuring from 10 to 20 mm in length and from 2 to 3 mm in breadth. When these fish are, in turn, consumed by larger carnivorous fish, the sparganum migrates to the tissues of the new host. When a raw or insufficiently cooked infected fish is eaten by a human or another susceptible host, the plerocercoid larva attaches itself to the mucosa of the small intestine and grows, in about 3 weeks, into an adult *D. latum*. Nonhuman hosts such as birds, bears, seals, cats, foxes, and wolves may also serve as a definitive host.

Most cases of diphyllobothriasis remain subclinical. Clinical manifestations may include weakness, abdominal pain, diarrhea, weight loss, salt craving, dizziness, anorexia, or exaggerated appetite. The mass of tangled proglottids, especially when more than one parasite is harbored, may produce intestinal obstruction. *D. latum* absorbs dietary vitamin $B_{12}$, and thus prolonged infection may lead to vitamin $B_{12}$ deficiency and a characteristic macrocytic, hyperchromic anemia. The diagnosis of diphyllobothriasis is made by demonstration of the characteristic eggs in the feces.

# HELMINTHS AND PROTOZOA INFECTING THE HUMAN INTESTINE

Helminths discussed in the preceding pages are responsible for the overwhelming majority of all intestinal helminthic infections in humans. However, a few other worms may be encountered with lesser frequency. Several species of hermaphroditic intestinal flukes are found in human populations with unique food and environmental exposures. *Fasciolopsis buski,* a fleshy, elongated-ovoid trematode flatworm, living in the small intestine of a human or porcine host is found in South and Southeastern Asia. Its ovoid operculate eggs, about 135 μm long, are discharged in the feces and hatch in water. Miracidia that escape from them penetrate appropriate snails, pass through different evolutional stages, and emerge again as cercariae, which then encyst on aquatic vegetation. Humans acquire the parasite by consuming raw or poorly cooked contaminated plants. In the small intestine, the flukes attach to the mucosa, producing inflammatory reaction and ulcers. The infection is usually asymptomatic but may give rise to abdominal pain, diarrhea, anasarca, and ascites. *Echinostoma* and related species can infect humans, and cases are most common in Southeast Asia where undercooked freshwater snails, clams, and fish are eaten. The adult fluke, measuring 2.5 to 6.5 mm, inhabits the small intestine of birds, mammals, and humans. The eggs are discharged in the feces. The life cycle of this worm involves two different intermediate hosts. Humans acquire the infection by ingesting the second intermediate host, usually a bivalve mollusk, fish, or amphibian. Low parasite burdens cause limited disease. More severe infections may be clinically indistinguishable from *Fasciolopsis. Heterophyes* and *Metagonimus* are similar organisms that represent over 10 species that can infect human, animal, or avian hosts. The most common are *Heterophyes heterophyes,* which is found in North Africa, Iran, and Turkey, and *Metagonimus yokogawai,* which is found in Southeast Asia. This fluke (1–2 mm long) lives in the small intestine of the definitive host. Eggs are passed in the feces, ultimately reaching water, where they are ingested by appropriate species of snails and hatch. Miracidia pass through various developmental stages and emerge again as cercariae that penetrate under the scales of various species of freshwater fish, where they encyst. The definitive host becomes infected by consuming raw or insufficiently cooked infected fish. The adult flukes may produce a mild inflammatory reaction at the attachment sites; intestinal symptoms occur only with heavy worm burdens. Eggs may also embolize to the heart or brain, causing local tissue damage. The different species of the nematode genus *Trichostrongylus,* ubiquitous parasites of herbivorous mammals, are reported with increasing frequency in humans. *Capillaria philippinensis* is a small intestinal nematode morphologically similar to *Trichuris trichiura* that is most prevalent in the Philippines but is also seen in the Middle East and Southeast Asia. *C. philippinensis* is acquired by consumption of infected freshwater fish that harbor the infectious larvae in muscle. *C. philippinensis* is capable of autoinfection through gut mucosa and can cause a hyperinfection syndrome, leading to diarrhea, malabsorption, wasting, and ascites. *Nanophyetus salmincola* is seen in the Pacific Northwest of the United States. Normally a parasite of mammals and birds, human infection is acquired by ingestion of infected salmonid freshwater fish or their eggs. Symptoms include abdominal pain, gas, and bloating.

OVA OF HELMINTH PARASITES AND PSEUDOPARASITES AND RHABDITIFORM LARVAE

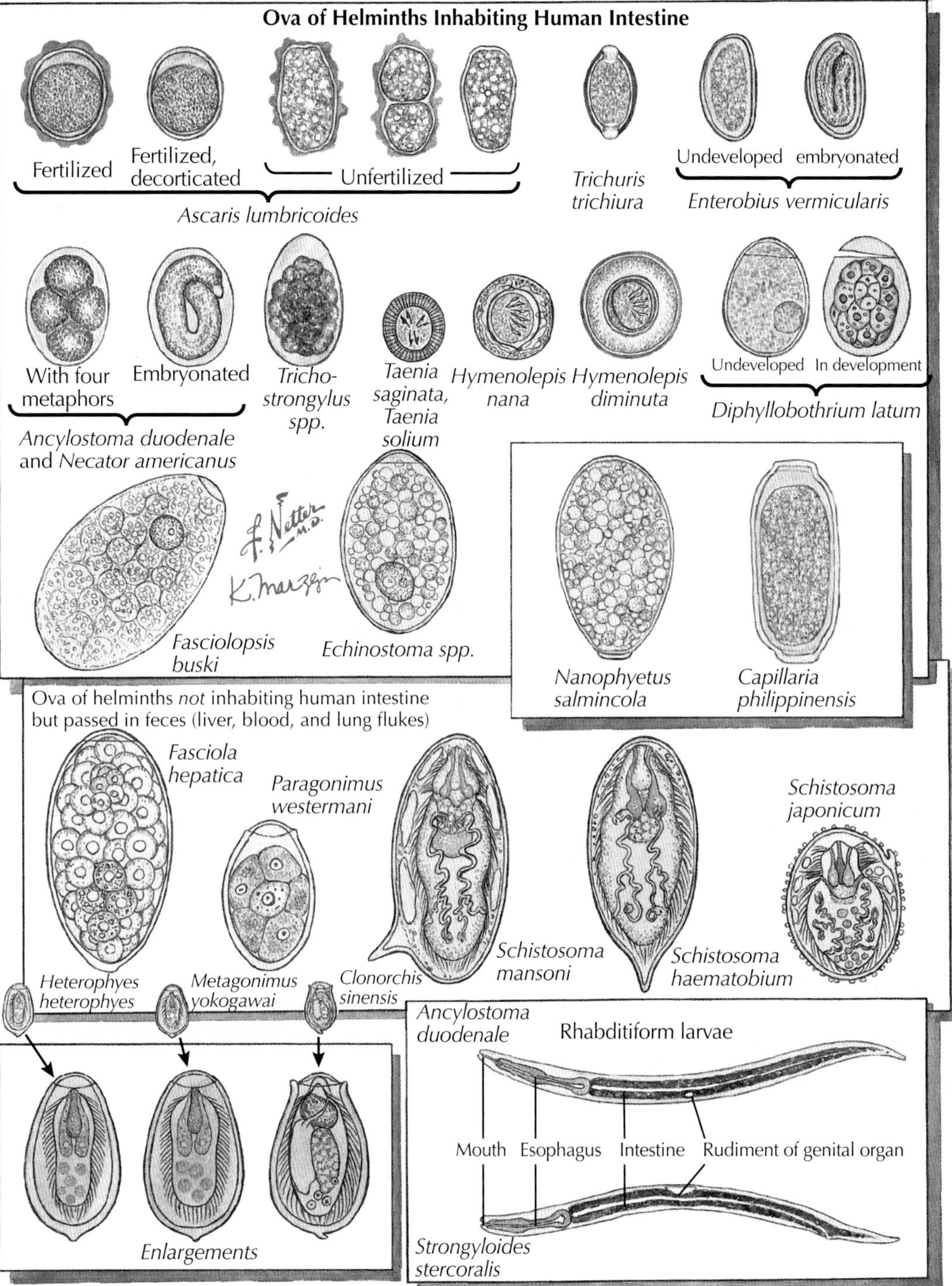


Intestinal helminthic infections, though eventually suspected on the ground of clinical symptoms or blood eosinophilia, are ultimately diagnosed by the identification of ova, larvae, adult parasites, or proglottids in the feces; scrapings from anal or perianal regions; gastric or duodenal aspirates; and, eventually, in other body fluids or tissues. A diagnosis of cysticercosis from *T. solium* may be made from radiologic studies showing characteristic cysticerci in the brain. For parasitologic fecal examination, many different methods are used. The simplest is direct microscopic examination of fecal material spread thinly on a slide. For detection of low-level infection, a number of concentration methods consisting of sedimentation, flotation, and centrifugation have been described. The search for parasitic eggs by microscopic examination of transparent tape that has been applied several times to the perianal skin is indicated mostly when *E. vermicularis* or *T. saginata* is suspected. Of all common helminthic infections, strongyloidiasis is the only one in which normally rhabditiform larvae, not ova, are found in freshly voided feces. These can be differentiated from those of hookworms (found only in stools that have been excreted some time before examination) chiefly by a shorter buccal

## Helminths and Protozoa Infecting the Human Intestine (Continued)

vestibule and larger rudimental genital organs. With liver, blood, or lung fluke infections, these eggs are discharged via the intestine or, in the lung-fluke parasitism, reach the intestine with the swallowed sputum and can be found in the feces. The ova of some phytoparasitic nematodes, particularly *Meloidogyne marioni,* which inhabits root vegetables such as radishes and turnips, may also be observed in the human feces, having been ingested with infected vegetables and released in the intestine, through which they pass undamaged.

The human intestine may be inhabited not only by helminthic but also by protozoan parasites. *Entamoeba histolytica* is the most important. Other species of amebae that live in the large intestine of humans and have been implicated with occasional symptomatic illness include *Blastocystis hominis, E. Bangladeshi, and E. moshkovskii.* The amebae *Endolimax nana, Entamoeba coli, E. dispar, E. hartmanni, E. polecki,* and *Iodamoeba bütschlii* are rarely associated with symptoms and are generally not considered pathogenic. These nonpathogenic amebae would be of very little consequence if it were not for the danger of confusion between them and *E. histolytica.* Their life cycle is similar to that of *E. histolytica* but they do not invade intestinal tissues. In the feces they appear as trophozoites or, more commonly, as cysts, because trophozoites usually perish soon after leaving the body. Identification of nonpathogenic amebae has been associated with poorer sanitary environments. The trophozoites of intestinal amebae can be identified and differentiated morphologically by their size, motility, form of pseudopodia, endoplasmic inclusions, and nuclear structure. The characteristics by which the cysts can be differentiated include the size, shape, number, and structure of nuclei; chromatoid bodies; glycogen vacuoles; and the presence or absence of a cyst wall. *Entamoeba histolytica* may be documented by direct examination of fecal samples or mucosal biopsy or by antigen detection in stool. Serologic assays may be positive with extracolonic manifestations.

*Balantidium coli* is the only known pathogenic ciliate parasite in humans. This large protozoon, usually 50 to 100 μm in length, inhabits the large intestine of pigs, monkeys, and humans. The trophozoites are actively motile and have oval bodies covered with short, delicate cilia. The granular endoplasm contains two contractile and several food vacuoles, a kidney-shaped macronucleus, and a micronucleus. The cysts are spherical or oval in shape and have a double-outlined wall that encloses a clearly differentiated *Balantidium.* In older cysts, however, the outline of the organism is lost, and all structures except granular cytoplasm, macronucleus, and a contractile vacuole disappear. Most individuals with balantidiasis are asymptomatic or have mild diarrhea. However, *B. coli* may invade the intestinal tissues and produce microperforations that may lead to bacterial sepsis or ulcerations similar to those caused by *E. histolytica.* Pathogenic flagellate protozoa that can be found in the human intestine include *Giardia duodenalis* and *Dientamoeba fragilis. Chilomastix mesnili, Enteromonas hominis, Retortamonas intestinalis,* and *Pentatrichomonas hominis* may inhabit the intestines but are not pathogenic and lead only to asymptomatic carriage. With the exception of *P. hominis* and *D. fragilis,* which are not known to form cysts, their life cycles includes a trophozoite and a cystic stage. The intestinal flagellates do not invade tissues. *G. duodenalis* adheres to intestinal

GIARDIA LAMBLIA AND OTHER PROTOZOANS

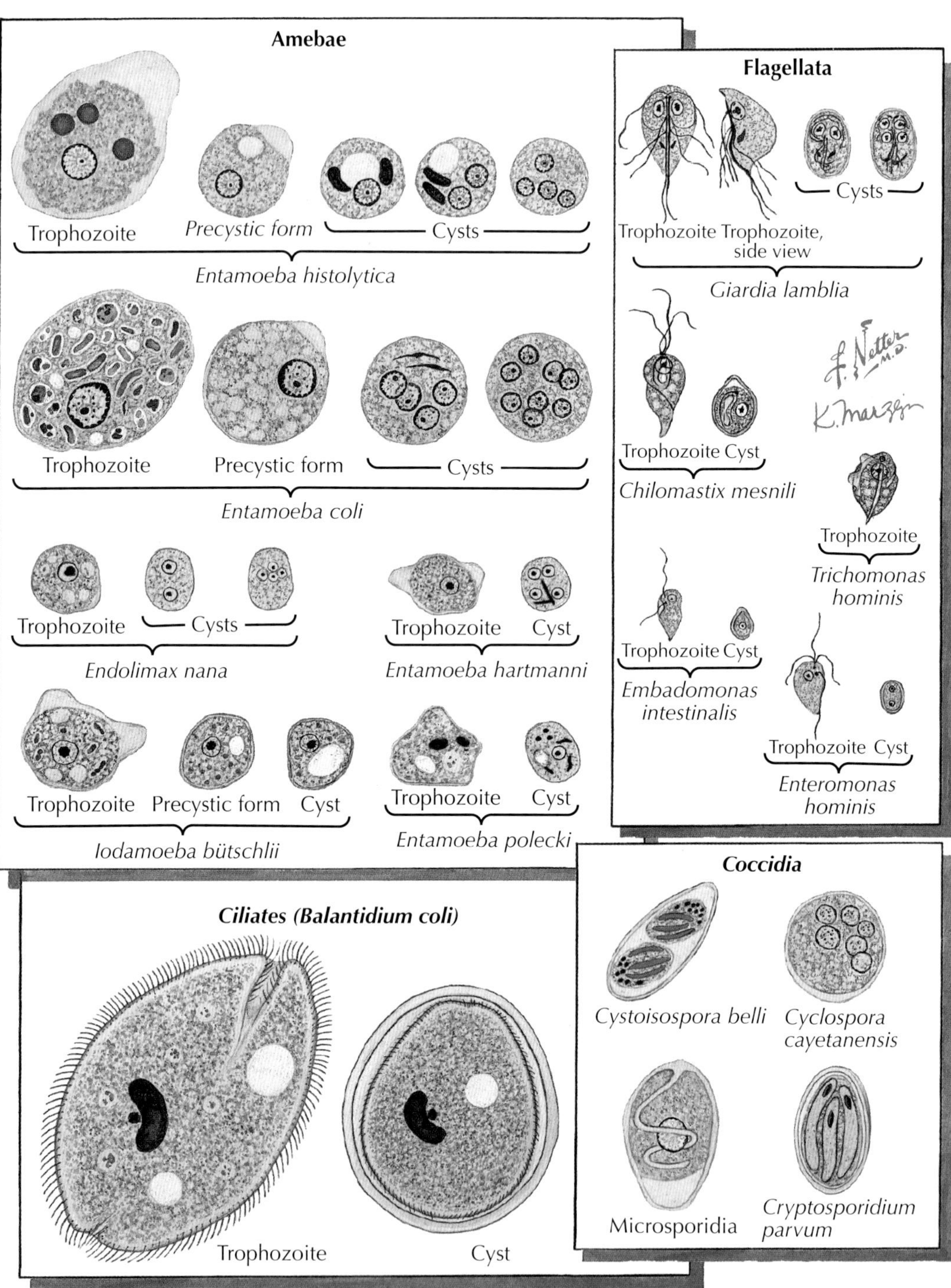


epithelium, leading to diarrhea, anorexia, and flatulence. This may be chronic in immunocompromising conditions and is often exacerbated by the onset of an acquired intestinal disaccharidase deficiency. The coccidian *Cystoisospora belli* is a cause of diarrhea in returning travelers from tropical and subtropical environments and a cause of chronic diarrhea in patients with AIDS. *Cyclospora cayetanensis* is found worldwide and usually causes asymptomatic carriage in indigenous hosts but has been associated with diarrhea in travelers returning from developing areas or from ingestion of imported contaminated foods. *Cryptosporidium parvum* and *C. hominis* are intracellular protozoan parasites that have worldwide distribution. They are acquired through direct person-to-person spread or from drinking water sources that have been contaminated by infected animals, usually cows or humans. Outbreaks have occurred in settings of contaminated public water sources. Symptoms include watery diarrhea, which may be debilitating in patients who are immunocompromised.

The diagnosis of intestinal protozoan infection is usually made by microscopic examination of the feces with identification of the trophozoite or cyst form of the organism using wet mount or iodine on fresh or concentrated specimens. Modified acid-fast stains will identify *Cystoisospora, Cryptosporidium,* and *Cyclospora.* In addition, cysts of *Cystoisospora* and *Cyclospora* will autofluoresce under ultraviolet light.

## AMEBIASIS

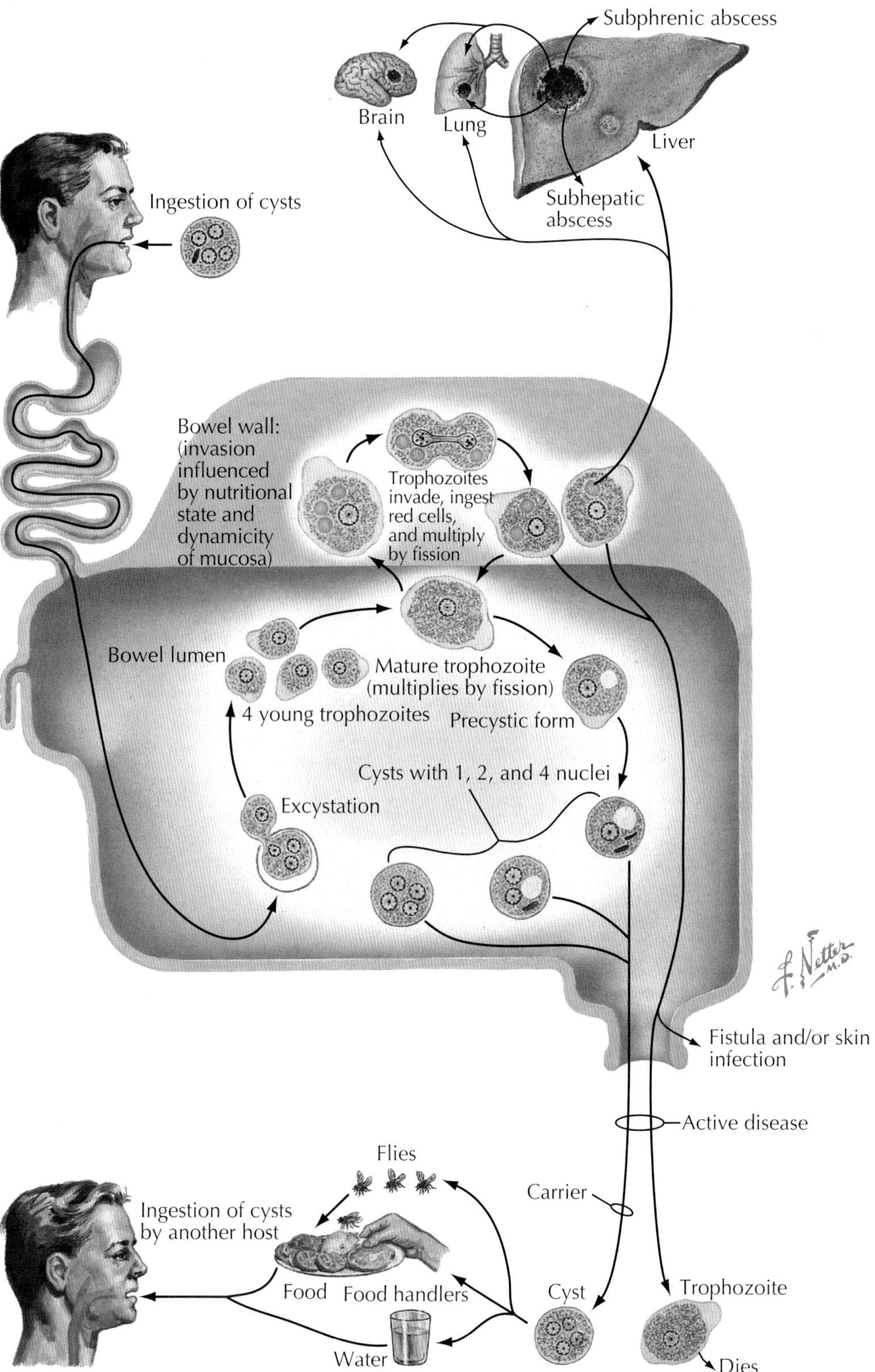


Amebiasis is caused by infection with *Entamoeba histolytica,* a protozoan of the class Rhizopoda and of the genus *Entamoeba*. Although more frequently observed in warm climates, amebiasis is ubiquitous. The prevalence has been estimated at about 10% of the global population, with increased incidence noted in Mexico, South Africa, South Asia, and Southeast Asia. The prevalence in North America is less than 3% but higher in certain demographics, including patients who are institutionalized and men who have sex with men, and in certain lower socioeconomic status geographic areas such as American Indian reservations. An increased incidence is related to poor sanitation.

The life cycle of *E. histolytica* is characterized by several stages. The motile and vegetative form, or trophozoite, multiplies by fission in the intestinal lumen and the tissues of the host and perishes when eliminated in the feces. It varies in size from 15 to 60 μm and is made up of two distinguishable portions of cytoplasm: the clear, glass-like ectoplasm and the finely granulated endoplasm, which contains the nucleus and ingested substances such as erythrocytes. The trophozoite moves by means of pseudopodia, formed by the ectoplasm, as may be observed microscopically in fresh, warm stool specimens. In cool stool, the motility is absent or very sluggish. In the second stage of the cycle, the mature trophozoite encysts and develops into the precystic form, which still may be equipped with pseudopodia. The precyst develops a cyst wall and matures into a cyst containing one, two, or four nuclei. The encystation occurs only in the intestinal lumen and never in other host tissues. Once cysts develop in the host, they are excreted with the stool. Cysts are the infective form of *E. histolytica* and are ingested via direct person-to-person transmission or fecal contamination of food and water. Ingested trophozoites are not infectious because they are degraded by the digestive gastric juices. In contrast, cysts are very resistant and survive in nature under the most unfavorable conditions. Transmission may be facilitated by poor hand hygiene during food preparation, direct fecal contamination of the environment, flies or other insects transmitting the organism from feces to food, or use of contaminated human excreta (night soil) for fertilizing vegetable crops. Transmission in residential facilities for the elderly or mentally disabled, prisons, and childcare settings have been described.

The organism passes through a tear in the cyst's membrane (excystation) in the distal small bowel, releasing a metacystic ameba that contains four nuclei. From each nucleus and accompanying cytoplasm a uninucleate trophozoite develops. Further division and development lead to eight uninuclear trophozoites. The trophozoite actively grows and divides and is the invasive form of the organism. It may invade the colonic mucosa to multiply either in the lumen or, usually, within the gut wall. In settings of diarrhea or dysentery, mature trophozoites may be excreted into the stool. With slower bowel motility and more formed stool, the trophozoites develop a cyst wall and undergo nuclear division to form quadrinucleate cysts prior to expulsion.

The pathogenicity of *E. histolytica* depends on many factors, with the degree of tissue invasion being the result of a complex balance between parasites and the environment offered by the host. *E. histolytica* exists as a spectrum of zymodemes based on electrophoretic isoenzyme patterns, with some zymodemes being associated with more symptomatic disease than others. Asymptomatic carriers, or "cyst passers," who have no or only slight symptoms, are the most important source of infection. *E. histolytica* may invade the large intestine, primarily in the cecum, sigmoid, and rectum. The small bowel is rarely affected, and then only in the terminal ileum. Invasion is facilitated by release of cytotoxic and proteolytic enzymes and phagocytosis of host cells. Host factors such as nutritional deficiencies, dietary intake, and stress contribute to invasion. The earliest lesions in the mucosa consist of pinhead-sized, hyperemic, and edematous areas or small yellow papules that evolve into ulcers. The ulcers may contain actively motile trophozoites in a viscous milieu of necrotic tissue. Inflammatory reactions around the ulcers are usually the result of secondary bacterial invasion. Amebic ulcers, smaller but deeper than the more diffuse ones caused by shigellae, spread in the submucosa, producing undermined edges and tunnels, which connect

## AMEBIASIS (Continued)

adjacent lesions. Amebae may be carried to the liver, lung, pleura, brain, skin, or pericardium by way of the bloodstream, rarely through the lymphatics, where they incite abscesses. Amebic invasion may cross tissue planes, leading to invasion of the intestinal muscular coat, intestinal perforation, or peritoneal involvement. Direct extension of lesions through the skin from contiguous sites such as liver abscesses or rectal or anal lesions may be seen. The incidence of extraintestinal amebiasis has decreased considerably, probably because of the availability of effective amebicides and antibiotics.

Most people infected by *E. histolytica* have no symptoms even though they may experience deep and extensive ulcerations. In others, amebic dysentery begins insidiously with vague abdominal sensations. The classical clinical picture of the acute form is characterized by mucous, bloody bowel discharges, tenesmus, abdominal pain, fever, and sometimes vomiting. More commonly, symptoms include chronic nonspecific gastrointestinal disturbances such as constipation alternating with bouts of diarrhea and abdominal tenderness that may be generalized or confined either to the lower or to the upper quadrants, combined with epigastric fullness after meals, nausea, malaise, aerophagia, and eructations.

An amebic infection should be considered in any person presenting with diarrhea of long-standing duration. The diagnosis is established by demonstrating the trophozoites or cysts in a freshly passed, still-warm fecal specimen. Trophozoites may degrade after 30 minutes of passage unless the stool is fixed or refrigerated. The passage of amebic cysts and trophozoites may be intermittent; collection of three samples over 6 days increases the sensitivity to 70% to 90% compared with a single stool collection. *E. histolytica* must be distinguished from other nonpathogenic or low-pathogenic ameba species that may be seen in clinical specimens. Rectosigmoidoscopy permits recognition of the pathognomonic, scattered, pinpoint ulcers or, in the early stages, of petechiae or yellowish elevations with hyperemic margins marking the site of future ulcers. Very rarely, large, undermined, oval-shaped ulcers are encountered. In the chronic stage the mucosa may appear normal or may have a granular surface with scattered red areas that bleed easily. Antigen detection in both serum and stool may be helpful for acute disease and can differentiate between *E. histolytica* and nonpathogenic ameba. Serology is useful in certain settings. Up to 35% of a population in highly endemic areas may have a positive serology because of past infection. Thus a positive test is most useful for diagnosis of amebiasis in returning expatriates who present with symptomatic disease after exposure to a highly endemic environment. A negative serology may help rule out amebiasis in areas of high prevalence.

The differential diagnosis of amebiasis may be broad because of the many other illnesses that present with diarrhea. Care must be taken in differentiating amebiasis from other infectious causes of acute bloody stools, including *E. coli, Salmonella, Shigella, Campylobacter, C. difficile,* and *Vibrio* as well as other protozoal infections and intestinal tuberculosis. Bacillary dysentery can be excluded by microscopic examination of the feces and bacteriologic techniques. Whereas in amebic dysentery the intestinal exudate is composed of mucus, erythrocytes, and very little cellular debris, in bacillary dysentery it is rich in neutrophils and phagocytic endothelial macrophage cells. Diverticulitis and noninfectious conditions such as ischemic bowel, UC, polyposis, and CD may also present similarly. In chronic amebic dysentery, amebic granuloma (or "ameboma"), resulting from an exuberant granulating fibroblastic response to repeated local amebic invasion, may easily be confused with malignant intestinal tumors or inflammatory granuloma of other origin. The clinical differentiation between a chronic amebic typhlitis and chronic appendicitis is difficult except by the success of antiamebic therapy. Diagnosis is further complicated by the fact that patients who have other compounding medical conditions noted above may also have symptomatic or asymptomatic amebic infection and may excrete trophozoites or cysts. Thus the identification of cysts or trophozoites in the feces may be unrelated to the acute medical issue.

HISTOLOGY AND SCOPE IMAGES

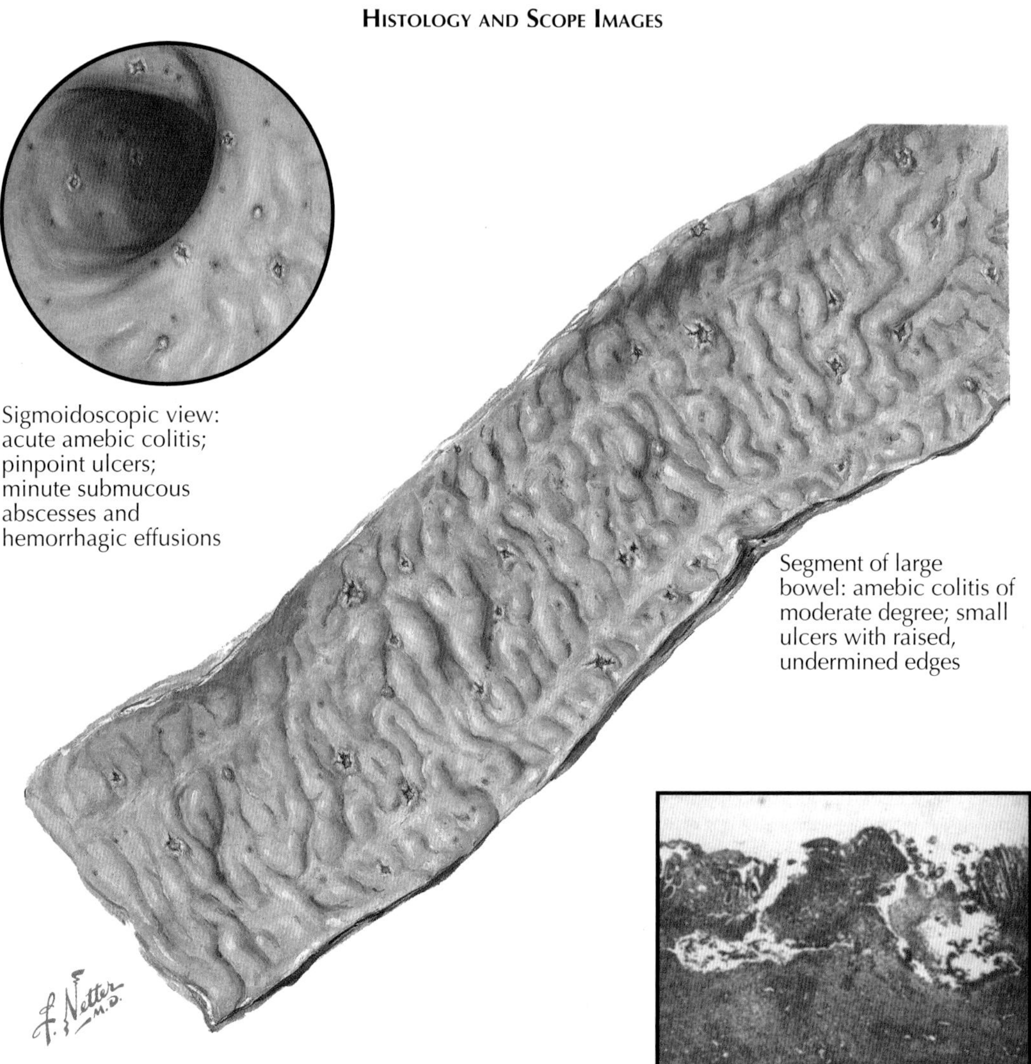


Sigmoidoscopic view: acute amebic colitis; pinpoint ulcers; minute submucous abscesses and hemorrhagic effusions

Segment of large bowel: amebic colitis of moderate degree; small ulcers with raised, undermined edges

Amebic ulcers with beginning submucous tunnel formation

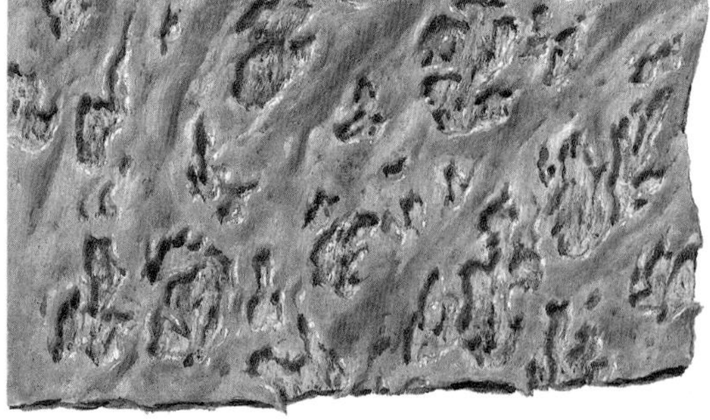

Severe amebic colitis—now rarely seen: large ulcerated areas resulting from confluence of smaller ulcers; ulcers have ragged, undermined edges; intervening mucosa congested

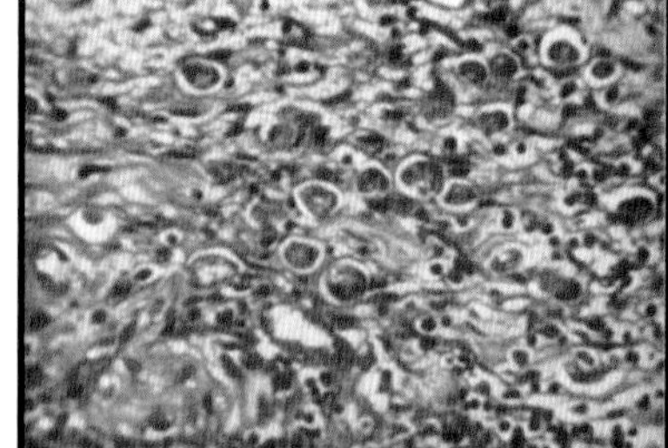

Numerous amebae in submucosa at edge of ulcer

## DISORDERS SEEN WITH HIV/AIDS

| HIV-Associated Gastrointestinal Pathogens | | | |
|---|---|---|---|
| **Pathologic Process** | **Small Bowel** | **Colon** | **Anorectal** |
| **Inflammatory** | HIV enteropathy | HIV enteropathy | |
| **Viral** | CMV | CMV<br>HSV | CMV<br>HSV<br>HPV<br>HHV8 |
| **Bacterial** | *Mycobacterium avium-intracellulare*<br>*M. tuberculosis* | *Bartonella*<br>*M. tuberculosis*<br>*C. difficile*<br>*Salmonella*<br>*Shigella*<br>*Campylobacter*<br>LGV | LGV<br>Chlamydia<br>Syphilis |
| **Parasitic** | *Cryptosporidium*<br>*Cystoisospora*<br>*Giardia*<br>*Microsporidia*<br>*Strongyloides* | | |
| **Fungal** | Histoplasmosis | *Cryptococcus*<br>Histoplasmosis | |
| **Neoplastic** | Kaposi sarcoma | Kaposi sarcoma<br>Lymphoma | Anal carcinoma |

HHV8 = human herpesvirus 8; HSV = herpes simplex virus; LGV = lymphogranuloma venereum.

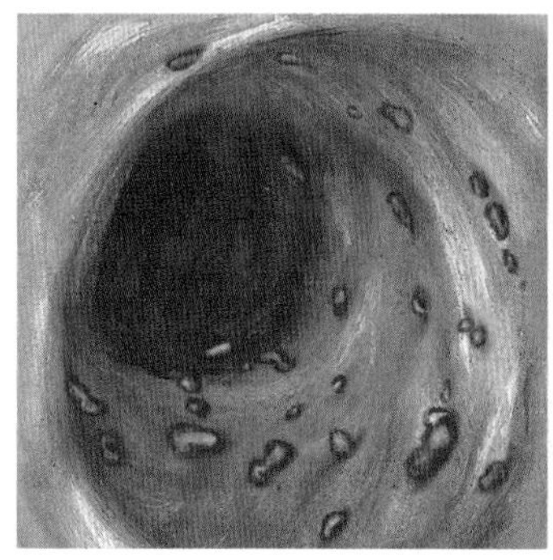

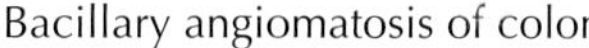
Bacillary angiomatosis of colon

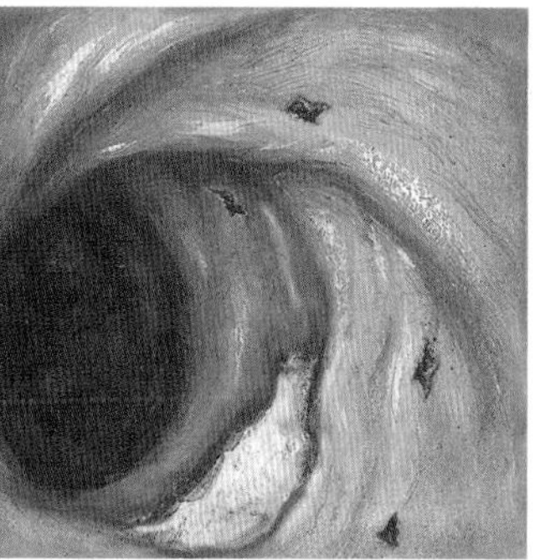
CMV ulcer, colon

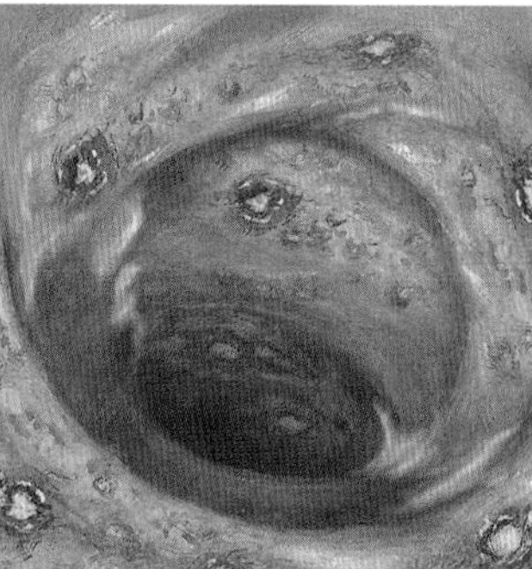
CMV colitis

The lower gastrointestinal system is a common location for complications and infections associated with HIV/AIDS. The spectrum of pathogens and conditions encountered mimics the HIV-negative population and may include bacterial, protozoal, fungal, viral, or neoplastic conditions. Additionally, infections in the individual who is HIV-positive may be due to unique exposure events and personal behaviors and/or due to progressive T-cell immune deficiency that may lead to exacerbation or more severe manifestations of infections that may occur in normal hosts. Patients with immune suppression from HIV/AIDS have an increased incidence and severity of disease caused by the protozoan pathogens *Cryptosporidium, Cystoisospora, Giardia, Microsporidia,* and *Strongyloides* and by the bacterial pathogens *M. tuberculosis, C. difficile, Salmonella, Shigella,* and *Campylobacter,* among others.

Cytomegalovirus (CMV) can have many manifestations in AIDS, including involvement of the entire GI tract, including the hepatobiliary tree. CMV colitis may be seen in patients with advanced HIV and in those with <50 CD4 cells cells/mL and is characterized by ulceration of the mucosa that can vary from punctate or shallow lesions to deep ulcers and necrotizing colitis. Diarrhea, abdominal pain, anorexia, weight loss, tenesmus, and watery diarrhea may be seen. Ulceration can lead to significant and life-threatening hemorrhage. The diagnosis is established by direct visualization of the lesions, with biopsy demonstrating CMV inclusions.

*Mycobacterium avium-intracellulare* causes a systemic illness with advanced AIDS that may have focal GI tract manifestations. Systemic symptoms of fever and weight loss are common. Mesenteric adenitis, abdominal pain, and diarrhea may be seen with gastrointestinal involvement. Endoscopy may reveal multiple raised nodules, ulceration, erythema, edema, or friability but may be entirely normal. The diagnosis is established by biopsy of the luminal wall demonstrating acid-fast bacilli. Blood cultures and stool smears and cultures for acid-fast bacilli may also aid in diagnosis.

*Bartonella henselae,* the agent of cat scratch fever, and *Bartonella quintana,* the agent of trench fever, may cause a syndrome of disseminated disease with liver involvement (peliosis hepatis) and angiomatous skin lesions. Cats are the reservoir for *B. henselae,* with transmission through direct contact such as bites or scratches or mediated by the bite of an infected flea vector. *B. quintana* has a human reservoir and is transmitted by the body louse. Focal involvement of colonic mucosa may lead to angiomatous lesions demonstrated on endoscopy.

*Histoplasma capsulatum* is the most common dimorphic fungus in patients with HIV. Although it causes a disseminated infection, focal gastrointestinal disease can be seen. It may cause focal diarrhea, abdominal pain, and weight loss. Pathologic findings include inflamed mucosa, ulceration, or polyps. The ileocecal region is most commonly involved. Diagnosis is made by demonstrating fungal hyphae in biopsy specimens. *Cryptococcus neoformans* and *C. gattii* may infect the colon, usually in the setting of disseminated infection. Biopsy reveals round fungal organisms surrounded by a clear halo of capsular material in focal abscesses or polyps, ulcerations, or strictures.

HIV-associated malignancies may occasionally involve the GI tract. Kaposi sarcoma is a multicentric proliferation of endothelial cells that can involve the viscera. Macroscopically, lesions are violaceous macules, papules, or polyps and are often seen in association with dermatologic lesions. Biopsy demonstrates characteristic spindle-shaped cells, atypical endothelial cells, and extravasated red cells. HIV-associated lymphomas are typically B-cell lymphomas that can occasionally affect the small or large intestine. HPV-related squamous intraepithelial lesions and squamous cell carcinomas of the anus or rectum may be seen in HIV-infected men who have sex with men.

AIDS enteropathy is a chronic diarrheal and malabsorption disease usually seen with advanced HIV and is thought to be due to direct or indirect effects of HIV on the enteric mucosa. It is characterized pathologically by villous atrophy, lymphocytic infiltration of the epithelium, crypt hyperplasia, and the absence of defined pathogens. HIV enteropathy is a diagnosis of exclusion and can be made only after other forms of diarrheal illness have been excluded.

## *CLOSTRIDIUM DIFFICILE* INFECTION

*Clostridium difficile* is a gram-positive, anaerobic, spore-forming bacillus that can cause colonic inflammation in patients with disturbance of the normal gut flora, especially as a result of antibiotic intake. After colonizing the bowel, the bacteria release toxin A (enterotoxin) and toxin B (cytotoxin), which cause mucosal inflammation. *C. difficile* is one of the most common causes of nosocomial infections, partly due to heat- and alcohol-resistant spores and widespread use of antibiotics. Transmission occurs via the fecal-oral route.

Recent antibiotic use is the strongest risk factor. Other risks include recent hospitalization, older age, history of *C. difficile* infection (CDI), underlying IBDs, use of immunosuppressive medications, or a weakened immune system. Proton pump inhibitors may also increase the risk due to suppression of gastric acid, although this is controversial.

Asymptomatic carriers are infected individuals who do not have symptoms but who may play an important role in the transmission of infection.

Most symptomatic patients present with abdominal pain, watery diarrhea (which is rarely bloody), anorexia, and fatigue. Patients may be dehydrated and/or have a fever. Abdominal tenderness is not uncommon.

Less than 5% of patients may present with fulminant colitis, which may lead to severe complications, including colonic perforation and toxic megacolon. It is important to know that diarrhea may be absent in severe disease when ileus is present.

The hypervirulent strain of *C. difficile* called NAP1 is associated with more severe disease.

Providers should only test for *C. difficile* infection in patients who have three or more loose stools in an hour with either a risk factor or exposure that predisposes them to infection. There is a high incidence of overdiagnosis and treatment for people without diarrhea who are asymptomatic carriers. Leukocytosis and electrolyte abnormalities, especially a rise in the creatinine level, can be present. Severe *C. difficile* infection is defined as having a white blood cell count over $15 \times 10^9$ cells/L or a rise in creatinine with normal kidney function to 1.5 mg/dL. Hypoalbuminemia and elevated lactate levels may be seen in severe cases. Stool examination may show fecal leukocytes or red blood cells.

The diagnosis of *C. difficile* can be challenging because many times people are colonized with a non-toxin-producing form. The first step should be to order a glutamine dehydrogenase test along with a toxin A/B assay. Glutamine dehydrogenase testing is sensitive, because all *C. difficile* species produce it, but not specific to find the pathogenic form. On the other hand, the toxin A/B assay is specific but not sensitive. If both are positive, the patient confidently has *C. difficile* infection. Likewise, if both are negative, the patient is not infected. If one of the two tests is positive, a nucleic acid amplification testing/polymerase chain reaction test looking for the toxin gene should be ordered to determine whether a patient is infected or not.

Sigmoidoscopy or colonoscopy may be considered in cases in which there is a high clinical suspicion for CDI with negative stool tests, atypical presentation with minimal diarrhea, or failure of response to treatment, but the procedures carry additional risks. The classic feature of CDI is the presence of yellowish-white raised plaques called *pseudomembranes* overlying the erythematous mucosa; in mild to moderate cases, however, the endoscopic evaluation may reveal normal mucosa or nonspecific colitis.

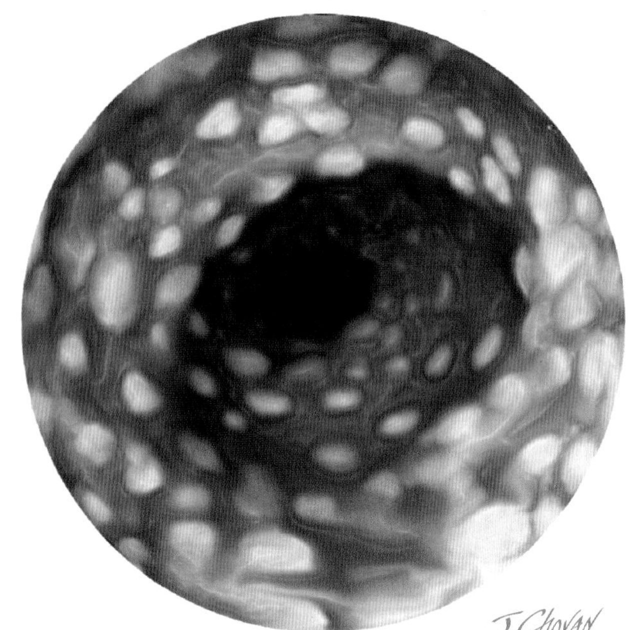

Pseudomembranous colitis

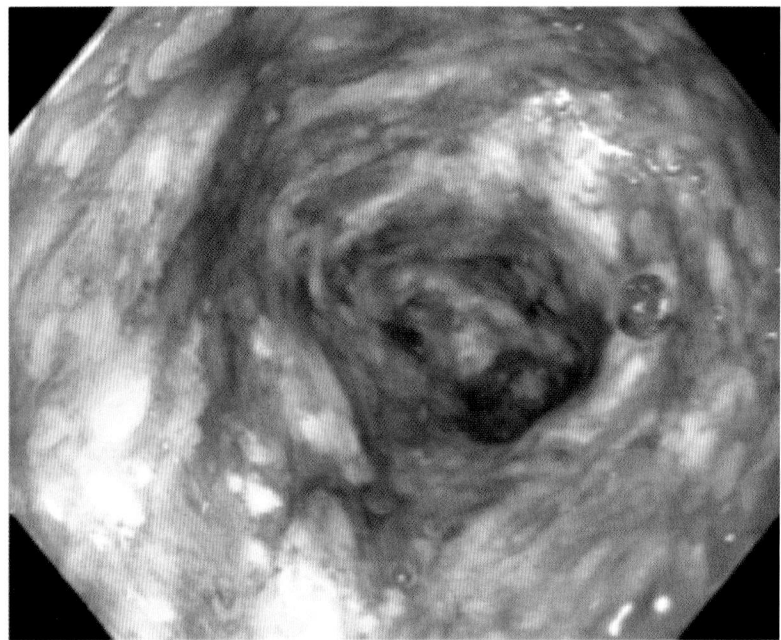
*C. difficile* colitis

Treatment is based on the severity of infection. Asymptomatic carriers usually do not require treatment. In symptomatic patients, fluid and electrolyte replacement should be considered, and the causative antibiotic should be discontinued, if possible. The most common antibiotics used for treating CDI include vancomycin, fidaxomicin, and occasionally metronidazole. Surgical intervention is required in fulminant cases with no response to medical treatment. Fecal microbiota transplant should also be considered for patients with severe and fulminant CDI refractory to antibiotic therapy, particularly in patients deemed poor surgical candidates.

Relapse occurs in 25% of patients because of reinfection or germination of the residual spores. Once the patient has one relapse, the risk for a second relapse increases to 45%. First recurrence of CDI is treated with either a tapered/pulsed-dose regimen of vancomycin or a course of fidaxomicin.

Bezlotoxumab is a human monoclonal antibody that binds to toxin B and prevents it from entering the gastrointestinal cell layer, hence preventing colonic cell damage. Bezlotoxumab can be considered for prevention of CDI recurrence in patients who are considered high risk for recurrence.

Most recent clinical guidelines recommend *against* probiotic use for prevention of CDI in patients being treated with antibiotics (primary prevention) as well as for prevention of CDI recurrence (secondary prevention).

Fecal microbiota transplantation (FMT) is highly effective in restoring gut microbiota diversity and hence treating recurrent CDI. FMT is recommended for patients experiencing their second or further recurrence of CDI. Although FMT can be delivered via fecal enema, infusion through nasogastric tube, colonoscopy, or capsules, delivery through colonoscopy or capsules is preferred because it is considered most effective.

Improving the antimicrobial prescribing practice, proper hand hygiene, isolating infected patients, and decontaminating the environment with solutions containing chlorine can decrease the transmission rate.

| Pathogen | Typical Presentation | Source | Treatment | Other Facts |
|---|---|---|---|---|
| **Bacterial Causes** | | | | |
| *Bacillus cereus* | Acute-onset diarrhea with vomiting | Reheated rice or other carbohydrate-dense foods | Supportive therapy | Symptoms present within hours of digestion |
| *Campylobacter jejuni* | Infectious, bloody diarrhea with severe abdominal pain that can mimic appendicitis and inflammatory bowel disease | Poultry is cited as the main source; however, it can be spread through drinking water or contact with other animal products. | Supportive therapy | Most common cause of invasive bacterial gastroenteritis. May be associated with Guillain-Barre syndrome. |
| *Clostridium difficile* | Colitis associated with antibiotics for another infection. Consequently, the antibiotics also kill the microbiome of the gut, allowing for *C. difficile* to colonize. Also known as pseudomembranous colitis or antibiotic-associated colitis | The most common antibiotics attributed to *C. difficile* infection are clindamycin, fluoroquinolones, cephalosporin family, and penicillin family of antibiotics. | Metronidazole is the preferred treatment, whereas oral vancomycin is reserved for severe cases. Both have been shown to have equal efficacy, with metronidazole being more cost-effective and having less chance for adverse outcomes | Oral vancomycin is first-line therapy in severe or complicated infections such as WBC >15,000 or when serum creatinine is 1.5x the patient's normal level. |
| *Enteroinvasive Escherichia coli* | Infectious, bloody diarrhea | Poorly cooked beef in addition to vegetables such as onions, bean sprouts, and spinach | Supportive therapy. Antibiotic therapy may result in hemolytic uremic syndrome (HUS). | O157:H7 is the major strain |
| *Noninvasive Escherichia coli* | Watery diarrhea | Naturally occurring *E. coli* of the GI gut flora picks up virulence factors, resulting in gastroenteritis. | Supportive therapy | Sometimes referred to as traveler's diarrhea |
| *Salmonella enteritidis* | Watery or mucous diarrhea | Eggs, peanut butter, uncooked poultry, and pet reptiles such as turtles | Supportive therapy | Most common cause of gastroenteritis from food poisoning |
| *Shigella* species | Infectious diarrhea seen with a high fever and bloody stools | Drinking water and food contaminated by feces | Supportive therapy, although some use antibiotics such as ciprofloxacin or trimethoprim-sulfamethoxazole (TMP-SMX). | High-risk populations are those with compromised immune systems or who have poor nutrition. The most common species is *Shigella flexneri*. |
| *Staphylococcus aureus* | Acute-onset diarrhea with vomiting | Cold cuts and dairy-based products left out too long such as cold salads with mayonnaise, deli meats, and milk | Supportive therapy | Symptoms present within hours of digestion |
| *Vibrio cholera* | Profuse, watery diarrhea usually described as "rice-water stool" | Contamination of a public water supply with feces | Supportive therapy with a major focus on volume repletion | Death usually results from dehydration. |
| *Yersinia enterocolitica* | Acute onset with vomiting and diarrhea (bloody or watery) that is also associated with terminal ileitis and pseudoappendicitis | Meat, water, or unpasteurized milk | Supportive therapy | Most common bacterial cause of gastroenteritis in developed countries |
| **Parasitic Causes** | | | | |
| *Cryptosporidium* species | Profuse watery diarrhea that can lead to dehydration. Commonly seen only in patients with immunocompromise | Fecal to oral spread | Immunocompetent patients usually need supportive therapy. Patients with HIV should first start on HAART therapy, with nitazoxanide used in select cases. | Most common parasitic infection |
| *Entamoeba histolytica* | Bloody diarrhea, although 90% of infections are asymptomatic | Fecal to oral spread | Metronidazole and a luminal agent such as paromomycin | |
| *Giardia lamblia* | The acute phase is frequently described as malodorous steatorrhea. Chronic infections usually are reported as loose stools resulting in weight loss and malabsorption. | Streams and daycare centers | Metronidazole | The most common infectious cause of chronic diarrhea |
| **Viral Causes** | | | | |
| Adenovirus | Watery diarrhea | Fecal to oral spread | Supportive care | |
| Astrovirus | Watery diarrhea most commonly seen in children up to the age of 7 but can occur in the elderly population | Fecal to oral spread | Supportive care | |
| Norovirus | Rapid onset of watery diarrhea that lasts approximately 48–72 hours and can be accompanied by vomiting | Fecal to oral spread. The most common sites for an outbreak are restaurants, hospitals, long-term care facilities, schools, daycare, and vacation spots such as cruises. | Supportive care | Most common viral cause in humans and usually seen in the winter season |
| Rotavirus | Watery diarrhea | Fecal to oral spread | Supportive care | A common cause of childhood diarrhea |

# Food Poisoning and Infectious Diarrhea

The Centers for Disease Control estimates that nearly one in six persons in the United States gets food poisoning annually, leading to 128,000 hospitalizations and nearly 3000 deaths. Causes of food poisoning can be split into three categories. The first includes illnesses caused by the ingestion of preformed toxins, such as *Bacillus cereus* and *Staphylococcus aureus*. These two forms of diarrhea will result in symptoms within the first 8 hours of ingestion. The second type includes bacterial diseases in which toxins are released after ingestion of bacteria, such as *Vibrio cholerae* and enterotoxigenic *E. coli*. The final category of infection includes invasive forms, such as *Campylobacter jejuni* and enteroinvasive *E. coli*, which can lead to systemic infection.

Food poisoning and other forms of infectious diarrhea can be caused by bacteria, parasites, and viruses. Causes of infectious diarrhea are almost always acute; however, some illnesses such as giardiasis can persist for longer than 14 days. A detailed social history is crucial with possible food poisoning and should focus on the patient's travel history, diet, and contact with sick persons. It is also important that the detailed history and physical examination focus on key elements that would suggest an infectious cause other than food ingestion. For example, a recent history of antibiotic therapy with clindamycin, penicillins, cephalosporins, or fluoroquinolones could suggest *C. difficile* infection, and a history of HIV/AIDS may add cryptosporidiosis to the differential diagnosis. Physical examination findings should rule out other gastrointestinal causes while assessing the volume status of the patient. Certain vital signs are important (e.g., hypotension strongly suggests severe diarrheal illness, and fever strongly suggests invasive diarrhea). It is important to report all causes of foodborne illness to the public health department.

Most causes of infectious diarrhea are viral and usually do not need further work-up. Typically, stool cultures are not recommended, unless a patient presents with hypovolemia, bloody diarrhea, six or more stools in a day, abdominal pain that has lasted for a week, age over 65 years, or immunocompromised status. A positive fecal leukocyte test will guide a practitioner to start empirical antibiotic treatment while stool cultures are pending. A negative fecal leukocyte test indicates that supportive therapy only is needed.

Most cases of infectious diarrhea need supportive care and will resolve spontaneously without therapy. First-line therapy is usually oral rehydration, which is a mix of sodium chloride, water, and glucose solution. Intravenous therapy should be reserved for patients with severe dehydration or inability to tolerate oral therapy. Antibiotic therapy is usually reserved for certain infections and is started empirically if the infection is thought to be systemic. Antibiotics are contraindicated in patients with enterohemorrhagic *E. coli* infection. This form of *E. coli* carries the virulence factor called the *Shiga toxin*, which has been shown to put patients at higher risk of hemolytic-uremic syndrome with antibiotic therapy.

# Ulcerative Colitis

## EPIDEMIOLOGY

Ulcerative colitis (UC) is one of two major types of IBDs; the other is CD (see Plate 3.69). UC leads to inflammation of the mucosal layer of the colon, which commonly involves the rectum but can extend proximally in a continuous fashion. The disease is more common in White populations and those of Eastern European and Ashkenazi Jewish descent. It is less common in those of Asian, Black, Native American, and Hispanic descent; however, new diagnoses are becoming more common for these populations. The incidence rates are rising in some newly industrialized countries in the Middle East and Asia.

## ETIOLOGY

Although the exact cause of IBD is unknown, it has been postulated that a dysregulated immune system may cause an inappropriate immune response to the antigenic component of bacteria that reside in the intestine of a genetically susceptible individual. Although the genetic susceptibility is less prominent in UC compared to CD, individuals with family history of UC in first-degree relatives are at higher risk for this disease.

Although no single factor has been proven as the consistent trigger, some environmental factors may also trigger the disease, such as infection, smoking cessation, high-fat/high-sugar diets, and taking nonsteroidal antiinflammatory drugs (NSAIDs). Given that the incidence is higher in northern locations compared with southern parts, lower sunlight exposure and vitamin D level may also be risk factors.

## MANIFESTATIONS

The disease course typically consists of intermittent flares alternating with periods of remission; however, a small percentage of patients may not be able to achieve remission. The symptoms of UC depend on the extent and severity of the disease. The most common symptoms of UC are diarrhea, rectal bleed, and abdominal pain. Tenesmus is also common due to rectal involvement. Other symptoms include nocturnal bowel movements, flatulence, incontinence, fever, weight loss, and symptoms associated with anemia. Malnutrition may occur from the increased diarrhea and the presence of inflammatory burden.

A severe and life-threatening complication of UC is toxic megacolon (see Plate 3.88). These patients have nonobstructing dilation (>6 cm) of the colon with signs of systemic toxicity, including fever, tachycardia, leukocytosis, and anemia. In these patients, the inflammation of the colonic wall typically extends beyond the mucosa. Dehydration, electrolyte abnormality, hypotension, and altered mental status may be present.

## LABORATORY FINDINGS, IMAGING STUDIES, AND ENDOSCOPIC EVALUATION

Laboratory findings in patients with UC depend on the severity of the disease. The blood tests may show hypochromic iron deficiency anemia, leukocytosis with a shift to the left, thrombocytosis, an elevated C-reactive protein and/or erythrocyte sedimentation rate, and hypoalbuminemia due to the colonic protein loss.

Radiologic tests, including *radiographs, barium enema* (enema should not be done during an acute presentation), and *CT scan,* are useful in evaluation of patients with known or suspected UC, but the findings are overall nonspecific. Images may show loss of mucosal pattern, ulceration, loss of haustration, ileus, colonic dilation, and perforation in advanced cases.

The colonoscopic findings in UC are nonspecific and biopsies are necessary to make the diagnosis. The endoscopic findings depend on the disease severity. Colonic mucosa may appear erythematous, granular, and friable, with loss of the normal vascular pattern and often with scattered hemorrhagic areas. In more advanced stages, the inflammatory process may evolve with the abscesses forming in dilated crypts, which discharge on the mucosal surface resulting in the formation of ulcers. The mucosa becomes darker red and more roughly granular and bleeds easily. A variable amount of mucus, blood, and pus may be seen in the lumen of the bowel. In the most severe active cases, the crypt abscesses burst through the wall of the crypt and spread in the submucosa, undermining areas of mucosa, which are deprived of a blood supply and subsequently are shed. In this way, extensive serpiginous ulcers are formed, often deep enough to expose the muscle coat; the remaining mucosa is edematous and partly undermined, leading to the appearance of pseudopolyps.

In nearly all cases of untreated UC, the rectum is involved in a continuous fashion. At presentation, the disease is limited to the rectum or rectosigmoid area in 30% to 50% of patients, while 20% to 30% have left-sided colitis and 20% have extensive colitis with disease extending proximal to the splenic flexure. In patients with more limited disease, the inflammation can extend more proximally later on. Mild terminal ileal inflammation may occur in patients with UC involving the entire colon. This is called *backwash ileitis* and is almost always associated with cecal inflammation. Cecal patch,

### Endoscopic Images and Histology

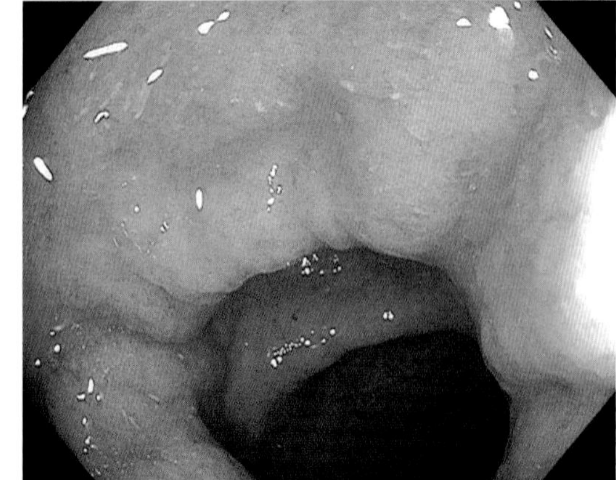

Mild ulcerative colitis

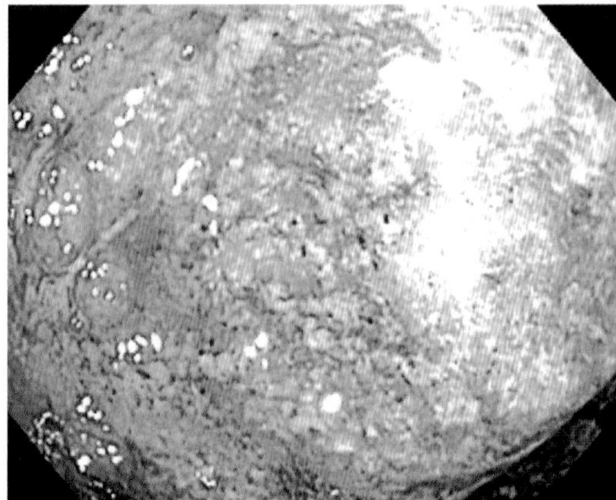

Moderate ulcerative colitis

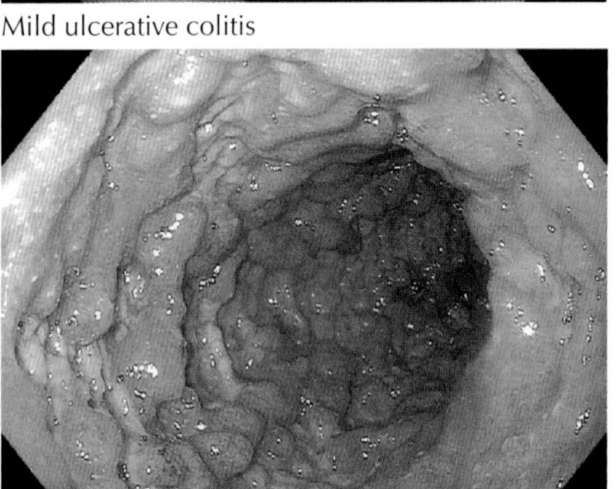

Severe ulcerative colitis

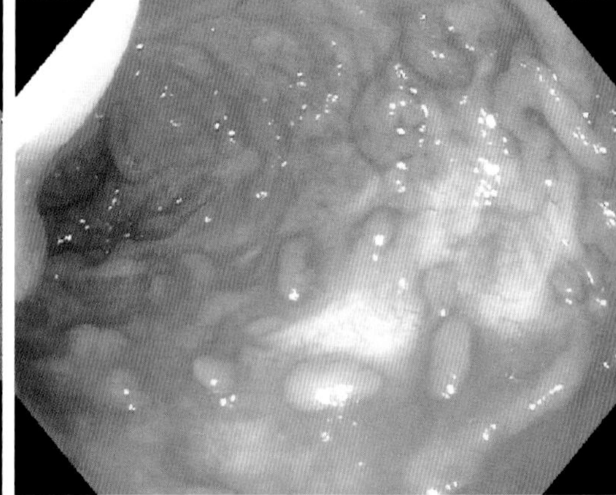

Pseudopolyps in ulcerative colitis

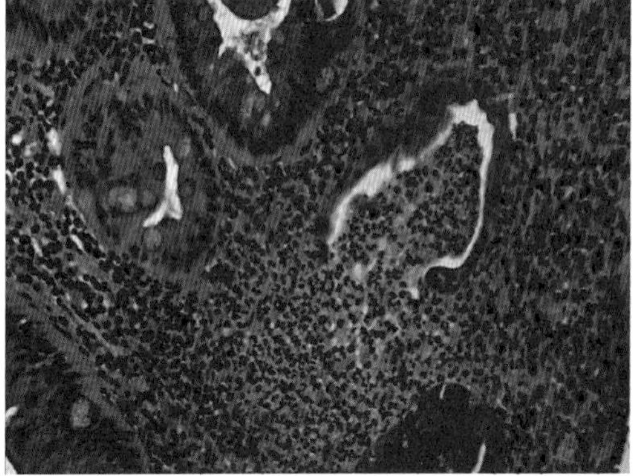

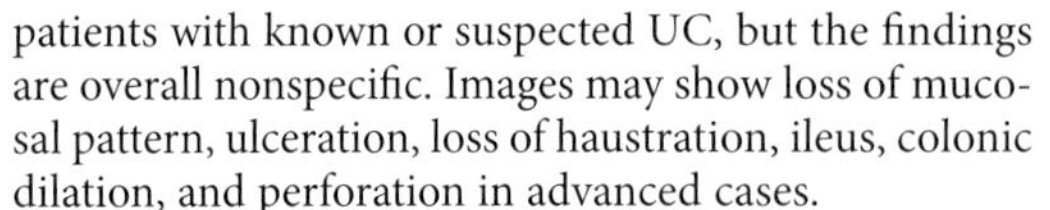

Active chronic colitis with crypt abscess characteristic of ulcerative colitis but not specific

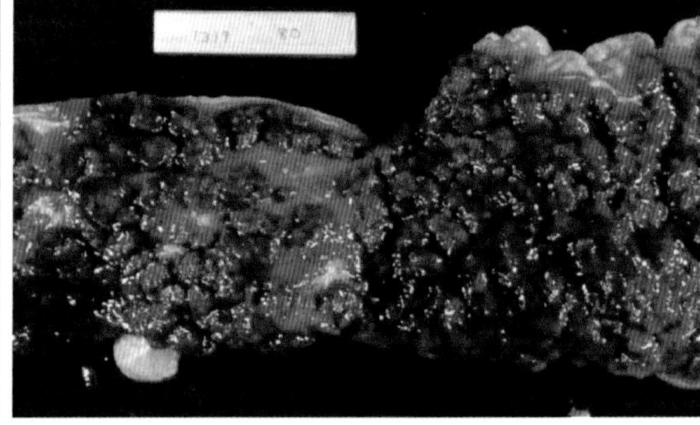

Ulcerative colitis, gross. Flat superficial ulcers with many inflammatory pseudopolyps.

## ULCERATIVE COLITIS (Continued)

a focal periappendiceal inflammation that is not contiguous with the disease in the left side, may be seen in a subset of patients with left-sided UC.

### PATHOLOGIC FINDINGS

Biopsy findings in patients with UC are nonspecific. Findings include chronic changes defined by Paneth cell metaplasia and crypt architectural distortion, with an increase in chronic inflammatory cells (lymphocytes and plasma cells), especially below the base of the crypts (so-called *basal plasmacytosis*). The presence of acute inflammation indicates disease activity and is characterized by neutrophil infiltration of the lamina propria, superficial ulcers, cryptitis, and crypt abscesses. Crypt abscesses are characterized by crypts filled with neutrophils and apoptotic debris.

### DIFFERENTIAL DIAGNOSIS

In addition to UC, one should always consider the following conditions in the differential diagnosis of patients presenting with abdominal pain, gastrointestinal bleeding, and intestinal ulcerations: Crohn colitis, infections of the colon (especially with *C. Campylobacter,* and *E. Coli* O157:H7 species, ameba, and cytomegalovirus), ischemic colitis, solitary rectal ulcer syndrome, NSAID-induced colopathy, diverticular-associated colitis, microscopic colitis, and radiation-induced colitis.

### COMPLICATIONS

UC can be associated with intestinal and/or extraintestinal complications.

#### *Intestinal Complications*

Although UC is a mucosal disease, the transmural extension of ulceration can result in loss of muscular tone and localized or extensive dilation of the colon in severe cases. This may result in toxic megacolon and possible perforation and peritonitis. Massive hemorrhage and occurrence of carcinoma are other intestinal complications of UC.

One of most dreadful complications of long-standing UC is epithelial dysplasia and colon cancer. Risk factors include extensive involvement, long duration of disease regardless of clinical activity, young age at onset, presence of primary sclerosing cholangitis (PSC), severe inflammation, and a family history of colorectal cancer. Surveillance colonoscopy is recommended after 8 years of having UC with the extent of more than rectal involvement because patients with proctitis may not be at increased risk for cancer. Compared with non–colitis-associated colorectal cancer, colitis-associated dysplasia and cancers are more often multiple and anaplastic, look minimally raised or nearly flat, and are uniformly distributed throughout the colon. Colitis-associated colorectal cancers do not follow the usual adenoma-cancer sequence.

#### *Extraintestinal Complications*

Extraintestinal complications occur in 20% to 25% of patients with IBD and are most likely the consequence of aberrant self-recognition and dysregulated autoantibodies against organ-specific cellular antigens shared by the colon and other organs. The most common

**ETIOLOGIC FACTORS, COMPLICATIONS OF INFLAMMATORY BOWEL DISEASES**

**Intestinal complications of ulcerative colitis and/or Crohn's disease**

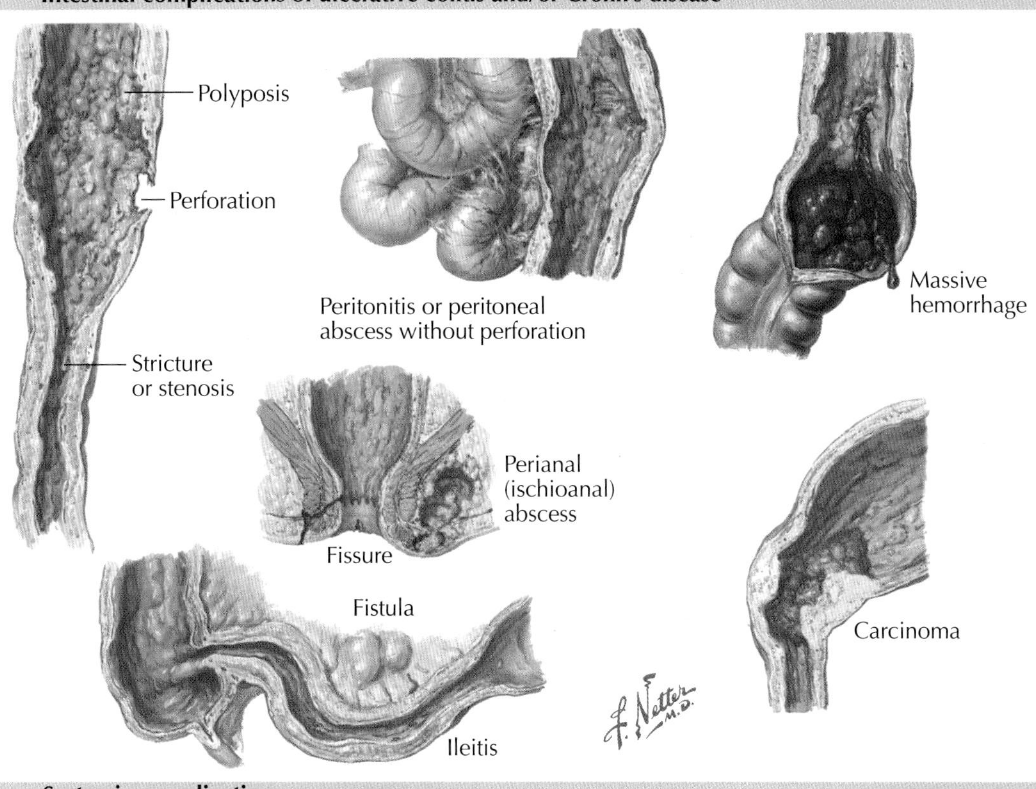


**Systemic complications**

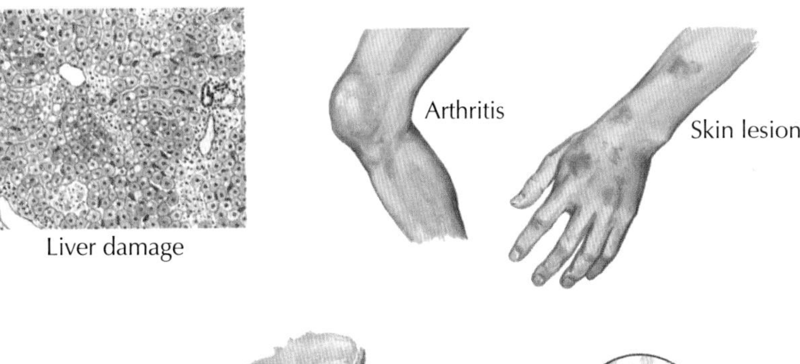


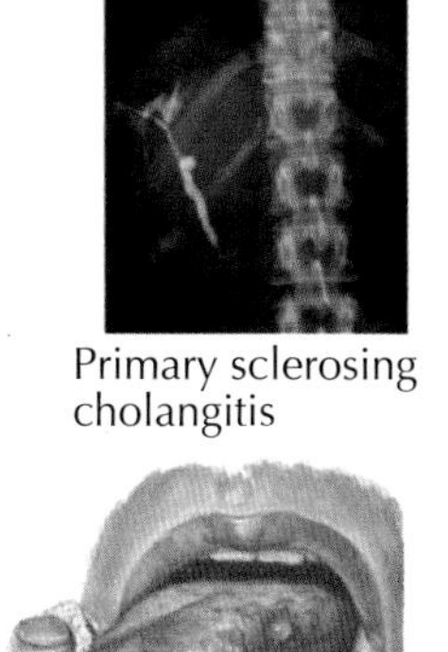


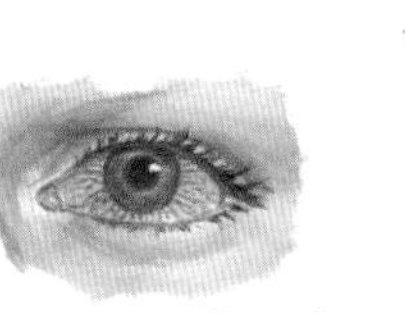


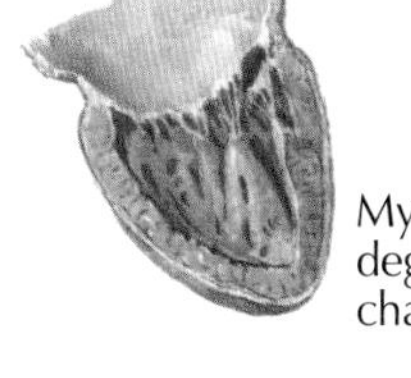


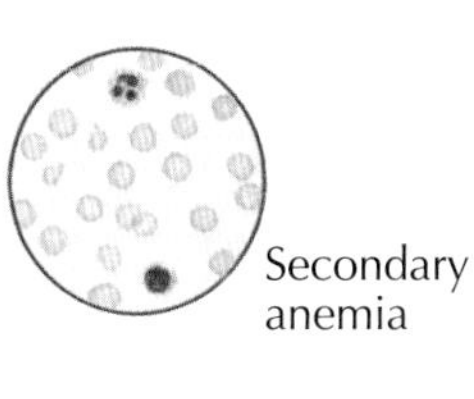


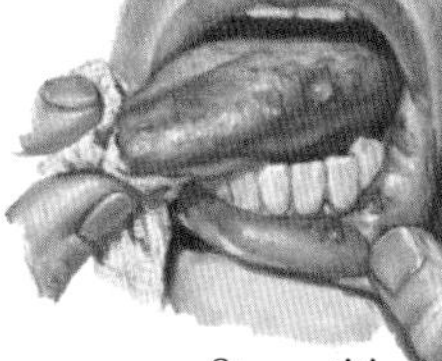


extraintestinal complications of UC include oral involvement with aphthous ulcerations, skin lesions (erythema nodosum and pyoderma gangrenosum), ocular manifestations (uveitis/iritis and episcleritis), hepatobiliary involvement (PSC), musculoskeletal involvement (arthropathy and osteoporosis), and hematologic consequences (anemia and thromboembolic diseases).

### MEDICAL AND SURGICAL TREATMENT

The goals of treatment of UC are inducing and maintaining steroid-free remission, improving the quality of life, and minimizing the risk of cancer. The choice of treatment depends on the severity and extent of the disease, prognostic factors, disease course during follow-up, and patient preferences.

#### *Medical Treatment*

Medical treatment usually is based on disease severity, which can range from mild, moderate, severe, to fulminant. In most cases, severity of symptoms is classified by stool frequency, presence of increased inflammatory markers, anemia, and symptoms of toxicity.

There are many different classes of medications available for treatment of UC. Sulfasalazine and 5-aminosalicylates (5-ASAs) given orally or rectally, or both, are the first-line treatment for mild disease and can be used for induction and maintenance of remission. The route of administration depends on the disease extent. Patients with mild proctitis or left-sided disease may be successfully treated with topical treatment (suppository/enema). The effect is usually seen in 2 to 4 weeks but may take longer. 5-ASAs do not have as many side effects as sulfasalazine; however, there is a rare risk of

## ULCERATIVE COLITIS (Continued)

nephrotoxicity with both of these medicines. Patients report intolerance toward sulfasalazine due to its common side effects, including dyspepsia, nausea, and vomiting. Pancreatitis, hepatotoxicity, bone marrow suppression, and anemia may occur less commonly.

*Steroids* are used for induction of remission in moderate to severe cases and can be given orally, rectally, or through an intravenous line. There are substantial adverse effects associated with the use of steroids, especially when they are taken in high doses and for extended periods of time. Side effects may include increased risk of infection, metabolic disturbances, psychiatric problems, cataracts, glaucoma, impaired wound healing, and metabolic bone disease. Steroid-sparing agents should be used to shorten the duration of therapy with systemic steroids. The extended-release *budesonide* has minimal side effects due to its high first-pass metabolism and should be considered in milder cases instead of more systemic steroids.

*Thiopurines (6-mercaptopurine* and *azathioprine)* are effective as steroid-sparing agents. Due to the slow onset of action, these agents are not recommended as monotherapy for induction of remission but can be considered in maintenance of remission or as dual therapy with tumor necrosis factor-α (TNF-α) inhibitors. Possible side effects include bone marrow suppression, increased risk of infection, allergic reaction, hepatotoxicity, pancreatitis, and increased risk of cancer including lymphoma.

*Biologics* are genetically engineered medications made from living organisms and their products, which interfere with the inflammatory response in patients with colitis. They can be used for induction and maintenance of remission in moderate to severe disease. Different classes of biologics for treatment of UC include TNF-α inhibitors (*infliximab, adalimumab,* and *golimumab*), α4β7 integrin inhibitor (*vedolizumab*) with gut-selective antiinflammatory activity, and interleukin 23 and 12 (IL-23 and IL-12) inhibitor (*ustekinumab*).

Biosimilars are biologic products that are highly similar to the reference drugs and are available for some of TNF-α inhibitors and can be used instead of the reference products. There is an increased risk of allergic reaction, autoimmunity, demyelinating disorders, worsening heart failure, psoriasis, infection (including opportunistic infection), and a possibly increased risk of cancer associated with the use of TNF-α inhibitors. *Vedolizumab* and *ustekinumab* have much more favorable safety profiles.

*Cyclosporine,* a *T-lymphocyte inhibitor,* is also a very effective agent for induction of remission in acute severe UC but unfortunately carries a significant risk of toxicity. Infection, seizures, hypertension, nephrotoxicity, and hyperkalemia are among the severe adverse effects with this medicine.

The newest medications for treating UC are small molecules. The two classes in this category are sphingosine 1-phosphate receptor modulator (*ozanimod*) and Janus kinase inhibitors (*tofacitinib and upadacitinib*). There is an increased risk of infection and cancer. Patients with cardiac risk factors and recent cardiac events are at higher risk for cardiac events when being treated with these agents.

**ILEOSTOMY**

Ileostomy site

Operative incision site

1. Ileum is divided. End of ileum with its mesentery is delivered through prepared stoma site.

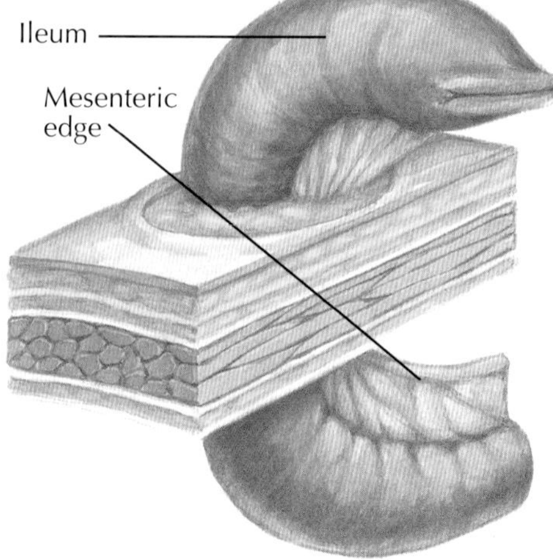


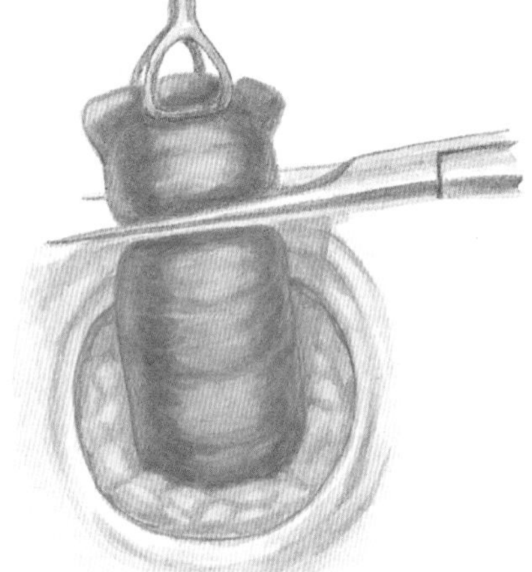

2. Stump of intestine is resected.

3. Final sutures (8–10) are placed through full-thickness bowel and dermis (avoiding epidermis) and are left untied.

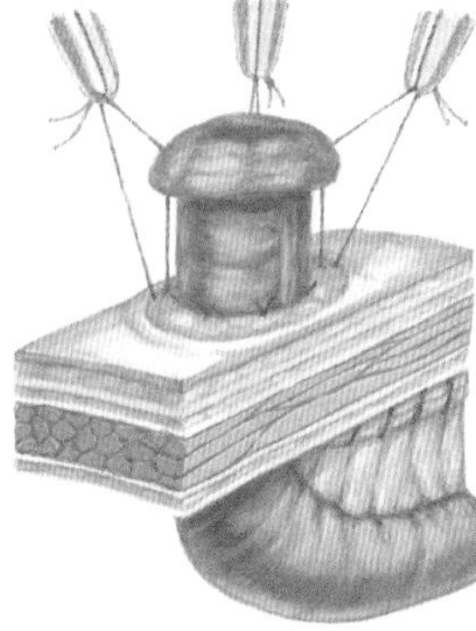

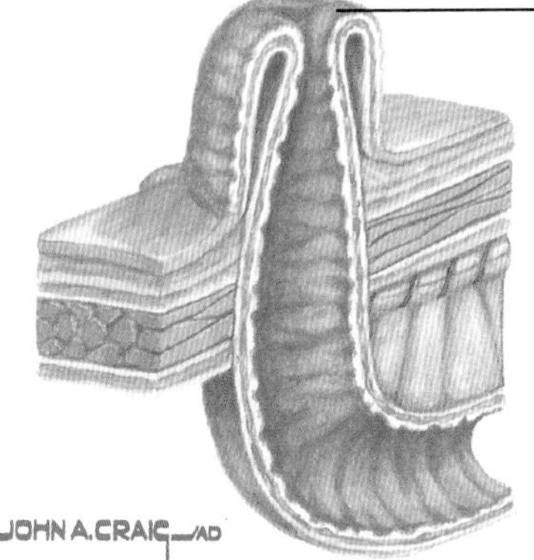


4. After all sutures are placed, progressive traction is applied, everting bowel to create the stoma. Skin and intestine edges are approximated and the sutures tied. Small slivers of Penrose drain may be placed in subcutaneous space during tying of sutures.

5. Final conformation protrudes above skin and is fitted with stoma appliance at end of procedure.

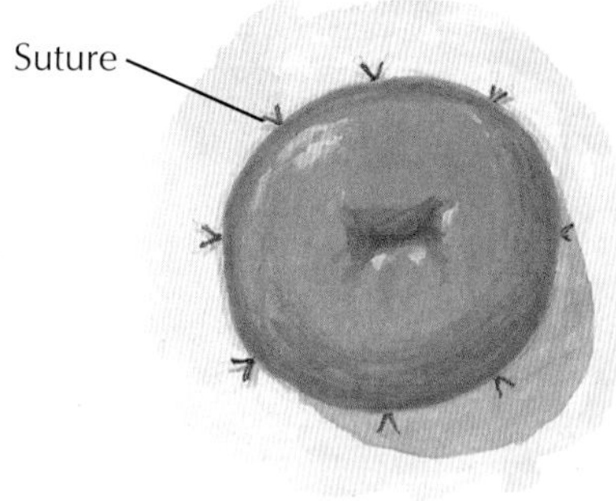


### *Principles of Surgical Treatment*

The indications for surgery in patients with UC are medically refractory disease, intolerable side effects of medical treatment, documented or strongly suspected cancer, unresectable high-grade or multifocal dysplasia, perforation, exsanguinating hemorrhage, and toxic megacolon. It is important to note the effect of health disparities on surgery. In one study of patients with UC between 1998 and 2003, Black and Hispanic patients were less likely to receive a colectomy than White patients.

Refractory extraintestinal manifestations of UC, which are related to disease activity, usually improve after colectomy.

The goal of surgery in patients with UC is to remove the diseased organ with minimal alteration of normal physiologic function and a good postoperative quality of life.

The following operations can be considered for patients with UC:

1. Proctocolectomy and Brooke ileostomy
2. Proctocolectomy and Kock pouch
3. Abdominal colectomy and ileorectal anastomosis
4. Total proctocolectomy with ileal pouch–anal anastomosis (IPAA)

Factors that need to be considered in choosing the type of surgery include the patient's age, comorbidities, body habitus, indication for surgery, and quality of the anal sphincter.

### *Total Proctocolectomy and End Ileostomy*

During the surgery, the entire colon and rectum are removed and a permanent ileostomy is created. The two types of end ileostomy include an incontinent or Brooke ileostomy and continent or Kock pouch ileostomy. End ileostomy is an especially appropriate choice for patients who are elderly, those with poor anal sphincter function, and patients with dysplasia or cancer in the lower rectum. Possible complications of

## ULCERATIVE COLITIS (Continued)

proctocolectomy are delayed perianal wound healing, impotence, retrograde ejaculation, and dyspareunia. The construction of the ileostomy can be difficult in obese patients.

A Brooke ileostomy involves pulling the ileum through the abdominal wall, turning it back, suturing it to the skin, and creating an inside-out ileum as the stoma. Most patients are suitable candidates for this type of operation, but unfortunately it scores the lowest in comparative quality-of-life studies between the four operations. It is one of the best options for patients who are elderly or have comorbidities. Disadvantages of this type of surgery include the need to wear an external appliance and risk of parastomal hernia.

A Kock pouch surgery involves the creation of an ileal pouch with a nipple valve, which is then connected to the skin of the lower abdomen. The stool is drained with a catheter as needed. The procedure can be considered in younger patients who do not wish to wear an external appliance. This type of surgery unfortunately carries a high complication rate, with a significant percentage of patients requiring reoperation. Nipple valve dysfunction resulting in difficulty with intubation and subsequent incontinence is a common problem. Other possible complications include fistula formation, ischemic changes, and pouchitis.

### *Abdominal Colectomy and Ileorectal Anastomosis*

This type of surgery should rarely be considered and only in patients whose rectal inflammation is under good control. Possible candidates include patients who are not suitable for IPAA but also refuse to have end ileostomy, presence of contraindication to ileostomy (e.g., ascites), or limited life expectancy. This type of surgery does not carry the usual complications of having a total proctocolectomy, such as impotence, because it does not require the mobilization of the rectum. The disadvantage of this surgical procedure is the risk of continued symptoms because of the retained inflamed rectal mucosa and the risk of dysplasia and cancer in this area.

### *Total Proctocolectomy With Ileal Pouch–Anal Anastomosis*

Total proctocolectomy with IPAA involves resection of the colon and rectum and formation of an IPAA. This can be done in one, two, or three stages, depending on the clinical scenario and the judgment and experience of the surgeon. In most cases with severe colitis, an ileostomy with subtotal colectomy is done as a first stage, followed by excision of the remaining rectocolic segment a few months later and creation of the IPAA.

This type of surgery preserves the anal sphincter function, with good postoperative quality of life, but complications are not uncommon, including pouchitis, small bowel obstruction, fistula, anastomotic leak, pelvic sepsis, and the negative effect on fertility and sexual function. Pouch excision or revision is required in some cases.

### *Pouchitis*

Pouchitis is nonspecific inflammation of the ileal pouch reservoir and is the most important long-term complication of total proctocolectomy and IPAA, occurring in approximately 15% to 50% of patients during long-term follow-up. Pouchitis typically occurs in patients with UC or indeterminate colitis but is rare in a patient who undergoes IPAA for familial adenomatous polyposis.

ILEAL POUCH–ANAL ANASTOMOSIS (IPAA) AND POUCHITIS

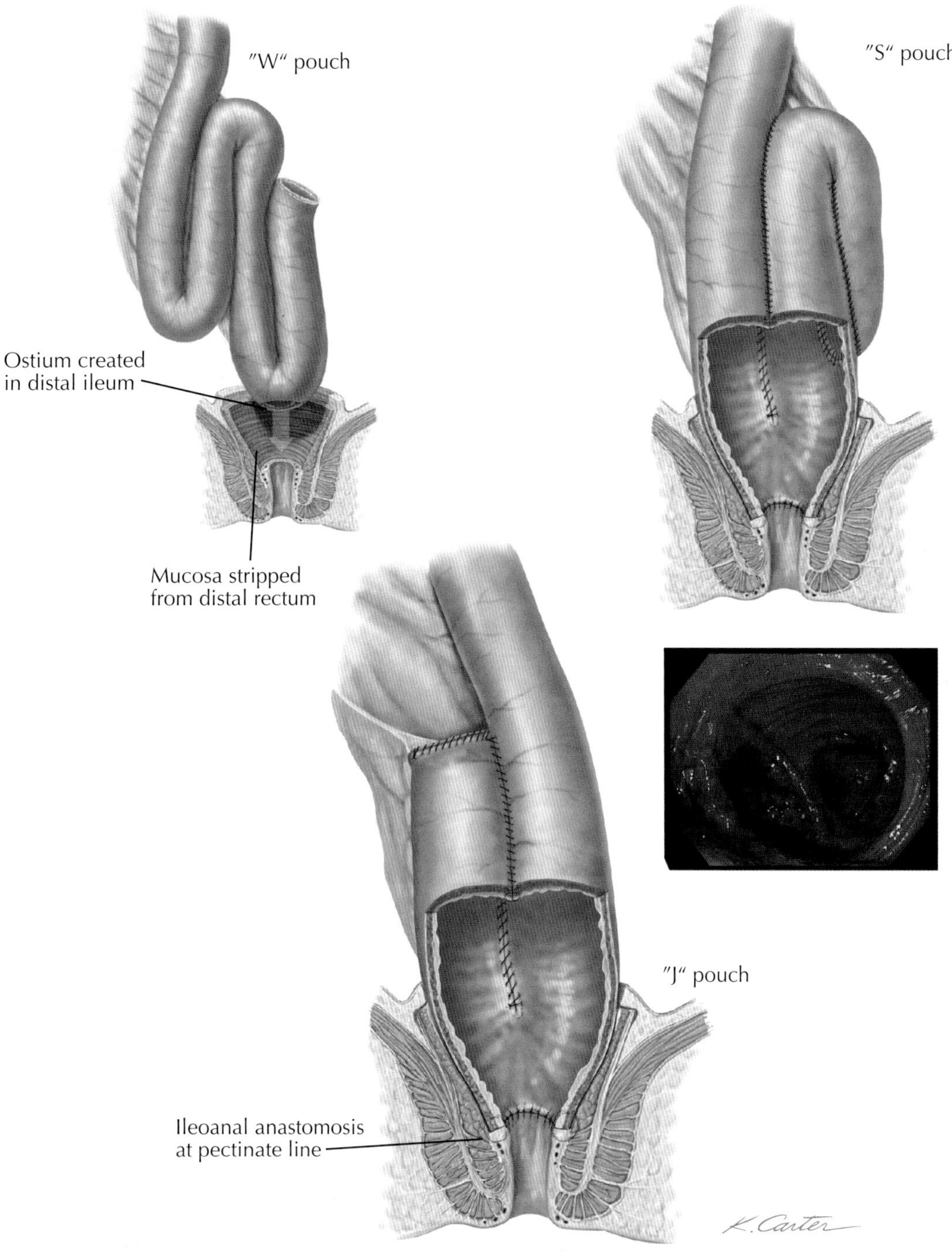


The cause is unclear but thought to be due to abnormal immune response to altered microbiome in genetically susceptible hosts. Risk factors include history of extensive disease; presence of extraintestinal manifestations, especially PSC; and young age at diagnosis. Obesity, NSAID use, and fecal stasis due to pouch stricture or functional outlet obstruction may also increase the risk of pouchitis.

Symptoms may include increased stool frequency, urgency, pelvic pressure, and incontinence. Patients suspected of having pouchitis should undergo endoscopic evaluation. Endoscopic findings are nonspecific and include erythema, friability, and erosions with or without ulcerations. Biopsies often show an acute inflammatory infiltrate superimposed on a background of chronic changes and chronic inflammatory cells, villous atrophy, and crypt distortion.

Differential diagnosis include postoperative complications especially during the first year after surgery, ischemic changes, irritable pouch syndrome, infection, cuffitis in the residual rectal mucosa, and CD. Radiologic assessment by means of pouchography with contrast, CT, or MRI may be considered in some patients, especially if symptoms are suggestive of alternate diagnosis.

Antibiotics such as ciprofloxacin or alternatively metronidazole should be used for the initial episode. Patients whose symptoms do not resolve in less than 4 weeks are considered to have chronic pouchitis. Refractory patients should be treated with budesonide, immunomodulators, biologics, or small molecules after thorough evaluation for an alternate diagnosis. Patients with antibiotic-dependent pouchitis will need cycling therapy with antibiotics.

# CROHN'S DISEASE

## EPIDEMIOLOGY

The incidence and prevalence of Crohn's disease (CD) vary among different studies evaluating patients in various geographic locations and with differing levels of socioeconomic status. The annual incidence is estimated to range from 5 to 20 per 100,000, with a prevalence of as high as 320 per 100,000 persons in Europe and North America. White persons and persons of Jewish Ashkenazi descent have a higher risk for developing the disease. Although there is a significant difference in the incidence rate of IBD among different racial and ethnic groups, with a higher rates in Whites, the rate is rising more rapidly in non-Whites. CD is more prevalent in North America and Western Europe, but the incidence of CD is noted to be rising in South America and Asia.

## ETIOLOGY

The cause is unknown, although the interplay of genetic, immunologic, and environmental factors exists. *NOD2/CARD15* on chromosome 16 and *IL23R* on chromosome 1 are the most studied susceptibility genes. There is a high concordance rate of about 50% among monozygotic twins.

Some environmental factors have been recognized as triggers for development of CD, the most important of which is cigarette smoking. NSAIDs and high dietary intake of fat and meat may also increase the risk, although the magnitude of this risk is very small. Physical activity and a high-fiber diet may have a protective effect against CD.

## MANIFESTATIONS

CD can involve any part of the GI tract, with the most common sites being small and large bowel, especially the terminal ileum and cecum. Transmural inflammatory changes can lead to progressive fibrosis with subsequent strictures or perforating disease with abscess and/or fistula formation. Perianal disease is not uncommon and may indicate a more aggressive clinical course. The disease course typically consists of intermittent flares alternating with periods of remission; however, some patients may not be able to achieve remission and continue to have active disease.

The location, severity, and phenotype of the disease dictate the individual's symptoms. Most patients present with abdominal pain and diarrhea, which is often nonbloody. Fever and weight loss are common. Patients with obstructive symptoms due to underlying stricture may experience abdominal distension and pain, nausea, and vomiting. Abnormal drainage of pus or fecal material can be seen if a fistula is present.

Abdominal tenderness, cachexia, abdominal or perianal mass, fistulae, and abscess are among the more common signs of CD. Affected children may have growth failure or delayed development of the secondary sex characteristics.

Extraintestinal manifestations can be present in a significant number of patients.

## LABORATORY TESTS, ENDOSCOPIC EVALUATION, AND IMAGING STUDIES

There is no specific laboratory test for the diagnosis of CD. Leukocytosis, thrombocytosis, and anemia are commonly present. Anemia can be due to iron deficiency, associated with chronic disease, or due to other vitamin deficiencies, including vitamin $B_{12}$ deficiency in patients with ileal involvement or resection. Hypoalbuminemia, low vitamin D levels, elevated C-reactive protein levels, and an abnormal erythrocyte sedimentation rate are other abnormalities that can be seen. The most common serologic markers associated with CD include antibody to the yeast *Saccharomyces cerevisiae* and the bacterial proteins outer membrane protein C (OmpC), I-2, and flagellin. These markers have limited diagnostic value as individual tests. Stool studies may reveal the presence of leukocytes and are negative for infectious pathogens in most cases.

Colonoscopy is the mainstay diagnostic tool for patients with terminal ileum and/or colonic involvement of CD. It not only allows direct visualization of the mucosa, but biopsy samples can be obtained during the examination. The terminal ileum should be evaluated during the colonoscopy. Endoscopic findings are nonspecific and include erythematous mucosa, shallow aphthous erosions/ulcers, punched-out ulcers, and skip lesions (intervening normal mucosa) with nodular mucosal changes resulting in a cobblestone appearance. Rectal sparing is common in CD. Endoanal ultrasound is a valuable tool in the evaluation of perianal disease.

### Crohn's Disease: Histology and Endoscopy

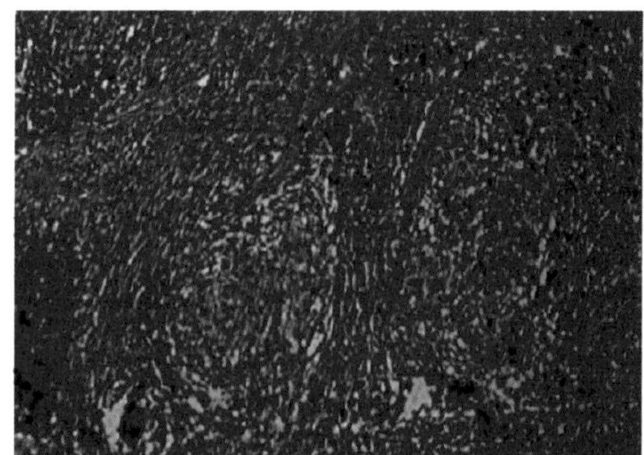
Epithelioid granulomatous reaction associated with chronic inflammation in the muscularis of colon in a patient with CD

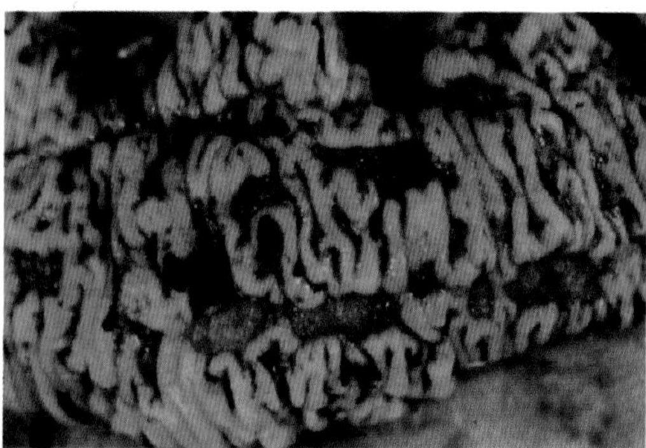
Linear deep fissure-like ulcer in the colon in a patient with CD

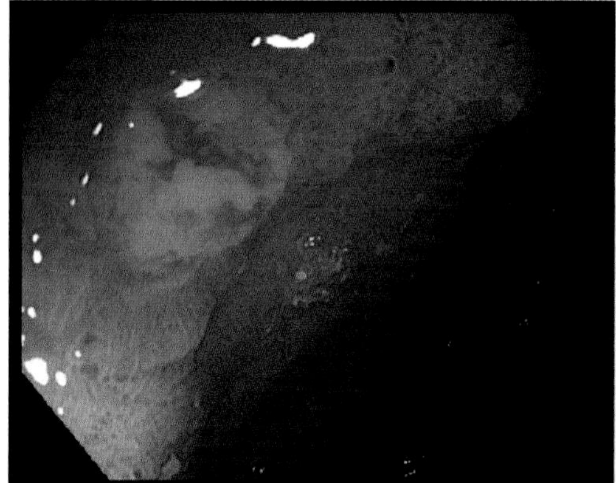
Crohn's ileitis

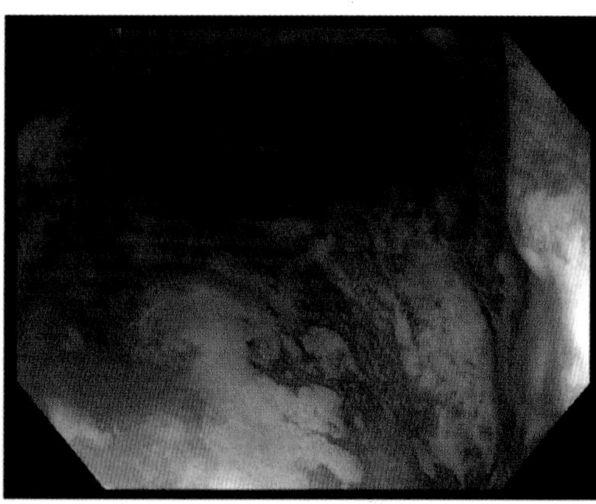
Crohn's colitis

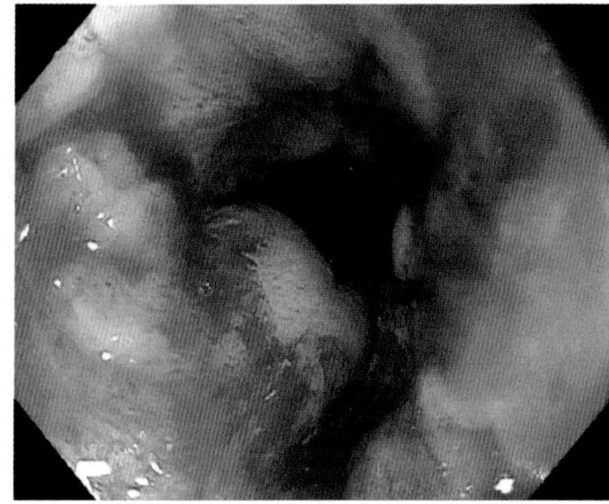
Crohn's stricture

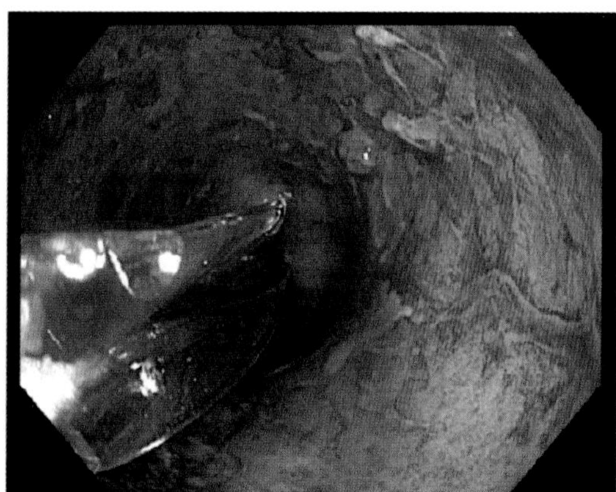
Balloon dilation of Crohn's stricture

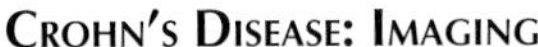

# CROHN'S DISEASE (Continued)

Esophagogastroduodenoscopy should be performed in patients with suspected CD who have upper GI symptoms. Mucosal erythema, erosions, ulcerations, and strictures may be seen.

Capsule endoscopy allows direct visualization of the small bowel mucosa without radiation exposure. There is a risk of capsule retention and subsequent bowel obstruction in patients who may have bowel strictures. The risk can be reduced by careful patient selection and use of a patency capsule study in advance.

Radiologic tests are useful when evaluating patients with known or suspected CD. Abdominal radiographs may help diagnose bowel obstruction or megacolon. Small bowel follow-through and air-contrast barium enema may detect mucosal disease, strictures, and fistulas. Transabdominal ultrasound (especially contrast-specific ultrasound) can help in the diagnosis of abscess and bowel wall thickening and has gained popularity in Europe. CT scan can also help in the diagnosis of bowel wall thickening, abscess, and strictures, and CT enterography allows for more detailed images of the small bowel wall by means of a special low-density contrast. MRI is another important radiologic tool. MR enterography is an excellent modality for evaluation of small bowel and has advantage over CT enterography with the elimination of the exposure to ionizing radiation. MRI of the pelvis is used when assessing for perianal diseases.

## PATHOLOGIC FINDINGS

In CD, pathologic changes may be seen throughout the entire GI tract from mouth to anus. Pathologic features are usually confirmatory but nondiagnostic. Findings include acute and chronic inflammation with neutrophilic and plasmacytic infiltration of the lamina propria, crypt distortion, and crypt abscess. Submucosal fibrosis can also be detected. Noncaseating granulomas may be found in up to 30% of patients but are not required for the diagnosis. These granulomas and transmural involvement are highly specific for the diagnosis of CD.

Mucosal biopsies from the same segment may show variable findings known as *skip lesions,* which are one of the features that distinguish CD from UC.

## DIFFERENTIAL DIAGNOSIS

Conditions that mimic CD include infectious disease, ischemic colitis, radiation enteritis/colitis, segmental colitis, diversion colitis, NSAID colopathy, other granulomatous colitides (e.g., sarcoidosis), and UC, among others.

## COMPLICATIONS

CD can be associated with intestinal and/or extraintestinal complications.

### *Intestinal Complications*

These may include bowel obstruction, enterovesical fistulae resulting in urinary tract infection and pneumaturia, enterovaginal fistulae with feculent vaginal discharge, and enterocutaneous fistulae with feculent soiling of the skin, intraabdominal or retroperitoneal abscess formation, and perianal involvement.

Patients with long-standing Crohn colitis who have more than one-third colon involvement are at increased risk for colon cancer.

**CROHN'S DISEASE: IMAGING**

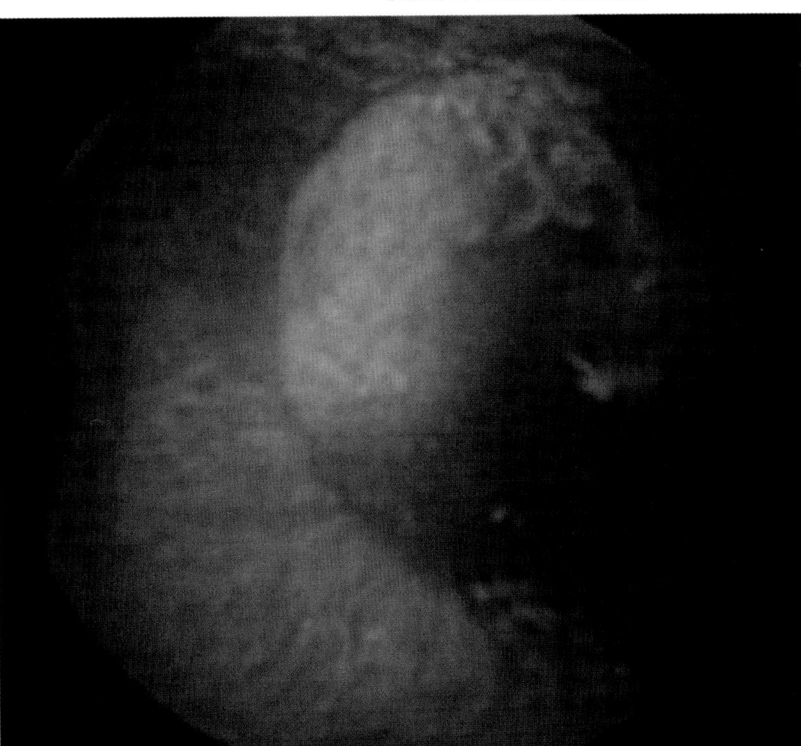

Capsule endoscopy in small bowel CD

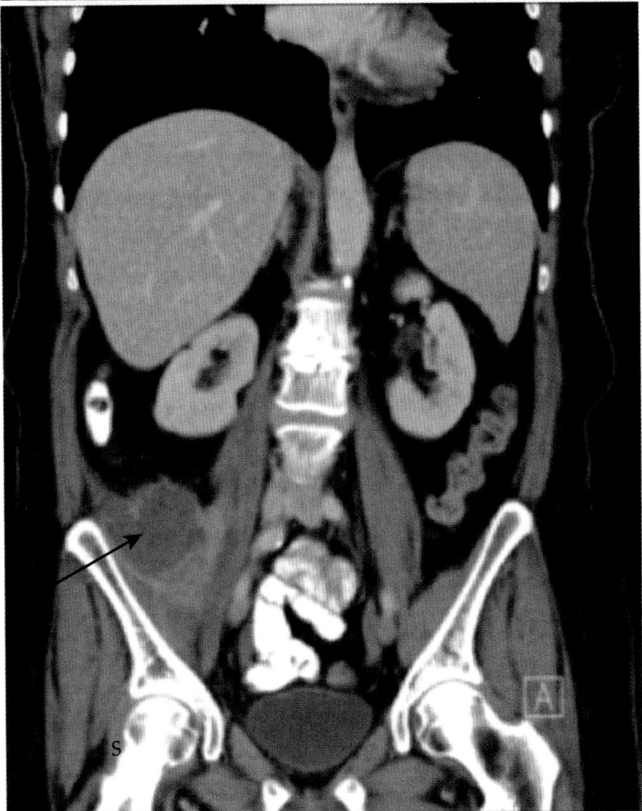


CT scan of right-sided psoas abscess

### *Extraintestinal Complications*

The most common extraintestinal complications include musculoskeletal involvement (arthropathy and osteoporosis), ophthalmologic manifestations (episcleritis and iritis/uveitis), skin lesions (pyoderma gangrenosum and erythema nodosum), urinary tract involvement (kidney stone), oral involvement by aphthous ulcers, biliary tract involvement (primary sclerosing cholangitis, cholelithiasis), and hematologic manifestations (hypercoagulable state and anemia).

## MEDICAL AND SURGICAL THERAPY

### *Medical Treatment*

The goals of medical treatment are induction and maintenance of remission with the least adverse effect from the medications and improvement of quality of life. The choice of therapy should be based on the disease extent, location, phenotype, and severity.

Several medications are used in treating CD:

*5-ASAs* and *sulfasalazine:* Although *sulfasalazine* can be used in patients with mild to moderate Crohn colitis,

## CROHN'S DISEASE (Continued)

oral *mesalamine* has not been shown to be effective compared with placebo despite being widely used in practice.

*Antibiotics:* The role of gut bacteria in the pathogenesis of CD has led to the use of antibiotics in these patients, with the most commonly used antibiotics being *metronidazole* and *ciprofloxacin.* Although antibiotics have a role in treatment of pyogenic complications, postoperative management, and perianal fistula with abscess, they should not be recommended for therapy of luminal disease. These medicines should be considered in combination therapy with biologics in treatment of perianal fistula without abscess but not as monotherapy.

*Steroids:* They are mostly used for treatment of flares. Controlled-release *budesonide* is effective and has fewer side effects than *prednisone* when mild to moderate inflammation is confined to the ileum and/or right colon. *Prednisone* can be used for treatment of moderate to severe CD, but it has substantial possible adverse effects, including, but not limited to, metabolic disturbances, increased risk of infection, metabolic bone disease, and psychiatric and ocular complications.

*Immunomodulators: Thiopurines (6-mercaptopurine and azathioprine)* and *methotrexate* are effective as steroid-sparing and maintenance treatment but have a slow onset of action and are not appropriate for induction of remission. They may also be used as adjunct therapy to reduce the risk of immunogenicity toward biologics. There may be a role for using *thiopurines* for prevention of postoperative CD.

Possible side effects for *thiopurines* include increased risk of infection, bone marrow suppression, allergic reaction, liver toxicity, pancreatitis, and increased risk of cancer including lymphoma.

Some of the side effects of *methotrexate* include nausea/vomiting, bone marrow suppression, hepatotoxicity, and pulmonary toxicity.

*Biologics:* These are genetically engineered medications made from living organisms whose products interfere with the patient's inflammatory response. This group of medicines has been used for induction and maintenance of treatment in moderate or severe disease.

Different classes of biologics for treatment of CD include TNF-α inhibitors (anti-TNF-α) including (*infliximab, adalimumab,* and *certolizumab*), *alpha-4 integrin* inhibitors (*natalizumab* and *vedolizumab*), IL-23 and IL-12 inhibitor (*ustekinumab*), and recently approved IL-23 inhibitor (*risankizumab*). These medications should be considered in the treatment of moderate to severe disease that has not responded to other therapies or as first-line therapy for patients with poor prognostic criteria. Biosimilars that are highly similar to the reference drugs are available for some of TNF-α inhibitors.

There is an increased risk of allergic reaction, autoimmunity, demyelinating disorders, worsening heart failure, psoriasis, infection (including opportunistic infection), and a possibly increased risk of cancer associated with the use of TNF-α inhibitors. *Vedolizumab, ustekinumab,* and *risankizumab* have much more favorable safety profiles.

*Natalizumab* has restricted application due to the reported cases of progressive multifocal leukoencephalopathy and should only be considered when alternative therapy is not available and patient is John Cunningham virus antibody negative and willing to have ongoing monitoring. This specific complication has not been reported with the use of *vedolizumab* because of its gut specificity.

### CROHN'S DISEASE: STRICTUREPLASTY

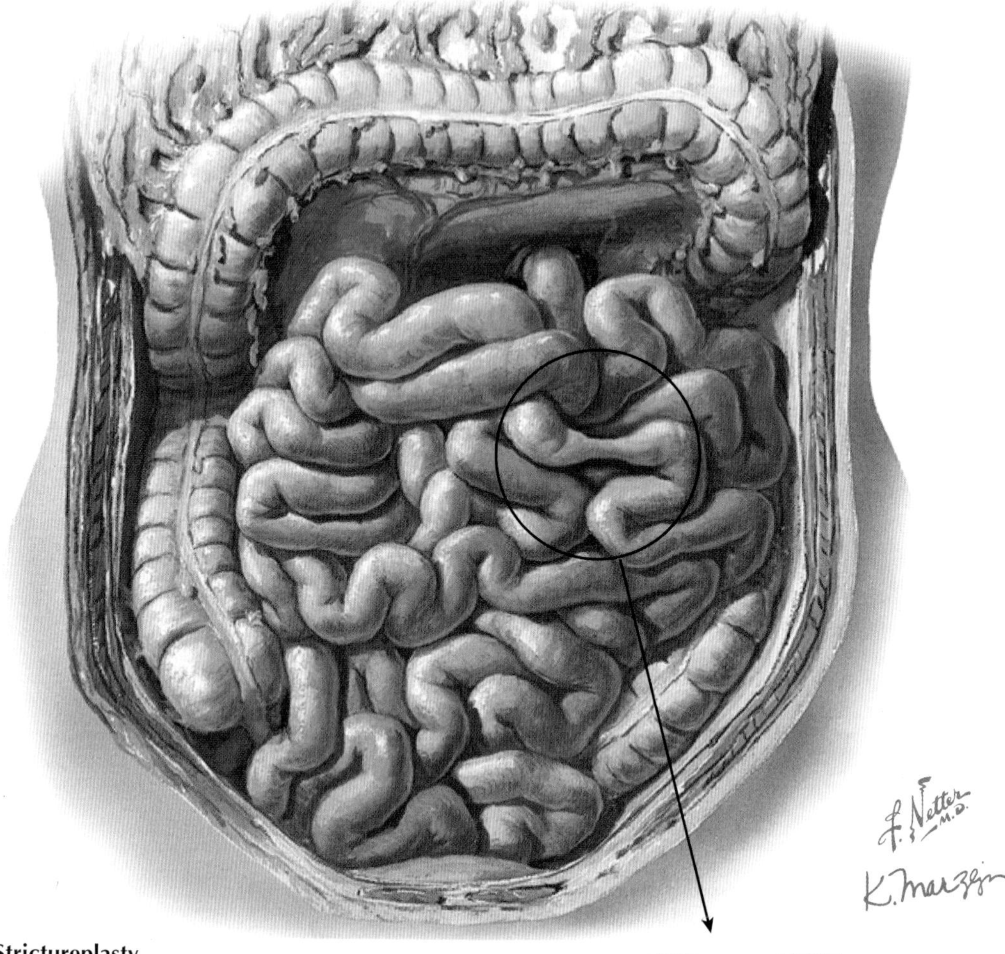


**Strictureplasty**
During this intervention, the narrow segment of the bowel is cut lengthwise and then sutured widthwise.

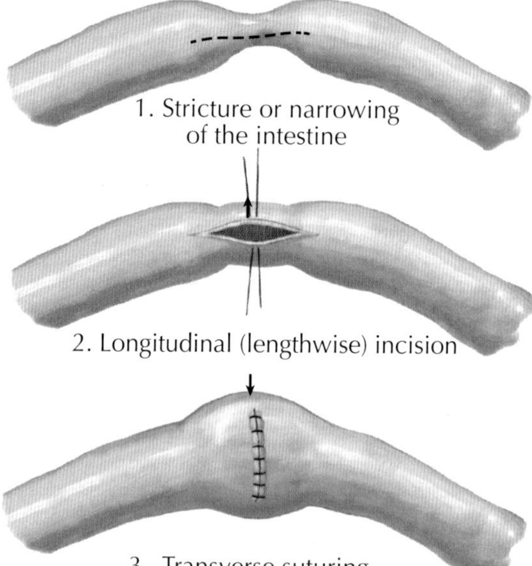


#### *Surgical Intervention*

Although advances in medical therapy have resulted in a lower rate of surgical resection, a 10-year cumulative risk of nearly 50% has been estimated in this population, with many requiring second or third surgeries.

The indications for surgical intervention include failed medical therapy, the presence of neoplastic complications, perforation, persistent or severe hemorrhage, abscesses not amenable to drainage by the radiologist, or cases with bowel obstruction nonresponsive to conservative management. Due to the concern over short bowel syndrome, bowel-sparing interventions, including balloon dilation or strictureplasty (the narrow segment of the bowel is cut lengthwise and then sutured widthwise), can be considered, particularly in patients with a history of previous significant bowel resections, a known history of short bowel syndrome, or the presence of multiple strictures over a long segment of small bowel. It is important to know that even after surgically induced deep remission, most patients with CD will require medical treatment to decrease the risk of recurrence.

# Microscopic Colitis

Microscopic colitis (MC) is an inflammatory disease and a relatively common cause of chronic diarrhea in older adults. There are two forms of MC, collagenous colitis (CC) and lymphocytic colitis (LC). These two subtypes are similar clinically but can be differentiated based on histology.

The incidence of MC has plateaued recently after a period of time of an increased incidence. The initial increase in the incidence has been attributed to a higher awareness resulting in more diagnostic colonic biopsies in patients with chronic diarrhea and increased use of the triggering medicines.

MC appears to be more prevalent in females than in males and has a mean age at diagnosis of 65 years. The sex difference is less striking in LC than CC.

The pathogenesis of microscopic colitis is unknown, but several potential mechanisms may play a role including deranged mucosal immune response to luminal factors, including bacterial products, bile salts, medications, and dietary antigens in a genetically susceptible individual. Myofibroblastic malfunction and abnormalities in collagen production may also be involved in the pathogenesis of CC. MC has been linked with an increased risk of some autoimmune conditions such as celiac disease, type 1 diabetes mellitus, rheumatoid arthritis, psoriasis, or thyroiditis, among others. Smoking and medications have been reported to be associated with an increased risk of MC. The most commonly reported medicines include NSAIDS, proton pump inhibitors, statins, and selective serotonin reuptake inhibitors.

Patients with MC can have variable disease course. The most common symptom is intermittent or chronic diarrhea. Patients may also experience abdominal discomfort or weight loss, urgency, bowel incontinence, and dehydration in more severe cases.

The physical examination usually does not reveal any specific abnormality. Blood tests are usually within normal limits but may also show hypokalemia, hypoalbuminemia, anemia, and an elevated erythrocyte sedimentation rate. Imaging studies are typically normal. Celiac disease, CD, IBS and infections (especially *giardiasis*) should be considered in the differential diagnosis of patients presenting with symptoms of MC.

Endoscopic evaluation to obtain colonic biopsies is the diagnostic method of choice. The colon typically appears normal but erythema and edema may be seen. The hallmark histologic feature for LC is intraepithelial lymphocytosis of at least 20 per 100 surface epithelial lymphocytes without a significantly thickened collagen band, whereas a thickened subepithelial collagen band of 10 μm or greater is pathognomonic for CC.

The goal of therapy is symptomatic improvement, because there is no increased risk of colon cancer in patients with MC, but the disease has an effect on the quality of life.

When managing patients with MC, it is important to review their medication list and discontinue the drugs that may have triggered the disorder if possible, based on chronologic relationship with the diarrhea onset.

**Lymphocytic colitis**

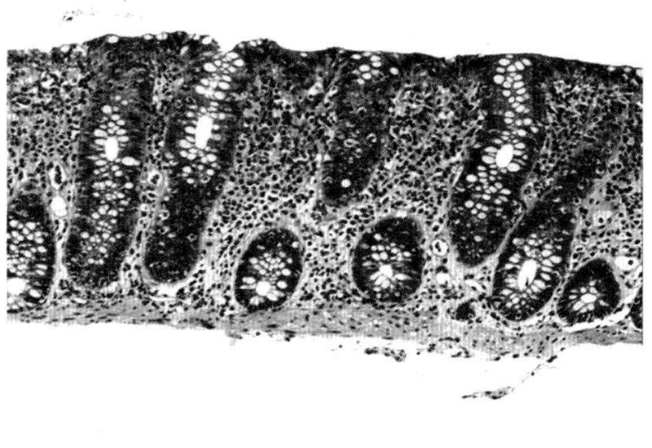

Low-power microphotograph of lymphocytic colitis that shows increased lymphocytic and round cell infiltration in the lamina propria. The crypts appear normal.

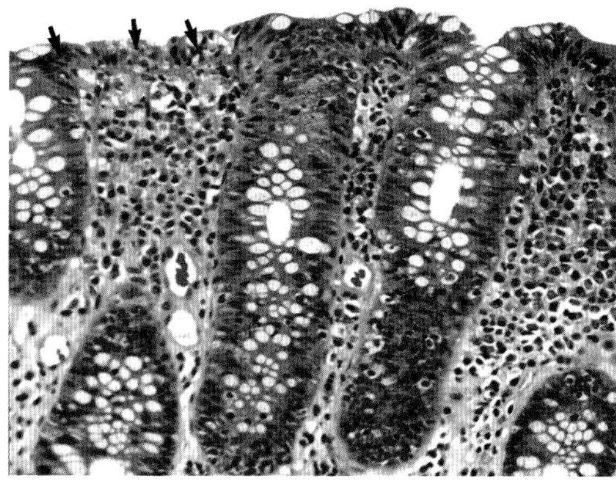

High-power microphotograph of lymphocytic colitis (same patient and biopsy as in figure at left). *Arrows* indicate the classic infiltrate of lymphocytes in the epithelium.

**Collagenous colitis**

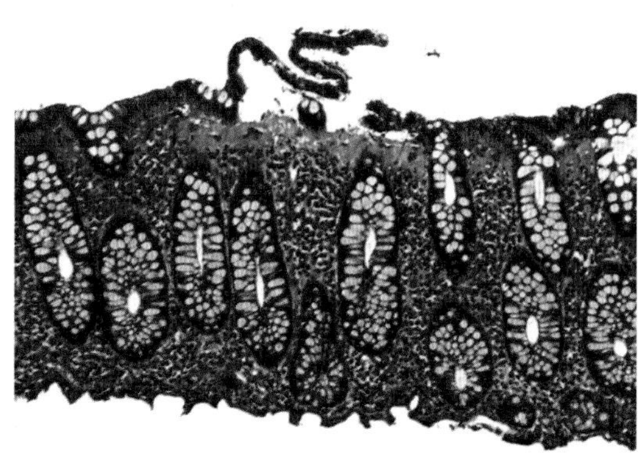

Colon biopsy specimen showing collagenous colitis (trichrome stain [blue]). Note the enlarged subepithelial collagen layer. *(Photomicrographs from Floch M. Netter's Gastroenterology. 2nd ed. Elsevier; 2009, courtesy Dr. Marie Robert.)*

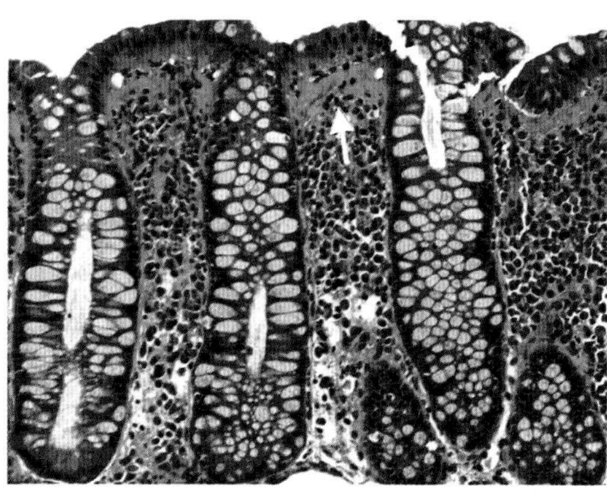

High-power microphotograph of collagenous colitis that shows an enlarged (pink) collagen layer and an increased lymphocytic infiltrate in the lamina propria. The *arrow* indicates a cellular element (fibroblast nucleus) entrapped in the enlarged collagen layer.

A trial of lactose-free diet and avoidance of excessive artificial sweeteners may be beneficial to exclude factors that can exacerbate diarrhea.

Antidiarrheal medicines can be used as the only therapy in patients with mild diarrhea or in combination with other therapies in more severe forms of the disease. In patients with moderate to severe symptoms or patients who have not been responsive to antidiarrheal medicines, budesonide, which is an oral steroid with low systemic bioavailability, is recommended. Initial therapy with budesonide is 9 mg daily for 6 to 8 weeks with a tapering regimen of 6 mg daily for 2 weeks followed by 3 mg daily for another 2 weeks. Longer duration may be needed in patients whose symptoms recur while tapering or after the therapy is stopped. Some patients may need maintenance therapy with low-dose budesonide. Unlike budesonide, there are limited data on the role of systemic steroids.

Bile salt–binding agents have a role in the management of MC and are more effective in individuals with bile acid malabsorption.

Mesalamine is currently not recommended for treatment of MC. The use of bismuth subsalicylate is also limited due to the risk of cumulative toxicity and limited data on its efficacy. Patients who do not respond to budesonide should be reevaluated for other etiologies for diarrhea. Treatment with immunomodulators (6-mercaptopurine, azathioprine), anti–tumor necrosis factor-α antibodies (infliximab, adalimumab), or alpha-4 beta-7 integrin inhibitor (vedolizumab) can be considered in refractory cases of MC.

Rarely, patients may need surgery as the last option if all medical therapies fail. Surgical therapy includes ileostomy, subtotal colectomy, and total proctocolectomy with ileal pouch–anal anastomosis.

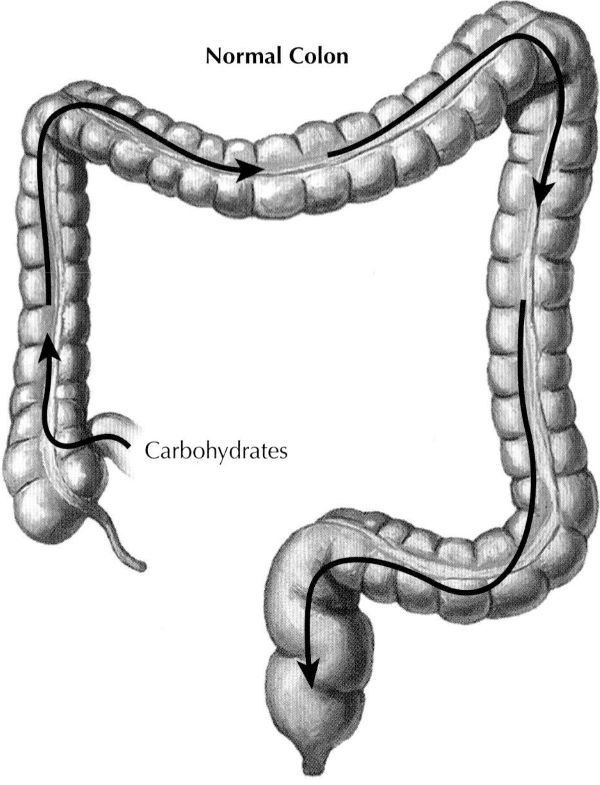


**Carbohydrates:**
- Metabolized by anaerobic metabolism
- Oxidized to short-chain fatty acids (butyrate, acetate, propionate) by colonocytes
- Serve as major fuel supply for mucosal cells
- Regulate transport of fluid and electrolytes
- Determine colonic motility and mucosal blood flow

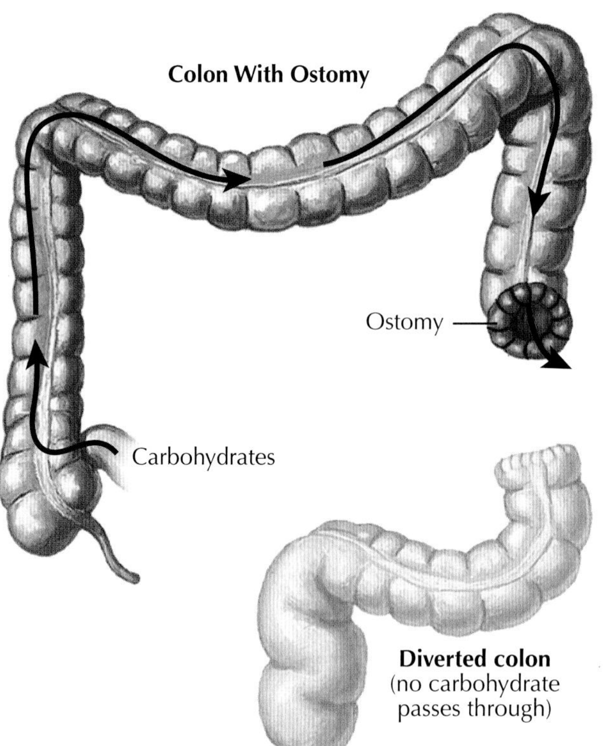


**Diverted colon:**
- Histologically difficult to distinguish from IBD, with cellular infiltrate throughout and hyperplasia of lymphatic follicles.
- Changes can be evident as early as a few months after surgery or much later and are seen histologically in 95%.
- 10% are symptomatic with rectal bleeding, tenesmus, pain, and discharge.

F. Netter M.D.

K. Marzen

## Diversion Colitis

Diversion colitis refers to nonspecific inflammation of the mucosa of a defunctionalized segment of colon. The cause is unclear, but it has been hypothesized that the disease may be due to bacterial overgrowth, the presence of harmful bacteria, nutritional deficiency, toxins, or a disturbance in the relationship between luminal bacteria and the mucosa. Some studies have shown that there is an increase in nitrate-reducing bacteria, which release nitric oxide into the colonic tissue; toxicity may result with higher concentrations of nitric oxide. Another proposed mechanism is ischemia due to a decrease in short-chain fatty acids.

Typically, diversion colitis is asymptomatic, but some studies have shown an incidence of 100% by 4 weeks to 3 years after surgery. When patients do present with symptoms, they may have lower abdominal discomfort, pelvic or anorectal pain, mucus discharge, tenesmus, bleeding, or low-grade fever. This presentation may be challenging to distinguish from that of IBD, so there may be difficulties in considering reanastomosis, particularly in patients with a history of IBD. There are isolated case reports of patients with severe symptoms requiring surgical intervention, but the incidence of significant symptoms was shown to be only 6% in a prospective study. Symptoms were shown to resolve once bowel continuity was restored.

The diagnosis is made clinically based on the history and symptoms, with some endoscopic and histologic findings to support it. On double-contrast barium enema, a variable distribution of lymphoid follicular hyperplasia may be noted, although this may also be present in IBD, colon carcinoma, or lymphoma. Mucosal friability and edema with aphthous ulcers and bleeding may be visible macroscopically on endoscopy. Diffuse granularity, mucous plugs, or erythema may be visible. Rectal volume has been shown to decrease by 35% at 1 month.

Symptoms have been successfully treated in a few studies with irrigation of the diverted segment with short-chain fatty acid enemas twice daily for 4 to 6 weeks. Others have shown a benefit of fiber, 5-aminosalicylic acid, and steroid enemas. When possible, restoration of continuity should be performed if other causes of inflammation are ruled out.

## Ischemic Colitis

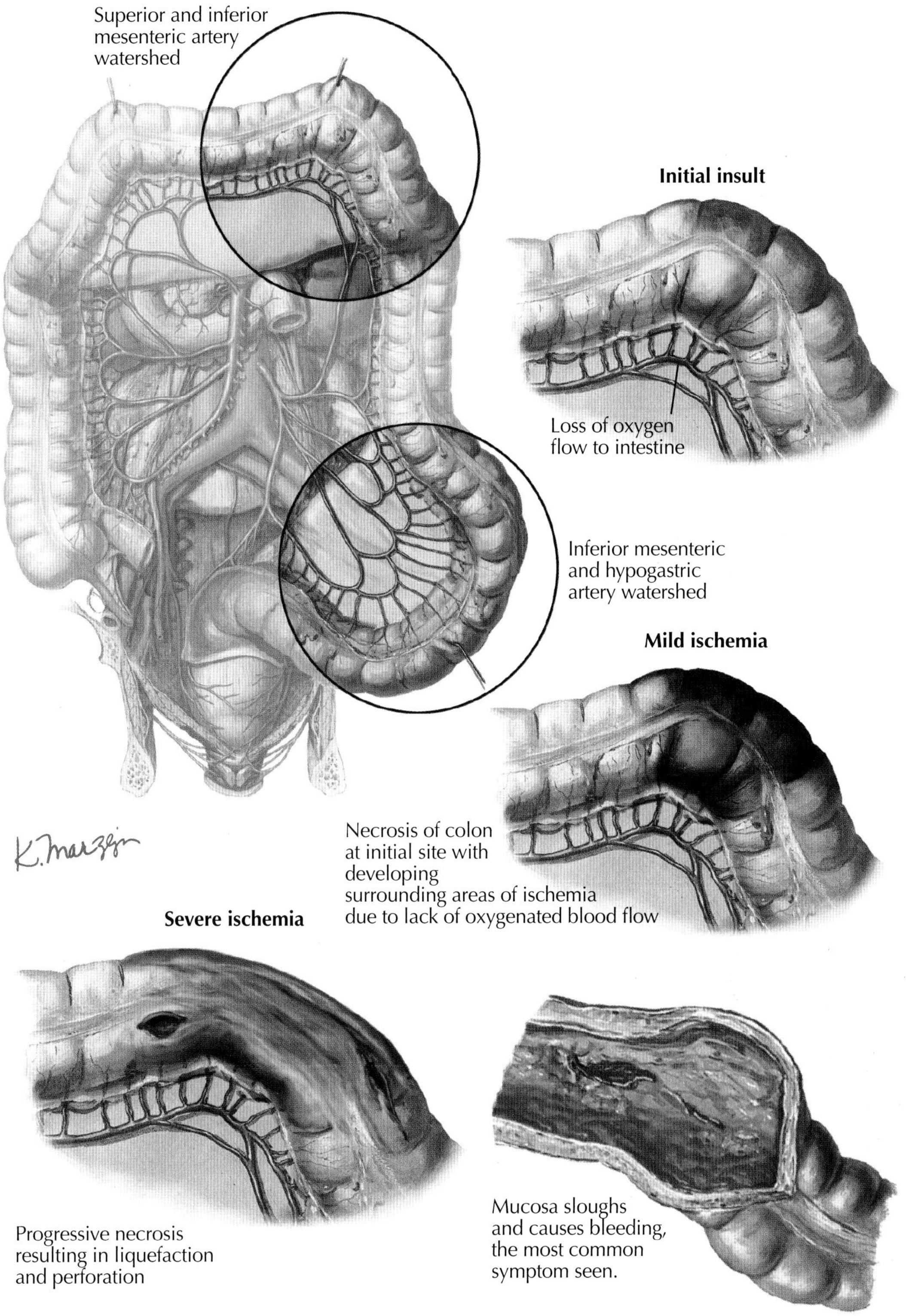

The blood supply of the colon includes the superior mesenteric artery, inferior mesenteric artery, and branches of the internal iliac arteries. Because of the redundant blood supply to the colon, the typical sites for ischemia are known as the "watershed" areas of the colon with singular or nonredundant supply, such as the splenic flexure and transverse colon. Although the mesenteric collateral circulation helps to promote redundancy, the artery of Drummond, running along the splenic flexure, serves as a conduit for communication of the superior and inferior mesenteric arteries. Up to 5% of the population has an underdeveloped or absent artery of Drummond, a condition that leads the splenic flexure to be a particularly susceptible area for ischemia. In contrast, the rectum has a rich blood supply from the mesenteric and iliac arteries, which renders it unlikely to succumb to ischemic injury.

Ischemic colitis is reported in 1 out of every 1000 to 2000 hospitalizations. The incidence of ischemic colitis increases with age and with comorbid risk factors of vascular disease. Approximately 90% of those who develop ischemic colitis are over 60 years of age. The most common triggers include hypotension related to sepsis, compromised left ventricular function, hypovolemia, vascular disease, and hemorrhage. A variety of medications can also result in a low-flow state and certain hypercoagulable states such as protein C deficiency, protein S deficiency, and antithrombin III deficiency, among other abnormalities. Strenuous exercise, including long-distance running, presumably from shunting of blood flow from the mesenteric vasculature to support muscle action is another cause. Finally, patients undergoing surgery, particularly cardiac surgery, are at increased risk.

Patients may present with abdominal pain, diarrhea, and/or tenderness on examination; bloody bowel movements are common, but rarely is massive bleeding a problem. Ischemic colitis is classified as either gangrenous (transient or chronic) or nongangrenous. Brandt and Boley have defined six types in a classification scheme as follows:

1. Reversible ischemic colonopathy
2. Transient ischemic colitis
3. Chronic ulcerative ischemic colitis
4. Ischemic colonic stricture
5. Colonic gangrene
6. Fulminant universal ischemic colitis

Laboratory markers of ischemia (e.g., lactate) are usually normal unless there is severe ischemia. Stool cultures for *Salmonella, Shigella, Campylobacter,* and *E. coli* O157:H7 should be obtained. The typical findings on radiography include bowel dilation, air-filled loops of bowel, and thumbprinting. Barium enema is another possible imaging method for diagnosis; however, it is contraindicated when there is suspicion of gangrene or perforation. CT scan may be the initial examination, yet there is no role for mesenteric biopsy unless there is a high suspicion of acute mesenteric ischemia with difficulty in distinguishing this disorder from ischemic colitis on presentation or when superior mesenteric artery occlusion may be considered with presentation of isolated involvement of the right colon.

Colonoscopy is the gold standard to visualize the mucosa, rule out other problems or causes of bleeding, and confirm the diagnosis. Findings on colonoscopy include a spectrum from petechial hemorrhages and edema to erythema or linear ulcerations or a dusky appearance with cyanosis as the disease severity advances. Chronic ischemia can result in strictures and fibrosis. Pathologic examination of biopsy specimens is nonspecific and may show crypt distortion, edema, ulceration, hemorrhage, thrombi, and/or necrosis.

The treatment is supportive, with fluid hydration, discontinuation of antihypertensive medications, bowel rest with nothing by mouth, oxygenation, and antibiotics. There is limited research on the indication for antibiotics. Approximately one-fifth of patients will develop peritonitis despite management and will require urgent surgery. Any necrotic segment of bowel should be resected. Judgment must be used as to whether an anastomosis is possible versus proximal ostomy creation.

Since COVID-19 was first identified in December 2019, reports have noted that up to 50% of patients had gastrointestinal symptoms upon presentation. Given the hypercoagulability associated with COVID-19 infection, some patients have been found to have ischemic colitis. Most cases have been noted to be limited to the left colon, although some were found to involve the right colon. Prompt recognition of this condition is important to facilitate appropriate treatment to attempt to limit mortality of this condition in these patients with already high morbidity and mortality rates.

Superior and inferior mesenteric artery watershed
Initial insult
Loss of oxygen flow to intestine
Inferior mesenteric and hypogastric artery watershed
Mild ischemia
Necrosis of colon at initial site with developing surrounding areas of ischemia due to lack of oxygenated blood flow
Severe ischemia
Progressive necrosis resulting in liquefaction and perforation
Mucosa sloughs and causes bleeding, the most common symptom seen.

**Environmental or ingested allergens**

Allergen

IgE

Granules

Mast cell

**Binding of allergen to surface IgE**

Allergen

**Degranulation of mast cells**

Release of histamine and leukotrienes

- Vasodilation
- Swelling/edema
- Itching
- Smooth muscle contraction
- Hypotension, shock

## ANGIOEDEMA

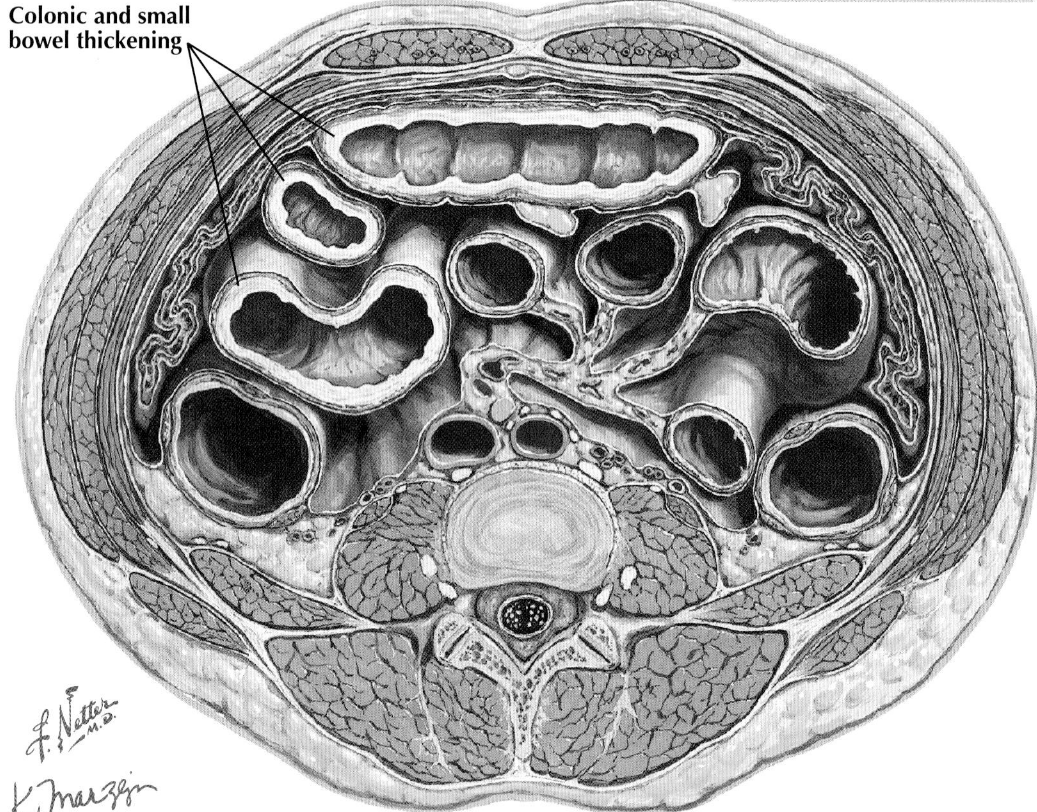


Angioedema is nonpitting edema that is localized and temporary. It can occur in any layer of skin or the walls of hollow viscera in the respiratory or GI tract. The presenting symptoms can range from life-threatening respiratory distress to abdominal pain with nausea and vomiting. Angioedema is classified based on etiologic findings. These classes include allergic angioedema, angiotensin-converting enzyme inhibitor–mediated angioedema, NSAID-mediated angioedema, hereditary angioedema, inherited angioedema with normal C1 esterase inhibitor, and angioedema with acquired C1 esterase inhibitor deficiency.

Angioedema results from a massive histamine release from mast cells or from increased accumulation of bradykinin due to increased production or decreased inactivation. Any allergen, ranging from food, to medication, to environmental causes, may cause allergic angioedema. Swelling can be associated with urticaria and pruritus. If allergens are ingested, they can cause abdominal pain and vomiting as well. Episodes typically resolve within 1 to 3 days after contact with the allergen. Angiotensin-converting enzyme inhibitor–induced angioedema occurs in 0.1% to 2.2% of patients taking these medications and typically develops within the first month of use, but the presentation can be delayed much longer. NSAID-induced angioedema has been reported in 0.1% to 0.3% of patients taking NSAIDs. The other types of angioedema are much more rare, and their pathophysiologic factors are not as well understood.

Diagnosis is difficult in these patients because they typically present to a specialist when symptoms have resolved. Patients with abdominal involvement may exhibit abdominal tenderness with or without rebound, with hypoactive or hyperactive bowel sounds, and, possibly, shifting dullness. CT scans may show edema of the intestines, with fluid accumulation in dilated bowel loops as well as ascites. Plain films may show signs of obstruction during an acute attack. Endoscopy can be useful in diagnosis, but care must be taken to observe for laryngeal swelling as well. Laboratory derangements, such as elevated serum tryptase and urine histamine levels, can detect IgE-mediated angioedema, and allergy testing can help identify the cause.

Abdominal symptoms may be related to other causes, and misdiagnosis may occur, particularly in the absence of associated skin or respiratory symptoms. Patients may undergo unnecessary surgery as a result, because the symptoms may be confused with those of ischemia or acute abdomen. Treatment varies by type but should begin with protecting the airway and giving fluid resuscitation. For allergic reactions, epinephrine and diphenhydramine will help reduce edema, and steroids may decrease the risk of relapse. If an inciting cause is identified, its avoidance is key to prophylaxis. Depending on the type, various new medications are available to treat acute attacks or prevent new ones. A multidisciplinary approach is necessary to evaluate and treat these patients successfully.

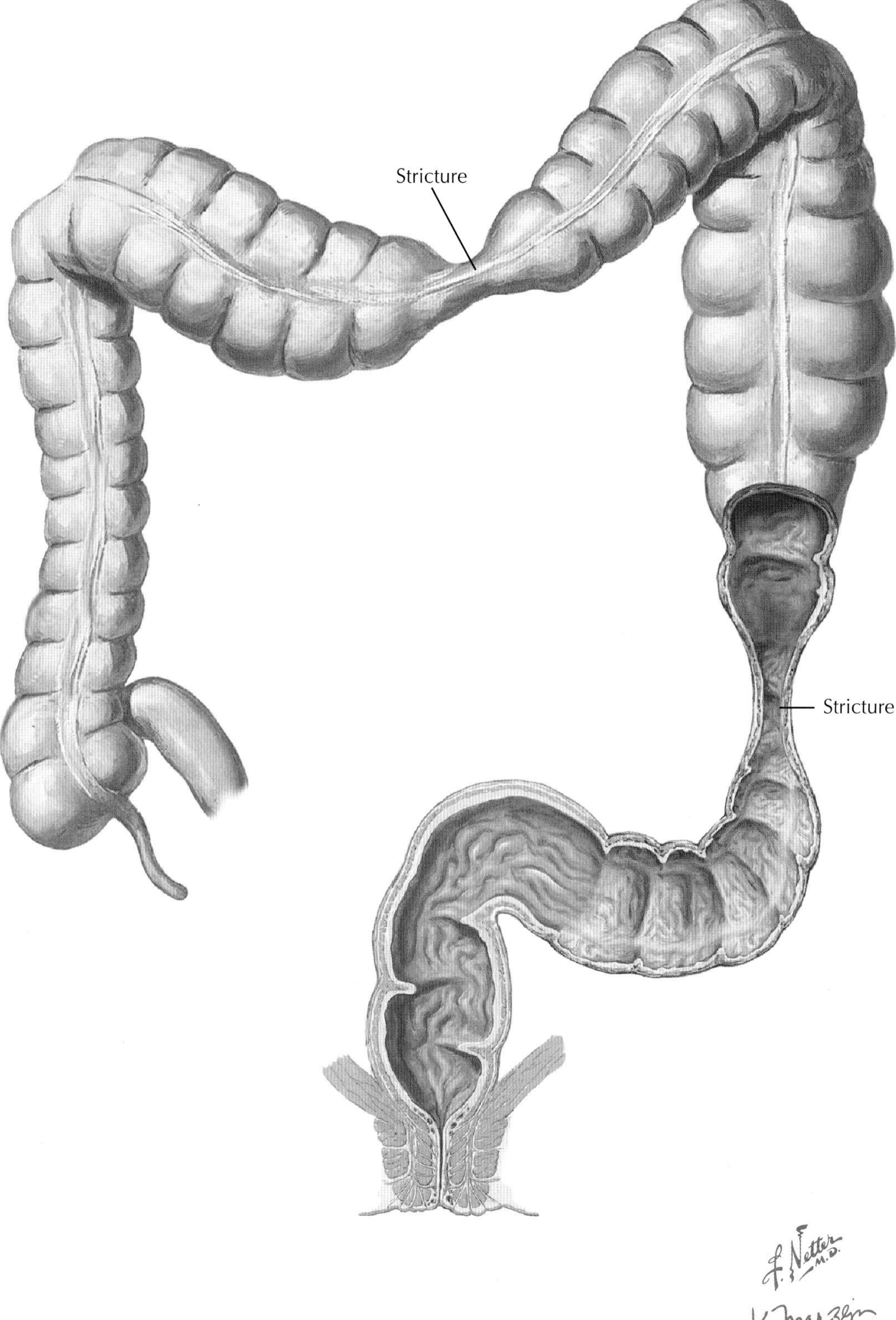


## Strictures From Use of Nonsteroidal Antiinflammatory Drugs

Colonic stricture resulting from use of NSAIDs, sometimes referred to as *colonic diaphragmatic disease,* is a rare entity. NSAIDs are widely used for pain relief, and given their availability over the counter, it is difficult to estimate the actual level of usage. Many side effects have been demonstrated, particularly in the upper GI tract, but given the availability of slow-release preparations, side effects have been seen in the lower GI tract as well.

Colonic strictures are most often seen in the seventh decade of life. Care must be taken to differentiate them from neoplasms, radiation enteritis, diverticulitis, IBD, ischemia, or other ulcerations. They appear to be more common in females, perhaps due in part to the fact that musculoskeletal diseases that require NSAID use are more common in females as well.

Presenting symptoms may vary from blood loss to mechanical obstruction. More typically, the presentation is chronic rather than acute due to obstruction or perforation. There may even be a delay in diagnosis for many years given the vague nature of symptoms. Literature review has shown that most reported cases occur in the ascending colon, probably because of the higher bioavailability of NSAIDs in this region. Diclofenac was the most common cause, likely due to widespread use. Variable lengths of use have been noted, with durations as short as 2 months leading to stricture formation. It is also unclear as to whether the route of administration is a factor, because strictures have been seen with local application of suppositories occurring in the rectum and in the ascending colon, implying some systemic response.

Colonoscopy is the most sensitive method for diagnosis and allows for direct visualization and biopsy. Radiologic contrast studies have lower sensitivity because lesions may not be large enough to be visible. Histologic study typically shows associated areas of ulceration and granulation, which may be attempts at healing with fibrosis.

Addition of misoprostol for a protective effect did not show any benefit in some studies. Sulfasalazine and metronidazole administration has shown some benefit, but discontinuation of NSAID use seems to be the most important treatment. Treatment with steroids and 5-aminosalicylic acid has shown some promise.

Because the strictures are irreversible, some intervention is required for treatment. Therapeutic endoscopy can be performed with dilation in certain cases. Surgical resection of the diseased colon with primary anastomosis should be considered as definitive treatment, but recurrence is common. Uncertainty remains as to whether there is a malignant progression; therefore regular follow-up is recommended.

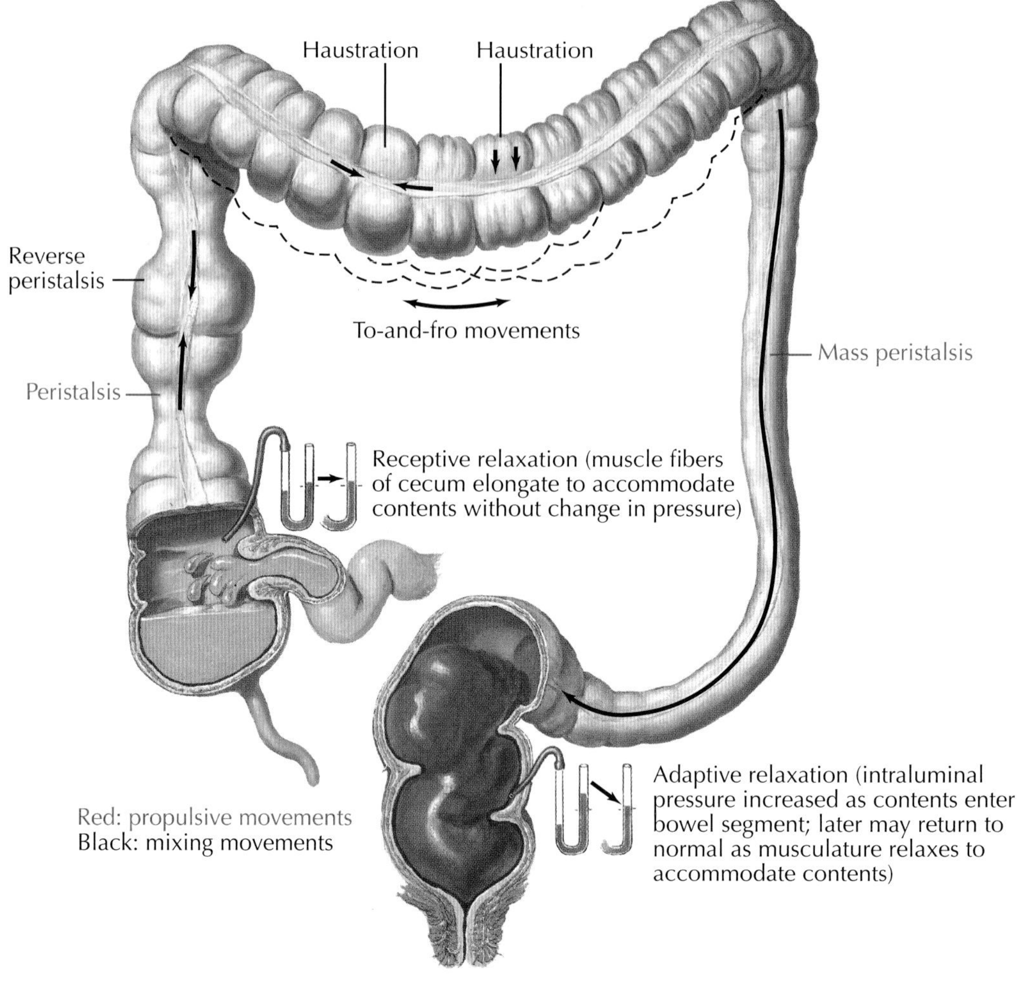


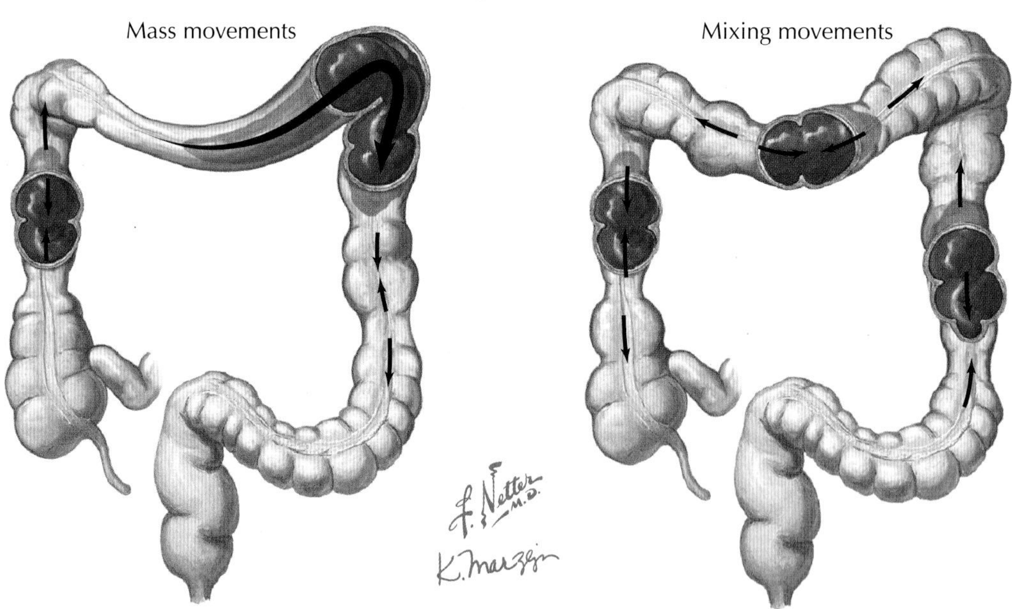


## MOTILITY OF LARGE INTESTINE

The large intestine's major functions are to absorb water and store and move feces into the rectum for future expulsion. The cecum and ascending colon carry out most of the absorption function, and the descending colon and sigmoid colon serve as the ultimate reservoir for the storage of feces. These functions are carried out in the setting of two main forms of colonic motor activity: the to-and-fro segmental contractions and the mass movements, which are facilitated by high-amplitude peristaltic contractions (HAPCs).

Approximately 5 gallons of fluid enters the large intestine daily to be absorbed. This function is facilitated by nonperistaltic and nonsynchronized contractions leading to the to-and-fro mixing without forward propulsion. The mixing movements improve nutrient absorption in certain segments. Contraction of the longitudinal muscular bands known as *taenia coli* shorten the bowel, forming pleats or haustrations. These structures allow chyme to be retained so there is enough time to absorb water and other nutrients. This function is aided by contractions of circular muscles that create small indentations within the haustra to stop material from escaping. As a result of this motility pattern, residue remains in the colon for approximately 30 hours, and bacteria inhabiting the large intestine can further break down this material.

The second form of motility pattern in the colon is that of HAPCs, which occur six to eight times daily in most individuals. These contractions occur spontaneously but may be in response to pharmacologic agents or to distension of the colon. HAPCs begin in the proximal colon and usually progress only to the midcolon, where fewer than 5% reach the rectum. These mass movements can transfer colonic contents toward the rectum in preparation for evacuation. Mass movements are a two-step process that begins with the colon creating a constrictive ring and then contracting in a squeezing motion toward the rectum. HAPCs can be reduced in slow-transit constipation and appear to be increased in IBS with diarrhea.

Conditions that distend the colon or irritate the mucosa, such as MC, may promote increased motor activity in the colon. The gastrocolic and duodenocolic reflexes are physiologic reflexes made in response to stretching or distension of the stomach or duodenum, resulting in increased motility of the colon and the urge to defecate.

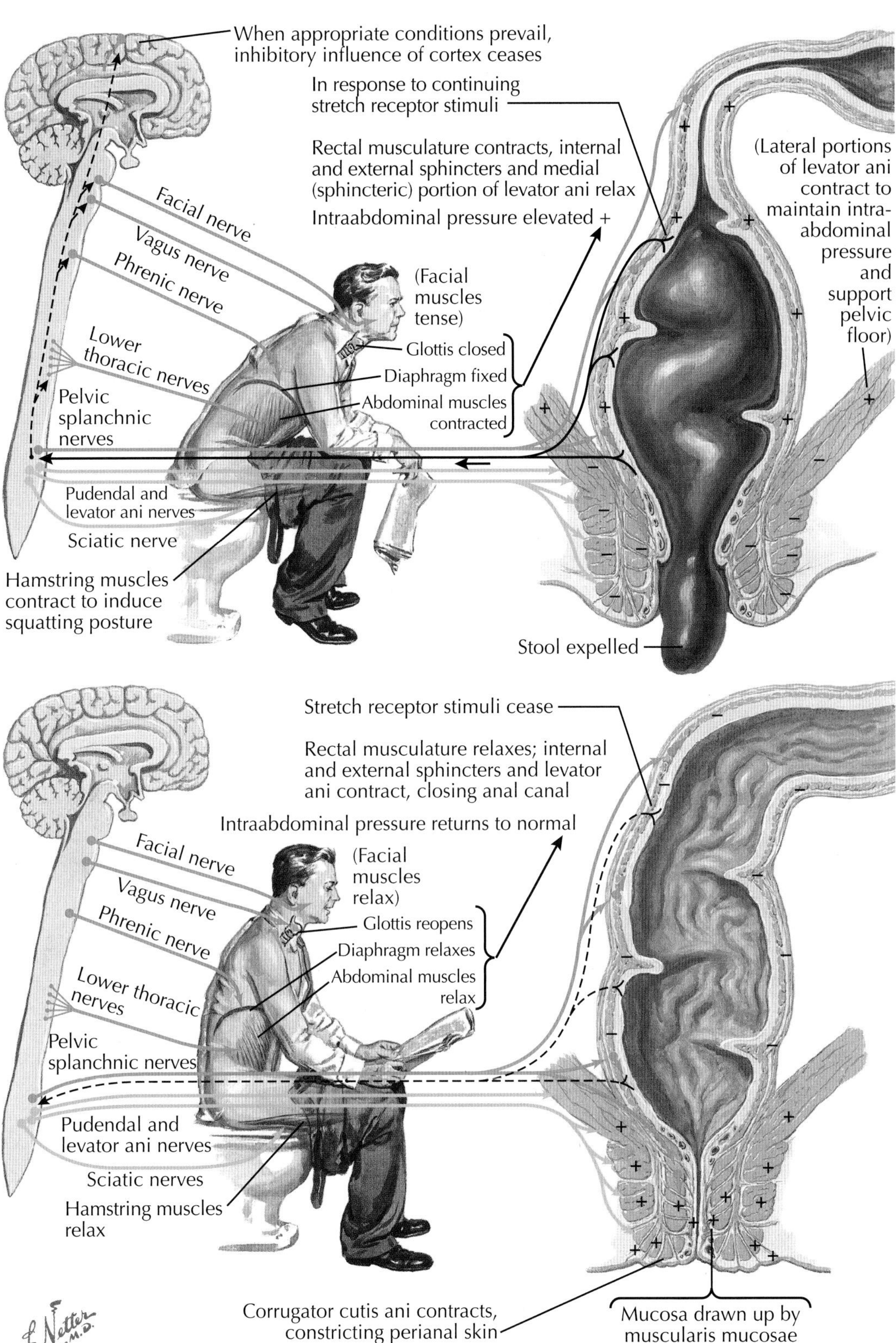


## NORMAL DEFECATION

Physiologic defecation is the step in which, after digestion and absorption, waste is expelled from the body as feces. Mass peristalsis moves feces from the right to left colon, where it eventually accumulates in the rectum. Rectal pressures at about 18 mm Hg lead to the release of the hormones vasoactive intestinal peptide and nitric oxide from stretch receptors of the pelvic splanchnic nerves. These hormones relax the internal anal sphincter and contract the external anal sphincter, preventing incontinence. At this point, the body is aware of the material in the rectum and can determine whether the urge is for flatus or solid or liquid feces. This phenomenon is known as *rectal sampling*. In healthy individuals, continence allows one to delay defecation until deemed appropriate as long as the pressure in the rectum does not exceed approximately 55 mm Hg.

Once the person chooses to defecate, the next step is the actual expulsion of waste. A squatting position can allow for an improved angle for fecal expulsion and the optimal generation of abdominal pressure during defecation. Another essential step is the relaxation of the puborectalis muscle, allowing for the rectoanal angle to be reduced from its resting state of 90 degrees. Once in the proper position, the person can voluntarily relax the external sphincter, controlled by the pudendal and levator ani nerves, to expel feces. Expulsion is further enhanced with contraction of the abdominal, diaphragmatic, and levator ani muscles. The body can also increase pressure via the Valsalva maneuver. This can be performed by closing one's mouth and attempting exhalation, which generates extra pressure for defecation. The body goes through similar motions during expulsion of flatus; however, the puborectalis muscle stays contracted. This allows one to expel gas without the loss of feces.

The frequency of what is accepted as normal defecation varies extensively. Most people get the urge to defecate daily, but others may have more than one daily bowel movement and some may have bowel movements less frequently, at only three times per week.

## 3D High-Resolution Anorectal Manometry With Balloon Expulsion Testing

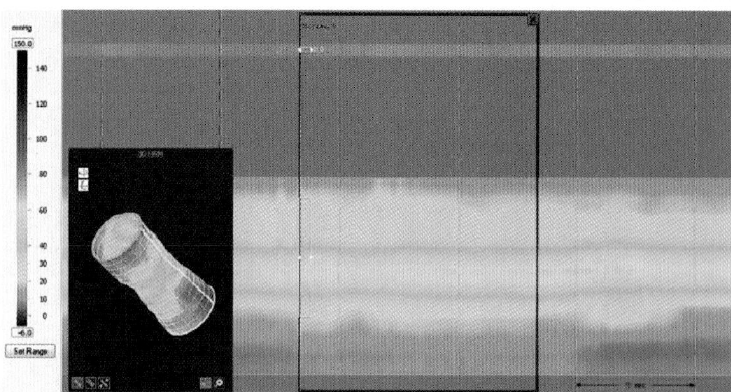
High-resolution anorectal manometry image of baseline resting pressures

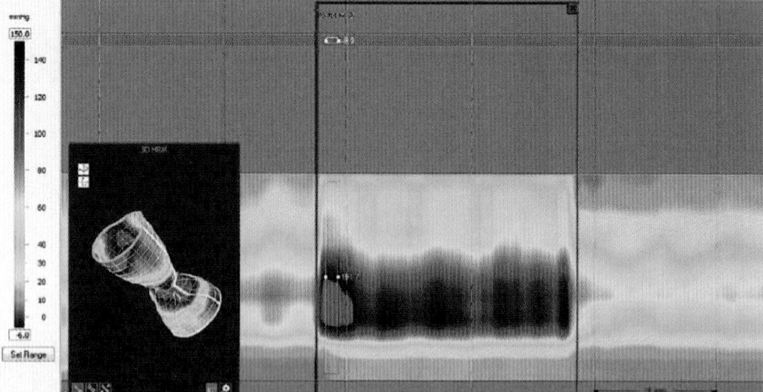
High-resolution anorectal manometry image during squeeze effort

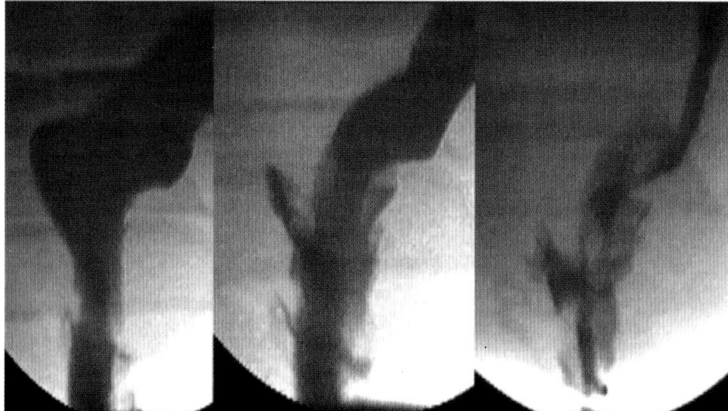
Defecogram showing progression of internal intussusception. *(From Fry RD, Mahmoud NN, Maron DJ, Bleier JIS. Colon and rectum. In: Townsend CM, ed. Sabiston Textbook of Surgery. 19th ed. Elsevier; 2012.)*

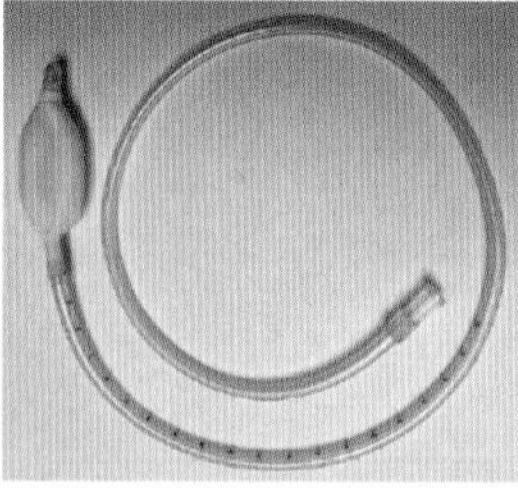
Balloon used for expulsion testing

| Test | Description | Used in the evaluation of |
|---|---|---|
| **Anorectal manometry** | Catheter with balloon or sensors placed in the rectum and measures physiologic parameters | Constipation, dyssynergic defecation, and fecal incontinence<br>Absence of rectoanal inhibitory reflex (RAIR) is seen in Hirschsprung disease |
| **Anal ultrasonography** | Small probe placed in anal canal to evaluate integrity of musculature | Constipation, dyssynergic defecation, and fecal incontinence |
| **Balloon expulsion study** | Patient places a balloon into the rectum and is asked to push it out | Pelvic floor dysfunction |
| **Barium enema** | Barium is inserted in the rectum under the visualization of fluoroscopy | Obstruction, colon cancer screening, incomplete colonoscopy, intussusception, volvulus, pseudoobstruction |
| **Colon transit study** | Patient swallows radiopaque capsules/markers with subsequent abdominal x-ray(s) | Colonic transit time |
| **Defecating proctography** | Patient is given a contrast-based enema and asked to defecate under fluoroscopic visualization | Obstructive defecation, fecal incontinence, rectal prolapse, dyssynergic defecation, rectocele or other structural abnormalities |
| **Electromyography** | Probes are placed along the anal sphincter that can directly measure myoelectric activity | Disorders of the anal sphincter and may be used in biofeedback therapy |
| **Pudendal nerve conduction study** | Electrode stimulates the nerve during a rectal examination to evaluate pudendal nerve terminal latency | Fecal incontinence due to pudendal neuropathy |
| **Scintigraphic studies** | Patient ingests a radiolabeled meal | More commonly used to evaluate disorders of gastric emptying. It can also be used to evaluate bile flow and small and large intestine transit times. |
| **Wireless capsule motility study** | Orally ingested, collects data and profiles of pH and temperature, and calculates transit times | Evaluation of transit times for the stomach, small bowel, and colon |

## Motility Testing

Motility problems with the colon can be associated with either acceleration (e.g., dumping syndrome) or slowing (e.g., gastroparesis, colonic inertia, or even retrograde movement, as in vomiting). The most common presenting symptoms for colonic dysmotility are nonspecific and may include constipation, pain, difficulty in defecating, or incontinence. In many cases, colonic motility testing is sought out when a practitioner suspects a certain disorder such as Hirschsprung disease, wants to monitor complications of an illness such as scleroderma, or seeks to further characterize chronic constipation, diarrhea, or malabsorption that has yet to be explained. The most common tests for the colon are scintigraphy, wireless motility capsules, and radiopaque marker studies.

Motility disorders of the rectum can be split into functional causes (e.g., fecal impaction, conditions like Alzheimer disease), those with increased or decreased rectal tone or those with sensory loss such as spinal cord injury, diabetic neuropathy, or pudendal nerve injury. In most cases, patients are identified to need anal motility studies based on history. Examples of patients who may benefit from motility testing are those with a history of spinal cord injury or malformations, multiple sclerosis, dementia, obstetric or other traumatic experiences, diabetic neuropathy, pudendal nerve damage, or other conditions such as pelvic floor dyssynergia. Anorectal manometry is the best test to evaluate fecal incontinence and suspected constipation from increased rectal tone. This form of testing is the treatment of choice as a mechanism of biofeedback therapy in dyssynergic defecation. Other motility tests for the rectum include ultrasonography, balloon expulsion, defecating proctography, MR defecography, electromyography, and pudendal nerve conduction studies.

# Pathophysiology of Defecation: Factors Affecting Normal Defecation

Dysfunctional defecation is a common problem, usually resulting from issues with continence, urgency, frequency, or the loss of discriminatory power of the colon. Common causes that lead to dysfunction of defecation include diet, diarrhea or constipation, laxative or other medication use, psychological factors, and neuromuscular problems. The following section provides a brief overview of conditions that may lead to dysfunctional defecation.

## NEUROLOGIC DISORDERS

Acute spinal cord injuries are defined as damage to the spinal cord that has occurred over the last 21 days. Overall, these injuries usually lead to delayed transit times and fecal incontinence. Fortunately, more than half of patients with spinal cord injuries will show some improvement in continence, yet it is nearly impossible to predict which patients will regain normal function. The effects of spinal cord lesions are best understood when they are split into acute and chronic issues affecting both colonic motility and defecation.

In acute spinal cord injuries, one can expect to find prolonged transit times of the entire GI tract, resulting in constipation, and many patients will also experience fecal incontinence. Chronic injuries, including conus medullaris and cauda equina lesions, continue to show increased colonic transit time along the transverse and descending colon; lesions of the sacral nerves appear to slow movement along the sigmoid colon. Lesions along the lumbar, thoracic, and cervical spine have shown mixed results, with some studies supporting slower transit times and others showing no changes compared with the general population. It is well accepted that lesions of the sympathetic nervous system are not associated with a change in colonic motility. Patients with long-standing spinal cord injuries will continue to have poor motility and function with constipation but may also develop diverticular disease, hemorrhoids, and volvulus.

Patients show no change in rectal tone with acute spinal cord injury but are no longer able to consciously contract the external anal sphincter. Chronic spinal cord injuries appear to greatly affect rectal tone; cauda equina lesions are associated with decreased tone, and supraconal injuries tend to increase both rectal tone and contractions. This makes supraconal lesions especially problematic and can lead to issues with expelling feces from the rectum. Many patients with this problem must undergo manual removal of feces for proper evacuation. Another problem that patients with supraconal spinal cord injury face is decreased sphincter tone. This becomes a problem with patients who are treated with too much fiber, resulting in frequent episodes of incontinence.

## TRAUMA

The other major condition that causes incontinence is damage to the muscles of the peritoneum from either physical trauma or damage to the nerve supply to that area. Third- and fourth-degree vaginal tears during birth can lead to damage of the external anal sphincter and puborectalis muscles, resulting in fecal incontinence. Painful lesions of the anal canal, such as ulcers, fissures, and thrombosed hemorrhoidal veins, impede defecation by exciting spasm of the sphincters and voluntary suppression to avoid pain.

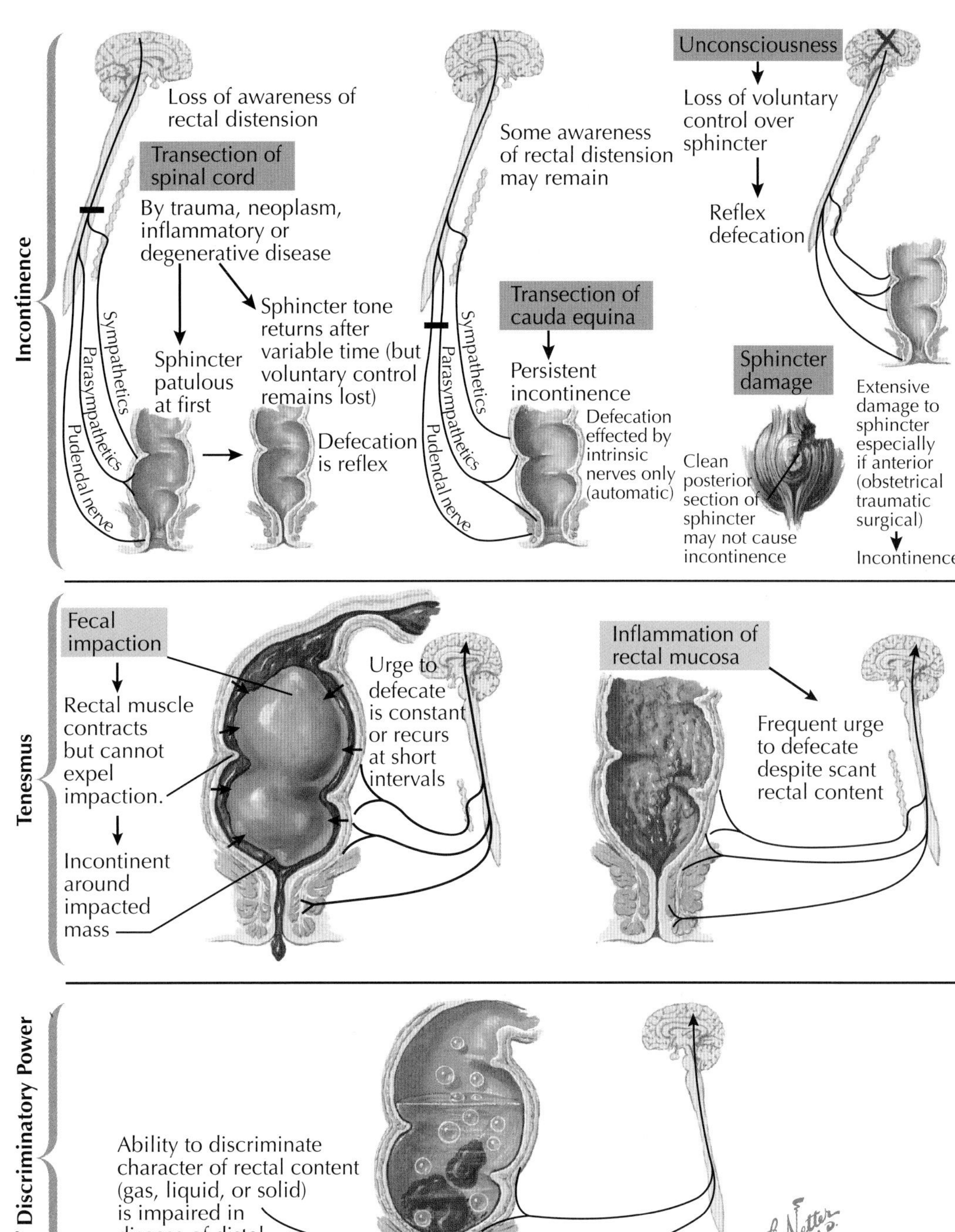


## MEGARECTUM

The presence of excretory material in the rectum is not in itself sufficient to excite the urge to defecate. The content must be sufficiently large to exceed the threshold of the distension stimulus characteristic for the individual. In many patients with regular bowel habits, digital examination may reveal a considerable mass of stool of varying consistency. The accumulation of a large amount of stool in a greatly dilated rectum occurs frequently with older age groups. This finding is suggestive of a loss of tonicity of the rectal musculature and high compliance. This condition, known as *megarectum* or *terminal reservoir syndrome,* may be due to a long-standing habit of ignoring or suppressing the urge to defecate, absence of sensation, or degeneration of nerve pathways concerned with defecation.

## MISCELLANEOUS FACTORS ASSOCIATED WITH DEFECATORY DYSFUNCTION

Diet is one of the major contributors for constipation or diarrhea. Medications such as iron or opioids are also notorious for causing chronic constipation, and laxatives and other medications such as erythromycin may cause diarrhea. *Tenesmus* is the recurrent or persistent urge to defecate, even after complete evacuation, and may represent a disorder of the rectum. This condition is usually exacerbated by rock-like stool that does not allow for the proper passage through the sphincters. This may be alleviated by rectal infusions of oil to render the stool more slippery, by surface-acting agents such as dioctyl sodium sulfosuccinate, or by digital evacuation. The constant urge to defecate in the absence of appreciable content in the rectum may be caused by external compression of the rectum, by intrinsic neoplasms, and, particularly, by inflammation of the rectal mucosa.

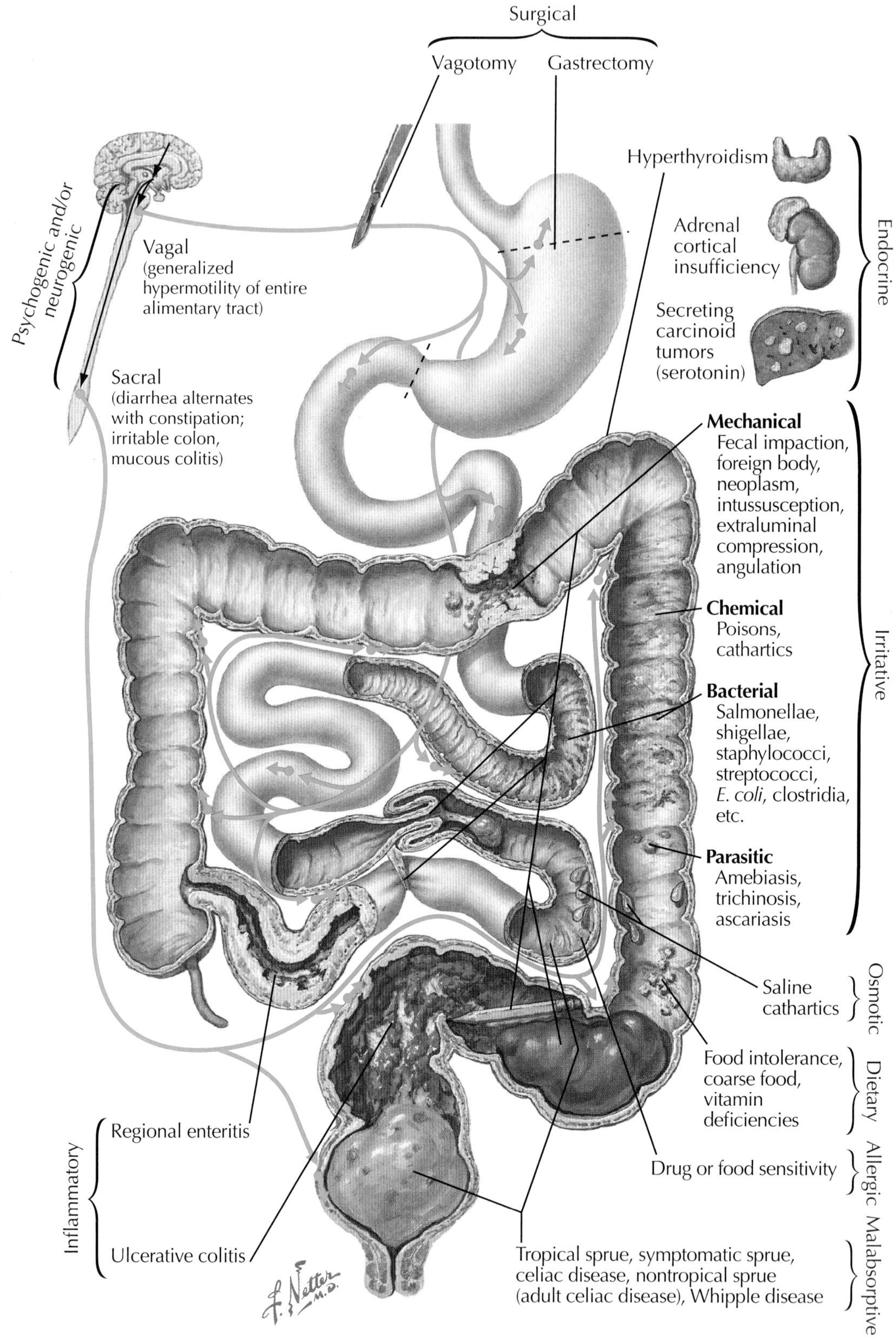

## DIARRHEA

The World Health Organization lists diarrheal diseases as the seventh leading cause of death and the leading cause of malnutrition for children younger than 5 years. Unfortunately, 760,000 children in this age group die each year from infectious causes of diarrhea that could be prevented with improved public health measures such as clean water, proper hygiene, and adequate hospital care.

Diarrhea is defined as three or more loose or watery stools in a 24-hour period and is usually subdivided further based on length of illness. An acute episode of diarrheal illness lasts less than 14 days, chronic diarrhea lasts at least 30 days, and persistent diarrhea has a duration between those of the other two forms. The most common cause of acute diarrhea is infection, with the most likely pathogen being a viral entity such as rotavirus or norovirus. Most cases of infectious diarrhea are clinically indistinguishable from one another and resolve spontaneously without medical intervention. As a practitioner, one should inquire about recent travel, diet, history of contact with another sick person, or antibiotic use to rule out food poisoning and other causes of infectious diarrhea. Patients who present with hypovolemia, bloody diarrhea, six or more stools in a day, and abdominal pain lasting for 1 week or patients who are either over the age of 65 years or immunocompromised should warrant further workup. A more detailed explanation of infectious diarrhea is described in its own section.

Chronic diarrhea is typically noninfectious and is separated into three broad categories based on the consistency of the stool as watery, fatty, or inflammatory. These three categories are nonexclusive and have considerable overlap with one another. Watery diarrhea can be further subdivided based on results from a fecal osmotic gap as an osmotic disorder (>125 mOsm/kg), secretory disorder (<50 mOsm/kg), or motility disorder (50–125 mOsm/kg). Osmotic diarrhea results in poor absorption of nutrients, leading to a solvent drag into the intestinal lumen. Common causes of osmotic diarrhea are laxative abuse or malabsorption disorders such as lactose intolerance or celiac disease. On the other hand, secretory diarrhea results from either active secretion or poor absorption of nutrients in the intestinal lumen. Causes of secretory diarrhea include endotoxins from bacteria such as *Vibrio cholerae,* endocrine problems, neuroendocrine disorders such as carcinoid tumor, or conditions affecting absorption such as postsurgical resection and colitis. Finally, motility disorders are those of hypermobility, such as irritable bowel syndrome–diarrhea predominant type (IBS-D) or others seen predominantly in children such as intussusception. Patients with IBS-D usually do not have symptoms at night, and their symptoms resolve with fasting.

Patients who present with fatty diarrhea may report foul-smelling stool, steatorrhea, or a film left in the toilet after defecation. Fatty diarrhea can result from either malabsorption or incomplete digestion. The differential diagnosis for disorders of malabsorption is extensive and can result from disorders of poor absorption such as celiac disease, medications, infections such as tropical sprue or Whipple disease, or even bacterial overgrowth. On the other hand, incomplete digestion may occur as a result of disorders of the pancreas, liver, or biliary system. Inflammatory diarrheal disorders can result from infectious agents, inflammatory bowel disease, or even malignant disease. This form of diarrhea usually is accompanied by leukocytosis, with bowel movements that are characterized as bloody with pus.

## Overview of Constipation

Constipation is the third most common gastrointestinal complaint in the United States, leading to 2.5 million ambulatory visits and 92,000 hospitalizations annually. The US healthcare system spends nearly 235 million dollars in the inpatient and ambulatory setting to treat constipation, along with hundreds of millions that are spent annually on over-the-counter laxatives for self-treatment. Constipation is a symptom-based diagnosis often defined as less than three bowel movements in a week. Patients more commonly define constipation related to symptoms such as difficulty defecating, incomplete evacuation, discomfort, pain, hard stools, or excessive straining. In the absence of alarm signs and symptoms, the workup can be limited once medications affecting bowel habits have been adjusted and management can be pursued. Patients most likely to report being constipated include those who are non-White, female, low-socioeconomic-status, and elderly.

Constipation is classified as being primary or secondary in origin. Practitioners should first try to identify an external or secondary cause of constipation that can explain a patient's current symptoms. Secondary constipation can be broadly organized into six categories: dietary and lifestyle options, medications, structural, neurogenic, metabolic, or other unclassified causes. Common unclassified causes of secondary constipation are a low-fiber diet, poor fluid intake in those who are dehydrated, inadequate time spent attempting defecation, lack of exercise, and depression. If there are no obvious secondary causes, the next step is to assess for primary causes of constipation such as functional constipation, IBS-C, slow-transit constipation, and pelvic floor dysfunction, which are all discussed in detail in later sections.

Workups for constipation should start with asking a patient about diet, exercise habits, and daily bathroom routine. Clinicians should always ask about new medications and alternative over-the-counter therapies the patient might be taking to help explain the symptoms. Another important consideration is to look for alarm symptoms such as unexplained gastrointestinal bleeding, unexplained weight loss, symptoms of colonic obstruction, or sudden bowel habit changes that could suggest malignancy. Laboratory tests such as a comprehensive metabolic panel or a thyroid panel can be ordered to rule out metabolic and endocrine causes when indicated. The physical examination should be focused and include a digital rectal examination to rule out gastrointestinal bleeding, stool impaction, or structural causes of constipation. Tests for colonic transit are reserved for patients who do not have pelvic floor dysfunction or defecatory dysfunction that has not responded to pelvic floor retraining.

Treatment for constipation is dependent on the root cause. One must first treat any underlying disease causing the constipation, such as giving thyroxin to a patient with hypothyroidism or removing an adjunct therapy.

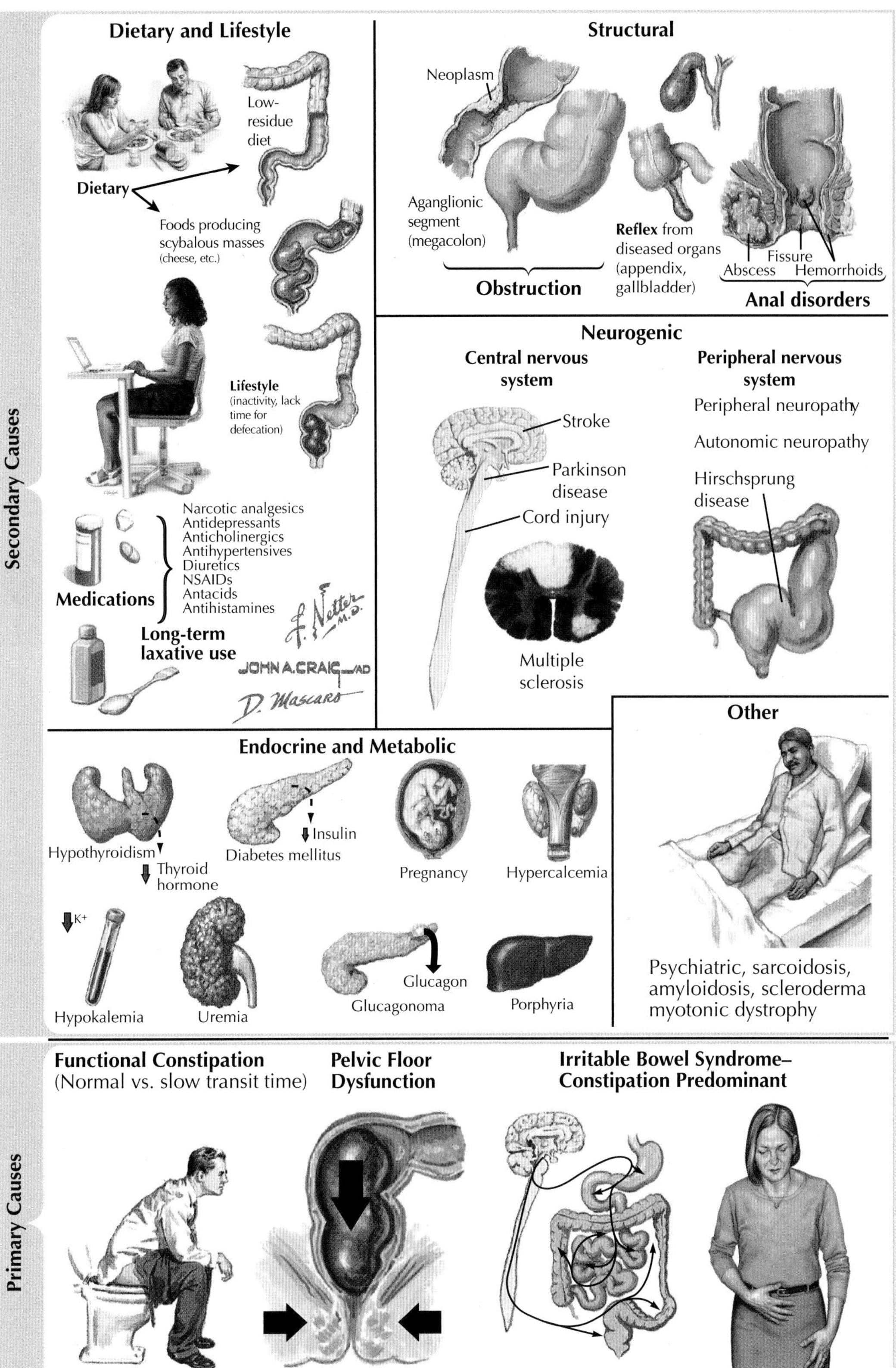


Less complicated causes of constipation are managed by encouraging a diet with 20 to 25 g of fiber daily and explaining behavioral modifications such as encouraging more time for toileting. Pharmacologic therapy, such as bulking agents, osmotic laxatives, stimulants, surfactants, and prokinetic drugs, should only be introduced if behavioral modifications fail. Biofeedback modification has shown success in selected pediatric patients and for adults with some neurogenic causes of constipation and those with dyssynergic defecation. Botulinum toxin has shown some success in those diagnosed with pelvic floor dysfunction. Surgery is rarely needed and is reserved for conditions such as Hirschsprung disease, malignant disease, fissures, and structural causes.

## FUNCTIONAL CONSTIPATION

Functional constipation (FC) is a cause of primary constipation as defined by the Rome IV criteria illustrated in Plate 3.84. FC is further subdivided by how long it takes food to go through the alimentary canal. The two classifications are normal-transit and slow-transit constipation. The most popular method to determine a transit time is a colon marker study. In this method, a patient is asked to swallow one or more capsules filled with radiopaque rings or markers and is then scheduled for an abdominal radiograph to determine what percentage of the markers remain. There are several different protocols for this study reported in the literature, but one suggests a diagnosis of slow-transit constipation when 20% or more of the markers are still present at 5 days. Other common modalities to measure transit time include scintigraphy and other capsule studies. It should be noted that the Bristol stool scale seems to correlate with transit where types 1 and 2 stool indicate slow transit (82% sensitivity) and types 6 and 7 best correlate with fast transit. FC can also occur in conjunction with pelvic floor disorders. It is important to note that IBS-C and FC are distinct diagnoses that present very similarly, except that IBS-C must include abdominal pain or discomfort as the prominent complaint.

Normal-transit constipation is the most common form of FC seen in the ambulatory setting. This condition has an increased incidence of associated depression compared with other forms of constipation. Although the transit time in the colon is not abnormal, patients will perceive being constipated due to issues with straining, decreased frequency, size of bowel movements, or hard stool. On the other hand, slow-transit constipation is the least common form of chronic constipation and can broadly be described as a pathologic condition resulting in ineffective propulsion of food contents through the GI tract. Some possible causes of ineffective propulsion are the loss of the interstitial cells of Cajal seen with increased age, decreased frequency and strength of colonic contractions, decreased morning colonic response, and loss of enteric or cholinergic neurons. There may be a subset of patients who present with idiopathic colonic inertia or who may experience postinfectious alteration of the motility of the colon and/or other parts of the GI tract.

Practitioners should first rule out secondary causes for all patients presenting with a new report of constipation and treat accordingly. If the practitioner can find no obvious secondary cause, primary forms of constipation such as FC, IBS-C, and pelvic floor dysfunction must be considered, with initial therapy targeted toward lifestyle modifications to improve defecation. A diagnosis of FC can be made once other causes of primary constipation have been considered. For patients refractory to empirical therapy, newer algorithms suggest that use of testing to determine transit times be pursued only after a defecatory disorder has been ruled out.

**Causes of slow-transit constipation**

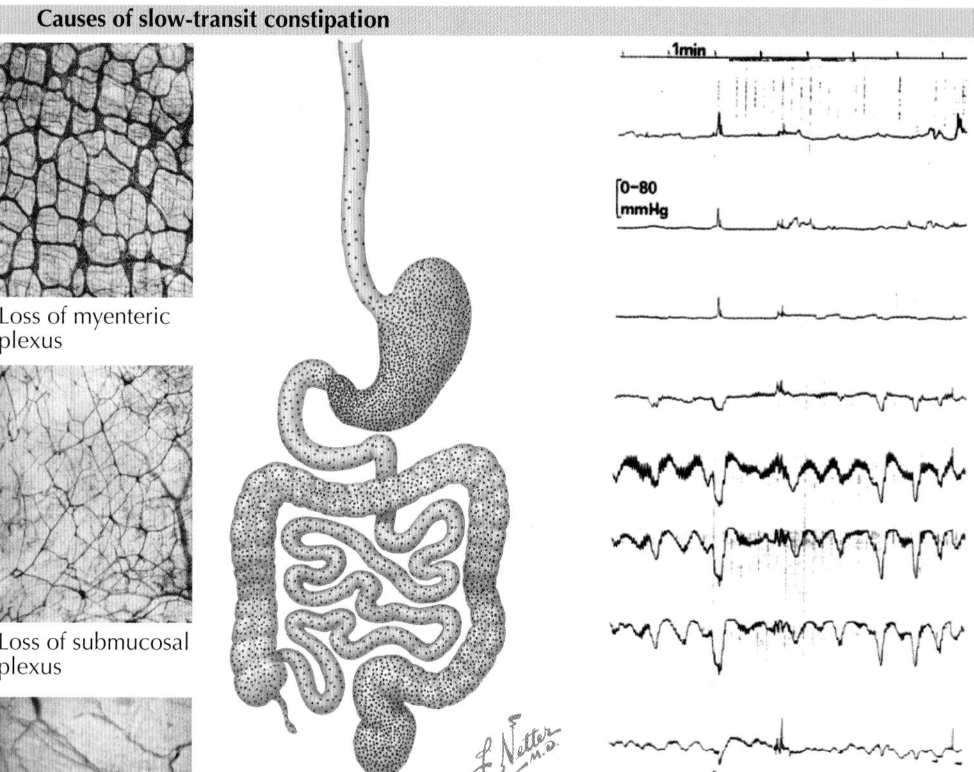


Loss of interstitial cells of Cajal with age

Relative concentration of ganglion cells in myenteric (Auerbach) plexus and in submucous (Meissner) plexus in various parts of alimentary tract (myenteric plexus cells represented by maroon, submucous by blue dots)

Low-amplitude propagated contractions (LAPC) decrease in frequency or strength of contractions.
*From Bassotti G, Iantorno G, Fiorella S, et al. Colonic motility in man: features in normal subjects and in patients with chronic idiopathic constipation. Am J. Gastoenterol. 1999;94(7).*

**Bristol stool form scale**

|  |  |
|---|---|
| Type 1 | Separate hard lumps, like nuts (hard to pass) |
| Type 2 | Sausage-shaped but lumpy |
| Type 3 | Like a sausage but with cracks on its surface |
| Type 4 | Like a sausage or snake, smooth and soft |
| Type 5 | Soft blobs with clear-cut edges (passed easily) |
| Type 6 | Fluffy pieces with ragged edges, a mushy stool |
| Type 7 | Watery, no solid pieces Entirely liquid |

*Bristol Stool Form Scale created by Heaton and Lewis at the University of Bristol. Originally published in Scand J Gastroenterol. 1997;32(9):920–924.*

After the exclusion of secondary causes that can affect motility, the first-line therapy for all patients with FC should be patient education, with emphasis on a healthy diet and better bowel habits, such as attempting defecation after meals. Patients with normal-transit constipation should be encouraged to eat a diet consisting of 20 to 25 g of fiber daily. Evidence shows that slow-transit constipation may become worse with increased fiber intake. Bulking laxatives are considered first-line therapy when increased fiber fails, but stimulant laxatives may have more success in patients with the slow-transit subtype. Medications with novel mechanisms targeting motility at the cellular level may be indicated. Finally, surgery is rarely indicated and reserved only for severe cases of slow-transit constipation.

**Biopsychosocial model for irritable bowel syndrome**

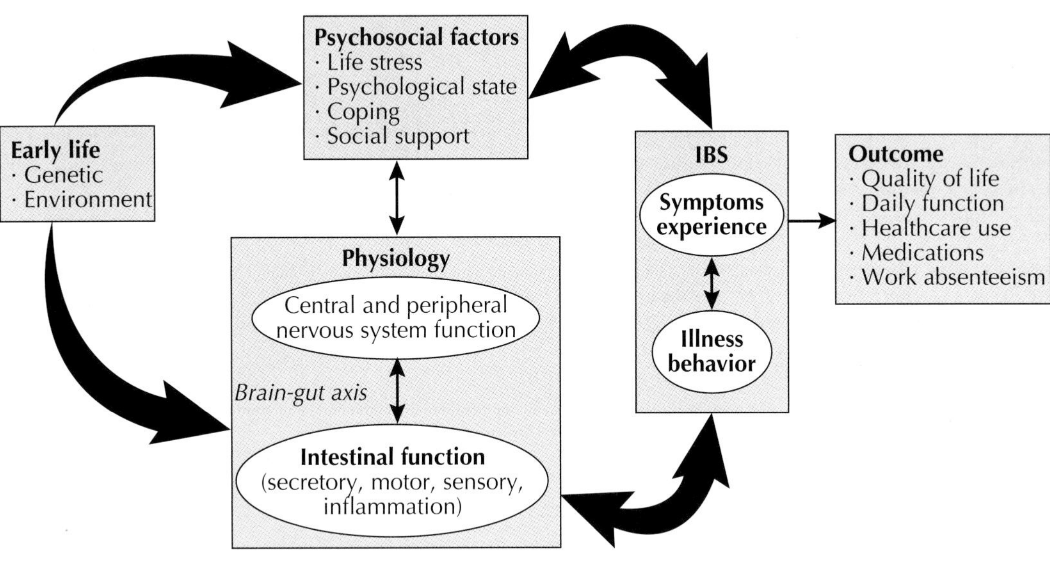


**Brain-gut axis**

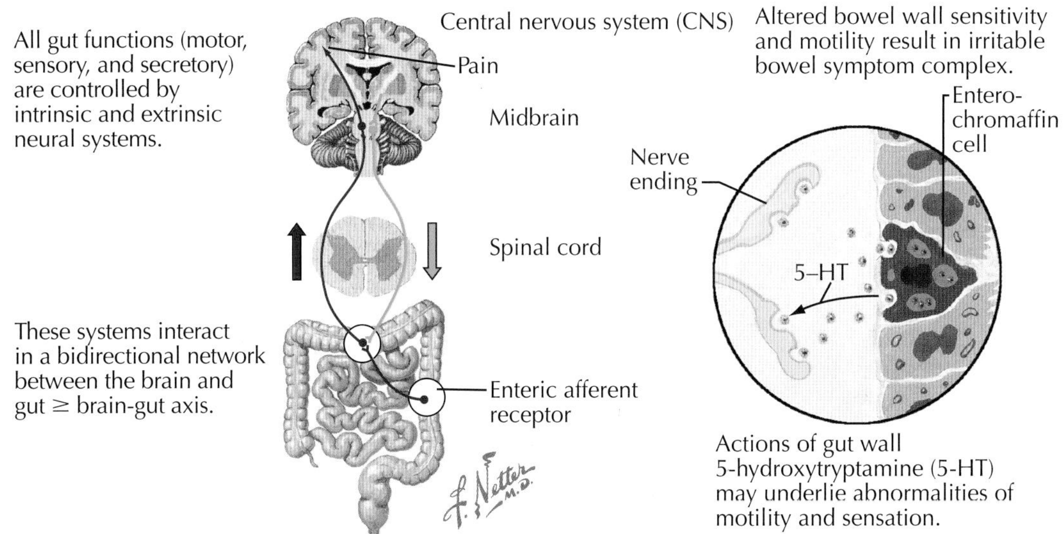

All gut functions (motor, sensory, and secretory) are controlled by intrinsic and extrinsic neural systems.
Central nervous system (CNS)
Pain
Midbrain
Spinal cord
These systems interact in a bidirectional network between the brain and gut ≥ brain-gut axis.
Enteric afferent receptor
Altered bowel wall sensitivity and motility result in irritable bowel symptom complex.
Entero-chromaffin cell
Nerve ending
5–HT
Actions of gut wall 5-hydroxytryptamine (5-HT) may underlie abnormalities of motility and sensation.
F. Netter M.D.


**Rome IV diagnostic criteria for IBS***

Recurrent abdominal pain on average at least 1 day/week in the last 3 months, associated with **two or more** of the following criteria:

1. Related to defecation
2. Associated with a change in frequency of stool
3. Associated with a change in form (appearance) of stool

*Criteria fulfilled for the last 3 months with symptom onset at least 6 months prior to diagnosis.

## Irritable Bowel Syndrome, Constipation Predominant

Irritable bowel syndrome, constipation predominant (IBS-C), is one of three primary causes of constipation. IBS has an estimated prevalence of 14.1% in the United States, with the constipation-predominant form seen more in females than males. Diagnosis is made using the Rome IV criteria. IBS is further subdivided into IBS-D, IBS-C, and a form that alternates between diarrhea and constipation (IBS-M). The predominant subtype can change over the course of a patient's life span. For the diagnosis of IBS to be made, the patient must have visceral pain that may be subjectively described as a bloating or cramping sensation.

Though the pathophysiology of IBS is not well understood, it is accepted that it involves problems associated with proper regulation of the brain-gut axis. The brain-gut axis is disturbed when one or more triggers affect the homeostasis of either the central or enteric nervous system, leading to visceral hypersensitivity, improper gut motility, and the development of symptoms associated with IBS. These triggers can range from psychological stress such as depression or anxiety, enteric infections, small bowel bacterial overgrowth, colonic dysbiosis, medications, food allergies, and abuse. Patients who are just recovering from an enteric infection are at a sixfold increased risk for developing IBS compared with the general population. Identification of these triggers may indicate which therapies will be more effective.

Diagnosis is made by taking a comprehensive history and performing a focused physical examination. Ordering laboratory tests is reserved for addressing any alarm signs and/or symptoms to rule out other likely causes for the patient's symptoms. The full differential diagnosis for IBS includes small intestinal bacterial overgrowth, celiac disease, lactose intolerance, diabetic gastroparesis, hyperthyroidism, carcinoid syndrome, inflammatory bowel disease, parasitic infections such as giardiasis, and colon cancer. In females, gynecologic problems may be a factor. All patients should be screened for alarm symptoms suggestive of other disease processes such as malignancy. Classically, patients who present to the clinic with IBS-C report constipation associated with significant abdominal pain that is relieved with defecation. As long as no alarm symptoms or physical examination findings are present, the diagnosis of IBS can be made using the Rome IV criteria, with no additional diagnostic workup. It is good to screen all newly presenting patients with IBS for a history of sexual, physical, or emotional abuse with sensitivity and available resources as necessary.

Without alarm signs and symptoms, the clinician can proceed to management. Management is tailored toward a patient's presenting symptoms. All patients should be offered formal education, allowing for enough time for patients to address any questions or concerns they have with this diagnosis. Clinicians should encourage regular exercise and healthy eating habits. Patients should try to ingest 20 to 25 g of fiber daily through their regular diet, although evidence is weak that this helps. In some patients, ingesting higher levels of fiber offers no additional benefit and may actually worsen symptoms. Cognitive-behavioral therapy has been shown to be effective for patients who develop IBS because of an underlying psychological condition such as anxiety. Laxatives approved to treat constipation include agents such as polyethylene glycol, lactulose, linaclotide, and lubiprostone, all of which can stimulate gut motility. The 5-hydroxytryptamine receptor 4 ($5\text{-HT}_4$) agonist prucalopride results in increased peristalsis and stimulates gut motility and is approved only for adults with FC with not enough evidence that it is effective in IBS-C.

## Pelvic Floor Dysfunction and Constipation

**Normal pelvis**

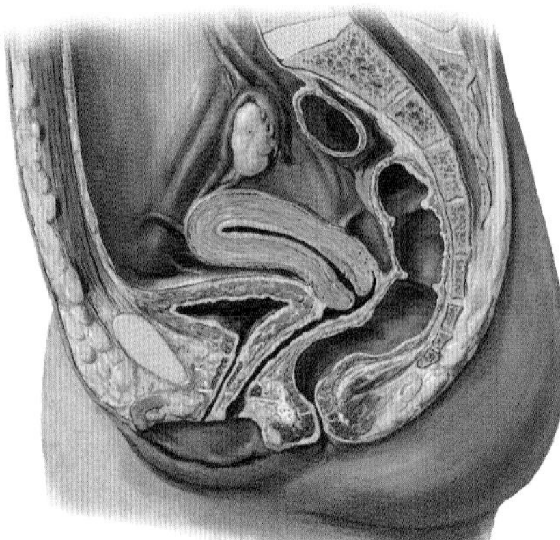

**Rome IV diagnostic criteria for functional constipation (must include two or more of the following)*:**

1. Straining during >25% of defecations
2. Lumpy or hard stools (Bristol scale 1–2) >25% of defecations
3. Sensation of incomplete evacuation >25% of defecations
4. Sensation of anorectal obstruction/blockage >25% of defecations
5. Manual maneuvers to facilitate more than >25% of defecations (e.g., digital evacuation, support of the pelvic floor)
6. Fewer than three spontaneous bowel movements/week
7. Loose stools rarely present without the use of laxatives
8. Insufficient criteria for irritable bowel syndrome

*Criteria fulfilled for the last 3 months with symptom onset at least 6 months prior to diagnosis.

**Rectocele**

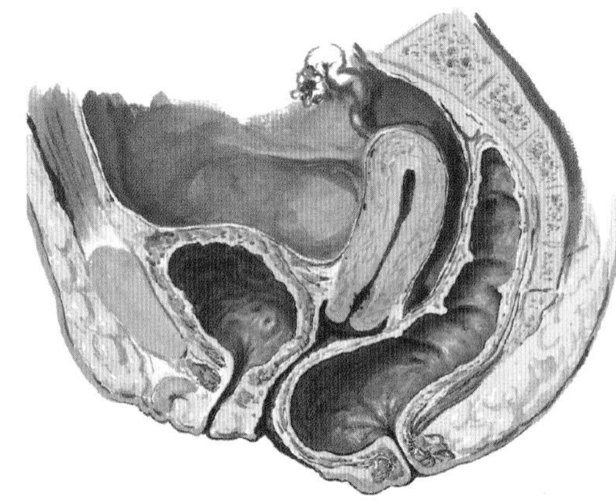

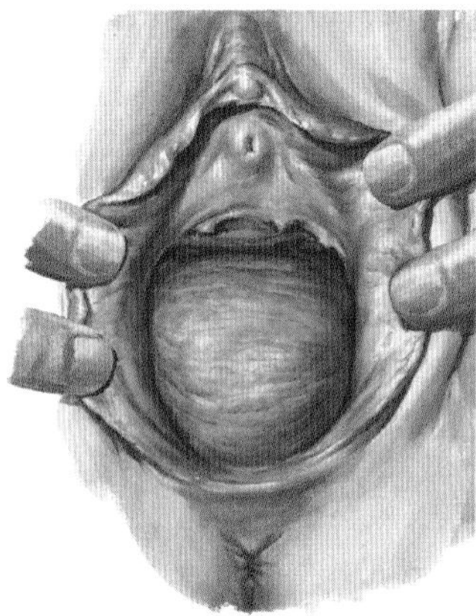

**Dyssynergic defecation and fecal impaction**

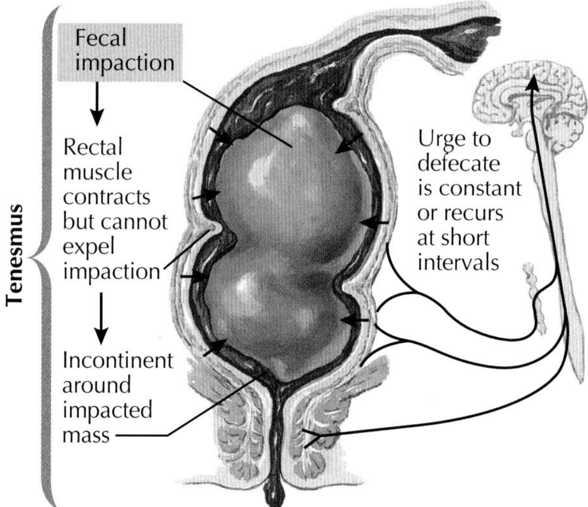


Fecal impaction, or a large amount of hard stool in the distal rectum obstructing the anal outlet. The presence of a fecal impaction can lead to encopresis as more proximal fecal matter seeps around the impacted fecal mass.

**Pelvic floor dysfunction syndrome**

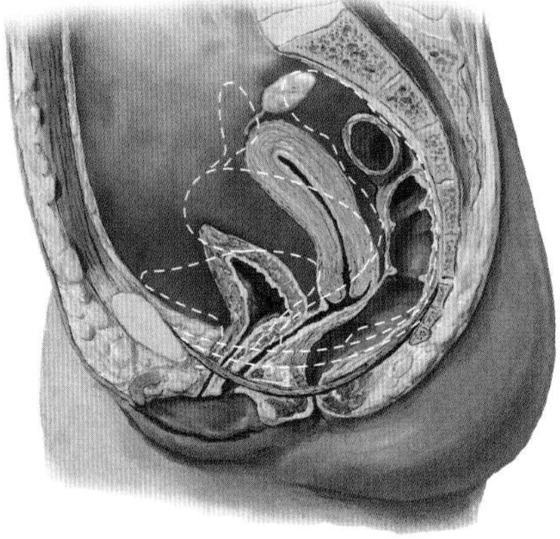

*Dashed lines* indicate normal position.

Constipation as a result of pelvic floor dysfunction may stem from a broad category of disorders that includes conditions such as dyssynergic defecation, descending perineum syndrome, stool impaction, and rectocele. Pelvic floor disorders are fairly common, with nearly 23.7% of all females experiencing at least one disorder.

*Dyssynergic defecation* is diagnosed by first meeting the Rome IV criteria for functional constipation in addition to the requirements listed at right. Patients may present with symptoms associated with straining on defecation, incomplete evacuation, and bloating and will demonstrate incomplete relaxation of the external anal sphincter when asked to bear down during the digital rectal examination or on manometry or electromyography. This diagnosis can be confirmed with physiologic testing such as anorectal manometer or balloon expulsion testing. Delayed colonic transit may also be seen on colon marker studies or with colonic transit scintigraphy; it may be difficult to determine whether this is secondary to outlet delay from the dyssynergia or an additional problem. For this reason, newer algorithms in the evaluation and treatment of constipation point out that transit studies are only performed after an expulsion problem is excluded.

The best treatment for dyssynergic defecation is biofeedback therapy using operant conditioning. This form of therapy uses an electromyogram or balloon probe placed in the patient's rectum and provides instant feedback related to muscle activity to overcome the dyssynergia through improved posture, more coordinated efforts for pushing, and improved sensation of stool during defecation.

*Descending perineum syndrome* is defined as a descent of the peritoneum of 3 cm or more upon defecation or 4 cm or more at baseline. Patients will present with constipation associated with dyschezia and straining. The best diagnostic examination is barium or magnetic resonance defecography, which demonstrates the necessary degree of descent to make the diagnosis. There is no current standard of therapy for descending perineum syndrome; most clinicians suggest biofeedback therapy to correct the excess straining or, in severe cases, isolated retroanal levator plate myorrhaphy surgery.

*Fecal impaction* is one of the most common causes of constipation in older adults and patients seen in the hospital setting and may be a sign of another underlying disorder such as dyssynergic defecation. Typically, patients have abnormal sensation with the accumulation of stool in the rectum, which can desiccate over time. Some patients present with diarrhea or fecal incontinence as liquid stool seeps around the impaction and through the anal canal. The diagnosis can usually be made by appreciating stool on digital rectal examination or seeing excess stool on diagnostic imaging with a radiograph or CT scan. Manometric testing will typically reveal abnormal sensation and high rectal compliance. The first step in management should be colonic decompression. A second therapeutic option should be the introduction of enemas or suppositories for relief. A good strategy is to keep the rectum clear with a regular bowel regimen, which may include a low-residue diet to decrease the mass of feces delivered to the colon.

A *rectocele* is a herniation of the colon into the anterior or posterior wall of the pelvis; weakness of the rectovaginal septum is generally accepted as the main cause. Females are at increased risk for rectoceles with advanced age. Factors that lead to pelvic floor muscle weakening can also result in a rectocele, including vaginal delivery, trauma during delivery, a history of straining, or prior rectal surgery. A rectocele must be at least 2 cm in size to be considered clinically significant. Bimanual rectal and pelvic examination can be used to make the diagnosis, and defecography is considered the gold standard test to determine the overall size and position. Generally, rectoceles are treated using a combination of diet modification, improved bowel habits, and biofeedback therapy. Surgery is reserved for rectoceles greater than 3 cm with coexisting vaginal prolapse or those who do not respond to initial medical therapy; one must recognize that outcomes from surgical interventions are disappointing. Another structural problem that can have functional consequences is *enterocele*, which is prolapse of the small bowel with pressure to the upper wall of the vagina; in some cases, there could be an effect on the large intestine or rectum.

## FECAL INCONTINENCE

Fecal incontinence is the unintentional and/or accidental loss of stool. Studies have shown that this condition is found in higher prevalence in those over 65 years of age, secondary to certain factors in the obstetric history, in those in poor general health, and in those with physical limitations. This condition alone can plague nearly 50% of all nursing home residents and leads to a significant financial burden to the healthcare system. The development of fecal incontinence in adults can be emotionally devastating. The associated stigma alone prevents many from seeking proper therapy to alleviate their symptoms.

Fecal incontinence can result from damage to the nerve supply or musculature responsible for sensing and controlling the anal sphincter muscles and puborectalis muscle. Neurologic conditions, such as spinal cord injuries, diabetes leading to peripheral neuropathy, and multiple sclerosis, can either weaken the muscles responsible for defecation or decrease the sensation of feces in the rectum. Another common cause of incontinence is a decreased storage capacity of the rectal vault. Conditions that fall into this category are adverse side effects from radiation therapy or surgery for UC and other conditions resulting in colitis. Increased compliance as seen in megarectum may also result in incontinence by liquid material seeping around a stool impaction.

Obstetric injuries are the most common cause of trauma leading to incontinence and deserve special attention. Disorders collectively known as *obstetric anal sphincter injuries* are the most common cause of fecal incontinence in females and result in a decreased desire for sexual intercourse and future childbearing. Certain adverse outcomes, such as third- and fourth-degree lacerations during vaginal delivery, can result in damage to both the pudendal nerve and surrounding musculature. Other risk factors putting females at higher risk of obstetric anal sphincter injuries are forceps delivery and improper fetal head position during delivery, large babies, and a long second stage of labor. Fecal incontinence may occur immediately after delivery, but development of fecal incontinence later in life may potentially be associated with degenerative changes over time related to pudendal neuropathy and/or muscle weakness. All healthcare professionals should ask about problems with both fecal and urinary incontinence after delivery to encourage early medical intervention.

The first step in evaluation of fecal incontinence is to take a detailed history that focuses on describing the nature of the symptoms in addition to how the disorder interferes with daily life. Physical examination, including a digital rectal examination, should determine whether the patient has a sphincter defect or other noticeable cause for incontinence. The digital rectal examination allows the practitioner to evaluate the overall resting tone of the internal anal sphincter. The external sphincter pressure can be assessed by asking the patient to voluntarily contract the anal muscles.

Anorectal manometry can assess sphincter strength, tone, and perception to sensation. If a patient has a suspected sphincter defect or obstetric trauma or is a good surgical candidate, the diagnostic workup should include anal ultrasound to evaluate the integrity of the musculature. Pelvic MRI has the best diagnostic yield for determining the integrity of the internal anal sphincter. Pudendal nerve terminal motor latency is another option for evaluating nerve integrity.

Medical therapy should be focused on the underlying cause of incontinence and is outlined in this plate. Biofeedback therapy uses operant conditioning to retrain patients to reduce episodes of fecal incontinence through a series of techniques using balloons or electromyography. Consideration of surgery must take into account many presenting factors and the cause. Sphincteroplasty is the best therapy for patients with identifiable sphincter defects and for those who are good surgical candidates. This technique tries to restore normal anal sphincter function but has variable long-term success. Other surgical techniques include dynamic graciloplasty, rectal augmentation, fecal diversion, and even artificial sphincter. Novel therapies include sacral or tibial nerve stimulation, radiofrequency, injectable bulking materials, and plug devices.

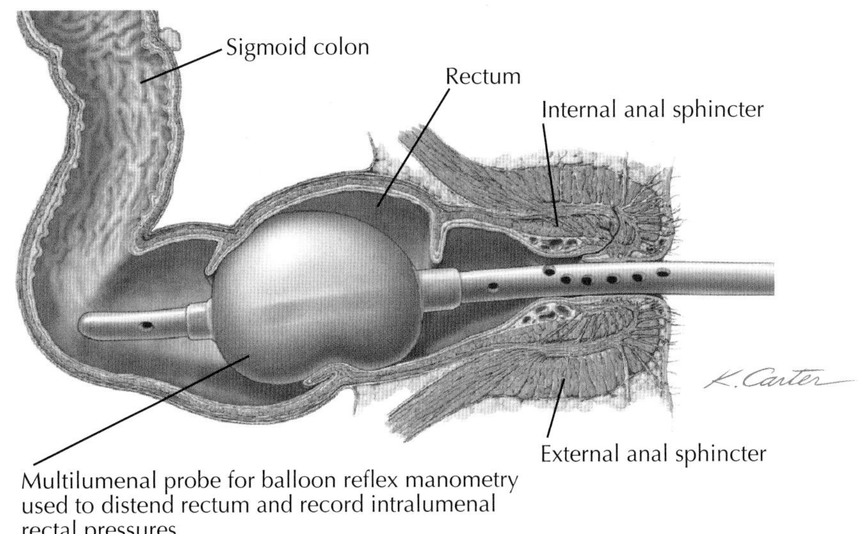


**Algorithm for the diagnosis and management of fecal incontinence**

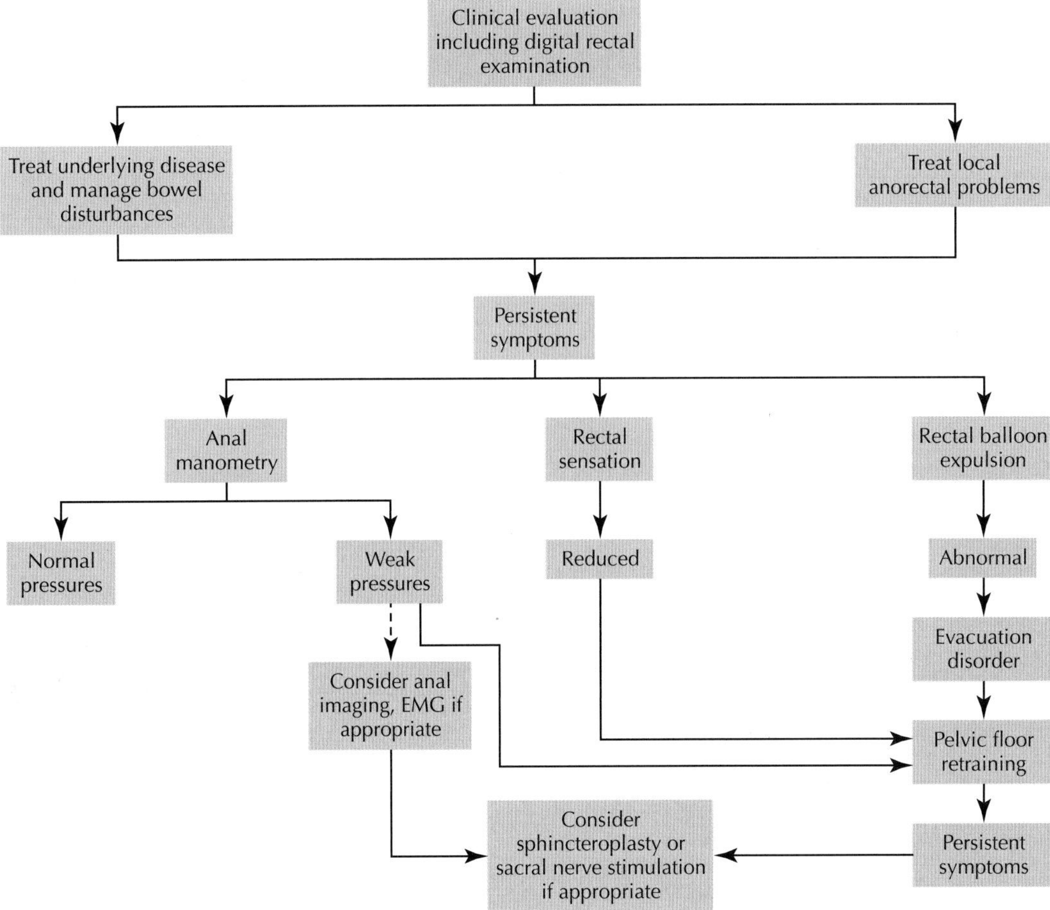


*From Whitehead WE, Bharucha AE. Diagnosis and treatment of pelvic floor disorders: what's new and what to do. Gastroenterology. 2010;138(4):1231–1235.*

# Medical Therapy for Motility Disorders

The following sections will address current treatment options available for constipation and diarrhea, including probiotic therapy.

## CONSTIPATION

A comprehensive summary of classes of medications used to treat constipation includes bulk laxatives (e.g., psyllium), surfactant laxatives (e.g., docusate), osmotic laxatives (e.g., polyethylene glycol), stimulant laxatives (e.g., bisacodyl), chloride channel activator 2 (e.g., lubiprostone), guanylate cyclase-C agonists (e.g., linaclotide), and mu-opioid receptor antagonists (e.g., methylnaltrexone and alvimopan). A 5-HT$_4$ agonist, tegaserod, was removed from the U.S. market by the Food and Drug Administration (FDA) because of an increased risk of adverse cardiovascular events. Other drugs not available in the United States are the 5-HT$_4$ agonists prucalopride, mosapride, and cisapride; mixed 5-HT$_4$ agonist and 5-HT$_3$ antagonist (e.g., renzapride); guanylate cyclase-C agonist (e.g., plecanatide); and bile acid resorption inhibitor (e.g., elobixibat).

Laxative abuse is a major problem in healthcare and is seen in both the inpatient and outpatient settings. Chronic laxative abuse can lead to electrolyte imbalances and acid-base disorders that result in cardiovascular and renal compromise and possible death. Patients who are at highest risk to develop laxative abuse are those who play sports with weight restrictions and or have a history of an eating disorder. The largest population at risk is middle-aged and older adults who hold the misconception that chronic laxative use is necessary to have a daily bowel movement. Patients should be educated on the dangers of chronic laxative use. Practitioners should encourage a diet of 20 to 25 g of fiber daily while promoting better toileting habits.

## DIARRHEA

Most cases of diarrhea are managed with supportive therapy and, if appropriate, antibiotics. Other medical therapies are generally reserved for symptomatic relief of severe diarrheal illness, IBS, and chronic diarrheal illness. The mu-opioid agonists loperamide and diphenoxylate are the most frequently used medications to treat both chronic and acute episodes of diarrhea. These medications are preferred over other mu-opioid agonists such as morphine and codeine because of their inability to cross the blood-brain barrier and affect the central nervous system. Loperamide is the most commonly used agent that works by slowing transit time through the alimentary canal. Another frequent medication used for diarrheal symptoms combines diphenoxylate with the anticholinergic drug atropine. The 5-HT$_3$ antagonist alosetron was an approved therapy for IBS until the FDA removed the drug from the market because of an association with ischemic colitis. Tricyclic antidepressants such as desipramine and nortriptyline have also shown promising results in reducing colonic transit time and generating more formed stool.

Laxatives

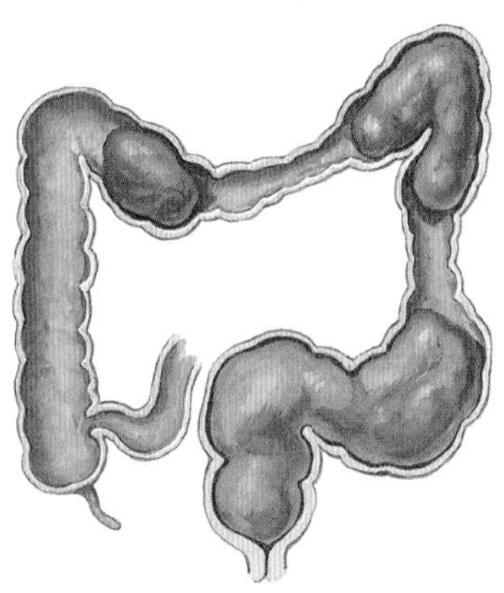

**Bulk agents** (bran, psyllium, methylcellulose) provide increased size, promote peristalsis by distension

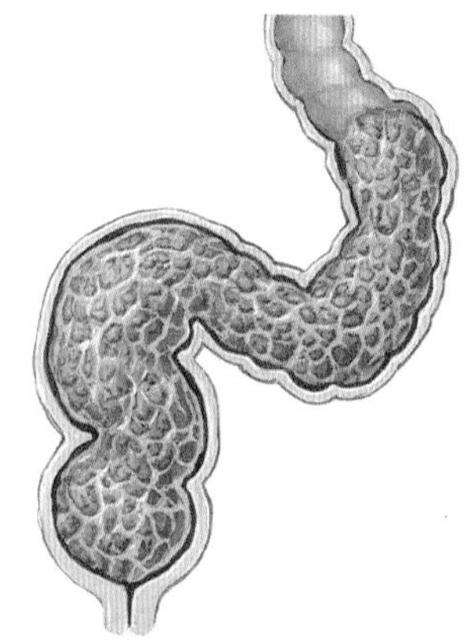

**Wetting agents** (dioctyl sodium sulfosuccinate) soften stool by coating and dispersion of component particles

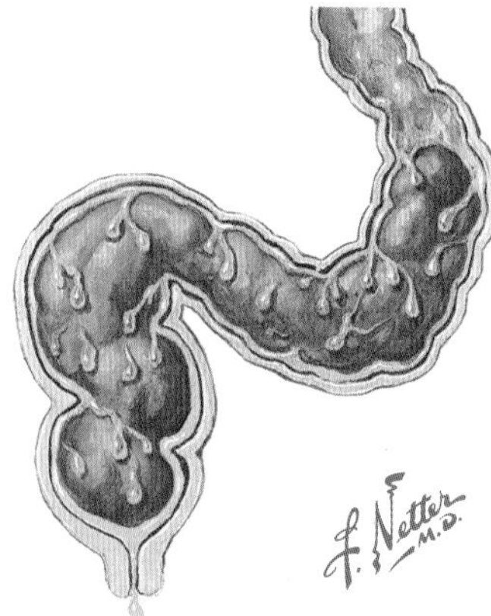

**Mineral oil** lubricates and mixes with stool to soften it

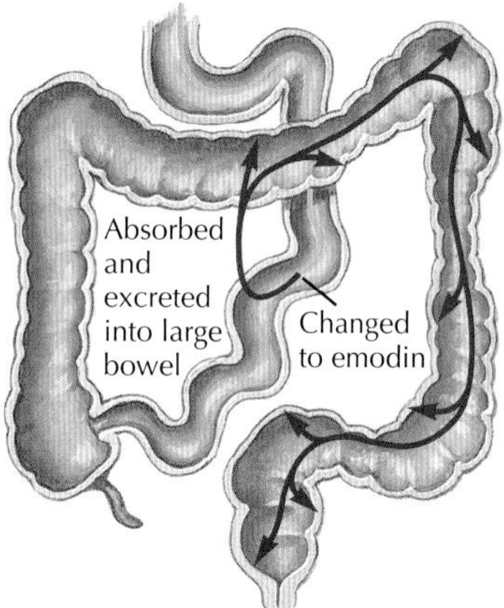


**Emodins** (cascara, senna, aloes) stimulate large bowel peristalsis and secretion by irritation

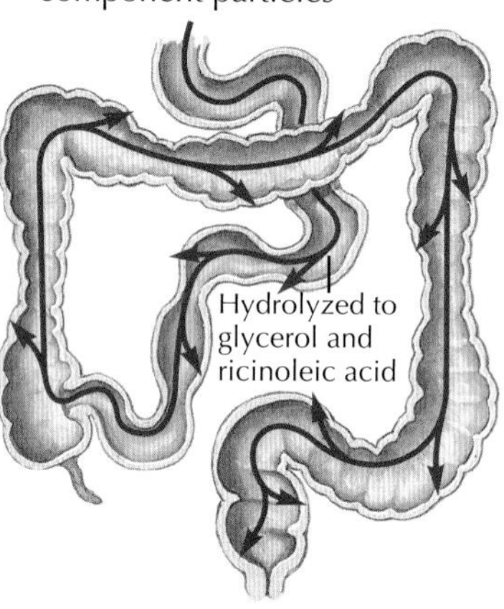


**Castor oil and derivatives** stimulate activity of small and large bowel by irritation

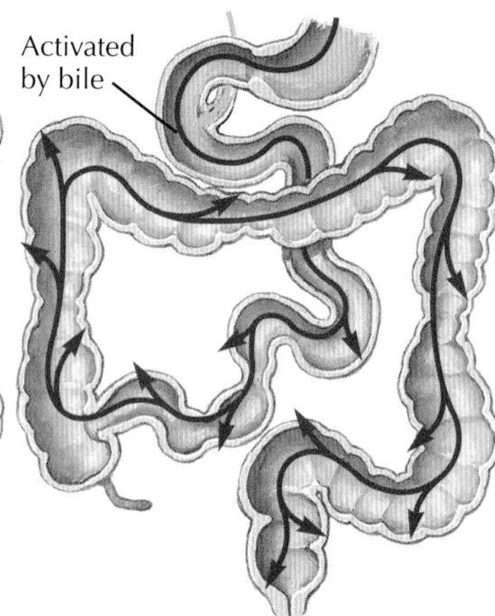


**Phenolphthalein** stimulates peristalsis and secretion by irritation; site of major action undetermined, probably widespread

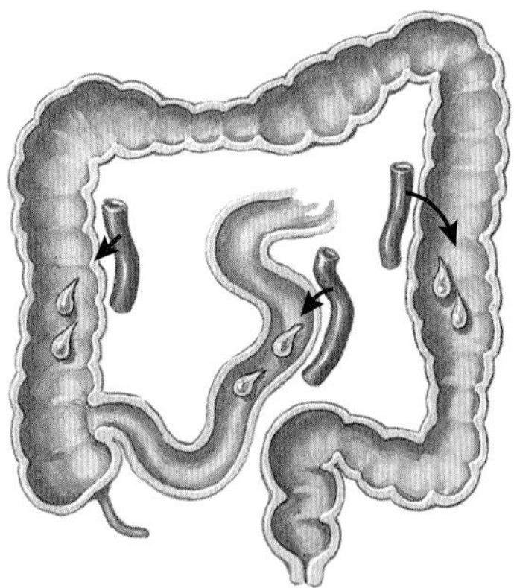

**Salines** (magnesium sulfate, citrate and hydroxide; sodium phosphate) draw and hold fluid in lumen osmotically, also have some irritant action

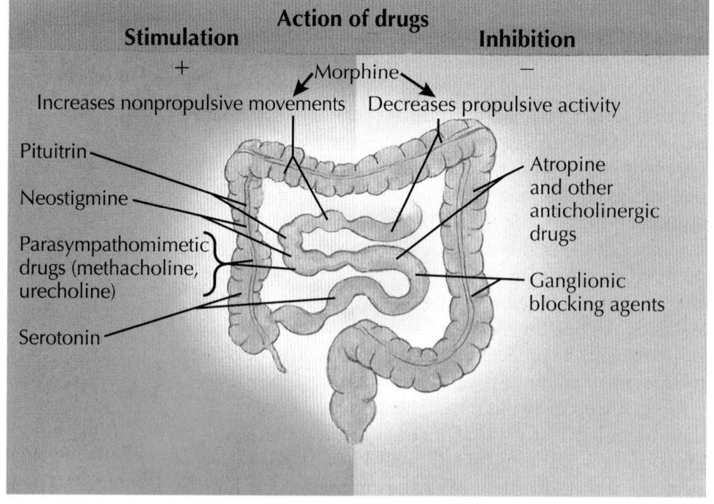


Other medical therapies available to treat diarrhea are those that work inside the lumen of the gut. Bismuth subsalicylate is a popular treatment for traveler's diarrhea and MC that has demonstrated both antimicrobial and antisecretory effects. Bile acid–binding agents (e.g., cholestyramine) may be the best therapy for those diagnosed with idiopathic diarrhea because it is hypothesized that some of these patients may have poor absorptive function of bile acids.

## PROBIOTICS

Some researchers theorize that disruption of the normal gut microbiome may result in bowel dysfunction. Growing literature supports the finding that probiotics can restore the normal microbiome of the body and might be useful in promoting bowel regularity. *Bifidobacterium infantis* has been shown to relieve gastrointestinal symptoms and improve motility; however, more research is needed on probiotics before they become mainstay therapy.

# Chronic Colonic Pseudoobstruction and Toxic Megacolon

The term *megacolon* refers to dilation of the cecum to greater than 12 cm or dilation of the sigmoid colon to 6.5 cm or more. Adverse events such as intestinal ischemia and perforation are directly related to size and how long a patient has had the megacolon. This condition is broken up into three different categories, with each described as simulating a mechanical obstruction in presentation with no evidence of true impediment or anatomic lesions. The first is acute colonic pseudoobstruction, or Ogilvie syndrome, which is discussed in greater detail on Plate 3.89.

*Chronic colonic pseudoobstruction* is a less common cause of distension of the colon. The most common cause in children is *Hirschsprung disease,* a condition characterized by the failure of normal migration of neural crest cells through the colon resulting in aganglionic bowel (see also Plate 3.28). This disorder is also found in babies born with Down syndrome and is strongly suspected when a newborn does not pass meconium in the first few days of life. The gold standard for diagnosis is rectal biopsy. Treatment involves surgical removal of the aganglionic bowel with approximation of the functionally normal bowel to the anus.

In the adult population, chronic colonic pseudoobstruction has primary and secondary causes resulting from an underlying neuropathy of the enteric nervous system, a myopathy of the smooth muscle of the bowel, or a problem with the interstitial cells of Cajal. Primary causes are either inherited or develop sporadically; secondary causes are generally acquired and a sign of advanced disease. Some secondary causes are connective tissue disorders (e.g., systemic scleroderma or systemic lupus erythematosus), infections (e.g., Chagas disease), metabolic disorders (e.g., diabetes, hypothyroidism), neuromuscular conditions (e.g., amyloidosis or Parkinson disease), and idiopathic myenteric ganglionitis. Use of certain medications (e.g., opioids and medications for Parkinson disease) may also be a secondary cause. For most patients, the cause of chronic colonic pseudoobstruction is never determined. Treatment is usually conservative, with medical therapy directed toward alleviating constipation.

*Toxic megacolon* is a serious secondary medical complication characterized by colonic distension of 6 cm or more shown on imaging in addition to systemic toxicity, as outlined in this plate. Diagnosis is made if a patient has three of four major criteria and at least one minor criterion. The major criteria are fever higher than 38.6°F, heart rate of more than 120 beats per minute, anemia, or a white blood cell count of more than 10,500/μL. The minor criteria are mental status changes, electrolyte imbalances, hypotension, and dehydration. The most common cause of toxic megacolon is irritable bowel disorder; the condition is seen more often with UC than with CD. Infections are the other common causes of this disorder, with pseudomembranous colitis caused by *C. difficile* being the most common one; there are also cases reported with *Campylobacter, Yersinia, Shigella,* cytomegalovirus, *Entamoeba histolytica, Aspergillus,* and *Cryptosporidium* infections. Less common causes are side effects from radiation therapy, colonic lymphomas, volvulus, ischemic bowel, and diverticulitis. The pathophysiologic characteristics of this condition are not yet fully understood; inflammation to the muscularis propria is thought to result in dilation of the smooth muscle. Nitric oxide may be one of the major contributors leading to the relaxation and dilation. Imaging studies such as radiography usually demonstrate a loss of haustrations in addition to the typical colonic dilation. This disorder is life-threatening and requires immediate medical attention that starts with placing a patient on intravenous fluids and bowel rest and the insertion of a nasogastric tube. High-dose steroids are the gold standard therapy for patients with UC who develop toxic megacolon. Surgical intervention is frequently needed and reserved for those who either do not respond to medical therapy or are very acutely ill.

## Chronic Colonic Pseudoobstruction/Megacolon

### Megacolon

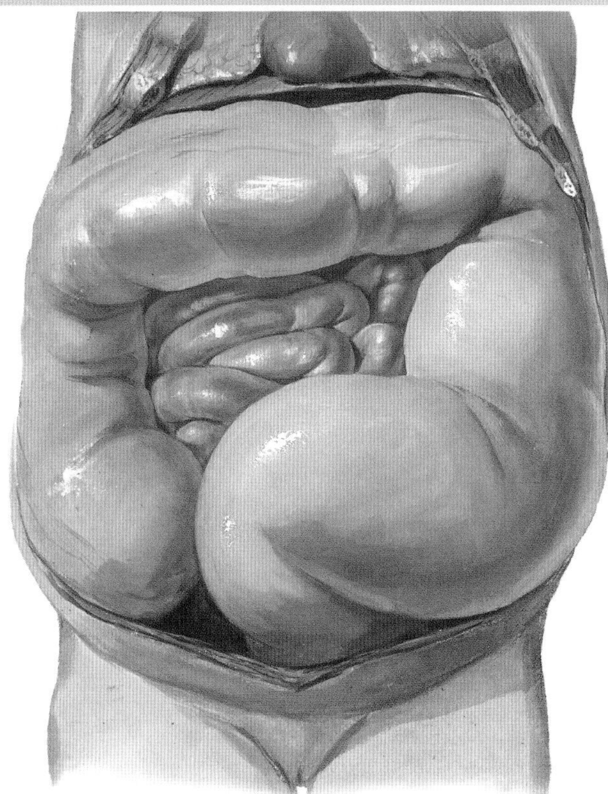

### Toxic megacolon

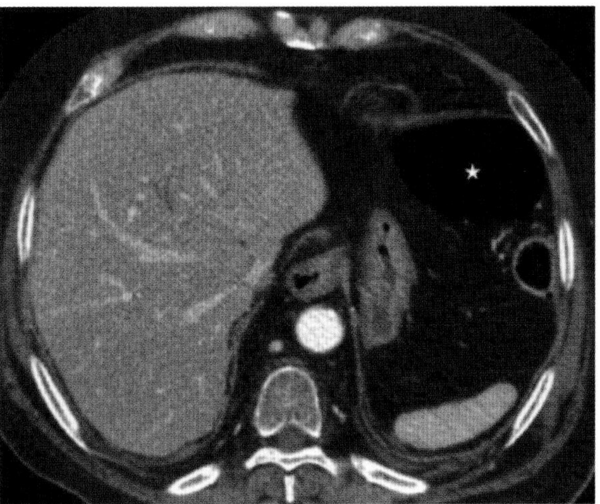

A 78-year-old man with toxic megacolon complicating acute colitis. Axial contrast-enhanced CT shows air-filled transverse colon distension (*star*) associated with colonic wall thinning.

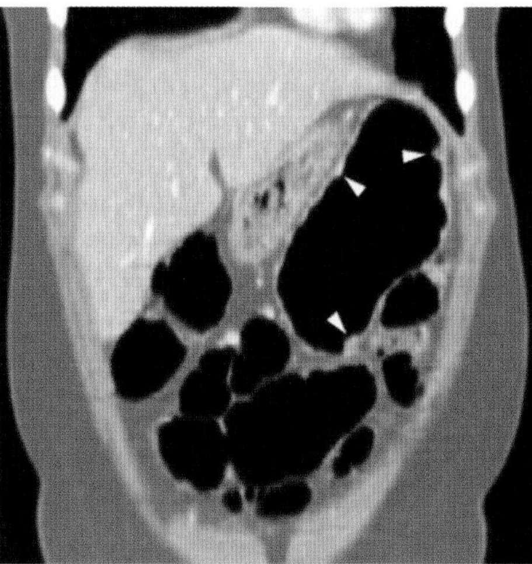

A 35-year-old woman with toxic megacolon complicating ulcerative colitis. Coronal contrast-enhanced CT scan with lung window setting shows abnormal haustral pattern of the dilated transverse colon and nodular pseudopolyps (*arrowheads*).

*From Moulin V, Dellon P. Toxic megacolon in patients with severe acute colitis: computed tomographic features. Clin Imaging. 2011;35:431–436.*

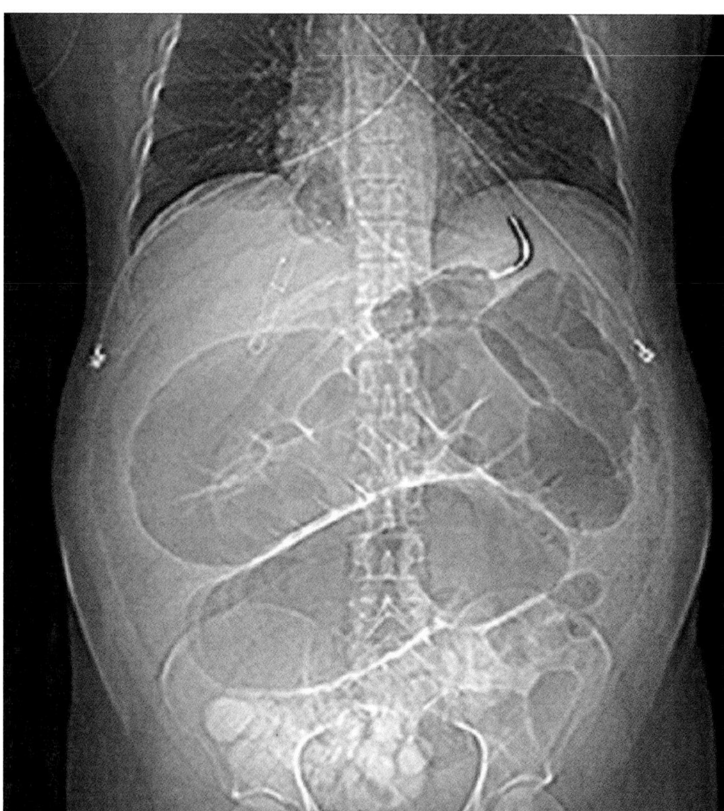

Abdominal CT scout view showing cecal distension of approximately 10 cm

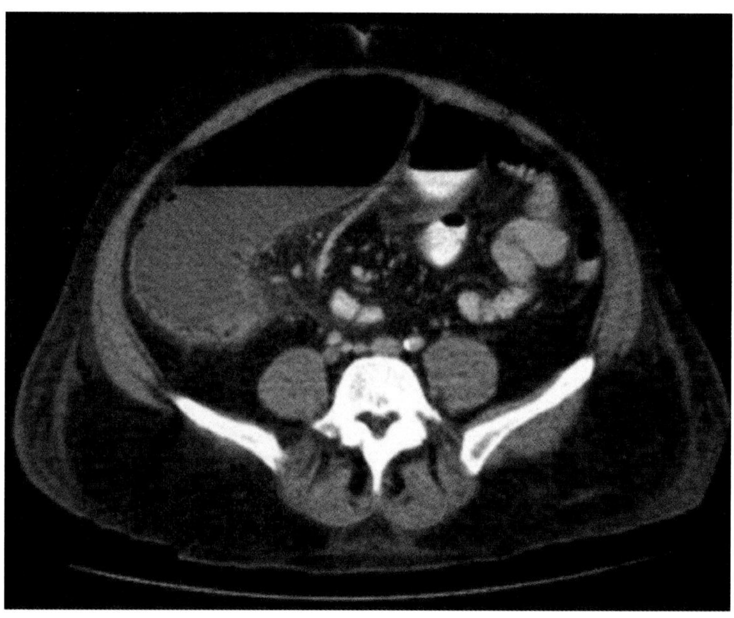

Abdominal CT suggestive of nonobstructive cecal distension

*From White L, Sandhu G. Continuous neostigmine infusion versus bolus neostigmine in refractory Ogilvie syndrome. Am J Emerg Med. 2011;29/5:576.*

## Ogilvie Syndrome

Ogilvie syndrome, also known as *acute pseudoobstruction of the colon,* presents with painless, progressive abdominal distension related to paralytic ileus of the large bowel. There is no mechanical obstruction as the cause of the distension, but significant dilation of the cecum can occur, compromising its blood supply and ultimately resulting in gangrene and perforation. Risk factors are trauma, infections such as pneumonia, obstetric/gynecologic conditions, myocardial infarction or congestive heart failure, neurologic conditions, or electrolyte imbalances; abdominal and pelvic surgery and orthopedic procedures may also be risk factors. The syndrome is thought to be related to sympathetic nervous overactivity, resulting in atony of the distal colon from interruption of the S2–S4 parasympathetic nerve fibers.

Patients typically present with nausea, vomiting, abdominal pain, constipation, or diarrhea after a few days of hospitalization for other causes. Those afflicted are usually males over age 60 years. On physical examination, patients are found to have a significantly distended abdomen and high-pitched bowel sounds. Laboratory studies may reveal electrolyte imbalances that may be related to a cause for the distension.

The diagnosis is supported by plain films, which show distension of all or part of the colon with loss of the haustral markings. Contrast enema can be performed to document the lack of a mechanical obstruction. Colonoscopy can be diagnostic and therapeutic as well. The possibility of bowel ischemia or perforation should be considered if there is localized tenderness, leukocytosis, metabolic acidosis, or clinical deterioration indicating sepsis. CT scan may be helpful to rule out any other cause for obstruction and can help differentiate between toxic megacolon and Ogilvie syndrome.

Patients should be resuscitated, with care taken to correct any metabolic or electrolyte imbalances. Serial physical examination and abdominal radiographs should be performed to determine whether colonoscopic decompression or surgical intervention is required. If colonic distension is less than 12 cm, conservative management can be continued. Nasogastric decompression may also be helpful in preventing swallowed air from worsening the condition. If there is concern for ischemia, surgery is warranted, with resection of any necrotic segment and proximal ostomy creation. If the bowel is intact, a cecostomy tube can be placed to relieve the distension.

Conservative management is successful in about half of the cases with no concerning signs on presentation. Spontaneous perforation occurs in about 3%, with a mortality rate of about 50%. Typically, the course resolves in 3 days. Endoscopic decompression is successful in 60% to 90% of cases but with a recurrence rate of up to 40%. Recurrence can be decreased with placement of a decompressive colonic tube. Neostigmine, a cholinesterase inhibitor, can produce colonic decompression in 80% to 100% of cases, with a recurrence rate of 5%. It may cause bradycardia, hypotension, or dizziness and is excreted by the kidneys, so caution should be taken in patients where this may be an issue. For patients without a contraindication, neostigmine should be considered as a first-line therapy prior to colonoscopy or surgical intervention.

# Colonic Involvement in Systemic Diseases

## DIABETES

Diabetes mellitus is a chronic metabolic disease in which there is an inability to regulate blood glucose levels. It affects virtually every organ system in the body, with the degree of involvement being dependent on the severity and duration of the disease. The majority of patients with diabetes mellitus report significant GI symptoms. Due to the rise in the disease prevalence, the number of patients with diabetes with GI involvement is also increasing.

The entire GI tract from the oral cavity and esophagus to the large bowel and anorectal region can be affected by diabetes. Thus symptoms experienced by the patient can vary widely. Common reports may include reflux, esophageal dysmotility, early satiety, nausea, vomiting, abdominal pain, diarrhea, constipation, and fecal incontinence (FI). This section discusses intestinal involvement, which may present as diarrhea, constipation, or FI. Patients with poorly controlled diabetes who have peripheral and autonomic neuropathy are at higher risk for having diabetic enteropathy

Diarrhea in patients with diabetes can be multifactorial. It can occur during the day but is more common at night. Autonomic neuropathy and fibrosis of the muscular layer of the bowel wall can result in altered motility and stasis. Intestinal stasis predisposes the patient to develop small intestinal bacterial overgrowth (SIBO), and decreased motility results in constipation, which may lead to overflow diarrhea and FI. Other etiologies for diarrhea in patients with diabetes include excessive use of artificial sweeteners, bile salt malabsorption, pancreatic insufficiency, celiac disease, MC, and side effects of medications such as metformin.

The first step when managing patients with diabetes with diarrhea is to review bowel habits, diet, and medications. Further testing for other causes including celiac disease, SIBO, pancreatic insufficiency, and infectious or inflammatory diseases should be considered. A stool osmotic gap can help differentiate between the types of diarrhea if the cause is unknown.

The goal of therapy in diabetic diarrhea is mostly symptom relief. Fluid and electrolyte replacement, correction of any other underlying etiologies when possible, and glycemic control are the mainstays of therapy. Antidiarrheal agents as needed are helpful for symptom relief. Fiber supplementation is beneficial in some patients, in the absence of gastroparesis. Patients with SIBO should be treated with antibiotics. Rifaximin, a poorly absorbed antibiotic, is the first choice when available. Clonidine, an alpha-2-adrenoreceptor agonist that stimulates intestinal fluid and electrolyte absorption, and octreotide, a somatostatin analog, should not be used routinely because of limited data.

Constipation is one of the most common GI symptoms in diabetic patients. Suggested causes are impaired gastrocolic reflex and neuronal dysfunction of the colon. As mentioned, patients with constipation may develop overflow diarrhea or incontinence. Colonic intestinal pseudoobstruction, megacolon, stercoral ulceration, and perforation due to severe constipation are rarely encountered.

Treatment is usually with conventional laxatives. Refractory cases may need further work-up including anorectal manometry and assessment of intestinal transit time. Prucalopride, a serotonin receptor agonist, can be an option in patients with concomitant gastroparesis, and linaclotide, a guanylate cyclase-C agonist, is helpful in patients with concomitant IBS.

As noted previously, diabetic neuropathy can lead in FI due to its effect on rectal sensation and reduced resting anal pressure due to dysfunction of the internal anal sphincter. Acute hyperglycemia may inhibit external anal sphincter in addition to decreasing rectal compliance, increasing the risk of incontinence. A typical presentation may be a patient with diabetes presenting with nocturnal soiling.

Management of diarrhea should be the first step of treatment because it can be a contributing factor to FI. Fiber supplementation and antidiarrheal agents are usually tried initially. Anorectal manometry and endoscopic ultrasound are diagnostic tools in patients with persistent FI. Biofeedback may help some patients via improving the rectal sensory threshold and increasing the anal sphincter tone. Patients with overflow FI should be treated for constipation. Other treatments for FI, such as sacral nerve stimulation, may benefit selected patients.

### Diabetes and Scleroderma

#### Diabetes

Autonomic neuropathy can affect bowel function with resulting diarrhea and/or constipation, urinary and fecal incontinence, and sexual dysfunction.

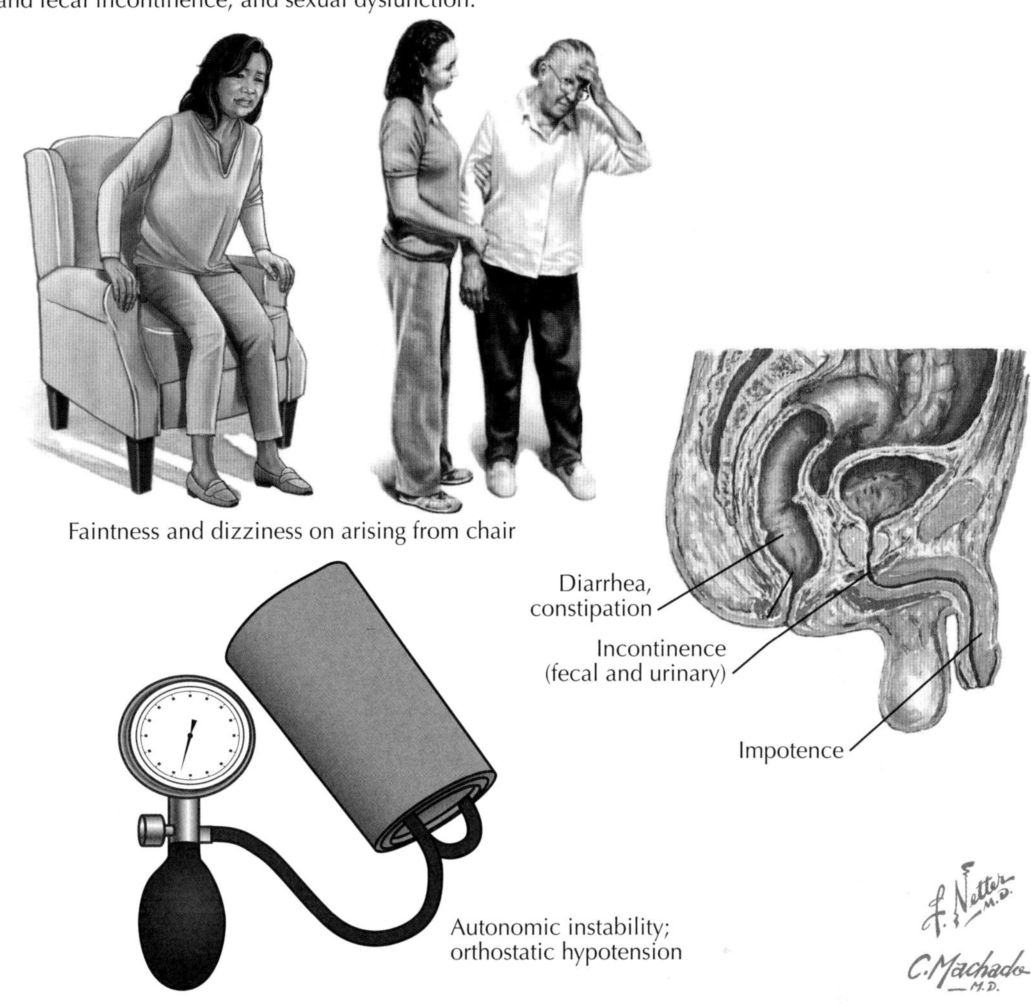


#### Scleroderma

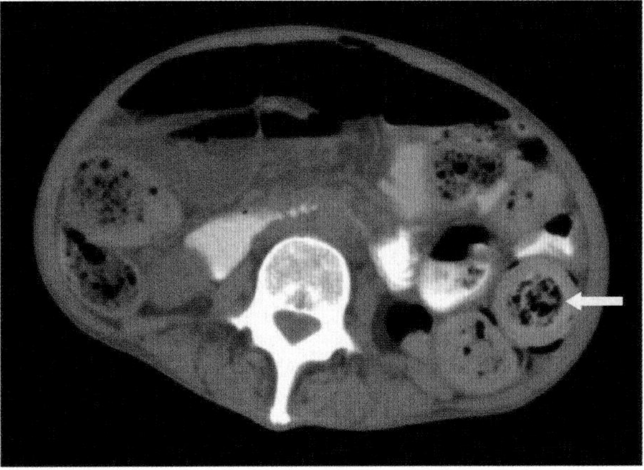

Noncontrast axial CT in soft tissue window from patient with scleroderma. Curvilinear collections of subserosal gas are present in the nondependent and dependent wall of the descending colon.

## Colonic Involvement in Systemic Diseases: Amyloidosis and Sarcoidosis

### AMYLOIDOSIS

Amyloidosis refers to the extracellular deposition of amyloid plaques, primarily composed of insoluble fibrils, altering the normal function of the affected organs. Involvement of the GI tract is commonly seen in systemic amyloidosis and is most often secondary to mucosal or neuromuscular infiltration.

Symptomatic patients may present with GI bleeding, protein-losing enteropathy, dysmotility, or malabsorption. Deposition of amyloid substances in the wall of small vessels causes frailty of the vessels and results in gastrointestinal bleeding. Mucosal lesions may be another etiology for bleeding in these patients. Patients with protein-losing enteropathy may present with diarrhea, hypoalbuminemia, edema, and ascites. GI tract dysmotility can predispose patients to nausea, vomiting, abdominal pain, diarrhea, constipation, bloating, and chronic intestinal pseudo-obstruction. Mucosal infiltration, bacterial overgrowth due to underlying dysmotility, and pancreatic insufficiency may result in malabsorption and weight loss.

Disorders known to be associated with amyloidosis include chronic inflammatory diseases such as inflammatory bowel diseases and plasma cell dyscrasia, as well as end-stage renal disease requiring dialysis. The underlying mechanism in dialysis-related cases is due to decreased renal clearance of large proteins with subsequent tissue accumulation. This is becoming less common with improved dialysis techniques.

The diagnosis is established by demonstration of amyloid in the biopsy specimen through special stains such as Congo red and thioflavin T, but unequivocal identification of amyloid requires electron microscopy.

Treatment is usually directed at the underlying cause of amyloidosis and symptomatic relief of the gastrointestinal manifestations.

AMYLOIDOSIS AND SARCOIDOSIS

**Amyloid deposit/sites and manifestations**

Skin
Alopecia
Nodular infiltrations
Purpura
Urticaria

Esophagus
Varices
Dysphagia

Liver
Hepatomegaly
Ascites

Pancreas
Diabetes mellitus

Stomach, intestines
Gastroparesis
Malabsorption
Diarrhea
Constipation

Peripheral nerves
Carpal tunnel syndrome
Areflexia
Sensory loss
Paresthesia
Autonomic dysfunction
(e.g., orthostatic hypotension)

Eyes
Conjunctival plaques
Vitreous opacities
Muscle weakness
Pupillary disorders
Proptosis
Amaurosis

Tongue
Macroglossia
Speech difficulty
Dysphagia

Larynx, trachea, bronchi
Hoarseness
Cough
Stridor
Dyspnea
Hemoptysis

Lungs
Nodules
(amyloidomas)
Pleural effusions

Heart
Enlargement
Conduction defects
Failure

Spleen
Splenomegaly

Kidneys
Proteinuria
Renal failure

Bladder, urethra
Hematuria

Joints
Arthritis

F. Netter M.D.

**Sarcoidosis**

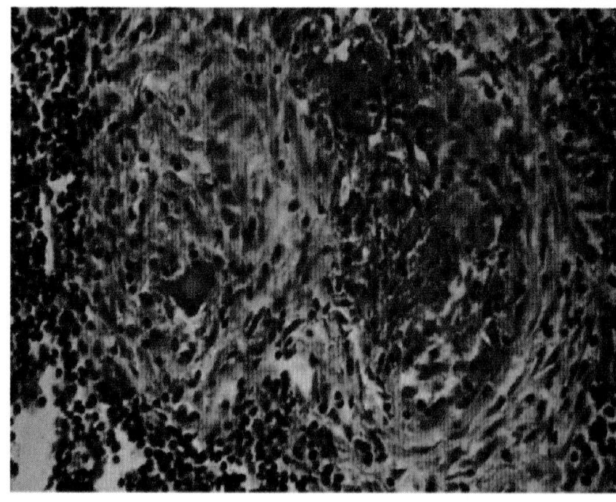

Sarcoid epithelioid granuloma in colonic wall consistent with sarcoidosis

### SARCOIDOSIS

Sarcoidosis is a systemic granulomatous disease characterized by the presence of noncaseating granulomas. The cause is unknown. Extrathoracic sarcoidosis has been reported in many organs, although extrahepatic gastrointestinal involvement is infrequent. There is an oral-anal gradient in cases with GI tract disease with the higher involvement of the esophagus, stomach, and duodenum. Involvement of the small bowel, colon, and rectum is extremely rare. When symptomatic, diarrhea and abdominal pain are the most common manifestations. Other presentations include weight loss, bleeding, and obstructive symptoms. Reported findings during endoscopic evaluation include erosions, polyps, nodules, strictures, and punctate bleeding sites.

The diagnosis is based on the presence of noncaseating granulomas in the biopsy specimen of the affected GI tract section and exclusion of sarcoid-like reactions caused by cancer or a foreign body and other causes of granulomatous diseases. While the presence of GI tract granulomas in patients who already have been diagnosed with sarcoidosis likely represents sarcoidosis of the GI tract, the diagnosis cannot be confirmed in the absence of granulomatous inflammation in at least another non-gastrointestinal organ.

Steroids are the mainstay therapy in symptomatic cases. Surgery may be required, especially in patients with life-threatening bleeding, for lesions mimicking colorectal cancer, and with presentation as acute appendicitis, perforation, and obstruction. Asymptomatic patients generally do not require treatment but should be monitored.

Relative regional incidence of carcinoma of large bowel

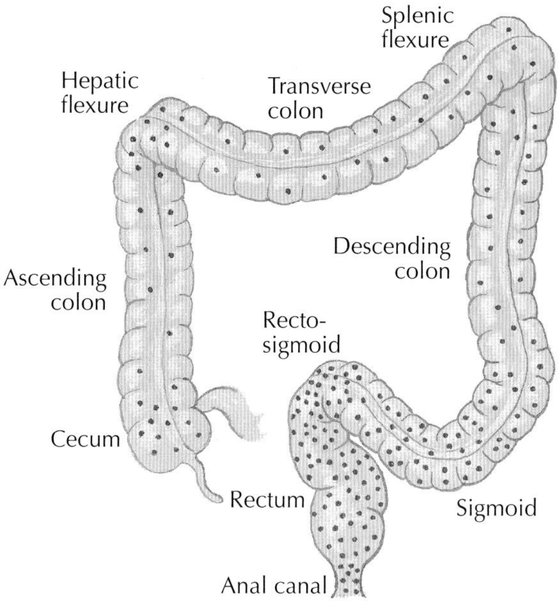

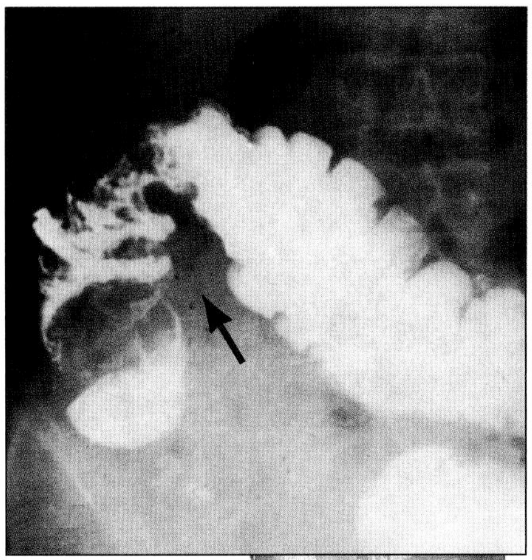

Contrast radiograph. Tumor in cecum (*arrows*).

Adenocarcinoma

Carcinoma of cecum

## Malignant Tumors of Large Intestine

Colorectal cancer is the third most common cancer in males and females in the United States. About 151,000 patients are diagnosed each year, with 52,000 deaths annually. The lifetime risk of developing colorectal cancer is 6%. The overall incidence and mortality rate have been declining for males and females over the last few decades. Colon cancer is three times more common than rectal cancer. Studies show an increasing incidence of right-sided colon cancers, a finding thought to possibly relate to environmental factors or increased screening leading to early detection of these lesions.

Colorectal cancers are believed to develop along the adenoma-to-carcinoma sequence. This has been found to result from chromosomal instability due to mutations in genes such as *APC, p53,* and *K-ras*. Others have been shown to be due to microsatellite instability, which results in aberrant DNA mismatch repair with mutations in *BAX, TGF-BIIR,* and *BRAF*. These tumors are typically more proximal and have a better prognosis. This is the pathway through which patients with Lynch syndrome develop cancer. Excessive gene methylation has also been implicated in the development of colorectal cancers.

Risk factors for the development of colorectal cancer are age over 50 years, a personal or family history of colorectal cancer or adenomas, or a personal history of IBD. Other factors like tobacco use, alcohol consumption, obesity, and red meat intake increase risk but not enough to affect screening recommendations. Sporadic cancers make up 75% of all colorectal cancers. Only 10% of cancers occur in those under age 40 years. Large villous lesions are most likely to harbor malignancy.

The mainstay of treatment for colorectal cancer is surgery. Adjuvant chemotherapy is administered to reduce the risk of distant recurrence. In patients with rectal cancer, neoadjuvant chemotherapy and radiation may be administered to improve resectability, aid in sphincter preservation, and reduce local and distant recurrence. Surgery is typically reserved for those patients in whom cure is possible with surgery or those who have symptoms such as obstruction or bleeding. With the effectiveness of neoadjuvant treatments, fewer patients require abdominoperineal resection and permanent colostomy.

The goal of surgery is to remove the primary tumor with adequate margins and regional lymph nodes. A margin of 5 cm is necessary to ensure that the tumor and potentially involved lymphatics are excised in the colon, and 2 cm has been found to be adequate for tumors of the rectum. Lymphatic vessels tend to follow the vascular pedicles, so resection typically follows these routes with the goal of harvesting a minimum of 12 lymph nodes with colon resections.

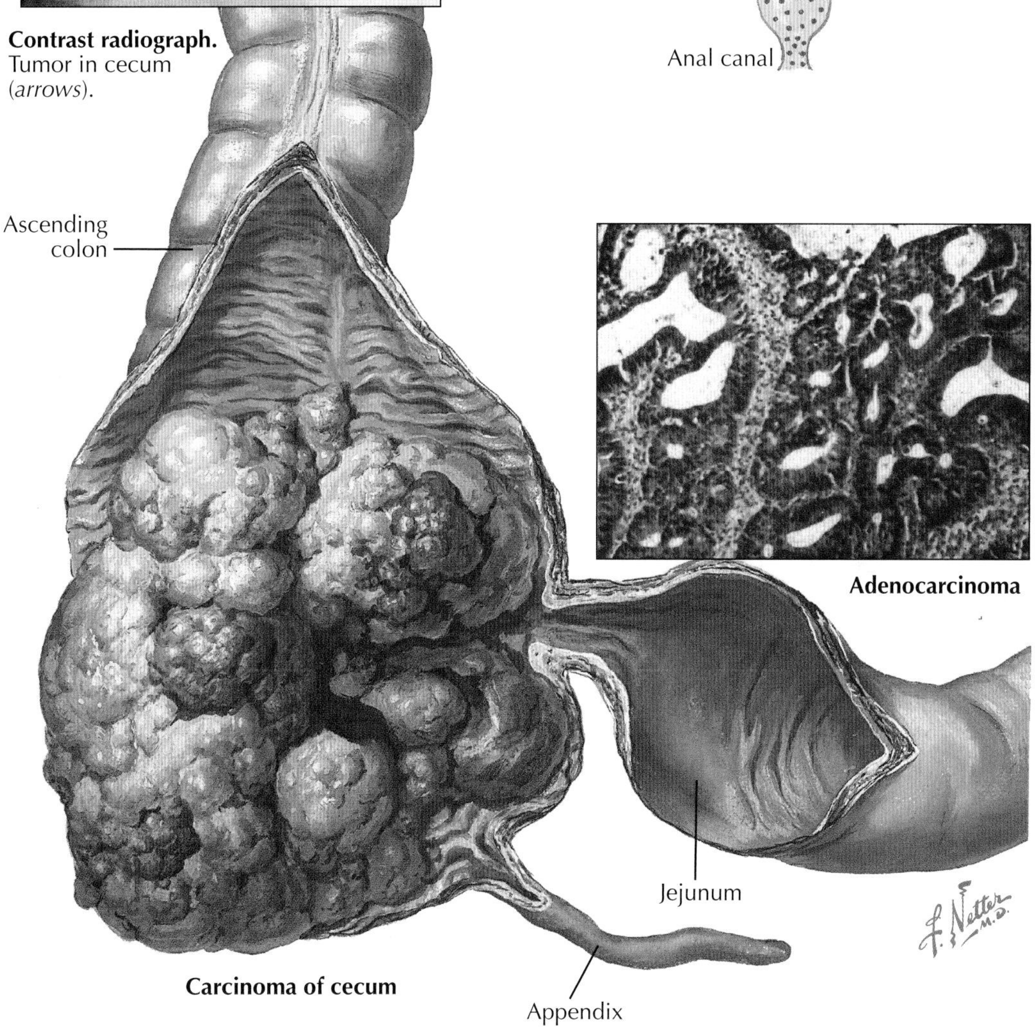

Some malignant polyps may be amenable to endoscopic removal if the cancer is confined to the head and stalk of the polyp. If completely removed, with clear margins and no high-risk pathologic features, patients can typically be observed, without the need for colectomy. For patients who have positive margins or high-risk features, such as lymphovascular or perineural invasion, poor differentiation, or single-cell infiltrate, a formal surgical resection is necessary.

For rectal cancers that are small (T1 or T2) or span less than one-third of the bowel circumference and have no evidence of lymph node metastasis, transanal excision may be an option. Cancers must be within 10 cm of the anal verge to be amenable to this method. The recurrence rates have been found to be higher than those with formal resection because local lymph nodes are not sampled with the excision and may be harboring disease.

## Malignant Tumors of Large Intestine (Continued)

Minimally invasive colectomy has been shown to be equivalent oncologically to open colectomy. This adds the benefit of smaller incisions, less discomfort, and a quicker postoperative recovery time.

Adjuvant chemotherapy has been shown to be effective in reducing risk by 33% compared with surgery alone. The basis for most treatment regimens is 5-fluorouracil with leucovorin. Oxaliplatin, a platinum-based compound, has shown greater activity when combined with 5-fluorouracil and leucovorin and has become the standard treatment regimen for patients with stage III colon cancer or high-risk stage II disease. This drug has no nephrotoxicity but does carry risks of neurotoxicity, myelosuppression, nausea, vomiting, and diarrhea. An oral version of 5-fluorouracil called *capecitabine* when combined with oxaliplatin is as successful in some patients.

The disease is more common in males, with a sex ratio of about 3:2. The neoplasms develop at any age but are most frequent between the ages of 50 and 70 years. It is important to realize that in about 10% of cases, the patients affected are under the age of 30 years, and most have not yet entered the second decade of life.

*Adenocarcinomas* are the most frequent malignant new growths of the large bowel. As a rule, only a single lesion is present, but multiple lesions are seen in 4% of patients. It is not rare for one or more benign adenomas to be found nearby or elsewhere in the colon, suggesting that the malignant lesion arose from a primary benign polyp. The possibility of cancer degeneration of benign adenomas is demonstrated by the following facts: (1) The incidence of benign adenomas in the different segments of the large bowel is the same as that of adenocarcinomas. (2) Follow-up of the untreated benign adenomas reveals malignant degeneration in a large number of cases. (3) Histopathologic studies of the adenomas reveal atypical cell arrangements, carcinoma "in situ," or invasive carcinoma in a fair percentage of cases. (4) In familial polyposis of the large intestine, the degeneration of one or more adenomas is frequently observed.

Chronic inflammatory conditions, such as UC and CD, are also considered to be lesions that may eventually give rise to malignancy. In UC, adenocarcinoma is observed in more than 5% of patients who have had the disease for 10 years or longer; some authors reported this occurrence in even more than 30% of their cases. The concern is for patients with pancolitis, particularly in UC but also in CD. UC limited to proctitis has no associated increase for colorectal cancer. Colorectal cancer seen in patients with IBD appears to progress from no dysplasia to indefinite dysplasia, low-grade dysplasia, high-grade dysplasia, and, finally, invasive adenocarcinoma. It is believed that colorectal cancer can arise without this process of step progression. The risk for colorectal cancer in these inflammatory conditions is associated with duration and a greater anatomic extent of colitis, degree of inflammation, and family history; in UC, the presence of primary sclerosing cholangitis is a risk factor. The molecular alterations recognized as responsible for sporadic colorectal cancer (chromosomal instability, microsatellite instability, and hypermethylation) appear to also play a role in the development of cancer in these inflammatory diseases.

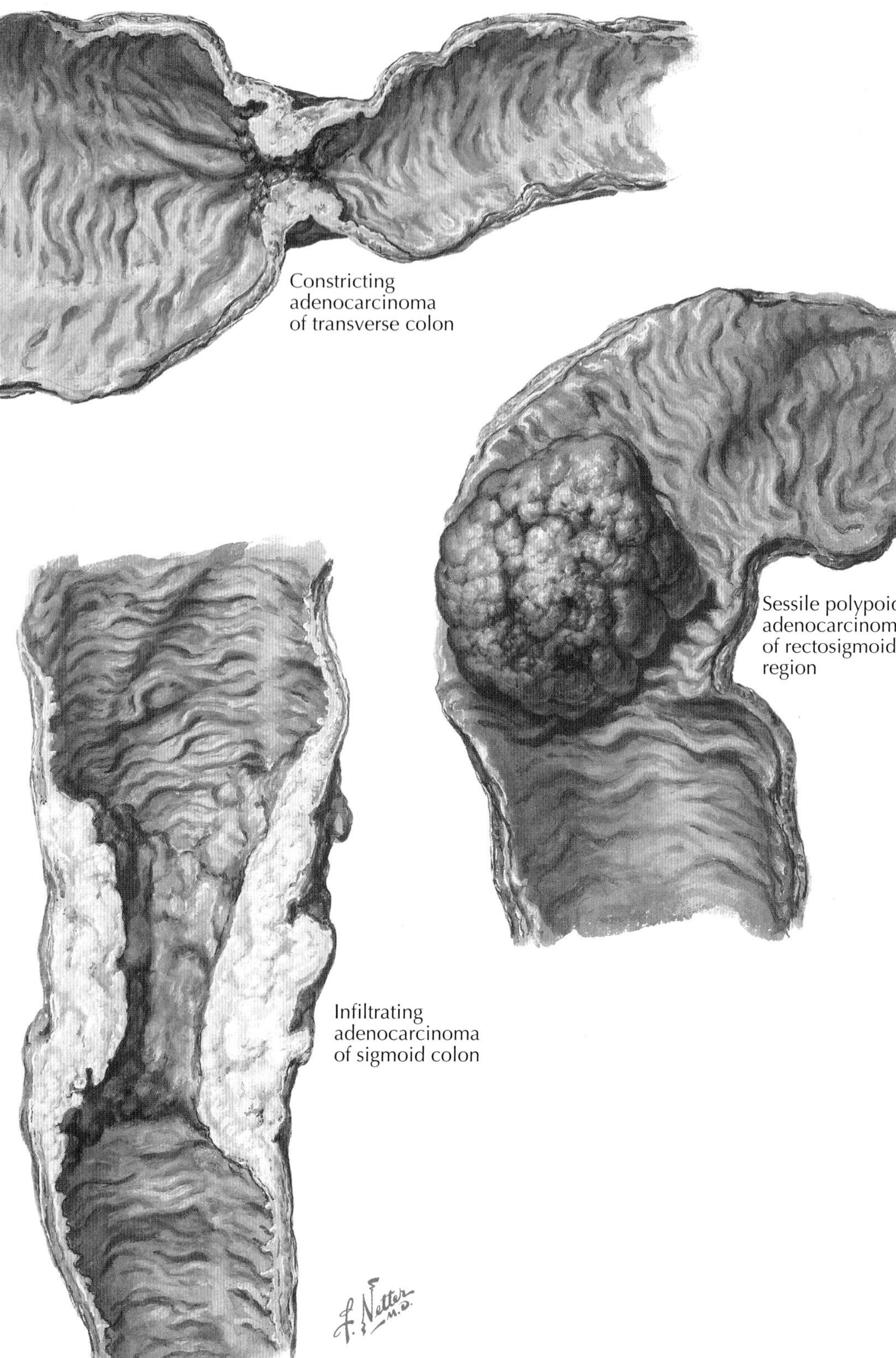


Adenocarcinomas of the large bowel occur usually as nodular proliferating or *scirrhous infiltrating tumors.* Both varieties may, occasionally, undergo mucoid degeneration *(colloid adenocarcinoma).* The nodular adenocarcinoma represents a bulky fungating mass, projecting into the lumen and becoming ulcerated rather speedily. In the well-differentiated tumor, one finds histopathologically well-formed glands lined by large columnar cells with darker-than-normal cytoplasm and vesicular, hyperchromatic nuclei showing mitoses here and there. In poorly differentiated tumors, the gland-like structures are much less in evidence; the cells vary in size and display mitoses relatively frequently. The scirrhous type of carcinoma infiltrates the bowel wall rather than projecting into the lumen. It tends to encircle the gut and give rise to stenosis. In this type of tumor, the fibrous elements predominate over the epithelial elements, producing an extremely hard,

## MALIGNANT TUMORS OF LARGE INTESTINE (Continued)

contracted mass. The carcinomas that have undergone mucoid degeneration display a gelatinous appearance, because of their rich content in mucinous material. A rare variety of tumor is the papillary adenocarcinoma, which presents, on its surface, villous processes and resembles the papilloma. Infection superimposed on a tumor may cause a suppurative process that may eventually spread and lead to formation of fistulous tracts, perforation, and peritonitis.

Malignant tumors of the large intestine present no pathognomonic symptoms. The difficulty of an accurate diagnosis is, in many cases, enhanced by the fact that the large bowel is frequently the site of other pathologic processes that resemble carcinoma in their main clinical manifestations. Moreover, the clinical features of carcinoma are often found to vary widely in different cases, the symptoms depending largely on the location and size of the tumor and the presence of complications such as ulceration, infection, and obstruction. Abdominal pain, diarrhea or constipation (or both), easy fatiguability, weight loss, and blood in the stools are the most common symptoms. With a tumor on the right side, patients may, in addition to the mentioned symptoms, report localized pain, nausea, loss of appetite, and occasional vomiting. Sometimes, the patient may palpate a mass in the right iliac fossa. Weakness, loss of weight, and severe anemia are, in many instances, the leading signs. Increasing constipation is conspicuous in patients with a tumor on the left side, although in such cases diarrhea (usually mild, either persistent or alternating with constipation) is characteristic of the early stages, in which a tumor should be suspected when blood and mucus are found in the stool. Because the lumen of the colon on the left side is somewhat smaller than on the right, the intestinal content is more consistent and formed and the tumors are more frequently of the scirrhous type; signs of intestinal obstruction become manifest with a left-sided cancer far more frequently and earlier than with a tumor on the right. Obstruction, of course, when present, dominates the clinical picture and dictates the management of the case.

When the tumor is located in the rectum, the prominent signs are discharge of blood mixed with mucus, tenesmus, and a frequent desire to defecate. Bleeding and persistent anal pain are the most important symptoms of malignant lesions of the anal canal.

For the diagnosis of malignant growth of the large bowel, the most important methods are digital examination and colonoscopy. Almost every case of rectal cancer can be easily detected by careful, methodical palpation of the entire rectal wall, from low down to as far up as possible. With a digital examination one feels the tumor as a bulky, indurated mass of irregular surface or as an ulcerated area, with a hard, raised, irregular border. Blood of a bright-red or dark-red color on the examiner's finger, sometimes mixed with mucus, and with a peculiar sickly, offensive smell, reinforces the suspicion of the presence of a carcinoma.

The rectum and terminal sigmoid should be visualized in every suspicious case. Such examination will reveal the characteristics of the growth, its size, its mobility, and the degree of obstruction of the bowel, if any is present. Biopsy should be taken to determine the histopathologic type and grade of the lesion. Sometimes, the histopathologic study of what seems to be a malignant tumor may reveal an amebic or other granulomatous inflammatory lesion.

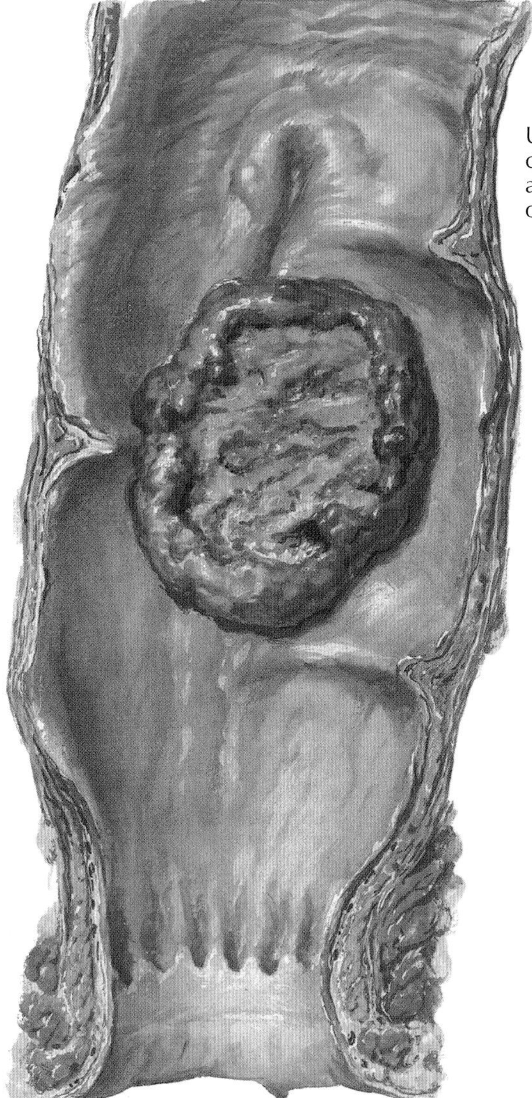

Ulcerated crateriform adenocarcinoma of upper rectum

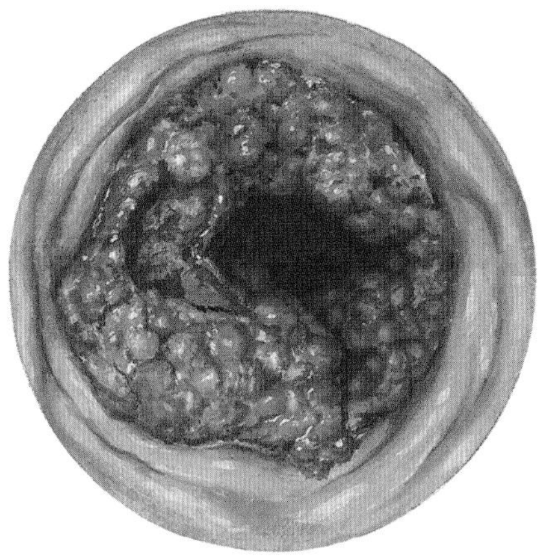

Adenocarcinoma completely encircling lower rectum (sigmoidoscopic view)

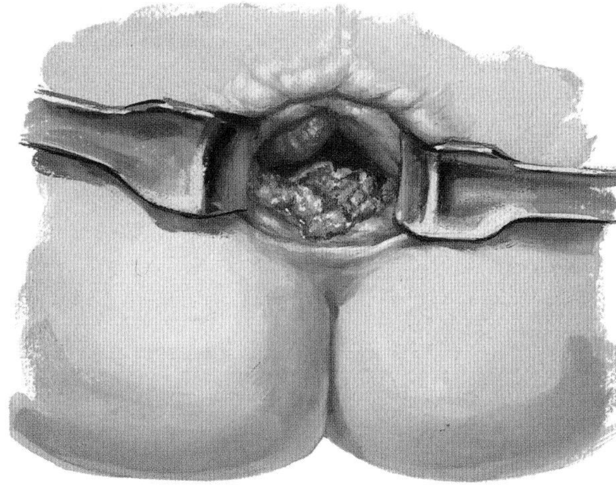

Epithelioma of anal canal

*Epitheliomas* of the anal canal are tumors that originated in the cutaneous coat and are nearly always of the squamous cell variety; only seldom is a basal cell type encountered. They appear as a piled-up nodule or as an ulcerated lesion with a soft or firm base and irregular, undermined edges. The growth may be very small, resembling a fissure, or it may show a greater extension and, eventually, involve the entire circumference of the anus.

Other malignant tumors that may occur in the large bowel, though very rarely, include carcinoids, leiomyosarcomas, fibrosarcomas, angiosarcomas, and lymphoblastomas.

Metastases of cancer of the large bowel occur in three ways: (1) by direct extension to contiguous structures, (2) via the lymphatics to regional and distant lymph nodes, and (3) through hematogenous dissemination to distant organs. The most common sites of metastases are the regional lymph nodes, the liver, the lungs, and the peritoneal cavity.

FAMILIAL POLYPOSIS

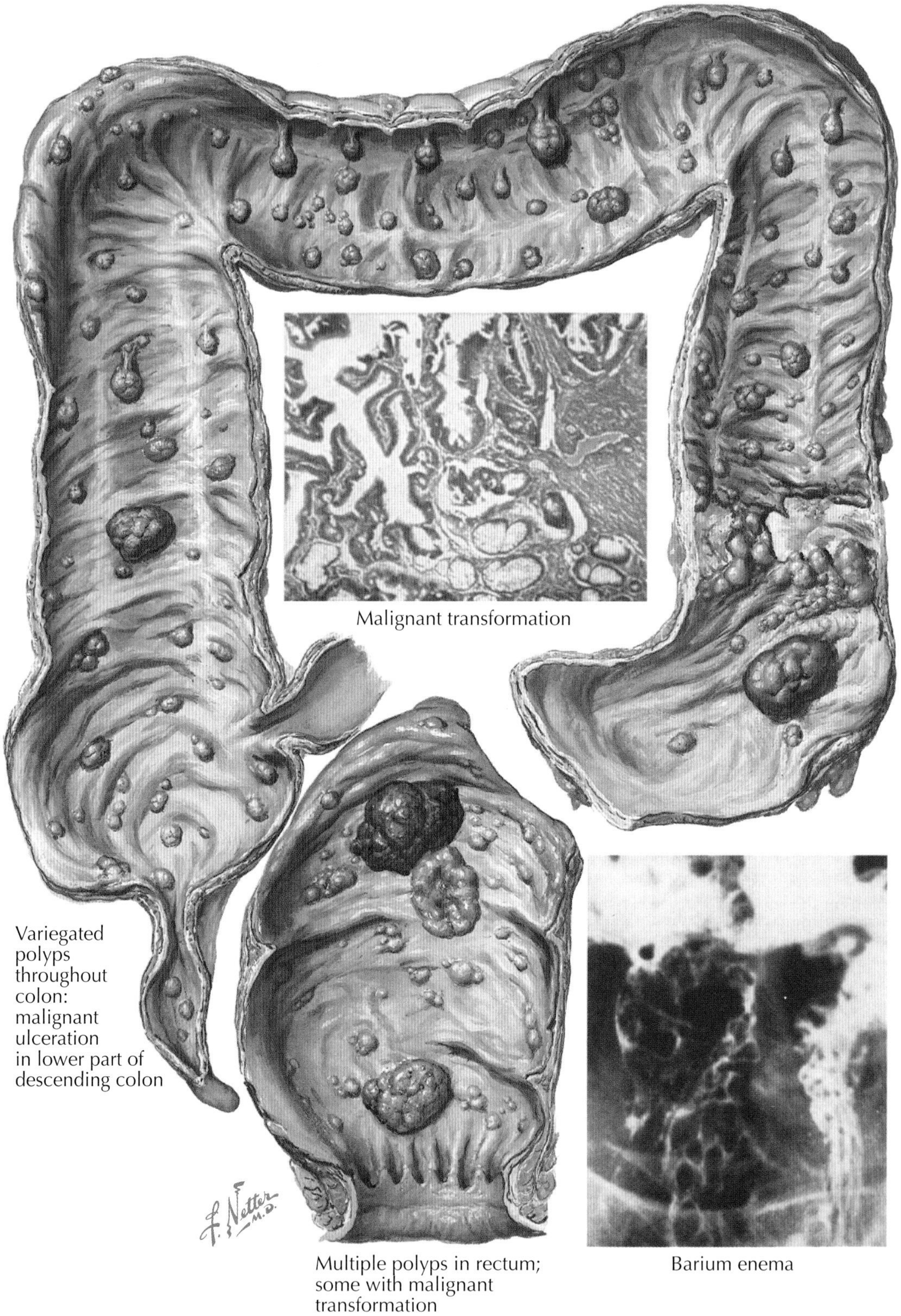

Malignant transformation

Variegated polyps throughout colon: malignant ulceration in lower part of descending colon

Multiple polyps in rectum; some with malignant transformation

Barium enema

## POLYPOSIS SYNDROMES

Various polyposis syndromes exist, which can be divided into adenomatous and hamartomatous polyposis syndromes. *Adenomatous polyposis syndromes* include familial adenomatous polyposis (FAP), attenuated familial adenomatous polyposis, *MUTYH*-associated polyposis, Lynch syndrome, and familial colorectal cancer type X. *Hamartomatous polyposis syndromes* include juvenile polyposis syndrome, Peutz-Jeghers syndrome, *PTEN* hamartoma syndromes (Cowden disease and Bannayan-Riley-Ruvalcaba syndrome), and Cronkhite-Canada syndrome. A *hereditary mixed polyposis syndrome* also occurs, which is characterized by formation of both hamartomatous and adenomatous polyps.

*Familial adenomatous polyposis* is an autosomal dominant disease, occurring in 1 of 10,000 live births. It is the second most common inherited colorectal cancer syndrome and has a variable presentation. Hundreds to thousands of polyps are seen throughout the colon, with a variety of extracolonic manifestations. The median age for adenoma formation is 17 years. If untreated, patients will develop colon cancer by age 40 years, with death by age 44 years on average.

FAP develops because of a germline mutation in the *APC* gene on chromosome 5q21. This leads to a loss of heterozygosity if the second copy of the *APC* gene is mutated or lost. Patients typically present without symptoms, but they are screened because of their family history. Approximately 10% to 30% of patients will have a de novo mutation in the gene and, therefore, no family history. Some patients have extraintestinal manifestations, such as osteomas, extra teeth, or congenital hypertrophy of the retinal pigment epithelium. Some may present with symptoms of polyposis, such as

MULTIPLE POLYPOSIS

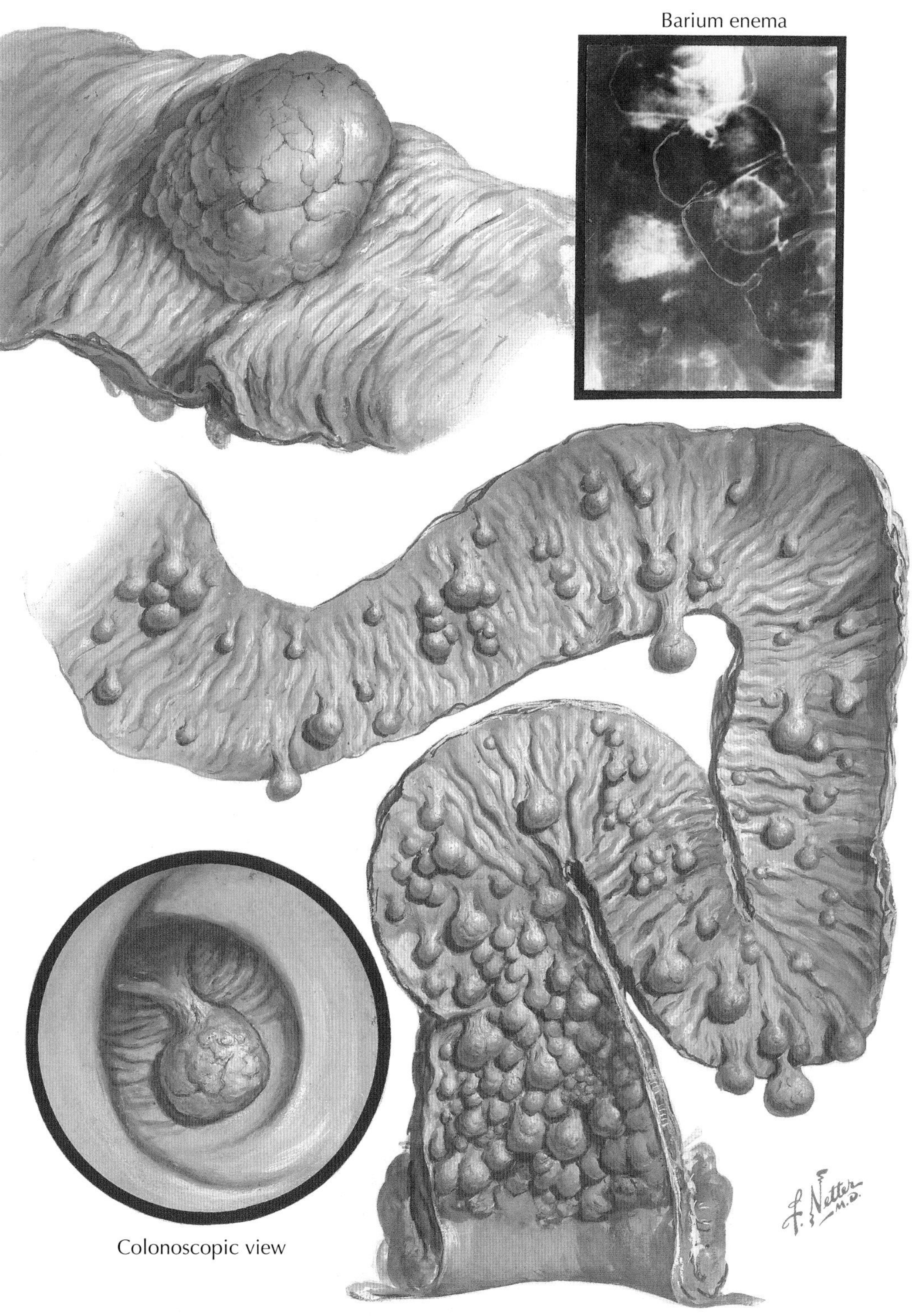


## POLYPOSIS SYNDROMES (Continued)

bleeding, change in bowel habits, or abdominal pain. When this occurs, malignancy is present in 60% of cases. The clinical diagnosis is made when at least 100 colonic adenomas are identified.

Chemoprevention is typically not recommended for those with multiple polyps, but it may be an adjunct to treatment to reduce the appearance of new polyps or cause existing ones to regress. This may delay the need for surgery in some patients. Sulindac has been shown to decrease the polyp burden by 35% to 44%. Celecoxib has been shown to reduce adenomas in as many as 30% of patients.

Prophylactic proctocolectomy is recommended for patients with FAP in early adulthood before they reach the early 20s. If the rectum is left in place, close endoscopic follow-up with ablation of any polyps is necessary because the incidence of cancer is 25% at age 20 years. Many patients will undergo an ileal pouch–anal anastomosis to avoid having a lifelong ostomy. These patients typically have five to six stools per day but decreased control, which can lead to functional limitations.

# Genetics of Colon Cancer

Colorectal cancer (CRC) is the third leading cause of cancer-related deaths in males and females in the United States. There are three different patterns of presentation of CRC, including (1) sporadic cancer, in which no family history or genetic predisposition is apparent (~70% of cases); (2) hereditary syndromes with or without polyposis including FAP and Lynch syndrome (<10% of cases); and (3) familial colorectal cancer, in which there is a family history of CRC but the pattern is not consistent with an inherited syndrome (up to 25%). These patterns rely on a sequence of genetic changes or mutations, which can either be inherited (*germline mutations*) or acquired (*somatic mutations*).

## Adenoma-Carcinoma Sequence

Adenocarcinomas constitute over 95% of all colorectal cancers. These cancers typically arise from abnormal growths called *polyps,* which develop when normal regulatory mechanisms for epithelial renewal are disrupted. *Conventional adenomas* and *serrated class lesions* represent the two main classes of precancerous lesions, with adenomas being the precursors of almost 70% of all CRCs and serrated class lesions the remaining 30%. *Advanced adenomas* are those with villous features, high-grade dysplasia, or size ≥1 cm. Within the serrated class, *sessile serrated polyps/adenomas* (SSPs) and *traditional serrated adenomas* are precancerous, whereas *hyperplastic polyps* typically lack malignant potential.

The classical pathway (conventional adenoma → adenocarcinoma) and the more recently described serrated/alternative pathway (serrated class lesion → adenocarcinoma) represent the two main pathways of colorectal carcinogenesis. Mutations in the *APC* tumor suppressor gene or *BRAF* oncogene are the initiating events leading to the development of adenomas and serrated polyps, respectively. Further genetic alterations are necessary for malignant progression.

## Molecular Basis of Colorectal Cancer

Vogelstein first described a multistep model of CRC development resulting from an accumulation of several genetic and epigenetic (i.e., in which the DNA sequence is not altered) alterations to key regulatory genes: oncogenes, tumor suppressor genes, and mismatch repair genes. This accumulation of alterations drives the initiation and progression of adenomas to carcinomas in sporadic and inherited forms of CRC. Three major molecular pathways to CRC development exist, including (1) the chromosomal instability (CIN) pathway, (2) microsatellite instability (MSI) pathway, and (3) CpG island methylator phenotype (CIMP) pathway. Molecular analysis of CRC allows for determination of prognostic biomarkers and influences management strategies and therapeutic decisions.

## Chromosomal Instability Pathway

Chromosomal instability refers to *gain of function* mutations and can result from the activation of oncogenes (e.g., *KRAS, BRAF*) or inactivation of tumor suppressor genes (e.g., *APC, TP53*) with resulting loss of heterozygosity (LOH). It is the most common type of genetic instability in CRC, and approximately 85% of CRCs develop via this pathway. This pathway typically involves the silencing of the *APC* gene, followed by oncogenic *KRAS* mutations, LOH of chromosome 18q, and, finally, deletion of chromosome 17p, which contains *TP53.* Loss of *p53* gene function, which is designed to help with DNA repair or induce apoptosis in cases of severe injury, promotes genomic instability and is a late event in the classical pathway, accompanying the transition from adenoma to carcinoma.

**Colonoscopy**

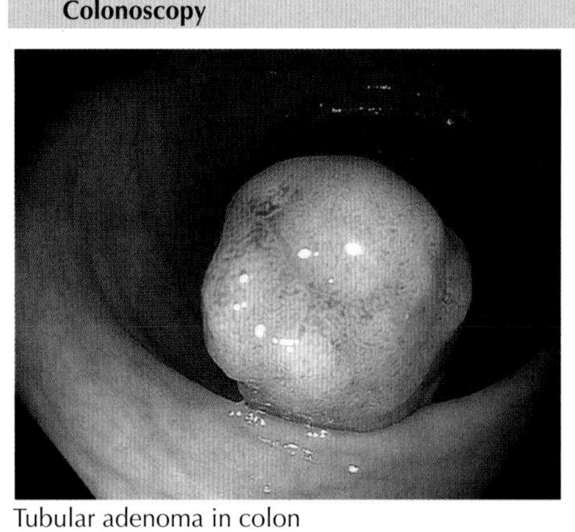

Tubular adenoma in colon

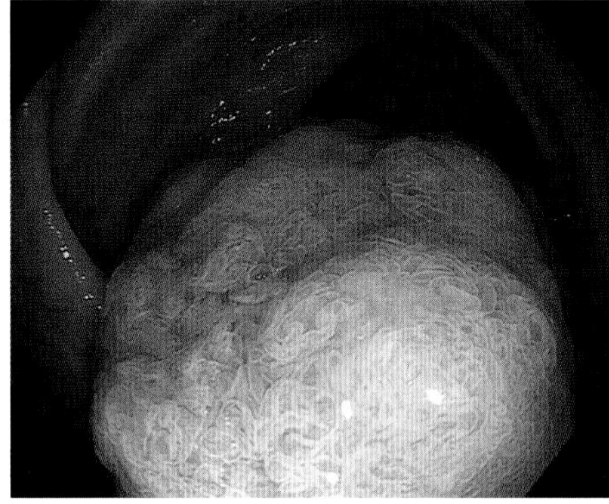

Tubulovillous adenoma

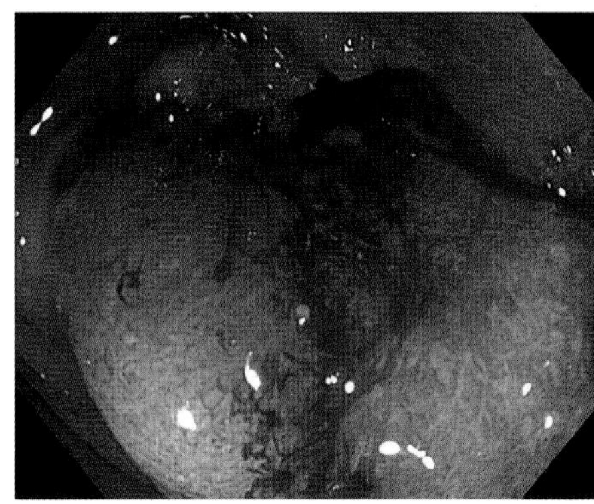

Adenocarcinoma of colon

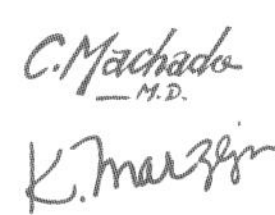


**Adenoma-carcinoma sequence**

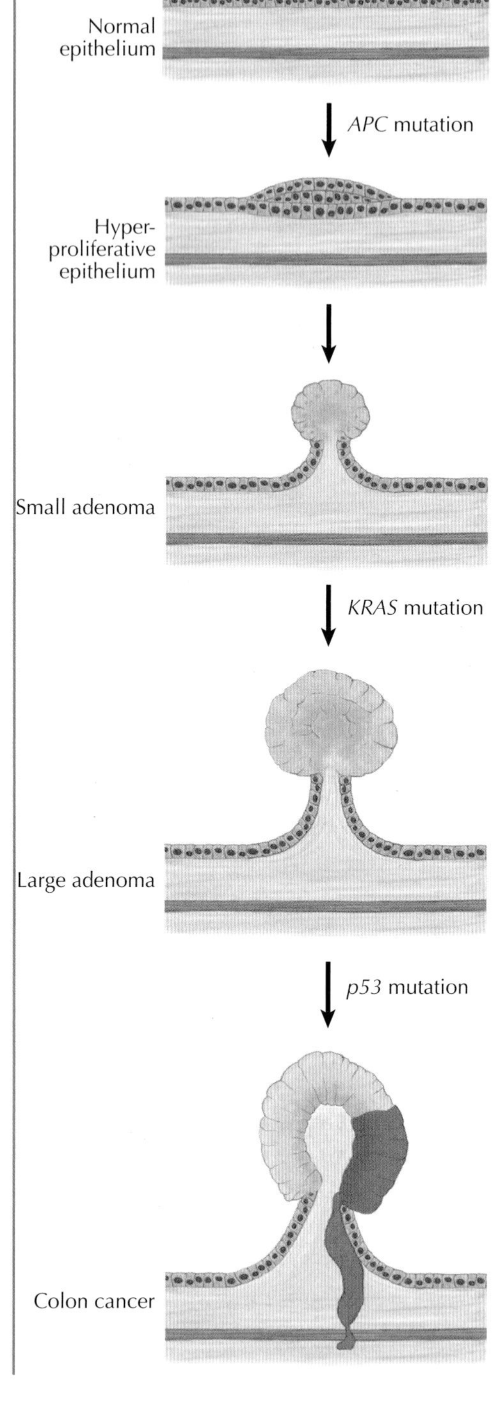


## Microsatellite Instability Pathway

Microsatellites, which are nucleotide repeat sequences throughout the genome, are another type of genomic instability. Although MSI is observed in nearly all CRCs that develop in patients with Lynch syndrome, high levels of MSI can also be seen in nearly 15% of sporadic CRC. Dysfunction of mismatch repair genes (e.g., *MLH1, MSH2, MSH6, PMS2*), which are involved in repair of DNA replication errors, is integral to the development of MSI. Such dysfunction can arise from either germline mutations, as seen in Lynch syndrome, or from epigenetic silencing of the *MLH1* gene via promoter hypermethylation, as seen in sporadic CRCs.

## CpG Island Methylator Pathway

CIMP+ tumors typically result from epigenetic alterations including DNA hypermethylation at promoter CpG islands of tumor suppressor genes leading to their silencing. CIMP-high status is commonly seen in conjunction with *BRAF* activation and hypermethylation of *MLH1,* which describe a large fraction of sporadic MSI-high tumors. SSPs are the predominant precancerous lesions in the CIMP pathway. This contrasts with the CIN pathway and Lynch syndrome in which adenomatous polyps are the precursor lesions to CRC.

# Colon Cancer Prevention

CRC is a major worldwide health problem. In the United States CRC is the third leading cause of cancer deaths in both males and females. Nonmodifiable risk factors for developing colon cancer include age, race and ethnicity, family history of CRC, presence of hereditary syndromes, and certain conditions such as IBD or diabetes. Modifiable risk factors include physical inactivity, smoking, alcohol consumption, obesity and overweight, poor dietary habits such as a diet with low fiber or high in red meats, and use of certain medications. Adequate intake of vitamin D and use of aspirin and other NSAIDs may reduce the risk of colorectal cancer. Signs and symptoms that might indicate the presence of CRC include unexplained anemia, blood in the stool, unexplained change in bowel habits or caliber of stool, and abdominal pain and may require further testing independent of the patient's age at presentation.

A focus on early secondary prevention screening improves detection and outcomes for colon cancer. Several screening tests exist, with colonoscopy being the gold standard for the detection of all precancerous lesions, and starts at age 45 for the average-risk patients. Its ability to detect both conventional adenomas and serrated class lesions (SSPs) (see Plate 3.97) is unmatched. Colonoscopy is the preferred CRC screening modality, although alternative tests may be considered if colonoscopy is not available or based on patient preference.

## ENDOSCOPIC TESTS

### Colonoscopy

Colonoscopy is highly sensitive for the detection of all types of precancerous and cancerous lesions. It plays a major role in cancer prevention via polypectomy. Drawbacks include the need for a vigorous bowel preparation, the risks associated with anesthesia and sedation, and procedural risks including perforation, postpolypectomy bleeding, and splenic injury. It should be noted that the quality of colonoscopy is highly dependent on the performing endoscopist, among other variables.

### Flexible Sigmoidoscopy

Flexible sigmoidoscopy has been shown to lead to a reduction in the incidence of distal colon or rectosigmoid cancers. Other advantages include its lower cost and associated risks, need for limited sedation, and less extensive bowel preparation compared with colonoscopy. The flexible sigmoidoscopy does not evaluate the ascending and parts of the transverse colon, leading to the possibility of missing more proximal cancers.

## STOOL-BASED TESTS

Previous guaiac-based fecal occult blood testing has largely been replaced by fecal immunochemical testing (FIT) because only one sample is required and it provides better detection of lower GI bleeding. Other advantages of FIT include its low cost, noninvasive nature, and good sensitivity for CRC detection (~80%). Disadvantages include poorer detection of more advanced lesions and SSPs along with the need for annual screening. FIT-fecal testing can also look for DNA which improves the sensitivity for CRC detection (~92%), giving it the highest one-time sensitivity for CRC among all noninvasive and nonradiologic screening tests. The FIT-fecal DNA test, a combination of FIT and markers of abnormal DNA, may be able to detect serrated lesions >1 cm in size. Its major disadvantages include increased cost and limited specificity with increasing age.

**Endoscopic tests**

Transverse colon

Left (descending) colon

Right (ascending) colon

Sigmoid colon

Rectum

Distribution of colorectal cancer

**Direct screening techniques are most reliable**

Examining up to 50 cm above anal verge can detect up to 40% of all colorectal cancers

60-cm flexible sigmoidoscope

Synchronous cancer

Colonoscope examination allows examination of complete colon

CT colonography allows for detection of larger (>1 cm) precancerous lesions.

JOHN A.CRAIG—AD

K. Marzen

**Stool-based tests**

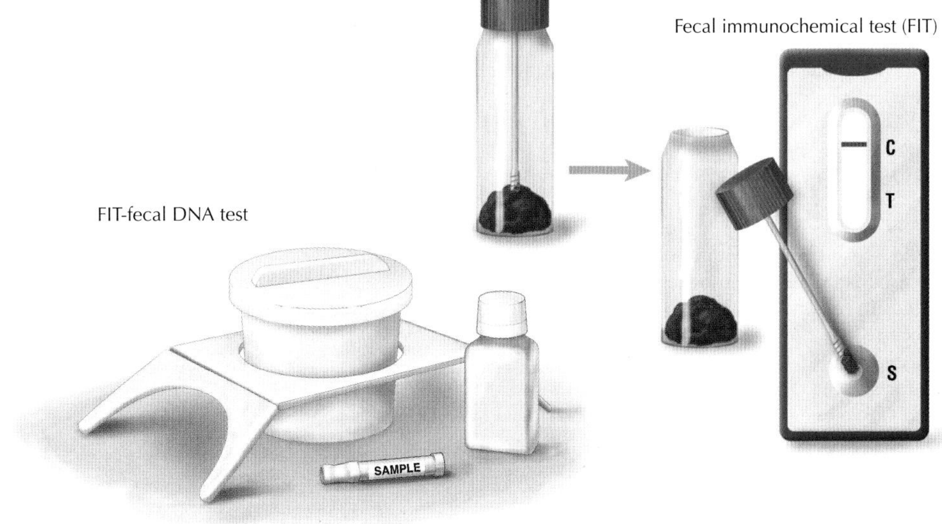


## OTHER TESTS

### CT Colonography

This imaging test has replaced double-contrast barium enema as the colorectal imaging test of choice. Its advantages include a high sensitivity for detecting precancerous lesions >1 cm (82%–92%) and lower risk for bowel perforation. Bowel preparation is still required, and there is limited ability to detect smaller (<1 cm), flatter, or serrated type polyps. Finally, the management of incidental extracolonic findings on CT and cumulative radiation exposure with repeated testing must be considered.

### Capsule Colonoscopy

Capsule colonoscopy allows for endoscopic imaging while avoiding the risks associated with an invasive procedure. There is good sensitivity (88%) for detecting adenomas >6 mm in size but, like many of these other modalities, it is not good at detecting SSPs. Like colonoscopy and CT colonography, extensive bowel preparation is required. This screening method may be used in patients with high procedural risk or in persons with a prior incomplete colonoscopy or suboptimal assessment.

### Septin9 Assay

This is the first FDA-approved serum-based test for colorectal cancer screening. Although this test is convenient, it is costly and has a poor sensitivity (<50%) for detecting CRC and limited ability to detect precancerous polyps.

# Colon Cancer Screening Guidelines

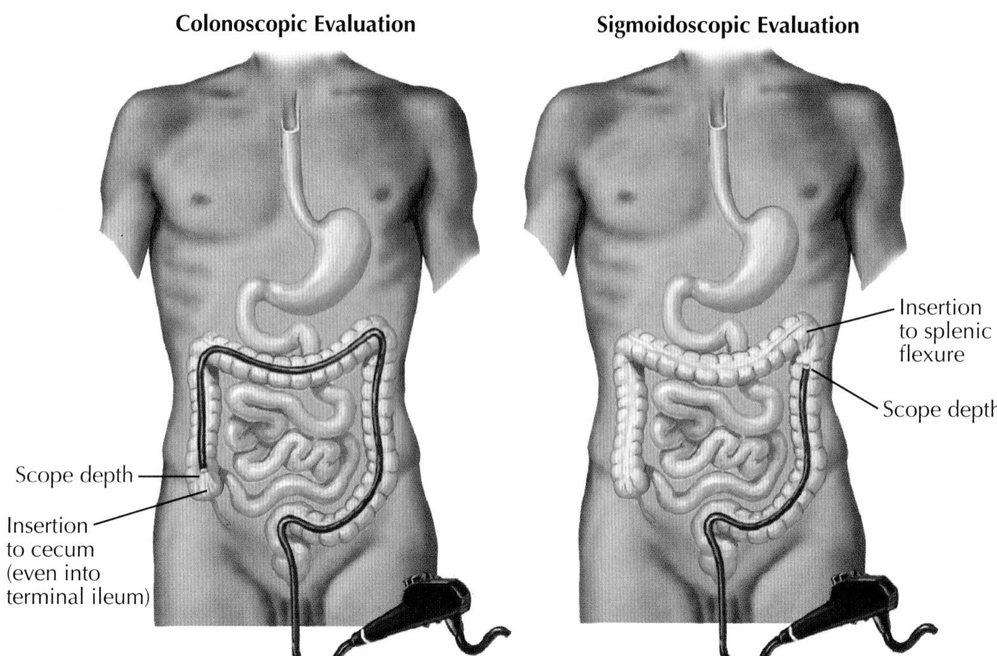


Sigmoidoscopy as shown on the right is a procedure that advances the insertion tube up to the splenic flexure. During colonoscopy the insertion tube is advanced to the right colon into the cecum. In many cases the terminal ileum is intubated to view the distal small intestine.

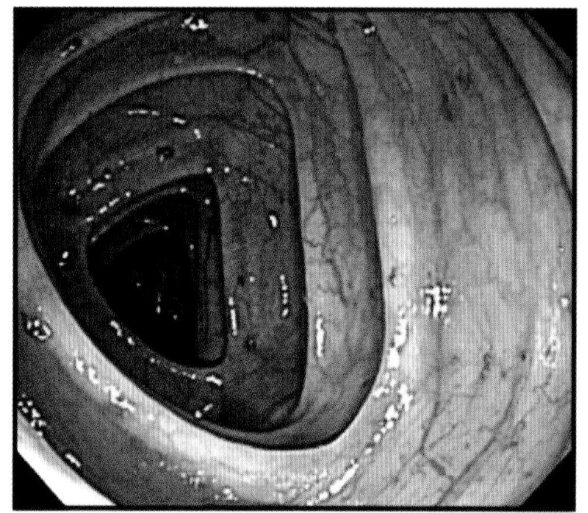

Normal transverse colon

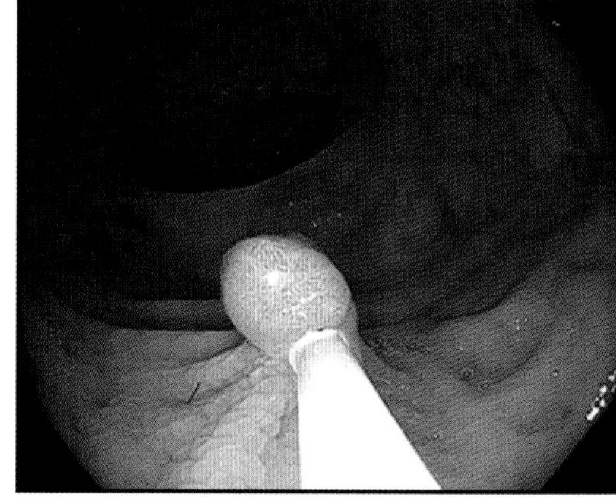

Polypectomy by cold snare

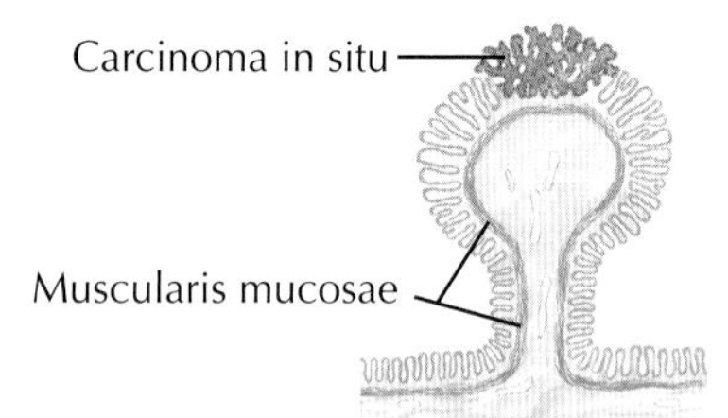


If carcinomatous involvement of polyp has not penetrated muscularis mucosae, it is classified as carcinoma in situ, and simple endoscopic removal by fulgurating snare is believed adequate.

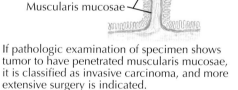

Invasive carcinoma

Muscularis mucosae

If pathologic examination of specimen shows tumor to have penetrated muscularis mucosae, it is classified as invasive carcinoma, and more extensive surgery is indicated.

Approximately 1 in 23 males and 1 in 25 females will develop CRC in their lifetime. Unlike with more inaccessible cancers, early detection and prevention of CRC can be achieved by screening with colonoscopy. Acceptance and availability of CRC screening have contributed to a decline in its incidence and mortality over the past several decades.

As described in Plate 3.98, multiple modalities are available for CRC screening, with the overall goal being a decrease in the incidence and mortality of CRC by identifying high-risk precancerous lesions including adenomas and serrated class lesions and early-stage CRCs. Cost analysis models have demonstrated the cost-effectiveness of any modality over no screening at all given the high costs of cancer treatment.

Although *organized screening* programs are advisable to improve adherence with CRC screening, screening in the United States is typically *opportunistic* in nature. Interactions between healthcare providers and patients lead to the selection of a certain screening test. Several approaches can be employed, including presenting a patient with the various screening options (*multiple options* approach), suggesting a preferred test first followed by another one if declined by the patient (*sequential testing* approach), or offering colonoscopy to those with risk factors (e.g. older age, male sex, smoker, obesity, diabetes) for precancerous lesions and other less invasive and costly screening tests to those with a predicted lower risk (*risk-stratified* approach). Although several GI societal guidelines advocate for a sequential testing approach with colonoscopy offered first given its high efficacy at preventing colorectal cancer and overall low absolute risk when performed by a skilled endoscopist, superiority of one approach over another has not been demonstrated. Regardless, any positive screening test other than colonoscopy warrants subsequent evaluation with a complete colonoscopy.

## CRC SCREENING MODALITIES

In 2021, the United States Multi-Society Task Force (USMSTF) grouped these screening tests into three tiers due to significant societal disparities in the performance and cost, with Tier 1 options including colonoscopy (every 10 years) and FIT (every year) being the preferred modalities for screening of average-risk patients. Tier 2 tests include CT colonography (every 5 years), FIT-fecal DNA (every 3 years), and flexible sigmoidoscopy (every 5–10 years). Capsule colonoscopy (every 5 years) comprises Tier 3. The Septin9 assay was not recommended given its inferior performance characteristics and high relative cost.

## AVERAGE-RISK PATIENTS

The 2021 USMSTF guidelines recommended that CRC screening of average-risk, asymptomatic patients begin at age 45 years. Subsequent studies have highlighted a rising incidence of CRC in individuals under age 50, leading several societies, including the USMSTF, to update prior recommendations, with 45 now the suggested age to begin CRC screening in all average-risk individuals.

Discontinuing CRC screening can be considered at age 75 in patients up to date with screening with negative prior testing (in particular, colonoscopy) or when life expectancy is less than 10 years. In patients without prior screening, CRC screening may be considered until age 85 dependent on the patient's overall clinical picture. Generally, the decision to pursue screening beyond age 75 should be an individualized one. Screening is not recommended after age 85.

## HIGH-RISK PATIENTS

A family history of CRC or advanced neoplasia is associated with an average twofold increase in CRC risk. The exact magnitude is dependent on several factors, including number of affected relatives and their age at diagnosis. Although a history of CRC in a first-degree relative (FDR) increases the risk of CRC regardless of the age at diagnosis, age 60 is recognized as a threshold for risk elevation.

Individuals with an FDR diagnosed with CRC/advanced polyp at age $<60$ years (or two FDRs diagnosed at any age) should begin screening with colonoscopy at age 40 or 10 years before the youngest affected relative, whichever is earlier. They should continue screening with colonoscopy every 5 years at minimum. Persons with a single FDR diagnosed with CRC/advanced polyp at age $\geq 60$ years should also start screening at age 40, although tests and intervals are as per the average-risk screening recommendations.

# Lower Gastrointestinal Bleeding

Acute lower gastrointestinal bleeding (LGIB) is defined as bleeding from the colon or rectum and is the cause of nearly 20% of all cases of GI bleeding. Typically, a patient presents with *hematochezia,* or the passage of red or maroon blood per rectum, although a minority of patients can present with *melena,* or black tarry stools, as can be seen in cases of more proximal LGIB involving the right-sided colon. Hematochezia can also be a manifestation of a brisk upper gastrointestinal bleed (UGIB) and, interestingly, this is the cause of approximately 15% of cases of presumed LGIB.

## CAUSES OF LGIB

Several etiologies of LGIB exist, with diverticular bleeding being the most common colonic cause of severe hematochezia among hospitalized patients. Ischemic colitis and internal hemorrhoids comprise the next two most common colorectal sources, with the latter being the leading cause of colonic bleeding in outpatient adults. Other etiologies include infectious or inflammatory colitis, vascular lesions (e.g., angiodysplasia, radiation telangiectasias), postpolypectomy ulcers, neoplastic lesions, or anorectal conditions (e.g., solitary rectal ulcer, rectal varices).

## INITIAL ASSESSMENT

The evaluation of a patient presenting with presumed LGIB consists of a focused history and physical examination along with routine laboratory tests to determine the possible etiology and severity of bleeding. Evaluation for risk factors portending poor outcomes should be done. These include hemodynamic instability, ongoing bleeding, advanced age (age >60), anemia, and significant medical comorbidities. Such factors may warrant closer monitoring in an intensive care unit setting and either radiologic evaluation or sooner colonoscopy after a rapid bowel preparation.

Efforts should be taken to ensure adequate hemodynamic resuscitation with intravenous fluids, and packed red blood cells should be transfused to maintain a hemoglobin >7 g/dL. A higher goal of 9 g/dL should be targeted in cases with significant cardiovascular comorbidities or massive bleeding. Prior to endoscopic evaluation and possible hemostasis, correction of underlying coagulation defects should be pursued and discussions with the appropriate specialty regarding reversal or holding of anticoagulant agents should be had. Aspirin for secondary cardiovascular prevention should not be discontinued.

As mentioned, brisk UGIB can also present with hematochezia, and in cases with associated hemodynamic instability, evaluation for an upper GI source should be pursued. A history of peptic ulcer disease, advanced liver disease or cirrhosis, or use of antiplatelet or anticoagulant medications raise the likelihood of this. An elevated blood urea nitrogen–to-creatinine ratio and positive nasogastric aspirate are indicative of a UGIB source, and upper endoscopy should be pursued prior to colonoscopy in these cases.

## COLONOSCOPY

In patients presenting with acute LGIB, colonoscopy should be pursued given its diagnostic and therapeutic capabilities. Through a careful assessment of the colon mucosa, the goal of colonoscopy is to identify a possible etiology of bleeding and perform hemostasis as necessary. The terminal ileum should also be examined to evaluate for more proximal (i.e., small bowel) sources of GI bleeding. Colonoscopy should ideally be performed once hemodynamic stability is achieved and a bowel preparation has been completed because this allows for adequate visualization and localization of the bleeding source while reducing the risk of bowel perforation. An examination without bowel preparation is not recommended. The timing of colonoscopy is dependent on the presence of high-risk clinical features and signs and symptoms of ongoing bleeding.

## NON-COLONOSCOPY INTERVENTION

In cases where upper endoscopy is negative and brisk ongoing LGIB precludes adequate hemodynamic resuscitation and tolerance of bowel preparation, angiography with embolization can be pursued for localization and treatment. This radiographic method relies on active bleeding and has the potential for serious adverse events including bowel ischemia. Tagged red blood cell scintigraphy and CT angiography are two other tests that may allow for localization of the bleeding site before angiography or emergent surgery, with CT angiography preferred given its widespread availability, increased accuracy, and expedience. Surgical consultation should also be obtained in cases with brisk ongoing LGIB, especially in patients with high-risk clinical features, in case surgical resection is eventually required after other therapeutic modalities have failed.

Common Etiologies of Lower Gastrointestinal Bleeding

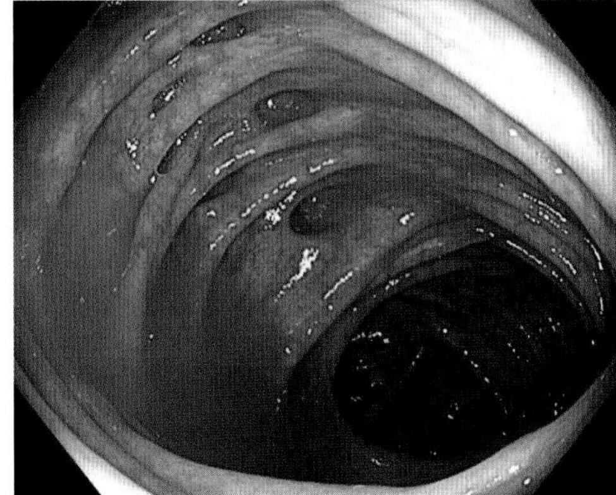

Diverticulosis

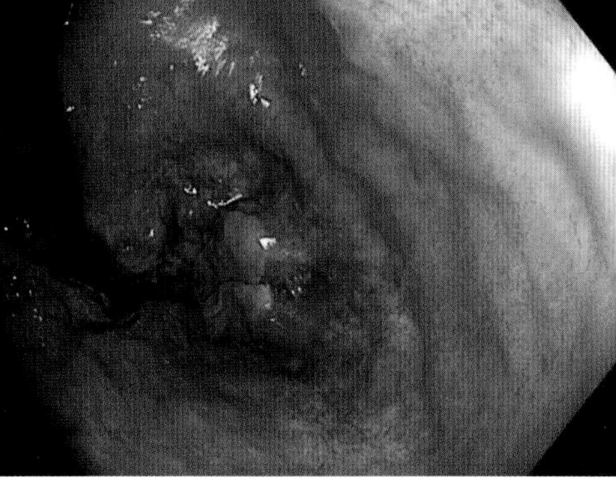

Internal hemorrhoids

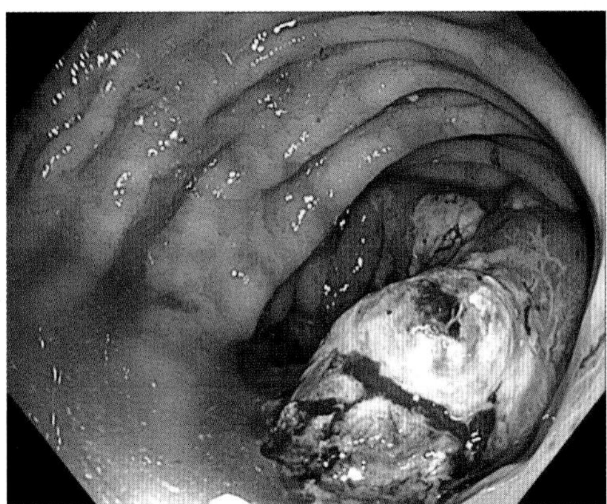

Colorectal cancer

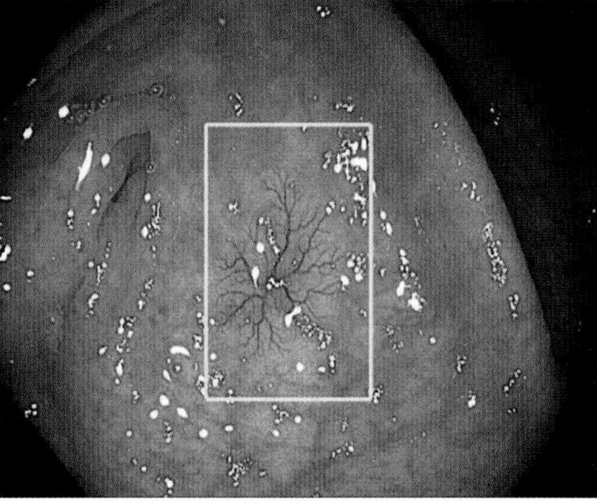

Angiodysplastic lesion

# SELECTED REFERENCES


### Section 1 Overview of Lower Digestive Tract

Deraco M, Elias D, Helm CW, et al. Management of peritoneal surface malignancy. In: Cameron JL, Cameron AM, eds. Current Surgical Therapy. 11th ed. Elsevier; 2014:245-251.

Levine EA, Stewart JH, Shen P, et al. Intraperitoneal chemotherapy for peritoneal surface malignancy: experience with 1000 patients. J Am Coll Surg. 2014;218(4):573-585.

### Section 2 Small Bowel

Kahraman G, Marur T, Tanyeli E, Yildirim M. Hepatomesenteric trunk. Surg Radiol Anat. 2002;23(6):433-435.

Yi SQ, Terayama H, Naito M, et al. A common celiacomesenteric trunk, and a brief review of the literature. Ann Anat. 2007;189(5): 482-488.

### Section 3 Colon

Alratrout H, Debroux E. Acute right-sided ischemic colitis in a COVID-19 patient: a case report and review of the literature. J Med Case Rep. 2022;16(1):135.

Ambartsumyan L, Smith C, Kapur RP. Diagnosis of Hirschsprung disease. Pediatr Dev Pathol. 2020;23:8-22.

Aniwan S, Harmsen WS, Tremaine WJ, et al. Incidence of inflammatory bowel disease by race and ethnicity in a population-based inception cohort from 1970 through 2010. Ther Adv Gastroenterol. 2019;12.

Brandt LJ, Boley SJ. Colonic ischemia. Surg Clin North Am. 1992; 72:203-229.

Burke KE, D'Amato M, Ng SC, et al. Microscopic colitis. Nat Rev Dis Primers. 2021;7:39.

Cairo SB, Rothstein DH, Harmon CM. Minimally invasive surgery in the management of anorectal malformations. Clin Perinatol. 2017;44:819-834.

Chen H, Cai Y, Liu Y, et al. Incidence, surgical treatment, and prognosis of anorectal melanoma from 1973 to 2011: a population-based SEER analysis. Medicine (Baltimore). 2016;95(7):e2770.

Chubak J, Whitlock EP, Williams SB, et al. Aspirin for the prevention of cancer incidence and mortality: systematic evidence reviews for the U.S. Preventive Services Task Force. Ann Intern Med. 2016;164: 814-825.

Coskun A, Erkan N, Yakan S, et al. Management of rectal foreign bodies. World J Emerg Surg. 2013;8:11.

Elagili F, Stocchi L, Ozuner G, Dietz DW, Kiran RP. Outcomes of percutaneous drainage without surgery for patients with diverticular abscess. Dis Colon Rectum. 2014;57(3):331-336.

Fearon ER, Vogelstein B. A genetic model for colorectal tumorigenesis. Cell. 1990;61:759-767.

Feuerstein JD, Cheifetz AS. Crohn disease: epidemiology, diagnosis, and management. Mayo Clin Proc. 2017;92:1088-1103.

Feuerstein JD, Ho EY, Shmidt E, et al. AGA clinical practice guidelines on the medical management of moderate to severe luminal and perianal fistulizing Crohn's disease. Gastroenterology. 2021; 160:2496-2508.

Feuerstein JD, Isaacs KL, Schneider Y, et al. AGA clinical practice guidelines on the management of moderate to severe ulcerative colitis. Gastroenterology. 2020;158:1450-1461.

Ghazanfar H, Kandhi S, Shin D, et al. Impact of COVID-19 on the gastrointestinal tract: a clinical review. Cureus. 2022;14(3): e23333.

Hall J, Hardiman K, Lee S, et al.; Prepared on behalf of the Clinical Practice Guidelines Committee of the American Society of Colon and Rectal Surgeons. The American Society of Colon and Rectal Surgeons clinical practice guidelines for the treatment of left-sided colonic diverticulitis. Dis Colon Rectum. 2020;63(6): 728-747.

Krishnan B, Babu S, Walker J, et al. Gastrointestinal complications of diabetes mellitus. World J Diabetes. 2013;4:51-63.

Laine L, Shah A. Randomized trial of urgent vs. elective colonoscopy in patients hospitalized with lower GI bleeding. Am J Gastroenterol. 2010;105:2636-2641.

Leggett B, Whitehall V. Role of the serrated pathway in colorectal cancer pathogenesis. Gastroenterology. 2010;138(6):2088-2100.

Lichtenstein G. Current research in Crohn's disease and ulcerative colitis: highlights from the 2010 ACG meeting. Gastroenterol Hepatol. 2010;6:3-14.

Lichtenstein GR, Loftus EV, Isaacs KL, et al. ACG clinical guideline: management of Crohn's disease in adults. Am J Gastroenterol. 2018;113:481-517.

Mahan ME, Toy FK. Rectal trauma. In: StatPearls [Internet]. StatPearls Publishing; 2022.

Meldgaard T, Olesen SS, Farmer AD, et al. Diabetic enteropathy: from molecule to mechanism-based treatment. J Diabetes Res. 2018;2018:3827301.

Meyer J, Orci LA, Combescure C, et al. Risk of colorectal cancer in patients with acute diverticulitis: a systematic review and meta-analysis of observational studies. Clin Gastroenterol Hepatol. 2019;17(8):1448-1456.e17.

Nguyen LH, Goel A, Chung DC. Pathways of colorectal carcinogenesis. Gastroenterology. 2020;158(2):291-302.

Pan W, Golstein AM, Hotta R. Opportunities for novel diagnostic and cell-based therapies for Hirschsprung disease. J Pediatr Surg. 2022;57(9):61-68.

Patel SG, May FP, Anderson JC, et al. Updates on age to start and stop colorectal cancer screening: recommendations from the U.S. Multi-Society Task Force on Colorectal Cancer. Gastroenterology. 2022;162(1):285-299.

Pena A, Hong A. Advances in the management of anorectal malformations. Am J Surg. 2000;180(5):370-376.

Rabbenou W, Chang S. Medical treatment of pouchitis: a guide for the clinician. Ther Adv Gastroenterol. 2021;14.

Rubin DT, Ananthakrishnan AN, Siegel CA, et al. ACG clinical guideline: ulcerative colitis in adults. Am J Gastroenterol. 2019;114:384-413.

Sewell JL, Velayos FS. Systematic review: the role of race and socioeconomic factors on IBD healthcare delivery and effectiveness. Inflamm Bowel Dis. 2013;19:627-643.

Shaukat A, Kahi CJ, Burke CA, Rabeneck L, Sauer BG, Rex DK. ACG clinical guidelines: colorectal cancer screening 2021. Am J Gastroenterol. 2021;116(3):458-479.

Song M, Garrett WS, Chan AT. Nutrients, foods, and colorectal cancer prevention. Gastroenterology. 2015;148(6):1244-1260.e16.

Strate LL, Gralnek IM. ACG clinical guideline: management of patients with acute lower gastrointestinal bleeding. Am J Gastroenterol. 2016;111(4):459-474.

Strate LL, Saltzman JR, Ookubo R, et al. Validation of a clinical prediction rule for severe acute lower gastrointestinal bleeding. Am J Gastroenterol. 2005;100:1821-1827.

Tyler JA, Welling DR. Historical perspectives on colorectal trauma management. Clin Colon Rectal Surg. 2018;31(1):5-10.

Wilkins T, et al. Diverticular bleeds. Am Fam Physician. 2009;80(9): 977-983.

Wood RJ, Levitt MA. Anorectal malformations. Clin Colon Rectal Surg. 2018;31:61-70.

Yamamoto R, Logue AJ, Muir MT. Colon trauma: evidence-based practices. Clin Colon Rectal Surg. 2018;31(1):11-16.

## E



## F



## G

## J



## K



## L

## M



## N

## Q



## R



## S